JOINT DISEASE IN THE HORSE

JOINT DISEASE IN THE HORSE

SECOND EDITION

Edited by

C. Wayne McIlwraith, BVSc, PhD, DSc (Purdue), Dr med vet (h.c. Vienna), DSc (Purdue) (h.c. Massey), Laurea Dr (h.c. Turin), D vet med (h.c. London), FRCVS, Diplomate ACVS, ECVS, & ACVSMR
University Distinguished Professor
Barbara Cox Anthony University Chair in
    Orthopaedics
Director Orthopaedic Research Center, Gail
    Holmes Equine Orthopaedic Research Center
College of Veterinary Medicine and Biomedical
    Sciences, School of Biomedical Engineering
Colorado State University
Fort Collins, Colorado

David D. Frisbie, DVM, PhD, DACVS, DACVSMR
Professor
Equine Orthopedic Research Center
College of Veterinary Medicine and Biological
    Sciences
School of Biomedical Engineering
Colorado State University
Fort Collins, Colorado

Christopher E. Kawcak, DVM, PhD, Diplomate ACVS & ACVSMR
Professor
Equine Orthopedic Research Center
College of Veterinary Medicine and Biomedical
    Sciences
Colorado State University
Fort Collins, Colorado

P. René van Weeren, DVM, PhD, Diplomate ECVS
Professor of Equine Musculoskeletal Biology
Department of Equine Sciences
Faculty of Veterinary Medicine
Utrecht University

ELSEVIER

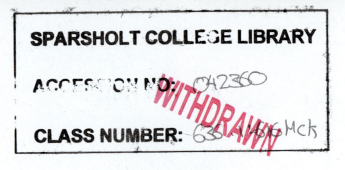

ELSEVIER

3251 Riverport Lane
St. Louis, Missouri 63043

JOINT DISEASE IN THE HORSE, SECOND EDITION   ISBN: 978-1-4557-5969-9
Copyright © 2016 by Elsevier Inc. All rights reserved.

Notices

Previous edition copyrighted 1996.

Library of Congress Cataloging-in-Publication Data

Joint disease in the horse / edited by C. Wayne McIlwraith, David D. Frisbie, Christopher E. Kawcak, P. René van Weeren. -- Second edition.
    p. ; cm.
  Includes bibliographical references and index.
  ISBN 978-1-4557-5969-9 (hardcover : alk. paper)
  I. McIlwraith, C. Wayne, editor. II. Frisbie, David D., editor. III. Kawcak, Christopher E., editor. IV. van Weeren, P. René 1957- , editor.
  [DNLM: 1. Horse Diseases. 2. Joint Diseases--veterinary. SF 959.J64]
  SF959.J64J385 2016
  636.1'089672--dc23
                                                      2015015062

Vice President and Publisher: Loren Wilson
Content Strategy Director: Penny Rudolph
Content Development Manager: Jolynn Gower
Content Development Specialist: Brandi Graham
Publishing Services Manager: Jeffrey Patterson
Project Manager: Bill Drone
Designer: Brian Salisbury

Working together
to grow libraries in
developing countries

www.elsevier.com • www.bookaid.org

Printed in China.

Last digit is the print number: 9 8 7 6 5 4 3 2 1

To Nancy, Myra, Erin, and Madelon for their continued participation in what we do, as well as their support and patience,

AND to the horse, whose unselfish efforts and willingness to serve have inspired much of the basic and clinical research reported in this text.

CONTRIBUTORS

Myra F. Barrett, DVM, MS, DACVR
Assistant Professor
Environmental and Radiological Health Sciences
Colorado State University
Fort Collins, Colorado

Pieter A. J. Brama, DVM, MBA, PhD, DECVS, DRNVA
Professor of Veterinary Surgery
School of Veterinary Medicine
Veterinary Science Centre
University College Dublin
Belfield, Dublin, Ireland

Janny C. de Grauw, DVM, PhD
Resident in Veterinary Anesthesiology
Faculty of Veterinary Medicine
Resident, Veterinary Anesthesiology (ECVAA)
Department of Equine Sciences
Utrecht University
Utrecht, The Netherlands

David D. Frisbie, DVM, PhD, DACVS, DACVSMR
Professor
Equine Orthopedic Research Center
College of Veterinary Medicine and Biological Sciences
School of Biomedical Engineering
Colorado State University
Fort Collins, Colorado

Laurie R. Goodrich, DVM, PhD, DACVS
Associate Professor in Equine Surgery and Lameness
College of Veterinary Medicine
Colorado State University
Fort Collins, Colorado

Kevin K. Haussler, DVM, DC, PhD, Diplomate ACVSMR
Associate Professor
Equine Orthopaedic Research Center
College of Veterinary Medicine and Biomedical Sciences
Colorado State University
Fort Collins, Colorado

Christopher E. Kawcak, DVM, PhD, Diplomate ACVS & ACVSMR
Professor
Equine Orthopedic Research Center
College of Veterinary Medicine and Biomedical Sciences
Colorado State University
Fort Collins, Colorado

Melissa R. King, DVM, PhD, DACVSMR
Assistant Professor
Equine Sports Medicine and Rehabilitation
Department of Clinical Sciences
College of Veterinary Medicine and Biomedical Sciences
Colorado State University
Fort Collins, Colorado

C. Wayne McIlwraith, BVSc, PhD, DSc (Purdue), Dr med vet (h.c. Vienna), DSc (Purdue) (h.c. Massey), Laurea Dr (h.c. Turin), D vet med (h.c. London), FRCVS, Diplomate ACVS, ECVS, & ACVSMR
University Distinguished Professor
Barbara Cox Anthony University Chair in Orthopaedics
Director Orthopaedic Research Center, Gail Holmes Equine Orthopaedic Research Center
College of Veterinary Medicine and Biomedical Sciences, School of Biomedical Engineering
Colorado State University
Fort Collins, Colorado

Kurt Selberg, MS, DVM, DACVR
Assistant Professor
Veterinary Biosciences and Diagnostic Imaging
Veterinary Teaching Hospital
University of Georgia
Athens, Georgia

P. René van Weeren, DVM, PhD, Diplomate ECVS
Professor of Equine Musculoskeletal Biology
Department of Equine Sciences
Faculty of Veterinary Medicine
Utrecht University

Natasha M. Werpy, DVM
Associate Professor
Department of Large Animal Clinical Sciences
College of Veterinary Medicine
University of Florida
Gainesville, Florida

vii

PREFACE TO THE FIRST EDITION

Lameness is the most important cause of wastage in racing horses as well as in horses that perform in other athletic events. Joint injury and joint disease are the most common causes of lameness, and together they represent a major part of the caseload for equine clinicians. Many medical and surgical treatments exist for various joint problems, but many of these treatments are controversial, particularly with regard to treatment selection and definitive treatment results. In recent years, much progress has been made in basic research in inflammatory and degenerative joint problems in the horse. In addition, prospective and retrospective studies have resulted in more realistic figures for the prognosis and treatment of many clinical entities. Much of the basic work in joint disease was originally done in laboratory animals, but more recently, considerable original work has been reported in the horse and *in vitro* work with equine tissue.

The purpose of this book is to define the current status of the rapidly changing area of developmental and degenerative joint disease, which is of significant clinical importance to the horse. We have been fortunate to obtain contributors who have done much of the original work. The principal objectives of this book are to present current scientific information on the basic joint pathobiology and translate it into practical, clinical usage for the equine clinician. At times, this can be difficult, and in some instances, only anecdotal information is available. The contents are designed to be of value to both researchers and clinicians.

Section I covers general principles in joint pathobiology and consists of eight chapters, written by contributors who have done original research in their areas. This section provides the necessary background information to effectively evaluate and interpret the diagnostic and surgical aspects of the diseases covered later. Section II presents the pathology, pathogenesis, and clinical diagnosis of traumatic and degenerative joint disease. Section III discusses the treatments available for traumatic arthritis and osteoarthritis, including physical therapy, nonsteroidal antiinflammatory drugs, intraarticular corticosteroids, hyaluronan, polysulfated glycosaminoglycan, other chondroprotective drugs, and surgery. In Section IV, osteochondritis dissecans, subchondral cystic lesions, infective arthritis, and other entities affecting joints are presented. Section V includes current research relative to equine joint disease that has not been presented previously. This includes the use of experimental models in the investigation of equine arthritis, chondrocyte culturing and explant culture systems, cellular responses and receptor mechanisms associated with bacterial lipopolysaccharide-induced joint damage, and finally, a summary by Dr. A. Robin Poole on the future direction of arthritis research.

In the time since the W.B. Saunders Company approached one of us (CWM) to write a book on equine joint disease, considerable new work has been undertaken and, fortunately, much of this is captured in timely fashion by the contributors.

It is the first time a book has been devoted to the subject of joint disease in the horse, and the amount of new information is impressive. With this book, we hope that clinicians now have a reference base with supportive data to provide more realistic answers to their clients and that the person involved in research becomes more aware of what work has been completed to date.

Three issues of semantics require mention. For consistency, we have chosen to use the word osteoarthritis instead of degenerative joint disease, which was previously used by the editors and others as a synonym for osteoarthritis. Osteoarthritis is the preferred term today in the nonequine literature and has been adopted in this text. With our international authorship, as second issue is the use of the term "infectious" versus "infective." As a British author has pointed out to us, infectious is frequently defined as "capable of being spread from one host to another with or without direct contact," thus, the equine influenza virus or equine herpesvirus could be regarded as an infectious organism. However, "infective" by usage is more restricted in its definition, and Churchill's Medical Dictionary suggests "capable of causing infection" as its only definition. Therefore, it is felt that in the case of infective arthritis, bacteria could not be regarded as infectious as in the case of respiratory viruses, although the bacteria could be regarded as infective because it is capable of causing infection. The editors and scrutineers are concerned about this distinction in Britain; whereas in American literature various terms (including septic) have been used synonymously. Both terms are used in this text according to the contributor's preference. Hyaluronic acid, sodium hyaluronate, and hyaluronan are also used interchangeably. It has been suggested that when the cation of polysaccharide is undetermined, the compound is properly referred to as hyaluronan; therefore, this term is used.

We would like to recognize the editorial and production staffs of the W.B. Saunders Company for their professional efforts on this project. We want to thank the authors for their excellent contributions, and Helen Mawhiney for secretarial assistance. We would also like to acknowledge Tom McCracken, Phil Guzzy, and Conery Calhoun of Biographics; and Jenger Smith and Charley Kerlee of CSU Multi-Media Instructional Development for their help with illustrations. Dr. McIlwraith gratefully acknowledges Drs. John F. Fessler and David C. Van Sickle for their early influence and mentoring in starting a career in investigating equine joint disease.

Finally, because many joint-associated (or orthopedic) problems remain to be solved for our equine patients, all royalties from this text will be used for ongoing research in our Equine Orthopedic Research Laboratory at Colorado State University.

C. Wayne McIlwraith

Gayle W. Trotter

PREFACE TO THE SECOND EDITION

As discussed in the preface to the first edition of this book, lameness is the most important cause of wastage in racing horses as well as in horses that perform in other athletic events. Joint injury and joint disease are the most common causes of lameness, and together they represent most of the caseload for equine clinicians. Many medical and surgical treatments exist for various joint problems, and there have been many advances in this area since 1996 as well as much clarification of the value of various treatments with evidence-based research. Whereas in 1996 we extrapolated much of our information from laboratory animal research and human studies, the majority of this text now provides evidence based on experimental and clinical research in the horse. This increases both the appropriateness of the findings and the clinical translation for the veterinarian.

The purpose of this book is to redefine the current status of the continually changing area of developmental and traumatic joint disease. We are fortunate to have contributors who have done much of the original work. New biologic therapies that are targeted against specific mediators that have been identified with different pathobiologic and biomechanical etiologies. These basics will be presented but limited to what is clinically relevant.

The text begins with a discussion of general anatomy and physiology of joints as well as biomechanics, followed by the pathogenetic pathways of traumatic arthritis and posttraumatic osteoarthritis and the pathologic manifestations of joint disease. Osteochondritis dissecans, subchondral cystic lesions, septic arthritis, and the effect of loading on joint tissues are then reviewed. The principles of diagnosis follow, with much increased detail on the current state-of-the-art in clinical examination and intraarticular injection (including simulations based on computed tomography) as well as in imaging, which has probably progressed the most in equine joint disease use in the 19 years since the first edition was published.

There is a chapter on synovial fluid and serum biomarkers, followed by separate chapters with discussion of the validation of the various treatment options including nonsteroidal antiinflammatory drugs, intraarticular corticosteroids, hyaluronan, polysulfated glycosaminoglycan, and pentosan polysulfate. Newer therapies that are presented for the first time include biologic therapies (including the autologous-conditioned serum products as well as the platelet-rich plasma products and mesenchymal stem cells). Various types of rehabilitation including underwater treadmilling as well as a careful discussion of oral joint supplements and their use in equine joint disease are also new materials included for the first time.

Chapters 20 through 26 then cover all details on pathogenesis, diagnosis, and treatment of the various joint entities by region including separate chapters on distal limb, fetlock, carpus, elbow and shoulder, tarsus, stifle, and hip. We conclude with a chapter on joint disease; both current research and future directions in joint disease that will continue to improve our ability to treat horses are featured.

ACKNOWLEDGMENTS

Much of the book has been written by the four of us, but we have had particularly critical contributions from Dr. Myra Barrett in both content and organization with the imaging parts of Chapter 9 as well as Chapters 20 through 26. Drs. Natasha Werpy and Kurt Selberg have also contributed to the imaging chapters; Dr. Janny de Grauw contributed to the chapter on synovial fluid and serum biomarkers; and Dr. Laurie Goodrich added her expertise to Chapter 27, and Dr. Jos Malda commented on Chapter 1 and Dr. van Weeren's part of Chapter 27. We also wish to acknowledge Lynsey Bosch for typing and patience and Paula Vanderlinden for typing and organization as we have prepared these manuscripts. We also thank Dave Carlson for the line drawings to go with the radiographs in Chapter 9 and the editorial and production staffs of Elsevier with special mention to Penny Rudolph who started this project; Brandi Graham for her great support, patience, and editing; and William Drone for copyediting.

Drs. McIlwraith, Frisbie, and Kawcak wish to acknowledge the incredible contributions and assistance of faculty and staff of the Orthopaedic Research Center and the more recent program of Equine Sports Medicine and Rehabilitation. This team has facilitated acquisition of much of the information in this book and will advance our knowledge for future editions. Dr. van Weeren also acknowledges the great contributions of the present and past members of his research team at Utrecht, with special mention of Dr. Pieter Brama, on whose research efforts a large part of the content of Chapter 8 is based.

In addition, Wayne, Dave, Chris, and René are fortunate to be married to experts in this or related areas. Dr. Nancy Goodman has been Wayne's major clinical mentor starting in 1983 and has given great professional and personal support. Dave Frisbie thanks Dr. Myra Barrett-Frisbie, and her major contributions to this text have been previously noted. Chris Kawcak is married to Dr. Erin Contino, who is a product of our Equine Sports Medicine and Rehabilitation program as well as our graduate research program and is soon to be a faculty member at Colorado State University. René van Weeren is married to Madelon Bitterling, who is both a human and an animal physiotherapist and an expert in veterinary ergonomics.

We would also like to recognize the funding agencies that have supported our research. This includes Grayson-Jockey Club Research Foundation, American Quarter Horse Association, United States Equestrian Foundation, and Morris Animal Foundation, as well as the National Institute of Health. Finances limit us answering many important relevant questions and, to support much of this work, we at the ORC owe it to our fantastic donors who contribute to answering these questions. These discretionary dollars have allowed a considerable amount of the research to be translated into clinical reality here.

CONTENTS

General Anatomy and Physiology of Joints

P. René van Weeren

The horse has always taken a special position among the species that have been domesticated by humankind. The horse was domesticated rather late, around 3500 BC,[1] millennia after such species as goat, sheep, and cattle. Unlike these other species, the main purpose of the horse's domestication was not the provision of edible products or products that could be somehow transformed into clothing, such as meat, milk, fur, or skin, but for a less tangible commodity: the combination of physical power and athletic capacity.

Horses have been the major power source for all Eurasian and Northern African civilizations since their introduction from roughly 3500 to 500 BC until the invention of the steam engine that started the Industrial Revolution in the late 1700s. The ultimate personification of the role of the horse in society is perhaps Bucephalus, the legendary horse of Alexander the Great, who conquered the vastest land empire the world has ever known. Bucephalus served Alexander who, according to legend, was the only person able to mount the stallion, from a young age to its death at the age of 30 after the battle of Hydaspes in what is now Pakistan, 2900 miles from its native Macedonia. There, Alexander named the city of Bucephala (present-day Jhelum) after him. After the Industrial Revolution horses still remained essential for many sectors of human society until after World War II, when the combustion engine definitively took over all traditional roles of the horse in warfare, transport, and agriculture. Some have predicted that the loss of its classic duties would make the horse into a zoo species,[2] but they were proven entirely wrong by the rapidly increasing popularity of the horse as a sports and leisure animal from the mid-1960s onwards. Over the millennia, humans and horses appeared to have bonded in a way that goes far beyond economic value or utility and is more profound than with any other domesticated species, with the exception of the dog. Though admittedly the equine industry is susceptible to the fluctuations of economic prosperity, this fascination for the equine species is not likely to disappear soon, if ever. This obviously guarantees the horse its privileged place in the big family of animal species with which humankind has surrounded itself.

Where the role of the horse in society has changed profoundly in the past century, the underlying reasons of its use and popularity have not changed at all. It is still the stamina of the animal and athletic capacity of its locomotor system that form the basis for almost all present-day use. The most critical body systems for athletic performance are the cardiorespiratory system and the musculoskeletal system. Within the latter system, joints are literally pivotal elements. It may not be surprising that orthopedic malfunctioning or other musculoskeletal disorders account for the vast majority of reasons to consult an equine vet.[3] Of the specific elements of the musculoskeletal system, joint disorders invariably rank first or second in importance (together with tendinopathies, depending on discipline). Most figures come from the racing industry,[4,5] but the relatively scarce data for sport horses also point in the same direction.[6,7] In a survey of U.S. horse owners in 1998 it was estimated that 60% of all lameness was related to osteoarthritis (OA) and approximately \$145 million was spent on veterinary bills relating to the problem.[8] In this respect, the clinical importance of joint disorders in the equine species is very comparable to the situation in humans where musculoskeletal disorders in general and articular pathologies in particular represent an enormous burden to society in terms of loss of quality of life and costs of healthcare with 151 million sufferers of OA worldwide.[9] For this and a number of important biologic reasons the horse is increasingly recognized as a suitable, if not the best, model for human joint disease.[10] This translational aspect of equine joint disease will be dealt with in more detail in Chapter 27, which discusses arthritis research and future directions in joint disease.

This first chapter gives a general introduction into the anatomy and physiology of the (equine) joint, as a basis for the understanding of the following chapters that address in detail specific disorders, diagnostic possibilities, and therapeutic interventions.

JOINT FUNCTIONS

Whereas the necessary stability of the equine musculoskeletal system is provided by the rigid bony components, joints permit motion of these bony components in relation to each other and, indirectly, the displacement of the entire individual with respect to the environment, that is, locomotion. To accomplish this, joints have to meet several requirements. They have to be as robust as the bony elements of the musculoskeletal system, as the forces generated by locomotion and other (athletic) activities are transmitted through joints as they are through bones. They also have to allow for smooth and as frictionless as possible motion of the bony ends that articulate with respect to each other. Lastly, they have a role, together with other structures, such as the digital cushion in the foot, to mitigate and dampen the accelerations and associated vibrations that are generated during the impact peak of the stride cycle at hoof landing. This latter aspect has been relatively well studied in the equine literature.[11,12]

All the aforementioned requirements that are at least partially contradictory (strength comparable to bone, smooth surfaces for supple gliding, and resilience for shock absorption) have to be accommodated in a single structure, which is a challenging task. As will be explained, nature deals with these challenges in an ingenious way, however, at the cost of flexibility and repair capacity. For reasons of clarity the components that make up a joint will be dealt with separately, but it is important to stress that a joint is more than a collection of tissues with separate characteristics and functions. There is common agreement nowadays that the joint should be seen as a complex multicomposite organ not unlike structures such as the liver, kidney or heart.[13,14] Within this organ the constituting elements act together to ensure proper joint function. There is a strong interplay of all these components in health and disease and mutual influencing of physiologic functioning; malfunctioning of the components will also inevitably affect the other constituents and hence performance of the entire joint at a shorter or longer term.

TYPES OF JOINTS

Joints can be classified in several ways. A gross division can be made between classification according to structural characteristics, that is, the type of tissue(s) that form the interface between the articulating bony parts of the skeleton, and classification according to function, or the degree and type of movement joints allow.

The currently used basic classification is three major categories, which are *fibrous joints* with the bone connected by dense connective tissue, *cartilaginous joints* where cartilage is the interface, and *synovial joints* in which there is a fluid-filled cavity.[15] In the horse, the articulations between the bodies of the vertebrae that make up the axial skeleton are fibrous joints, with the exception of the articulation between the first and second cervical vertebrae (C1-C2), which is a synovial joint. A cartilaginous joint has an interface consisting of hyaline or fibrous cartilage; examples are the human intervertebral

disk and the symphysis of the pubic bones in both humans and horses. In synovial joints there is no structural connection between the bony parts of the skeleton, but both ends are capped with hyaline cartilage and articulate by gliding over each other although contained in a joint capsule that is filled with synovial fluid, a viscous liquid. A sliding bearing in mechanical engineering basically functions according to the same principle.

In a functional sense, there are several other ways to classify joints. A common way is according to the degree of motion they permit. Although the following nomenclature is currently seen as obsolete,[15] it is still widely used and will hence be mentioned here. A *synarthrosis* is a joint permitting little mobility. Most of these joints are of fibrous nature, such as the sutures that connect the bony components that make up the skull. *Amphiarthroses* are joints that permit more, but still very limited, mobility. They are generally of either fibrous or cartilaginous nature, with the intervertebral joints (again with the exception of C1-C2) as the best examples. Finally, *diarthrodial joints* permit maximal motion. These are always synovial joints and their motion is limited by periarticular or intraarticular structures such as capsules or ligaments, but not by the nature of the joint. Virtually all joints of the appendicular skeleton of the horse are diarthrodial joints.

Other functional classifications are based on the degrees of freedom a joint has. Any three-dimensional body in space has six potential degrees of freedom within the global coordinate system: three translations along the x, y, and z axes of the coordinate system, and three rotations around these axes. In aeronautical terms these rotations are indicated as pitch, yaw, and roll. In joints, translations of bony parts with respect to each other are limited (but may occur, for instance in the middle carpal joint), but rotations can be substantial and may comprise rotations around more than one axis, as is the case in the hip joint. The horse has evolved as a flight-and-fright animal specialized in fast motion, for which reason most of the joints of the appendicular skeleton are largely monoaxial, permitting excursions that are basically restricted to flexion-extension in the sagittal plane.

This chapter is limited to the general anatomy and physiology of diarthrodial joints only, as the other joint types in the horse hardly, if ever, give rise to clinical problems.

EMBRYONIC JOINT DEVELOPMENT

The axial and limb skeleton is derived from the embryonic paraxial and lateral plate mesoderm, which is the precursor tissue of, among other tissues, the hyaline cartilage that is found in diarthrodial joints. The mesenchymal progenitor cells, originating from the lateral plate mesoderm, differentiate into chondrocytes that form a cartilaginous skeletal anlagen as precursor for the later bony skeleton and connecting diarthrodial joints.[16] Joint formation occurs when cells at the future joint site start to flatten and form a region that is distinct from the adjacent cartilaginous areas.[17] This zone, once morphologically distinct, is called the *interzone*. The cells in this zone lose their chondrogenic phenotype and cease the expression of collagen type II. The interzone is further characterized by the expression of growth/differentiation factor 5 (Gdf5), Wnt9a, double cortin, and versican, whereas matrilin-1 is not expressed anymore.[16,18] The importance of the interzone for joint formation has been demonstrated unequivocally by the experimental removal of the interzone from the elbow joint in chicken embryos, which led to the fusion of the humerus with the radius and the ulna in the absence of joint formation.[19]

The moment when interzone development starts during embryonic development varies per species. Recently, equine embryonic development has been mapped in detail using magnetic resonance imaging.[20] When taking the day in which ovulation was first detected as day 0 of pregnancy and hence of embryonic life (E0), it has been shown that at E40 the interzone is fully formed and consists of three distinct layers: the inner interzone (II) that will develop into the joint cavity, intraarticular structures, and articular cartilage, and two adjacent outer interzones, which are precursors to the epiphyseal growth cartilage and will eventually turn into bone.[21] Using laser capture microdissection to harvest tissue samples from outer and inner interzones, respectively, it was shown that the mRNA expression patterns of both tissue types varied markedly for genes related to chondrogenesis. Further, several genes involved in cell adhesion, transcription regulation, and various signaling pathways were expressed differentially. The top 25 genes expressed more in the outer than in the intermediate interzone were mostly associated with endochondral ossification, cartilage, and growth plate matrix composition. Examples are genes for matrilin-1 and 3, BMP5, and Col2al. They also partake in Wnt/b-catenin signaling, bone morphogenetic protein (BMP) signaling, and sonic hedgehog signaling, which are essential regulatory pathways for chondrogenesis and osteogenesis.[21] This information is important for the further development of regenerative techniques for articular lesions in which the full recovery of the original structure and function is still a major challenge (see also Chapter 27).

PRINCIPLES OF JOINT ANATOMY

Figure 1-1 presents a semischematic and simplified drawing of a diarthrodial joint. The basic structures common to all synovial joints are layers of articular cartilage covering the ends of the articulating bones that together constitute the joint, subchondral bone beneath this cartilage, synovial fluid that surrounds the articulating bone ends, and some structure that restrains the synovial fluid within the joint. This latter structure will often be a joint capsule, but other structures may serve this purpose as well, as is the case of the proximal interphalangeal joint that has no capsule but in which the synovial fluid is retained by the ligamentous and tendinous structures that surround the joint. Additional structures that serve principally to stabilize the joint and to restrict motion in unwanted directions are collateral or other periarticular ligaments, intraarticular ligaments, such as the cruciate ligaments in the femorotibial joint, and menisci, as in the femorotibial

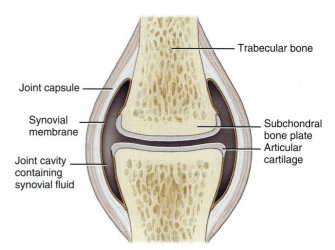

FIGURE 1-1 Schematic representation of a diarthrodial joint. (Adapted from: De Grauw J.C. (2010). Molecular monitoring of equine joint homeostasis. Thesis, Utrecht University.)

and temporomandibular joints. These constituting structures of the joint will be discussed separately in the following paragraphs.

Articular Cartilage

The functional characteristics of a construction are largely determined by the interplay of the material properties of the building blocks or components that construction is made of and the way these components are arranged and interconnected, that is, the architecture of the construction. For structured tissues, such as articular cartilage or bone, this is similar. However, as in all living tissues, the situation is more complex as cellular action, driven by a wide variety of cues and effected through various signaling pathways, determines tissue homeostasis and the response to external stimuli. If that response can somehow not cope with the demands made by these stimuli, pathology may ensue.

The major components of the extracellular matrix (ECM) of articular cartilage are collagen, proteoglycans (PGs), and water. Water content varies from 70% to 80%, depending on age. The other components account for approximately 50% (collagen) and 35% (PGs) on a dry weight basis. The remaining 15% consists of about two thirds (10% of total dry weight) of glycoproteins (substances such as proteinases and inhibitors of these, growth factors, specific molecules such as fibronectin, lubricin, cartilage oligomeric protein [COMP], etc.) Minor fractions are minerals (3%), lipids (1%), and miscellaneous components (1%).[22] The cellular component of articular cartilage is relatively small and accounts for approximately 1% to 12% volume percentage, depending on the location within the joint and the depth in relation to the surface.[22]

Layered Composition of Articular Cartilage

Whereas cartilage macroscopically is seemingly a homogeneous tissue, there are large differences in structure and composition from the surface down to the transition to the subchondral bone. Classically, four layers or zones are discerned, although the transitions between these layers are gradual rather than abrupt, apart from the last layer. These layers are the superficial zone, the intermediate zone, the deep zone, which together form the hyaline part of the cartilage, and the very distinct layer of calcified cartilage that forms the interface between the resilient hyaline cartilage and the rigid subchondral bone (Figure 1-2). The superficial layer is characterized by flattened chondrocytes, densely packed type II collagen fibrils running parallel to the surface, a relatively small amount of PGs, and high water content.[23] The middle or transitional zone has lower water content, more PG, and a lower density of collagen. The zone is further characterized by rounded chondrocytes dispersed irregularly in the ECM. The deep zone has the lowest collagen content, the highest

concentration of PG but the lowest percentage of water of any zone, and chondrocytes arranged in columns perpendicular to the subchondral bone. This zone is separated from the calcified layer by the so-called tidemark that is commonly described as a single, hematoxyphil line up to 10 μm in thickness.[24] However, the situation is less simple than that, as the tidemark has been shown to be a complex three-dimensional structure that dips at places through the entire calcified zone to abut onto subjacent bone or marrow spaces.[25] This means that there are places with direct contact between hyaline cartilage and subchondral bone. There are other differences in the architecture and chemical composition of the various zones that will be dealt with in the following sections that go into more detail on these subjects.

Collagen

The principal collagen of articular cartilage is the fibrillar collagen type II. This type of collagen consists of three identical proteins consisting of approximately 1000 amino acids each, the so-called α_1-chains that are wound around each other in the form of a right-handed triple helix. The collagen molecule is assembled intracellularly as proform with so-called propeptides at both the N (amino-) and C (carboxy-) terminals. These propeptides are cleaved once the molecule is in the extracellular space by proteinases to deliver the final collagen molecule (Figure 1-3). The α_1-chains consists of approximately 330 glycine-X-Y repeats in which X and Y are often proline or hydroxyproline, but they can also be other amino acids. The N- telopeptides and C-telopeptides, which are nonhelical, are important sites for the formation of cross-links by which collagen molecules can be linked to each other and to other molecules. Collagen type II molecules typically assemble into large fibrillar structures. These large collagen fibrils are of crucial importance for the mechanical properties of articular cartilage and have a function that can

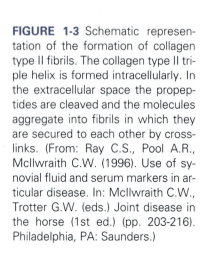

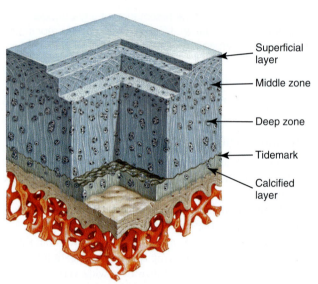

FIGURE 1-2 Semischematic drawing of the zonal composition of articular cartilage, sitting on the compact subchondral plate and the underlying trabecular bone.

FIGURE 1-3 Schematic representation of the formation of collagen type II fibrils. The collagen type II triple helix is formed intracellularly. In the extracellular space the propeptides are cleaved and the molecules aggregate into fibrils in which they are secured to each other by cross-links. (From: Ray C.S., Pool A.R., McIlwraith C.W. (1996). Use of synovial fluid and serum markers in articular disease. In: McIlwraith C.W., Trotter G.W. (eds.) Joint disease in the horse (1st ed.) (pp. 203-216). Philadelphia, PA: Saunders.)

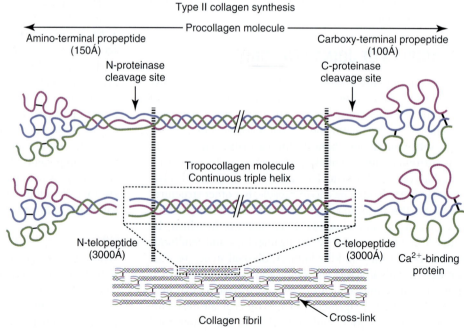

be compared to the steel rods in steel-reinforced concrete. They are arranged in a typical three-dimensional arcade-like structure that was described for the first time in 1925 by Benninghoff and is schematically represented in Figure 1-4.[26] The real situation can be visualized using advanced microscopic techniques, such as high-resolution helium ion microscopy[27] (Figure 1-5). In the classic Benninghoff pattern,

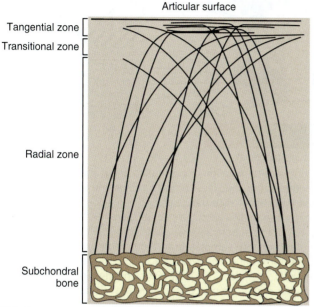

FIGURE 1-4 Schematic representation of the configuration of the collagen network within articular cartilage, showing the arcade-like structure originally described by Benninghoff (1925). (From: Van Weeren P.R., Firth E.C. (2008). Future tools for early diagnosis and monitoring of musculoskeletal injury: biomarkers and CT. Vet Clin North Am Equine Pract, 24(1), 153-175.)

collagen fibrils arise from the calcified layer and then course perpendicularly to the tidemark towards the articular surface through the deep cartilage layer. In the intermediate layer, the fibrils start to arch and hence change direction. The top of the arcade is positioned just under the articular surface in the superficial zone where fibrils can also be found running parallel or tangential to the surface (see Figure 1-4). The orientation of the fibrils can be made visible using special microscopic techniques based on the use of polarized light (Figure 1-6). Quantification of these images is possible through the calculation of the so-called orientation index,[28] a parameter describing the average angle of the collagen fibrils in relation to the articular surface. Whereas the arcade configuration is valid for mature joints, it has been shown that in joints from fetuses or neonatal animals this configuration does not yet exist in its final form. In these young individuals the predominant alignment of the collagen fibrils is parallel to the surface.[29] Modeling of the definitive Benninghoff arcade structure takes place in the juvenile period, triggered by mechanical loading[29] with important consequences for the biomechanical behavior of the cartilage.[30] Further, the exact form of the arcades may be not identical for all joints as it relates to the predominant direction of joint loading. It has been shown for instance that in the equine metacarpophalangeal joint the direction of the fibrils in the deep cartilage layer is less perpendicular to the surface than could be expected based on the classic Benninghoff configuration. This may have to do with the large range of joint motion in the loaded position, which will result in a relatively large contribution of tangential forces to overall loading.[31]

Structural coherence and extra strength to the collagen network are provided by cross-links that connect the α_1-chains within the same collagen molecule, but also connect different collagen molecules and different collagen fibrils.

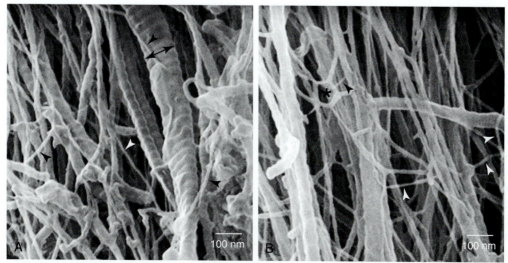

FIGURE 1-5 High-resolution helium ion microscopy images from the middle deep zone show a wide range of fibril diameters (A, B; double-head arrow, 126 nm; arrowheads 5 to 11 nm) and fibril connections (B, asterisk). (From: Vanden Berg-Foels W.S., Scipioni L., Huynh C., et al. (2012). Helium ion microscopy for high-resolution visualization of the articular cartilage collagen network. J Microsc, 246(2), 168-176.)

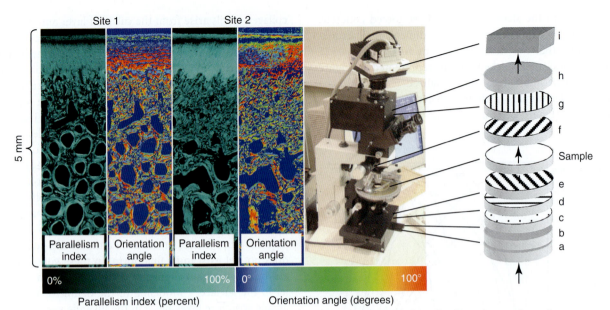

FIGURE 1-6 The use of polarized light microscopy for the determination of orientation angle and parallelism index. Collagen fibrils run parallel to each other in the deep layer of the cartilage and in the superficial layer, indicated by a white color. In the transitional zone they arch and hence lose their parallel arrangement (dark color). The orientation is perpendicular to the calcified layer (90°) in the deep zone (red color), changing to tangential (0°) in the superficial layer (blue color), with angles in between in the transitional zone. The pictures are from samples from the dorsoproximal margin (site I) and the central fovea (site II) of the proximal articular surface of the equine proximal phalanx. (From: Holopainen J.T., Halmesmäki E., Harjula T., et al. (2008). Changes in subchgoondral bone mineral density and collagen matrix organization in growing horses. Bone 43(6), 1108-1114.)

Cross-link formation is one of the so-called posttranslational modifications of collagen and is the last chemical modification occurring during the formation of the primary collagen structure. There are various types of cross-links. Common covalent cross-links are the pyridinoline cross-links that form between lysyl and hydroxylysyl residues in the collagen network in a largely irreversible process (lysylpyridinoline [LP], cross-links and hydroxylysylpyridinoline [HP] cross-links, respectively, the last being more abundant in articular cartilage). They have a major influence on the structural and hence on the biomechanical characteristics of the collagen network.[32] A special category of cross-links is formed through the process of nonenzymatic glycation. Collagen molecules have an exceptionally long lifetime once incorporated into the ECM of cartilage, which makes them susceptible to the accumulation of advanced nonenzymatic glycation end products (AGEs) via the Maillard reaction.[33] This process results in increased cross-linking, such as pentosidine formation from lysine, sugar, and arginine moieties. Pentosidine is one of the few Maillard cross-links of which the structure has been elucidated and can be used as a sensitive marker for the process of nonenzymatic glycation.[34] As the accumulation of AGEs depends on the turnover rate of a protein or tissue, it can be used as a measure for the metabolic rate of that structure.[35]

Apart from collagen type II, many other collagens can be found in the ECM of articular cartilage. Some, but not all, of these are fibrillar and some have a structural role. The exact role is not known of all collagens. Minor collagens that form, together with collagen type II as a copolymer, the fibril network of developing cartilage, are collagens IX and XI. Other minor collagen species that can be found in extracts of articular cartilage are types III, VI, XIII, and XIV. Collagen type X is restricted to the hypertrophic zone of cartilage actively undergoing the process of endochondral ossification.

The nonfibrillar collagen IX molecules are attached to the surface of the collagen type II fibrils. They are more abundant in juvenile articular cartilage (approximately 10% of total collagen), which is characterized by collagen type II fibrils that are on average smaller in diameter than in mature cartilage, in which the concentration of collagen IX is about 1% of total collagen.[36] Seven cross-linking sites have been described on the collagen IX molecule that interact with collagen II and other collagen IX molecules.[37] Collagen XI is a fibrillar collagen that is located in the core of the collagen II fibrils and of which the molecules are primarily cross-linked to each other in a head-to-tail manner (Figure 1-7). They are believed to form a template that constrains the lateral growth of collagen II fibrils.[38] Also collagen XI is more prominently present in juvenile tissue (approximately 10%) than in mature cartilage (approximately 3%).[36] Both collagens IX and XI are critical to the correct functioning of the collagen network in articular cartilage.

Collagen type III is a fibrillar collagen consisting of a homotrimer of α_1(III) chains that functions as a copolymer of collagen I in many tissues and is known to be prominent at sites of healing and repair of many tissues, including tendons.[39]

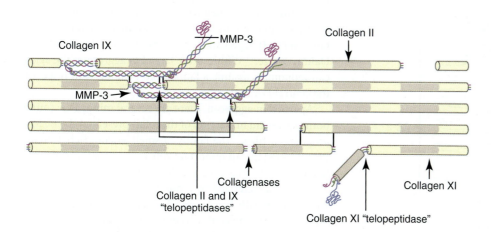

FIGURE 1-7 Known and speculated sites of cleavage peptide bonds of collagens, necessary for either degradation or lateral growth, within the collagen heteropolymer that forms the backbone of the collagen network. (From: Eyre D.R., Weis M.A., Wu J.J. (2006). Articular cartilage collagen: an irreplaceable framework? Euro Cells Mater, 12, 57-63.)

In articular cartilage a small, but significant amount of collagen III can be found, mostly in the matrix surrounding the chondrocytes. Recent studies indicate that the molecule may function as a covalently bound (to collagen II) modifier of the fibril network and may, as in other tissues, have a role in the response of the tissue to damage.[39] Collagen type VI is a nonfibrillar collagen that can be found in the matrix of most tissues, including articular cartilage, at low concentrations (<1%). It is predominantly localized within the pericellular matrix and is a structural component of the chondron. Chondron is the name for the *ensemble* of the chondrocyte and its pericellular microenvironment, which is generally considered the primary structural, functional, and metabolic unit of hyaline cartilages.[40] Collagen VI can self-assembly into a filamentous network and is more concentrated in fibrocartilage than in hyaline cartilage.[41] Collagens type XII and XIV are members of the so-called FACET (fibril-associated collagen with interrupted triple-helix) collagen subfamily. They are not covalently bound to the large collagen II network and their function is largely unknown.[41]

Collagen X has a special position in articular cartilage. The molecule is specific for cartilage of juvenile individuals in which an active process of endochondral ossification is ongoing. It is synthesized by hypertrophic chondrocytes and may make up to 18% of the total amount of collagen in the hypertrophic region of the epiphyseal growth cartilage in growing animals. It has a role in the regulation of matrix mineralization and the compartmentalization of matrix components.[42] Collagen X is expressed by clinically affected cartilage in mature patients with, for example, OA, where it is associated with enhanced mineralization, or other cartilage disorders,[43] where it may interfere with the normal interaction between collagens, which may result in ECM dysregulation.[44]

Proteoglycans

The other main component of cartilage ECM, apart from water, is formed by PG aggregates, which are interspersed between the collagen fibrils and connected to them either directly or via hyaluronan (hyaluronic acid) molecules. The PGs form a group of composite molecules featuring a protein (hence: *proteo*) and a sugar (hence: *glycol*) component. In the case of cartilage the PGs feature some number of chondroitin sulfate side chains, which are part of the so-called lectican family.[45] The family includes aggrecan, versican, neurocan, and brevican. The best researched and by far most abundant and emblematic member of this family in articular cartilage is aggrecan. Various forms exist and the aggrecan molecule may lose several parts when the animal ages or when pathology occurs, but the typical aggrecan monomer consists of a large core protein to which several hundreds of glycosaminoglycan side chains are attached (see Figure 1-8). The core protein has an amino (N-) terminal side and a carboxy (C-) terminal of which the former is normally connected via a link protein to another component of the ECM, mostly hyaluronan. Three distinct globular domains have been identified. The N-terminal G1 domain anchors the aggrecan molecule to hyaluronan via the link protein. The G2 domain is unique to aggrecan and is known to be highly conserved, but it has (as yet) no known function. The C-terminal G3 domain links the PG aggregates to the ECM.[46] This domain is not without importance, as in man hereditary disorders have been described, among which autosomal dominant familial osteochondritis dissecans, because of missense mutations in the aggrecan C-type lectin repeat in this domain.[46]

Between the G2 and G3 domains the glycosaminoglycan side chains attach to the aggrecan core protein. Keratan sulfate (KS) is a glycosaminoglycan consisting of repeats of disaccharides of galactose and sulfated or nonsulfated N-acetylglucosamine. Chondroitin sulfate (CS) is composed of disaccharide repeats of glucuronic acid and sulfated or nonsulfated N-acetylgalactosamine. The KS side chains are attached closest to the G2 domain, and the CS chains are situated more towards the terminal G3 domain (see Figure 1-8). Up to 30 KS and 100 CS side chains may be bound to a single core protein.[47] The sulfate groups in both side chains are highly hydrophilic because they are negatively charged. These groups account for the high viscosity of the molecules the CS and KS chains form part of, such as the aggrecan monomers. The molecular configuration of the aggrecan monomer is neither uniform nor stable over time. The length of both the core protein and the side chains tends to decrease with advancing age,

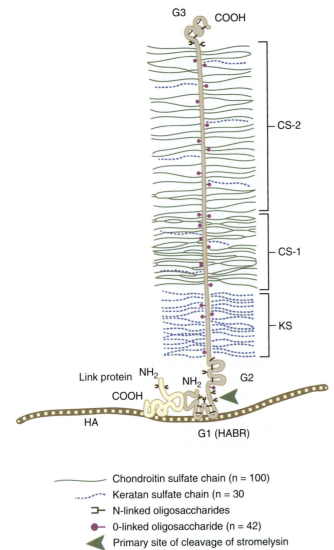

— Chondroitin sulfate chain (n = 100)
····· Keratan sulfate chain (n = 30)
⊐⊏ N-linked oligosaccharides
●— 0-linked oligosaccharide (n = 42)
◀ Primary site of cleavage of stromelysin

FIGURE 1-8 Schematic presentation of an aggrecan molecule, consisting of a core protein that is bound to hyaluronic acid (HA) by a link protein. To the core protein a large number of side chains consisting of sulfated glycosaminoglycans is attached. These are keratin sulfate (KS) and chondroitin sulfate (CS) side chains. Globular domains 1 (hyaluronic acid binding region [HABR]), 2 and 3 are indicated. (From: Ray C.S., Pool A.R., McIlwraith C.W. (1996). Use of synovial fluid and serum markers in articular disease. In: McIlwraith C.W., Trotter G.W. (eds.) Joint disease in the horse (1st ed.) (pp. 203-216). Philadelphia, PA: Saunders.)

which affects both nanostructure of the cartilage ECM and the nanomechanical properties of the tissue[48] (Figure 1-9).

The aggrecan monomers bind with their G1 domains via a link protein with hyaluronan or hyaluronic acid (HA). Hyaluronan is also a glycosaminoglycan, but it is not sulfated. The molecule consists of repeats of the disaccharides glucuronic acid and N-acetyl glucosamine. Hyaluronan is a major component of the ECM of articular cartilage (Figure 1-10), but it can also be found in free form in synovial fluid. As the aggrecan monomers are strongly negatively charged through the sulfate groups of their CS and KS side chains and

hence attract water, they will repel each other. Consequently, strongly water-binding PG aggregates will form that may contain over 100 aggrecan monomers and may be about 2.10^7 Dalton in size.[49] Within these large PG aggregates the aggrecan monomers assume a fan-shaped position with respect to the central HA molecule.

Apart from aggrecan, there are several minor PGs (minor both in size and in fraction of the total) present in the ECM of articular cartilage. The family of small leucine-rich proteins/PGs (SLRPs) has an important role in the creation and maintenance of the structure and function of articular cartilage. They are characterized by a number of repeats of around 25 amino acids with leucine residues at conserved locations.[50] Some of these molecules have CS or dermatan sulfate side chains, making them into proper PGs. Others have not and are actually proteins, hence the double meaning of the "p" in the abbreviation SLRP. The most well-known SLRPs in articular cartilage are decorin, biglycan, fibromodulin, lumican, and chondroadherin. An important function of several SLRPs is the regulation of fibrillogenesis, as they bind to collagens during fibril formation via their leucine-rich repeat domain.[51,52] Biglycan and decorin are known to bind via their core protein to filaments of collagen type VI.[53] In combination with members of another group of noncollagenous proteins called matrilins, which bind to triple helical collagen, links are provided that interconnect the entire ECM network and thus provide structural coherence. Fibromodulin and lumican also affect fibrillogenesis and seem to share many functions.[50] Chondroadherin is abundant in cartilage but also present in bone where it decreases the production of cytokines that activate osteoclasts, such as the interleukins IL-1 and IL-6.[50] The other SLRPs are also involved in many signaling pathways. An example is the role of biglycan in the regulation of inflammation through its function as an endogenous ligand of the innate immunity toll-like receptors TLR-4 and TLR-2 in macrophages.[52]

Noncollagenous Proteins

Apart from the major components (collagen and PGs), the ECM of cartilage contains numerous other components, including a number of noncollagenous proteins. The matrilins have already been mentioned. Another well-known constituent of the ECM is COMP, a member of the thrombospondin family, also called trombospondin 5. The COMP molecule has five identical subunits that can all bind to (different) collagen molecules. It is thought that COMP can bring five collagen molecules together, thus facilitating assembly of the matrix. It does not bind to established collagen fibrils but seems to act predominantly at an early stage of fibril formation. In mature ECM it has a more stabilizing role through its binding with collagen type IX and matrilins.[50]

The Cellular Component of Articular Cartilage

Mature articular cartilage has long been considered a tissue containing a single cell type only: the chondrocyte. Relatively recently it has become clear, however, that, as in many tissues, there is a population of progenitor cells.[54] The presence

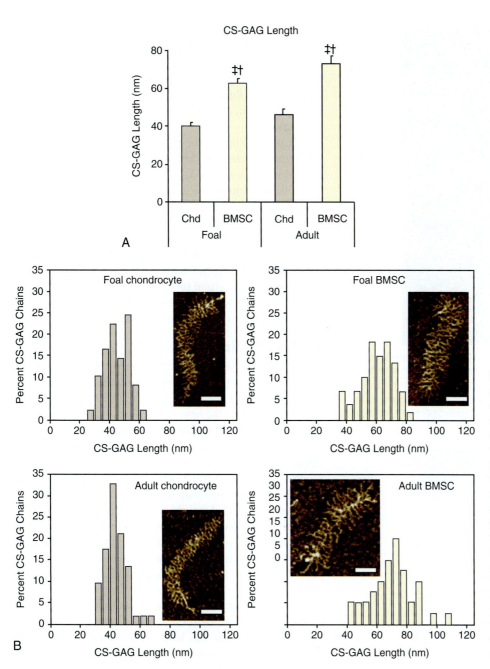

FIGURE 1-9 Aggrecan CS-GAG chain quantification. Aggrecan extracted from chondrocyte (Chd) and BMSC-seeded peptide hydrogels after 21 days of culture with TGF-β1. **(A)** Average CS-GAG length per molecule. Mean ± sem; n=28 to 35 aggrecan molecules; ‡ vs foal chondrocyte; † vs adult chondrocyte; p<0.05. **(B)** Histograms of CS-GAG distribution on the single pictured molecule. Scale bar=100 nm. (Reproduced with permission from Kopesky P.W., Lee H.Y., Venderploeg E.J., et al. (2010). Adult equine bone marrow stromal cells produce a cartilage-like ECM mechanically superior to animal-matched adult chondrocytes. Matrix Biol, 29(5):427-438.)

of articular cartilage progenitor cells (ACPCs) has been demonstrated in many species, including the horse.[55] These cells are potentially very interesting for the field of cartilage regeneration.[55,56] The amount of ACPCs is tiny in relation to the number of chondrocytes, which themselves represent only a small fraction of the total volume of articular cartilage (approximately 1% to 12%[22]).

Cell density is higher in lighter species; for example, small laboratory species such as rats and mice have relatively high cell density compared to larger species such as humans or horses. This may be caused by the relatively larger fraction of total cartilage thickness that is taken up by the superficial (cell-denser) layer in their cartilage. This feature that is specific for these small species may limit their value for translational studies on cartilage repair.[57]

Chondrocytes are of mesenchymal origin and can be seen as differentiated fibroblasts, a stage to which they tend to dedifferentiate rapidly when cultured in a monolayer without specific precautions. This dedifferentiation does not occur when cultured in the form of small pieces of the entire cartilage layer (explants) or in the three-dimensional environment of alginate beads.[58] This indicates that the spatial configuration of their environment is important for maintaining the phenotype. In the natural situation chondrocytes are located within small holes or lacunae within the ECM (Figure 1-11). The interaction of the chondrocyte with the ECM is complex. Chondrocytes have cytoplasmic processes that extend into the interterritorial region and may serve to sense changes in the (biomechanical) environment. Unlike cells in many other tissues, chondrocytes appear not to be connected with each

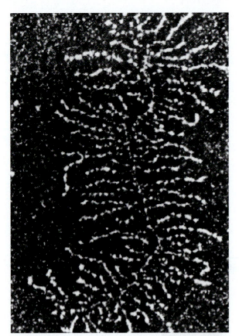

FIGURE 1-10 Electron microscopic image of aggregate of hyaluronan core molecule with aggrecan monomers attached to it. (Source: Rosenburg L, Hellman W, Kleinschmidt AK: Electron microscopic studies of proteoglycan aggregates from bovine articular cartilage, J Biol Chem 250:1877, 1975.)

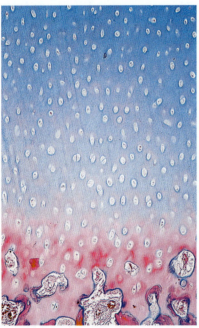

FIGURE 1-11 Microscopic picture of middle and deep layer of articular cartilage with part of the subchondral bone, showing the relative paucity of chondrocytes in relation to the ECM and the position of the cells within lacunae. The specimen is from a 5-month-old foal, explaining the lack of a clear tidemark and the incomplete mineralization of the subchondral bone. For microscopic pictures of mature cartilage, see Figure 1-16. Azan × 100. (From: Van Weeren P.R., Barneveld A. (1999). The effect of exercise on the distribution and manifestation of osteochondrotic lesions in the Warmblood foal. Equine Vet J, 31(suppl 31), 16-25.)

other, probably because of the large intercellular distance. The ECM affects cell adherence dynamics by influencing the formation of focal adherence complexes, especially the recruitment of cytoskeleton-associated molecules like vinculin.[59] Extracellular matrix-derived molecules such as laminin, fibronectin, and collagen play an important role in this interaction.[59]

The morphology of the chondrocyte differs with the distance from the cartilage surface. Whereas chondrocytes in the deep layer have a rounded shape, those in the superficial layer have a flattened appearance. This is not unlike the situation in tendons where the type 1 tenocytes that are predominant in mature, healthy tendons appear spindle-shaped and are very elongated; whereas, type 2 tenocytes or tenoblasts, as predominantly seen in juvenile or repair tissue, have a rounded appearance with plump, ovoid nuclei.[60] As in tendon, different cell shapes are related to different metabolic profiles, with the rounded cells being metabolically more active. This is also evident in the various layers of articular cartilage.

Subchondral Bone

The subchondral bone supports the overlying cartilage and is connected with it through a layer of calcified cartilage. Typically, subchondral bone consists of a layer of compact bone directly adjacent to the layer of calcified cartilage and trabecular bone at greater distance from the joint cavity. In humans, it has been shown that the subchondral bone plate is thin (around 10 μm) in most locations, but may be much thicker in others, such as below the center of the tibial plateau, where it reaches a thickness of up to 3 mm. In the thin areas the bone was constructed mainly of appositional layers continuous with trabeculae, and haversian canals were seldom seen; in the thicker areas it was composed primarily of a network of osteons that might be irregular in case of articular pathology.[61] This conformation has mechanical consequences: The compact subchondral plate provides firm support, but has some rigidity that may become substantially more in case of sclerosis; in contrast the trabecular component provides some elasticity. Bone has long been known to respond to mechanical loading, a mechanism that was first proposed by the German physician Julius Wolff in the late nineteenth century and has since been known as Wolff's law. This law states that bone will adapt to the loading to which it is subjected.[62] The morphology of the bone will change through remodeling, which will translate as thickening of compact bone as found in the cortices of the long bones and in the subchondral plate. In the epiphyseal and metaphyseal parts of bone and, as part of the epiphyseal bone, in the layers underneath the subchondral plate, this process will produce changes in thickness and architecture (configuration) of trabecular bone. These changes in bone composition and structure are effectuated by the anabolic and catabolic activities of osteoblasts and osteoclasts, respectively. Bone is, in contrast to the avascular articular cartilage, a richly vascularized tissue with intensive metabolic activity and an often high rate of tissue turnover. Given the responsiveness of bone to loading, distinct and characteristic differences in subchondral bone configuration can be supposed to exist, as there are distinct and quantitatively substantial topographical differences in loading over a given joint surface. This indeed is the case. Branch et al.[63] showed a repeatable pattern of subchondral bone thickness in the distal tarsal bones of horses without hind limb lameness, reflecting similar loading patterns across joints. The effect may be joint-dependent and is most probably not seen until a certain threshold is passed. In a study on the effect of treadmill exercise on subchondral bone density, exercised horses showed a higher subchondral bone density in the metacarpal bones, but not in the carpal bones.[64] In a developmental sense it has been shown that different exercise regimens can induce substantial differences in the biochemical composition of the subchondral bone of juvenile horses.[65-68]

Biomechanically, the subchondral bone plays an important role in the attenuation of the forces generated by locomotion and athletic activity. Although much less deformable than the overlying cartilage, the subchondral plate has been shown to be approximately 10 times more deformable than the cortical shaft of long bones.[69] It follows that changes in the rigidity of the subchondral bone will have repercussions for the mechanical loading of the articular cartilage. This consideration, together with the fact that sclerosis of the subchondral bone (and hence a decrease of elasticity of the subchondral plate) is a hallmark of OA, has led to the theory that subchondral bone sclerosis may be an initiating factor rather than a secondary sign of OA.[70,71] Whereas current opinion sees articular cartilage as the tissue where OA initiates, it is clear that the degenerative and reactive processes in the cartilage layer and in the subchondral bone are intricately linked and influence each other from the very early stages of the disease onwards.[72]

An important difference between the cartilage layer and the subchondral bone is the avascular and aneural character of the former versus the very rich vascularization and innervation of the latter. The abundant vascularization of subchondral bone allows for an extensive response of the tissue to both physiologic and pathologic stimuli. In the case of the latter this will translate as the formation of sclerosis, osteophytes, and fibrocartilaginous repair tissue in those cases where subchondral bone becomes exposed in the joint cavity because of deterioration of the cartilage layer. The nerve supply of the subchondral bone is one of the main vehicles of pain perception in the case of joint disease, together with the nerves that connect to nociceptors in the joint capsule and intraarticular and extraarticular ligaments (see the section on innervation of articular tissues).

Joint Capsule

The capsules of most joints grossly consist of two distinct layers. The outer layer of the joint capsule is made up of relatively stiff fibrous tissue. It is often tightly connected to extraarticular structures such as collateral ligaments and mainly serves mechanical stability. Apart from this, it hosts a great number of proprioceptive nerve endings that provide information on actual joint position to the brain. The inner layer of the capsule, which is the actual lining of the joint cavity, often called

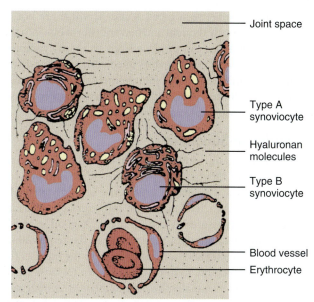

Joint space

Type A synoviocyte

Hyaluronan molecules

Type B synoviocyte

Blood vessel

Erythrocyte

FIGURE 1-12 Semischematic drawing of the synovial membrane. The subintimal layer is highly vascularized and the lack of a basement membrane facilitates passage of small molecules to the synovial cavity. The synoviocytes have both secretory and phagocytic properties. The main molecule that is secreted is hyaluronan. (From: Frisbie D.D. (2012). Synovial joint biology and pathobiology. In: Auer J.A., Stick J.A. (Ed). Equine surgery (4th ed.) (pp. 1096-1114). St. Louis, MO: Elsevier-Saunders.)

the *synovium* or *synovial membrane*, consists itself of two layers: the intimal and the subintimal layers (Figure 1-12). The subintimal layer is made up of loose connective tissue and is very well vascularized (the source of hemorrhage during arthroscopic surgery) and innervated (see the paragraph on the innervation of articular tissues). The intimal layer is the layer directly lining the joint cavity. This is a very thin layer, one to four cells thick without a basement membrane; the cells are located within a loose and porous bed of collagen fibrils and other matrix proteins. This lack of basement membrane and the immediate presence of a large number of blood vessels facilitate the passage of plasma components from the blood to the synovial cavity. In fact, synovial fluid is often described as an ultrafiltrate of blood plasma, in the sense that all but the larger molecules (the estimated size limit is 10 kDa[22]) can move freely from the blood to the synovial cavity (and vice versa). This does not mean that synovial fluid is formed by a largely passive process. There is a large excretory activity of the cells that constitute the intima, the so-called synoviocytes. Classically, they have been divided into two major categories. Type A are macrophage-like synoviocytes that are mostly involved in phagocytic actions. Type B are fibroblast-like synoviocytes that are mainly responsible for production and excretion into the synovial fluid of proteins and other molecules such as hyaluronan, the nonsulfated glycosaminoglycan macromolecule that is both a major component of the cartilage ECM and a principal component of synovial fluid, determining to a large extent the viscosity of this fluid.[73] An intermediate type C exists that is currently thought to be a transitional form between types A and B, which are not as distinct as previously thought and may transform one into the other.[74] All cell types can produce large arrays of cytokines, growth factors, and inflammatory mediators, making them crucial in the maintenance of joint homeostasis (see the relevant paragraphs on synovial fluid and tissue homeostasis), and giving synovitis a pivotal role in joint pathology.

Intraarticular Structures

Some joints contain intraarticular structures such as various ligaments or menisci. The purpose of these is to provide either mechanical stability or to improve joint geometry to realize a more even loading of the joint surface, avoiding excessive peak pressures at certain areas. A good example of this is the functioning of the menisci in the femorotibial joints. In both horses and humans damage to the menisci (or [partial] meniscectomy in humans) is known to cause cartilage damage and eventually the development of OA because of the altered pressure distribution, leading to a substantial increase in loading of certain areas.[75,76] The intraarticular structures are for the larger part collagenous in nature with collagen type I being their principal component (as in most ligamentous structures of the musculoskeletal system). Some of the structures that are frequently designated as intraarticular, such as the cruciate ligaments of the femorotibial joint, are in fact not located within the synovial cavity and thus strictly speaking not intraarticular. They still have, however, an important role in joint stability (as other periarticular structures such as collateral ligaments and the tendons of certain muscles that function as such, e.g., the shoulder joint). Failure of intraarticular structures may have important consequences for joint stability and result in severe pathology. Also, these structures are innervated and may give rise to substantial pain when damaged; for example, when meniscal flaps that may result from partial tears become entrapped between joint surfaces. Although these structures are important for providing mechanical stability, they do not seem to play a major role in joint homeostasis in either physiologic or pathologic conditions.

Synovial Fluid

The basis of synovial fluid is blood plasma, as outlined above. It is macroscopically also yellowish in color, but its rheological properties are much different because of the high hyaluronic acid content, giving it a highly viscous character. The cellular component is limited, normally not surpassing 500 cells/mm³, and consists mainly of lymphocytes and other bone marrow-derived mononuclear cells, including a limited number of macrophages under physiologic conditions. The rapid and relatively unhindered exchange between blood plasma and the synovial cavity allows the efficient supply with nutrients and the removal of waste products from the avascular cartilage. This exchange seems to be driven by both hydrostatic pressure differences and colloid osmotic pressure differences between plasma and synovial fluid.[22] Normal locomotion plays an important role in generating these hydrostatic pressure differences, as they are largely dependent on joint angle.

Intraarticular pressure is mostly subatmospheric (-2 to -6 cm H_2O)[77] and favors ultrafiltration into the joint, but may also vary with joint position.

Innervation of Articular Tissues

Articular cartilage is a rather unique tissue in that it is both aneural and avascular (at least in mature individuals). As a consequence, damage to the cartilage layer will not immediately be detected, which explains why initially minor cartilage damage may silently progress for a long time before becoming clinically manifest in an already advanced stage of OA. The other articular tissues, subchondral bone, the joint capsule, extraarticular and intraarticular ligaments, and menisci are innervated, some of them quite densely. In articular tissues there are four types of afferent receptors.[78] Type 1 receptors are low-threshold mechanoreceptors that have thinly encapsulated end organs of medium size (80 to 100 μm), which are connected to medium-sized myelinated nerve fibers. They are present in the fibrous joint capsule but not in the synovial membrane and have mainly a proprioceptive function. Type 2 receptors are large encapsulated end organs (280 to 300 μm), which are connected to 9- to 12-μm myelinated nerve fibers. These are low-threshold mechanoreceptors that typically reside at the junction of the fibrous joint capsule and the subsynovial adipose tissue, thus in closer proximity to the joint cavity than the type 1 receptors. The type 2 receptors can adapt rapidly and are activated only when the joint is in motion. In this way they act as dynamic proprioceptive sensors. Type 3 receptors are relatively large (approximately 150 by 600 μm). They are thinly encapsulated end organs that are located near the bony insertions of intraarticular and periarticular ligaments. They have a high threshold and usually are inactive under static conditions and during limited passive movement. However, these receptors become activated when joint motion reaches its physiologic limits. They have both mechanoreceptive and nociceptive potential and in fact act as safety mechanisms. These receptors are connected to very rapidly conducting myelinated fibers. Type 4 receptors, also known as polymodal nociceptors, consist of free nerve endings of afferent nonmyelinated C-fibers or small myelinated A-delta fibers. They are abundant in the entire joint capsule, can be found in limited numbers within the synovial membrane, and are also densely present in the periosteum directly adjacent to the joint margins. These receptors are high-threshold nociceptors that respond to thermal and chemical, but also mechanical, stimuli. The chemical stimuli (such as those evoked by inflammatory mediators) may augment the responsiveness to mechanical stimuli and in this way sensitize the joint, causing hyperalgesia as well as allodynia.

PRINCIPLES OF JOINT PHYSIOLOGY

The proper functioning of a joint depends on the correct interplay of its constituting elements that have been discussed above. To achieve this, all components will have to be in a state characterized by stable homeostasis in which anabolic and catabolic processes are equilibrated and match the biomechanical challenges posed to the joint. Whereas the joint must be seen as a functional entity like any other organ, its constituents (cartilage, subchondral bone, synovial membrane, and sometimes intraarticular structures) vary widely in their metabolic characteristics and turnover rate. This greatly affects the capacity for natural repair of the various tissues and thus the impact of damage to these. The key issue in joint homeostasis is whether tissue integrity and with it biomechanical functionality can be maintained or not. If this is not the case, the resulting tissue damage will further impair joint functionality and hence result in a loss of the capacity to withstand biomechanical loading, inevitably leading to further structural damage and the initiation of a vicious circle of relative overloading and joint deterioration, finally ending in the development of chronic joint disorders such as OA. If joint homeostasis and biomechanical resistance start to fail and consequently structural damage ensues, the mechanism of pain perception becomes of great importance. Pain is one of the most important, if not the most important, clinical sign of chronic joint disease and the main reason why this is so invalidating in both horses and humans.

Finally, it is important to realize that joints are not standalone units. Instead, they form an integral part of the entire musculoskeletal system that provides the body with structure and power for locomotion and athletic activities.

Tissue Homeostasis

Articular cartilage has always been regarded as a very static tissue, but it is now known that, similar to any other tissue, it undergoes constant remodeling through anabolic and catabolic processes, albeit the rate of change for some components of the ECM may be very different from that of most other tissues. Turnover time of PGs is variable and ranges in mature individuals from approximately 300 days for overall turnover in canine articular cartilage to around 20 years for the long-lived globular hyaluronic acid-binding domain of aggrecan in humans.[79] This may seem long, but observations based on the synthetic rate of hydroxyproline have indicated an even much lower turnover rate of the collagenous component of the matrix, with an estimated turnover time of up to 350 years for human femoral head cartilage.[80] As the collagen fibers form a three-dimensional scaffold that restrains the swelling pressure generated by PGs (see earlier), they are crucial to provide the articular cartilage with its overall mechanical properties. The deformation behaviors of articular cartilage have been modeled mathematically, confirming that disruption of the three-dimensional collagen network plays an important role in changing the mechanical properties as seen in case of cartilage degeneration.[81] The extremely long turnover time of collagen type II and the related incapacity to restore the collagen network make the restoration of the network very difficult, which is a crucial factor in the bad healing capacity of (mature) cartilage. In 1743 this gave rise to the famous observation by William Hunter that *"an ulcerated cartilage is universally allowed to be a very troublesome disease; that it admits of a cure with more difficulty than a carious bone; and that, when destroyed, it is never recovered."*[82]

Remodeling of the Extracellular Matrix

The chondrocyte, as the only cell type found in normal articular cartilage, produces all ECM components. Collagen molecules are manufactured intracellularly in the form of procollagen and are subsequently extracellularly modified by enzymatic cleavage of the C- and N-terminal propeptides before being integrated in the collagen network, which is critical for maintaining the strength and resilience of sound and functional articular cartilage. As pointed out earlier, the collagen network is basically a copolymer of the collagens II, IX, and XI. It is the chondrocyte that controls the assembly of this network and directs its remodeling when prompted by changing biomechanical challenges or damage. Classically, collagen cleavage is thought to be mainly effectuated by the collagenases, matrix metalloproteinases (MMPs)-1, -8 and -13, of which MMP-13 is most efficient at cleaving collagen type II.[83] The cleavage takes place at the so-called ¾ site, producing ¾- and ¼-length cleavage products. However, the effects of these enzymes were established when challenging in vitro cultures of cartilage with catabolic cytokines, principally interleukin-1 (IL-1), which is generally seen as the major cytokine driving the development of OA[84,85] (see also Chapter 3). The question is whether or not these enzymes are also the most important ones for the turnover and remodeling of the collagen network under nonpathologic conditions. It has been shown in genetically modified mice that expression of type I collagen lacking a functional sequence at the ¾ site did not lead to a pathologic phenotype at birth and later tissue changes were mild.[86] It has therefore been suggested that telopeptide cleavages may be instrumental in the initiation of fibril depolymerization, which would be possible if they occur in the sequence between the cross-links and the triple helix. They might in this way also create the possibility of selectively removing collagen IX molecules to permit lateral growth of fibrils.[36]

The other major structural component of articular cartilage is formed by the PGs, of which the large aggrecan aggregates are the most important representatives. Aggrecan can be cleaved between the G1 and G2 domains (see Figure 1-8) by MMP-3, also called stromelysin. Other MMPs found in the joint that act, among other targets, on PGs are the gelatinases MMP-2 and -9.[87] A well-known cleavage site of aggrecan is between glutamic acid 373 and alanine 374.[88] The nature of the enzymes responsible for this action (the "aggrecanases") has long remained elusive, but they are now known to belong to the so-called ADAMTS (a disintegrin and MMP with thrombospondin motif) family.[89] The enzymes ADAMTS-4 and -5 (aggrecanases 1 and 2) both play a role in aggrecan degradation in human articular cartilage,[90] with deletion of active ADAMTS-5 preventing the occurrence of cartilage damage in mice, suggesting that, at least in this species, this enzyme is more important under pathologic conditions than ADAMTS-4.[91]

The action of MMPs in the joint can be regulated in three manners. First, production can be regulated through transcription. As MMPs are produced in an inactive proform, activity can also be regulated by the degree to which these proforms are transformed into active MMPs, for example, through the action of certain cytokines. Lastly, active MMPs may form clusters with so-called TIMPs (tissue inhibitors of MMPs), leading to their inactivation.[92] As this bond is reversible, these MMPs may rapidly regain an active status once the bond is dissolved under the influence of certain stimuli. The last two mechanisms explain why MMP activity can increase very rapidly after an insult to the joint. In pathologic conditions there is an increase in the activity of many MMPs, which makes these enzymes potential targets for molecular therapies. However, it should be realized that they play an important role in the maintenance of joint homeostasis in healthy joints. In human articular cartilage there is a slight excess of TIMPs in relation to MMPs in healthy joints, and this equilibrium is disturbed in case of pathology.[93] Therefore, therapeutic targeting of MMPs certainly has potential, but, given the widespread effects that MMPs exert on natural processes in many parts of the body, including the joint, it seems that total inhibition is not the way to go and that targeted MMP modulation is more promising.[92]

Cues for the Chondrocytes

The role of the chondrocyte as the sole source of the major ECM components in articular cartilage is undisputed, but not all the exact mechanisms through which the maintenance of tissue homeostasis is realized have been elucidated. The balance between anabolic and catabolic growth factors and cytokines is important in this respect, but also mechanical loading plays a role and most probably both mechanisms are mutually influencing each other. In studies on the regulation of chondrogenesis it has been shown that the effects of dynamic compressive loading alone (i.e., in the absence of exogenous growth factors) were relatively minimal and much less than the effects of application of growth factors alone.[94] This may implicate that the right growth factor/cytokine environment is primary to the effects of mechanical loading (which are substantial once this condition has been met). However, this refers to research on cartilage formation, which is different from maintenance of homeostasis in existing cartilage. It may well be that in a physiologic situation where an appropriate cytokine/growth factor balance is present, it is the mechanical loading that produces the primary cues for the maintenance of tissue homeostasis.

Growth factors with a known anabolic effect on articular cartilage include transforming growth factor-β (TGF-β) and insulin-like growth factor-1 (IGF-1). TGF-β stimulates PG synthesis by chondrocytes and expression of collagen type II; possibly it downregulates matrix degrading enzymes.[95,96] It may therefore counteract the effects of the major catabolic cytokine IL-1.[97] However, not all effects of TGF-β are seen as positive, as it may also stimulate osteophyte formation when used over a longer period.[98] IGF-1 is important for the maintenance of ECM homeostasis in articular cartilage through the stimulation of matrix production and inhibition of degradation.[96] Chronic deficiency of IGF-1 and growth hormone (which induces its production) leads to OA-like lesions in rats.[99]

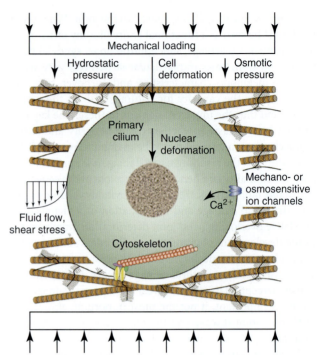

FIGURE 1-13 Schematic drawing depicting the mechanisms of mechanically induced chondrogenesis. Joint loading results in both direct cellular and nuclear deformation and in change of biophysical factors, such as osmotic and hydrostatic pressure and fluid flow. (From: O'Conor C.J., Case N., Guilak F. (2013). Mechanical regulation of chondrogenesis. Stem Cell Res Ther, 4(4), 61.)

Bone has long been known to respond to mechanical loading,[62] but all musculoskeletal tissues are highly sensitive to their mechanical environment and all respond to some degree or another. Articular cartilage is no exception. This is most evident in the juvenile phase when growth and development prevail[100] (see also Chapter 8), but seems less obvious in mature individuals where the ECM of cartilage is characterized by very long turnover times and extensive remodeling appears no longer possible. Still, there is compelling evidence that the chondrocyte is very sensitive to mechanical stimuli and these may well be the principal cues for tissue homeostasis and maintenance under physiologic conditions, as suggested above. The regular loading of articular cartilage provokes important changes in the biomechanical environment of the chondrocyte, both directly and indirectly. Directly, loading of the cartilage will lead to deformation of both nucleus and cell, eliciting a cellular response. Indirectly, there are changes in hydrostatic pressure, osmolality and, related to these, flow of interstitial fluid. This is schematically depicted in Figure 1-13. These physical events may have direct and indirect effects. Changes in flow of interstitial fluid will have effects on nutrient supply and waste removal, but may also be a stimulus for the activation of metabolically active substances such as TGF-β.[101] The chondrocyte possesses a so-called primary cilium (Figure 1-13). This organelle was described long ago,[102] but it has more recently become clear that it may have an important role in chondrocyte mechanotransduction.[103] The molecular pathways along which mechanotransduction is regulated in chondrocytes have not been investigated in detail, but there is growing interest.[94] Various ion channels have been implicated, including calcium and potassium signaling.[104]

Joint Lubrication

To realize a smooth, gliding motion there needs to be some form of lubrication between the moving parts of the joint that come into contact with each other or their surroundings. These are the articular surfaces with respect to each other and with respect to the other structures that line the synovial cavity, (i.e., the joint capsule and the eventual intraarticular structures, such as menisci and ligaments). Two different mechanisms are involved in joint lubrication: boundary lubrication and fluid-film lubrication. Boundary lubrication takes place at all gliding surfaces within a joint, and fluid-film lubrication is an additional form of lubrication between the articular surfaces.

In boundary lubrication there is direct contact between the gliding surfaces and there are specific lubricating substances or molecules that adhere to these surfaces and form a protective layer, preventing excessive wear and tear.[105] In diarthrodial joints, hyaluronan (HA) and mucinous glycoproteins with multiple O-linked $\beta(1-3)$Gal-GalNAc oligosaccharides, which are products of the PRG4 gene and of which superficial zone protein (SZP) or lubricin is the best known, are the most important boundary lubricants.[106] Hyaluronan is the principal boundary lubricant for the synovial membrane.[107] Both HA and lubricin play a role in the lubrication of cartilage surfaces. These substances are critical for correct functioning of healthy joints and their levels are often decreased in pathologic conditions.[108,109]

There are various forms of fluid-film lubrication. The lubricated surfaces can retain their shape and remain entirely separated from each other by the fluid film when moving over each other, as is the case with *hydrodynamic lubrication* (Figure 1-14A). If one or both surfaces have some elasticity and deform it is called *elastohydrodynamic lubrication* (Figure 1-14B). In case there is no motion between the surfaces, the lubricating fluid can be squeezed out because of the compressive forces, which is then called a *squeeze film* (Figure 1-14C), or it can remain trapped between the surfaces, in which case it is *hydrostatic lubrication*. In the joint, lubrication between the articular surfaces is thought to follow several of these pathways, depending on the actual situation in biomechanical sense (type of activity, speed of motion). The situation in a joint is more complex than in most applications of technical engineering, as not only will both surfaces deform under load, but interstitial fluid entrapped within the ECM will be squeezed out (see also following paragraph) and add to the synovial fluid already present around the articular surfaces. Further, there are high-motion and low-motion joints and either more static or more dynamic actions with higher or lower intensity may be performed by the musculoskeletal system. This will result in large variations in both absolute load, direction of loading (i.e., relative contribution of compressive and shear forces), and speed with which the articular surfaces

Fluid film

Surfaces completely separated by a fluid film

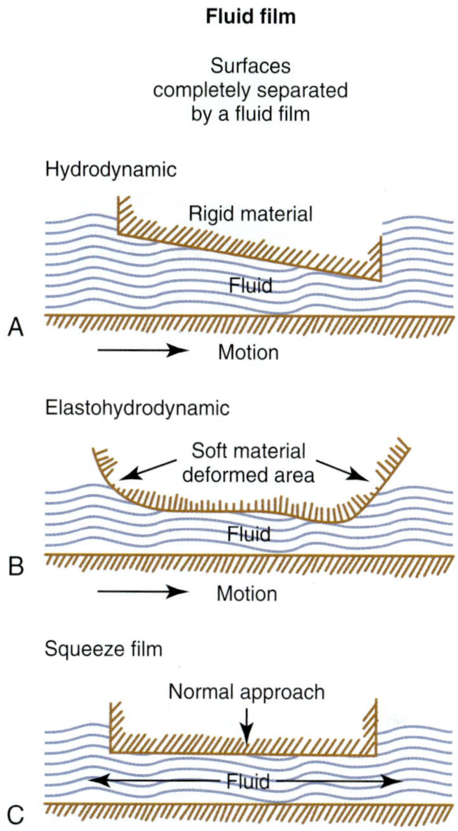

FIGURE 1-14 Various forms of fluid-film lubrication; **(A)** hydrodynamic lubrication between nondeformable surfaces; **(B)** elastohydrodynamic lubrication where one or two of the gliding surfaces are deformable; **(C)** squeeze film lubrication where under static compression the fluid film between the surfaces is squeezed out. A fourth form is hydrostatic lubrication, also a static condition in which the fluid film cannot escape. (From: Walker P.S., Dowson D., Longfield MD., et al. (1968). "Boosted lubrication" in synovial joints by fluid entrapment and enrichment. Ann Rheum Dis, 27(6), 512-520.)

move in relation to each other. These factors all influence behavior of the ECM of cartilage and the rheologic properties of the synovial fluid, which is a viscous, non-Newtonian thixotropic fluid.[110] This means that the viscosity of synovial fluid will diminish with increasing joint motion. To describe the complicated way of lubrication of synovial joints the term "boosted lubrication" was coined,[105] but this terminology did not stick.

Functional Biomechanics

Articular cartilage is a biomechanical tissue par excellence. As stated earlier, its main functions are providing both strength and resilience, together with a surface that makes smooth gliding of the cartilage-capped bony ends of the joint possible. The combination of strength and resilience, which are material characteristics that are difficult to reconcile in engineering, is made possible by the specific architecture of the cartilage in the form of the collagen network with the entrapped PG aggregates, of which aggrecan is the most important (Figures 4, 5, and 9). Because of their high degree

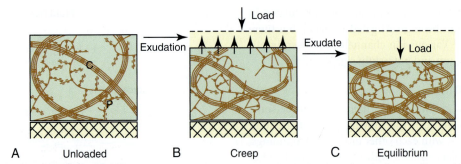

| A | Unloaded | B | Creep | C | Equilibrium |

FIGURE 1-15 Schematic representation of the sponge-like behavior of articular cartilage. **(A)** In the unloaded situation the negatively charged sulfate groups of the proteoglycans (p) that are attached to the collagen network (c) draw water into the network, making it swell. The swelling is restricted by the collagen network and an equilibrium results in which the collagen network is under intrinsic tension. When an external load is applied **(B)**, water will be squeezed out of the extracellular matrix until a new equilibrium is reached **(C)**. When the load is released, the mechanism acts reversely. Regular joint loading will thus result in a regular flow of interstitial fluid through the ECM, permitting nutrient and waste products transport. (Redrawn from Myers ER, Mow VC: Biomechanics of Cartilage and its Response to Bromechanical Stimuli. IN Hall BK (ed): Cartilage, Vol. 1, New York, Academic Press, 1983. IN McIlwraith CW and Totter GW: Joint Disease in the Horse. 1st ed, Philadelphia, 1996, WB Saunders.)

of sulfation and consequent negative charge chondroitin and keratin sulfate are highly hydrophilic. They will attract water, leading to swelling of the ECM. However, the expansion of the ECM is restricted by the collagen network as the collagen fibrils are very stiff, basically nonelastic structures. In this way an intrinsic pressure is generated within the ECM, maintained by the balance of osmotic pressure and restraint by the collagen fibrils. If such a system is loaded, hence subjected to external forces (that will normally act in either compression or shear mode or more often a combination thereof), the cartilage will yield as water will be squeezed out, caused by the increase in the forces counteracting the osmotic forces. When the external forces are released or diminished, the opposite will occur and water will be drawn again into the ECM (Figure 1-15). Articular cartilage is thus a viscoelastic tissue. If either the hydrophilic properties of the PG component or the integrity of the collagen network are compromised, this mechanism will not work properly anymore, resulting in loss of resilience and strength and hence in higher vulnerability to further damage.

The biomechanical concept of articular cartilage, as a combination of hydrophilic PG aggregates within the constraints of a strong collagen network providing both good resilience and high compressive stiffness (shear resistance being largely taken care of by the superficial collagen fibers that are arranged parallel to the surface), requires a homogeneous tissue. This is most probably the reason why articular cartilage is avascular and aneural, as the presence of this type of structures would have a big influence on the pressure distribution pattern within the tissue because of the creation of interfaces of tissue components with completely different biomechanical properties. This is not a problem in most tissues, but it is in cartilage. Seemingly, the same argument would hold for bone, but bone can be and is a composite tissue in which one component provides the biomechanical strength; whereas the other components (that are shielded by the rigidity of the

mineralized osteoid of bone) have no biomechanical function. In a resilient tissue, such as cartilage, this is not possible.

The lack of blood vessels drives the need for other means of transport of nutrition and waste products. This need is met by the pumping action of intermittent loading of the cartilage ECM caused by locomotion and athletic activities, which has been compared to the squeezing and relaxation of a submerged sponge, causing influx and efflux of the liquid surrounding the sponge (see Figure 1-15). Cartilage is thus maintained by what might be called assisted diffusion from the synovial fluid. The distance over which this type of diffusion can take place is limited, however, which might explain why cartilage thickness does not increase isometrically with increasing weight when comparing various species and why lighter species have a relatively higher cellular density compared with heavier ones (Figure 1-16).[57] There are indications that the heavier types of dinosaurs, which are the largest land creatures that have ever lived, had blood vessels in their cartilage.[111] This may have solved the diffusion problem. It is not known, however, if and how this conformation affected the biomechanical functionality of their cartilage.

Because of anatomic and geometric particularities, joints are not loaded evenly over their surface. Different areas are subjected to different magnitudes and types of loading. These may include low-level constant loading, intermittent loading, and very high-impact loading, or more compressive loading in a low-motion joint as opposed to a large amount of shear loading in a high-motion joint. These variable loading conditions can only adequately be met by cartilage that possesses different mechanical properties at different sites.[112] This issue has been investigated in the equine fetlock joint and most extensively on the proximal articular surface of the proximal phalanx. By taking biopsies from a large number of predefined sites and subsequently analyzing these biochemically, Brama et al. showed substantial differences between different sites on the joint surface.[113] The two most distinct sites were the dorsal

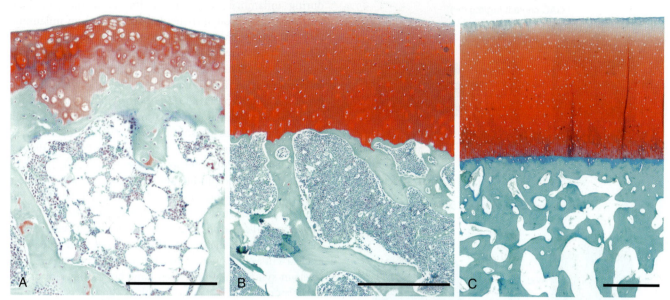

FIGURE 1-16 Safranin-O staining (stains glycosaminoglycans red) of osteochondral tissue of the (A) rat, (B) Barbary macaque, and (C) white rhinoceros. Scale bars indicate (A) 200 μm, (B) 400 μm, and (C) 1000 μm. Cartilage of heavier species is thicker, but the increase is not isometrical. Cartilage of heavier species is similar in cell density, but lighter species have more cell-dense cartilage. (From: Malda J., de Grauw J.C., Benders K.E.M., et al. (2013). Of mice, men and elephants: the relation between articular cartilage thickness and body mass. PLoS ONE 8(2), e57683.)

margin and the central part of the fovea of the proximal articular surface of the proximal phalanx (Figure 1-17). These are areas that are subjected to entirely different loading patterns. The central fovea is loaded at every instance the horse is on its feet, independent of athletic activity, whereas the dorsal joint margin is nonweight-bearing under most circumstances, but is quite heavily loaded when there is severe hyperextension of the metacarpophalangeal joint, as occurs during strenuous exercises such as galloping and jumping. The relationship between the loading pattern and the biomechanical composition became clear in another study of the same groups where, in an ex vivo setting, limb loading as occurring during athletic activity was mimicked and intraarticular pressure measured using pressure-sensitive films.[114] Results showed that high intermittent loading was related to high collagen content with a high level of cross-linking; less intense but more consistent loading was associated with higher PG content (Figure 1-18). Later biomechanical studies confirmed that this topographic heterogeneity in a biochemical sense indeed represented differences in biomechanical properties of the tissue.[115]

The topographic variation in biochemical and biomechanical properties is not genetically determined, but develops for the larger part in the early phase of life, that is, during the first year after birth in the horse, with most changes in the first 5 months of life. Biomechanical loading is an important cue in this development[100]; this issue is discussed in more detail in Chapter 8.

Pain Perception in Joints

Pain transmission through afferent fibers is more complex than it may seem with peripheral sensory neurons functioning as afferent conductors, but at the same time also exerting important efferent functions mediated by neuropeptides.[116] Neuropeptides are small molecules that are synthesized in the dorsal root and autonomic ganglion neurons and then transported via the axon to peripheral nerve terminals. They can induce the release of other mediators, such as cytokines, prostaglandins, and nitric oxide. They are relatively potent, but usually have a limited range of action, both in space and time, as they are chemically labile. In healthy or regenerating tissue, they may have growth factor-like functions,[117] meaning that they also play a role in maintenance of joint homeostasis. Well-known neuropeptides include substance P (SP), calcitonin gene-related peptide (CGRP), vasoactive intestinal polypeptide (VIP), neuropeptide Y (NPY), and somatostatin (SOM).[116] Neuropeptides play an important role in the complex mechanisms that modulate and mitigate nociceptive input. An example is VIP, which is thought to be important for the augmentation of responsiveness to mechanical stimuli in case of joint inflammation.[118]

In joint disease, numerous pathologic processes can contribute to the joint pain experienced by affected subjects; the precise tissue origin of pain is rarely identified in the individual patient (Figure 1-19). The sensory innervation of the subchondral bone, marginal periosteum, synovial membrane, and joint capsule will contribute to a variable extent to pain perception and associated loss of function. Within the joint tissues several pathologic processes may be at the origin of pain, such as subchondral bone exposure, remodeling, marrow edema (causing a rise in intraosseous pressure), and marginal periosteal activation related to osteophyte formation.[78] Synovitis is an important factor generating pain through joint

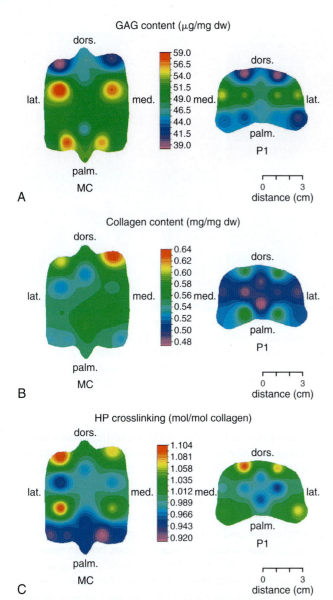

FIGURE 1-17 Distribution of glycosaminoglycans (GAG), collagen, and HP-cross-links over the proximal articular surface of the proximal phalanx and the distal articular surface of the third metacarpal bone. *Dors.*, Dorsal; *GAG*, glycosaminoglycan; *HP*, hydroxylysyl pyridinoline; *lat*, lateral; *MC*, distal third metacarpal bone; *med.*, media; *palm.*, palmar; *P1*, proximal first phalanx. (From: Brama P.A.J., TeKoppele J.M., Bank R.A., et al. (2000). Topographical mapping of biochemical properties of articular cartilage in the equine fetlock joint. Equine Vet J, 32(1), 19-26.)

effusion, swelling, and/or fibrosis that will activate mechano-receptors in the joint capsule, and through direct chemical stimulation of nociceptors.

Pathways and Mediators of Pain in the Joint

Nociception will in most cases be stimulated or enhanced by inflammation. In this context, the somewhat complex and mutually influencing interrelationship between mechano-ceptors and nociceptors needs to be pointed out: mechano-receptors can become sensitized by chemical stimuli released during inflammatory processes, but mechanical stimulation may also, through tissue damage, lead to an inflammatory response with release of pro-nociceptive mediators. In inflammation, pain originates from the chemical stimulation of nerve afferents by a variety of endogenous mediators. Interleukin-1β and TNF-α are the two major cytokine players in the pathogenesis of OA.[119] Both cytokines increase the synthesis of inflammatory mediators that are involved in pain perception, such as prostaglandin E_2 (PGE_2), by stimulating cyclo-oxygenase (COX)-2, microsomal PGE synthase-1 (MPES-1), and soluble phospholipase A_2 ($SPLA_2$). They further upregulate the production of nitric oxide via inducible nitric oxide synthetase (iNOS).[120] Relatively little work has been done on the exact identification of pain-related mediators in joint disease. Prostaglandins have always been seen as the major pain mediators in arthritis,[121] but their role is not as clear-cut as it may seem. In a horse study comparing PGE_2 levels in synovial fluid between lame horses that did or did not respond to an intraarticular block, there was no significant difference. However, when comparing the levels of these lame horses (blocking to a low 4-point or 6-point perineural nerve block) to those of sound horses, lame horses were found to have significantly higher and more variable PGE_2 levels than the sound control horses.[122] The other branch of the arachidonic acid cascade, the pathway that leads via 5-lipoxygenase (LOX) to the formation of leukotrienes, may play a role in nociception in joints, too. Leukotriene B_4 (LTB_4) has been shown to be implicated in hyperalgesia in joints of mice.[123] In the horse, LTB_4 levels were increased in animals suffering from osteochondrosis (OC) and may be involved in the extensive joint distension that is often seen in OC.[124] However, lameness in these patients is uncommon and thus far no link between LTB_4 and joint pain in the horse has been established. Various neuropeptides have been identified as direct pain mediators in joint disease in humans. These include NPY, serotonin, and CGRP.[125,126] In the horse, substance P was the only mediator that could be directly linked to outcome of intraarticular analgesia,[122] but it could not be related to radiographic OA status of a joint in another study.[127] As radiographic OA status is more a measure of cumulative damage to the joint than of actual pain, this was perhaps not to be expected. More recently, other families of cytokines, such as kinins and chemokines, have been implicated in the generation and maintenance of chronic pain in joints (for an overview see Miller et al.[128]). None of these possible mediators have as yet been investigated in the horse except for bradykinin, which showed a strong correlation with lameness and joint hyperalgesia in chemically induced synovitis.[129] The concentration, however, was not related to the outcome of intraarticular analgesia.[122]

The Joint as an Integral Part of the Body

Whereas the joint should be seen as an organ that is composed of the variety of structures and tissues outlined above, this organ itself is a constituting element of the entire body. Joints are integral parts of the musculoskeletal system and their functioning is partly determined by the other

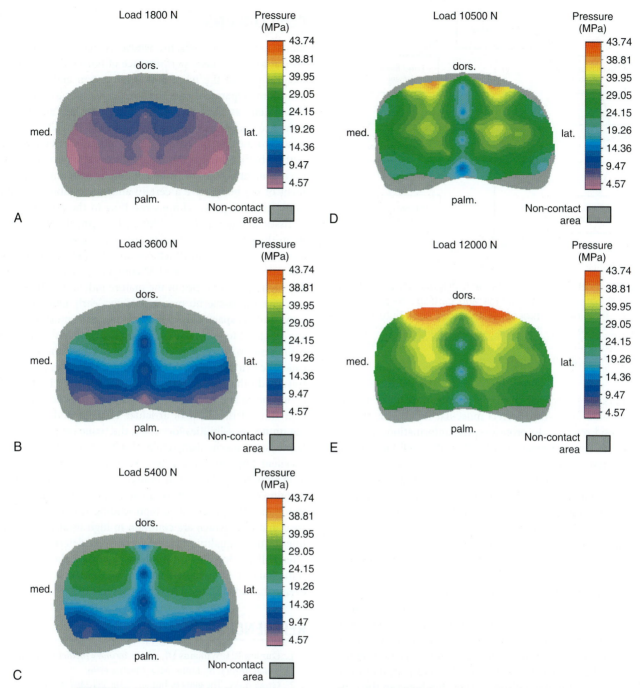

FIGURE 1-18 Topographic distribution patterns of pressures (MPa) on the proximal articular surface of the proximal phalanx measured in an ex vivo setting under varying loads based on peak vertical forces measured in a 600-kg horse during stance (1800 N), walk (3600 N), trot (5400 N), canter (10,500 N) and jumping a low (80 cm) fence (12,000 N). *Dors.,* Dorsal; *lat.,* lateral; *med.,* medial; *N,* Newton; *MPa,* megapascal; *palm.,* palmar. (From: Brama P.A.J., Karssenberg D., Barneveld A., et al. (2001). Contact areas and pressure distribution on the proximal articular surface of the proximal phalanx under sagittal plane loading. Equine Vet J, 33(1), 26-32.)

components of this system. The importance of muscular support for joint function and the prevention of instability that might lead to tissue damage can hardly be overemphasized. In the rehabilitation of human patients, who have suffered from trauma resulting in the loss of joint stability, for example, cruciate ligament damage in the knee joint, physical exercises to strengthen the musculature around the joint, which may

to a certain extent take over the stabilizing function of ligaments, have a prominent place.[130] In equine medicine, many joint disorders affect the more distally located joints of the limbs, which are not surrounded by musculature. However, it is known that a comparable change in functional stabilization can take place around the vertebral column, in this case from the deeper musculature (principally the multifidus muscle)

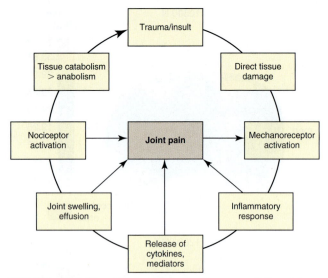

FIGURE 1-19 Simplified schematic diagram of the vicious cycle of osteochondral damage and cartilage degeneration in OA, showing key processes that may contribute to joint pain associated with the disease. (From: Van Weeren P.R., de Grauw J.C. (2010). Pain in osteoarthritis. Vet Clin North Am Equine Pract, 26(3), 619-642.)

to the more superficial layer (the longissimus dorsi muscle among others).[131] Also, correct muscular function is critical for a good response to proprioceptive information, which is needed to ensure proper joint loading. It is well known that fatigue may negatively affect this mechanism, resulting in a loss of coordination with loss of accuracy in the direction of joint loading and higher risk of injury as a consequence.[132] The issue of muscular function and strength is dealt with in more detail in Chapter 18.

Joints communicate with the rest of the body via the great infrastructural networks, the neural system, and the cardiovascular system. As alluded to earlier, important proprioceptive information is gathered in joint-related structures, principally tendons, ligaments, and the joint capsule, and used as input for (involuntary) corrections of position. Also, pain is perceived and the nervous system may actively influence joint homeostasis through neurotransmitter emission into the joint cavity. As synovial fluid is an ultrafiltrate of blood plasma, there is a direct relationship between the general circulation and the intraarticular environment. Noxious factors may reach the joint via the circulation, as is the case in joint sepsis based on hematogenous infection (see also Chapter 7), but also in more generalized immune-mediated disorders that may become manifest in joints. It is now known that the joint disorders that are frequently seen in obese people are not merely caused by increased biomechanical loading, but also by the generalized low-grade inflammation that is a hallmark of obesity.[133] Microvesicles have received much attention recently as an important transport medium in the body.[134] Not much is known yet about their possible role in joint homeostasis and disease, but their presence in equine synovial fluid and their ability to interact with chondrocytes have recently been demonstrated.[135]

CONCLUSIONS

Joints are complex organs, whose correct functioning is critical for the athletic performance of horses. They form an integral part of the musculoskeletal system and cannot be considered separately from the other constituting elements of this system, as there is an intricate relationship and mutual influence. The degree to which they are challenged is directly related to the demands made on the musculoskeletal system, putting both equine and human athletes at high risk for the development of joint disorders. Joints, as with any other element of the body, have a certain anabolic/catabolic balance under physiologic conditions resulting in the establishment of tissue homeostasis. In addition, the joint has a peculiarity in the presence of articular cartilage, a tissue that is both aneural and avascular, which has an extremely high ECM to cell ratio, and of which the ECM components have exceptionally high turnover times in the mature individual. These factors give the tissue no means to detect early damage and a very limited capacity for repair, making it the most likely tissue of a joint to fail. Tissue homeostasis in articular cartilage is the result of a complex equilibrium in which the anabolic/catabolic cytokine/growth factor balance plays an important role, as do the mechanical stimuli that are perceived by the chondrocyte and have various origins. Despite the long turnover time of the ECM of articular cartilage and the resulting limited possibilities for repair, the tissue can, through its homeostatic mechanism, retain a high degree of integrity and excellent functional characteristics over prolonged periods, as evidenced by the almost impeccable state of the joints of certain very senior people or horses. However, in many cases traumatic events, repetitive high loading resulting in heavy wear and tear (which are common in high-level athletes), or inferior tissue quality will create pathologic deterioration that often will develop into OA. In these cases the delicate homeostatic balance is disrupted, leading to a chain of pathologic events that are discussed in other chapters of this book.

REFERENCES

1. Dunlop RH, Williams DJ, eds. *Veterinary medicine. An illustrated history.* St. Louis, MO: Mosby; 1996.
2. Grogan JW. The gaits of horses. *J Am Vet Med Assoc.* 1951;119:112–117.
3. Loomans JBA, Stolk PW, van Weeren PR, et al. A survey of the workload and clinical skills in current equine veterinary practice in The Netherlands. *Equine Vet Educ.* 2007;19(3):162–168.
4. Rossdale PD, Hopes R, Wingfield Digby NJ, et al. Epidemiological study of wastage among racehorses 1982 and 1983. *Vet Rec.* 1985;116(3):66–69.
5. Williams RB, Harkins LS, Hammond CJ, et al. Racehorse injuries, clinical problems and fatalities recorded on British racecourses from flat racing and national hunt racing during 1996, 1997 and 1998. *Equine Vet J.* 2001;33(5):478–486.
6. Murray RC, Dyson SJ, Tranquille C, et al. Association of type and sport and performance level with anatomical site of orthopaedic injury diagnosis. *Equine Vet J.* 2006;38(suppl 36):411–416.

7. Sloet van Oldruitenborgh-Oosterbaan MM, Genzel W, van Weeren PR. A pilot study on factors influencing the career of Dutch sport horses. *Equine Vet J.* 2010;42(suppl 38):28–32.

8. Anonymous. *Lameness and laminitis in US horses. National animal health monitoring systems 2000.* Fort Collins, CO: veterinary services – centers for epidemiology in animal health; 2000.

9. Anonymous. *Orthoworld.* the orthopaedic industry annual report. 2009-2010; 2010.

10. McIlwraith CW, Frisbie DD, Kawcak CE. The horse as a model of naturally occurring osteoarthritis. *Bone Joint Res.* 2012;1(11):297–309.

11. Lanovaz JL, Clayton HM, Watson LG. In vitro attenuation of impact shock in equine digits. *Equine Vet J.* 1998;30(suppl 26):96–102.

12. Willemen MA, Jacobs MW, Schamhardt HC. In vitro transmission and attenuation of impact vibrations in the distal forelimb. *Equine Vet J.* 1999;31(suppl 30):245–248.

13. Samuels J, Krasnokutsky S, Abramson SB. Osteoarthritis. A tale of three tissues. *Bull NYU Hosp Joint Dis.* 2008;66(3):244–250.

14. Saris DB, Dhert WJ, Verbout AJ. Joint homeostasis. The discrepancy between old and fresh defects in cartilage repair. *J Bone Joint Surg Br.* 2003;85(7):1067–1076.

15. Dyce K, Sack WO, Wensing CJG. General anatomy. In: Dyce K, Sack WO, Wensing CJG, eds. *Textbook of veterinary anatomy (4th ed.).* St. Louis, MO: Saunders Elsevier; 2010:16.

16. Jenner F. *On the genesis of articular cartilage. Embryonic joint development and gene expression – implications for tissue engineering.* Thesis. Utrecht University; 2013.

17. Koyama E, Shibukawa Y, Nagayama M, et al. A distinct cohort of progenitor cells participates in synovial joint and articular cartilage formation during mouse limb skeletogenesis. *Dev Biol.* 2008;316(1):62–73.

18. Pitsillides A, Beier F. Cartilage biology in osteoarthritis – lessons from developmental biology. *Nat Rev Rheumatol.* 2011;7(11):654–663.

19. Holder N. An experimental investigation into the early development of the chick elbow joint. *J Embryol Exp Morphol.* 1977;39:115–127.

20. Jenner F, Närväinen J, Villani M, et al. Magnetic resonance microscopy atlas of equine embryonic development. *Equine Vet J.* 2014;46(2):210–215.

21. Jenner F, IJpma A, Cleary M, et al. Differential gene expression of the intermediate and outer interzone layers of developing articular cartilage in murine embryos. *Stem Cells Dev.* 2014;23(16):1883–1898.

22. Todhunter RJ. Anatomy and physiology of synovial joints. In: McIlwraith CW, Trotter GW, eds. *Joint disease in the horse (1st ed.).* Philadelphia, PA: Saunders; 1996:1–28.

23. Aydelotte MN, Kuettner KE. Differences between subpopulations of cultured bovine articular chondrocytes. I. Morphology and cartilage matrix production. *Connect Tissue Res.* 1988;18(3):205–222.

24. Gannon FH, Sokoloff L. Histomorphometry of the aging human patella: histologic criteria and controls. *Osteoarth Cart.* 1999;7(2):173–181.

25. Lyons TJ, McClure SF, Stoddart RW, et al. The normal human chondro-osseous region: evidence for contact of uncalcified cartilage with subchondral bone and marrow spaces. *BMC Musculoskelet Disord.* 2006;7:52.

26. Benninghoff A. Form und Bau der Gelenkknorpel in ihren Beziehungen zur Funktion. Zweiter Teil: der Aufbau des Gelenkknorpels in seinen Beziehungen zur Funktion. *Zsch Zelforsch Mikroskop Anat.* 1925;2:783–862.

27. Vanden Berg-Foels WS, Scipioni L, Huynh C, et al. Helium ion microscopy for high-resolution visualization of the articular cartilage collagen network. *J Microsc.* 2012;246(2):168–176.

28. Rieppo J, Hallikainen J, Jurvelin JS, et al. Practical considerations in the use of polarized light microscopy in the analysis of the collagen network in articular cartilage. *Microsc Res Technol.* 2008;71(4):279–287.

29. Van Turnhout MC, Haazelager MB, Gijsen MAL, et al. Quantitative description of collagen structure in the articular cartilage of the young and adult equine distal metacarpus. *Anim Biol.* 2008;58:353–370.

30. Van Turnhout M, Kranenbarg S, van Leeuwen JL. Contribution of postnatal collagen reorientation to depth-dependent mechanical properties of articular cartilage. *Biomech Model Mechanobiol.* 2011;10(2):269–279.

31. Brama PAJ, Holopainen J, van Weeren PR, et al. Effect of loading on the organization of the collagen fibril network in juvenile equine articular cartilage. *J Orthop Res.* 2009;27(9):1226–1234.

32. Eyre DR, Wu JJ. Collagen structure and cartilage matrix integrity. *J Rheumatol.* 1995;22:82–85.

33. Monnier VM. Toward a Maillard reaction theory of ageing. *Prog Clin Biol Res.* 1989;304:1–22.

34. Vlassara H, Li YM, Imani F, et al. Identification of galectin-3 as a high-affinity binding protein for advanced glycation end products (AGE): a new member of the AGE-receptor complex. *Mol Med.* 1995;1(6):634–646.

35. Verzijl N, DeGroot J, Bank RA, et al. Age-related accumulation of the advanced glycation end product pentosidine in human articular cartilage aggrecan: the use of pentosidine levels as a quantitative measure of protein turnover. *Matrix Biol.* 2001;20(7):409–417.

36. Eyre DR. Collagens and cartilage matrix homeostasis. *Clin Orthop.* 2004;427(suppl):S118–S122.

37. Eyre DR, Weis MA, Wu J. Articular cartilage collagen: an irreplaceable framework? *Euro Cell Mater.* 2006;12:57–63.

38. Blaschke UK, Eikenberry EF, Hulmes DJ, et al. Collagen XI nucleates self-assembly and limits lateral growth of cartilage fibrils. *J Biol Chem.* 2000;275(14):10370–10378.

39. Wu JJ, Weis MA, Kim LS, et al. Type III collagen, a fibril network modifier in articular cartilage. *J Biol Chem.* 2010;285(24):18537–18544.

40. Poole CA. Articular cartilage chondrons: form, function and failure. *J Anat.* 1997;91(Pt 1):1–13.

41. Eyre DR. Collagen of articular cartilage. *Arthritis Res.* 2002;4(1):30–35.

42. Shen G. The role of type X collagen in facilitating and regulating endochondral ossification of articular cartilage. *Orthod Craniofac Res.* 2005;8(1):11–17.

43. Gao ZQ, Guo X, Duan C, et al. Altered aggrecan synthesis and collagen expression profiles in chondrocytes from patients with Kashin-Beck disease and osteoarthritis. *J Int Med Res.* 2012;40(4):1325–1334.

44. Boos N, Nerlich AG, von der Wiest I, et al. Immunohistochemical analysis of type-X-collagen expression in osteoarthritis of the hip joint. *J Orthop Res.* 1999;17(4):495–502.

45. Ruoslahti E. Brain extracellular matrix. *Glycobiology.* 1996;6(5):489–492.

46. Aspberg A. The different roles of aggrecan interaction domains. *J Histochem Cytochem.* 2012;60(12):987–996.

47. Paulsson M, Mörgelin M, Wiedemann H, et al. Extended and globular protein domains in cartilage proteoglycans. *Biochem J.* 1987;245(3):763–772.

48. Lee H-Y, Han L, Roughley P, et al. Age-related nanostructural and nanomechanical changes of individual human cartilage aggrecan monomers and their glycosaminoglycan side chains. *J Struct Biol.* 2013;181(3):264–273.

49. Lohmander S. Proteoglycans of joint cartilage. Structure, function, turnover and role as markers of joint disease. *Baillière's Clin Rheumatol.* 1988;2(1):37–62.

50. Heinegård D. Proteoglycans and more – from molecules to biology. *Int J Exp Pathol.* 2009;90(6):575–586.

51. Hedbom E, Heinegård D. Binding of fibromodulin and decorin to separate sites on fibrillar collagens. *J Biol Chem.* 1993;268(36):27307–27312.

52. Schaefer L, Iozzo R. Biological functions of the small leucine-rich proteoglycans: from genetics to signal transduction. *J Biol Chem.* 2008;283:21305–21309.

53. Wiberg C, Hedbom E, Khairullina A, et al. Biglycan and decorin bind close to the n-terminal region of the collagen VI triple helix. *J Biol Chem.* 2001;276(22):18947–18952.

54. Dowthwaite GP, Bishop JC, Redman SN, et al. The surface of articular cartilage contains a progenitor cell population. *J Cell Sci.* 2004;117:889–897.

55. McCarthy HE, Bara JJ, Brakspear K, et al. The comparison of equine articular cartilage progenitor cells and bone marrow-derived stromal cells as potential cell sources for cartilage repair in the horse. *Vet J.* 2012;192(3):345–351.

56. Mobasheri A. Identification and phenotypic characterisation of chondroprogenitor cells for the repair of equine articular cartilage. *Vet J.* 2012;192(3):260–261.

57. Malda J, de Grauw JC, Benders KEM, et al. Of mice, men and elephants: the relation between articular cartilage thickness and body mass. *PLoS ONE.* 2013;8(2):e57683.

58. Domm C, Schünke M, Steinhagen J, et al. Influence of various alginate brands on the redifferentiation of dedifferentiated bovine articular chondrocytes in alginate bead culture under high and low oxygen tension. *Tissue Eng.* 2004;10(11-12):1796–1805.

59. Schlie-Wolter S, Ngezahayo A, Chichkov BN. The selective role of ECM components on cell adhesion, morphology, proliferation and communication in vitro. *Exp Cell Res.* 2013;319(10):1553–1561.

60. Stanley RL, Goodship AE, Edwards B, et al. Effects of exercise on tenocyte cellularity and tenocyte nuclear morphology in immature and mature equine digital tendons. *Equine Vet J.* 2008;40(2):141–146.

61. Clark JM, Huber JD. *The structure of the human subchondral plate. J Bone Joint Surg [Br].* 1990;72(5):866–873.

62. Wolff J. *Das Gesetz der Transformation der Knochen.* Berlin: Hirschwald; 1892.

63. Branch MV, Murray RC, Dyson SJ, et al. Is there a characteristic distal tarsal subchondral bone plate thickness pattern in horses with no history of hindlimb lameness? *Equine Vet J.* 2005;37(5):450–455.

64. Kawcak CE, McIlwraith CW, Norrdin RW, et al. Clinical effects of exercise on subchondral bone of carpal and metacarpophalangeal joints in horses. *Am J Vet Res.* 2000;61(10):1252–1258.

65. Brama PAJ, TeKoppele JM, Bank RA, et al. Training affects the collagen framework of subchondral bone in foals. *Vet J.* 2001;162(1):24–32.

66. Brama PAJ, TeKoppele JM, Bank RA, et al. Biochemical development of subchondral bone from birth until age eleven months and the influence of physical activity. *Equine Vet J.* 2002;34(2):143–149.

67. Brama PAJ, Firth EC, van Weeren PR, et al. Influence of intensity and changes of physical activity on bone mineral density of immature equine subchondral bone. *Equine Vet J.* 2009;41(6):564–571.

68. Van de Lest CHA, Brama PAJ, van Weeren PR. The influence of exercise on bone morphogenic enzyme activity of immature equine subchondral bone. *Biorheology.* 2003;40(1-3):377–382.

69. Mankin HJ, Radin EL. Structure and function of joints. In: McCarthy DJ, ed. *Arthritis and allied conditions: a textbook of rheumatology. (12th ed.)* Philadelphia, PA: Lea & Febiger; 1993:189. [cited by Frisbie, 2012].

70. Radin EL, Rose RM. Role of subchondral bone in the initiation and progression of cartilage damage. *Clin Orthop.* 1986;213:34–40.

71. Radin EL. Subchondral bone changes and cartilage damage. *Equine Vet J.* 1999;31(2):94–95.

72. Burr DB. The importance of subchondral bone in osteoarthrosis. *Curr Opin Rheumatol.* 1998;10(3):256–262.

73. Henderson B, Pettipher ER. The synovial lining cell: biology and pathobiology. *Semin Arthritis Rheum.* 1985;15(1):1–32.

74. Frisbie DD. Synovial joint biology and pathobiology. In: Auer JA, Stick JA, eds. *Equine Surgery. (4th ed.)* St. Louis, MO: Elsevier-Saunders; 2012:1096–1114.

75. Arno S, Hadley S, Campbell KA, et al. The effect of arthroscopic partial medial meniscectomy on tibiofemoral stability. *Am J Sports Med.* 2013;41(1):73–79.

76. Fowlie J, Arnoczky S, Lavagnino M, et al. Resection of grade III cranial horn tears of the equine medial meniscus alter the contact forces on medial tibial condyle at full extension: an in-vitro cadaveric study. *Vet Surg.* 2011;40(8):957–965.

77. Knox P, Levick JR, McDonald JN. Synovial fluid – its mass, macromolecular content and pressure in major limb joints of the rabbit. *Q J Exp Physiol.* 1988;73(1):33–45.

78. Caron JP. Neurogenic factors in joint pain and disease pathogenesis. In: McIlwraith CW, Trotter GW, eds. *Joint disease in the horse. (1st ed.)* Philadelphia, PA: WB Saunders; 1996:71–80.

79. Maroudas A, Bayliss MT, Uchitel-Kraushansky N. Aggrecan turnover in human articular cartilage: use of aspartic acid racemisation as a marker of molecular age. *Arch Biochem Biophys.* 1998;350(1):61–71.

80. Maroudas A, Palla G, Gilav E. Racemization of aspartic acid in human articular cartilage. *Connect Tissue Res.* 1992;28(3):161–169.

81. Duan X, Wu J, Swift B, et al. Texture analysis of the 3D collagen network and automatic classification of the physiology of articular cartilage. *Comput Methods Biomech Biomed Engin.* 2015;18(9):931–943.

82. Hunter W. Of the structure and diseases of articulating carti-lages. *Phil Trans R Soc London*. 1743;9:514–521.

83. Dahlberg L, Billinghurst RC, Manner P, et al. Selective enhancement of collagenase-mediated cleavage of resident type II collagen in cultured osteoarthritic cartilage and arrest with a synthetic inhibitor that spares collagenase 1 (matrix metalloproteinase 1). *Arthritis Rheum*. 2000;43(3):673–682.

84. Berenbaum F. The quest for the Holy Grail: a disease-modify-ing osteoarthritis drug. *Arthritis Res Ther*. 2007;9(6):111.

85. Goldring MB, Otero M. Inflammation in osteoarthritis. *Curr Opin Rheumatol*. 2011;23(5):471–478.

86. Krane SM, Byrne MH, Lemaître V, et al. Different collagenase gene products have different roles in degradation of type I collagen. *J Biol Chem*. 1996;271(45):28509–28515.

87. Clegg PD, Burke RM, Coughlan AR, et al. Characterisation of equine matrix metalloproteinase 2 and 9; and identification of the cellular sources of these enzymes in joints. *Equine Vet J*. 1997;29(5):335–342.

88. Sandy JD, Flannery CR, Neame PJ, et al. The structure of aggrecan fragments in human synovial fluid. Evidence for the involvement in osteoarthritis of a novel proteinase which cleaves the Glu 373-Ala 374 bond of the interglobular domain. *J Clin Invest*. 1992;89(5):1512–1516.

89. Tortorella MD, Burn TC, Pratta MA, et al. Purification and cloning of aggrecanase-1: a member of the ADAMTS family of proteins. *Science*. 1999;284(5420):1664–1666.

90. Song RH, Tortorella MD, Malfait AM, et al. Aggrecan degradation in human articular cartilage explants is medi-ated by both ADAMTS-4 and ADAMTS-5. *Arthritis Rheum*. 2007;56(2):575–585.

91. Glasson SS, Askew R, Sheppard B, et al. Deletion of active ADAMTS-5 prevents cartilage degradation in a murine model of osteoarthritis. *Nature*. 2005;434(7033):644–648.

92. Clutterbuck A, Harris P, Allaway D, et al. Matrix metallo-proteinases in inflammatory pathologies of the horse. *Vet J*. 2010;183(1):27–38.

93. Dean DD, Martel-Pelletier J, Pelletier JP, et al. Evidence for metalloproteinase and metalloproteinase inhibitor imbalance in human osteoarthritic cartilage. *J Clin Invest*. 1989;84(2):678–685.

94. O'Conor CJ, Case N, Guilak F. Mechanical regulation of chondrogenesis. *Stem Cell Res Ther*. 2013;4(4):61.

95. Edwards DR, Murphy G, Reynolds JJ, et al. Transform-ing growth factor beta modulates the expression of col-lagenase and metalloproteinase inhibitor. *EMBO J*. 1987;6(7):1899–1904.

96. Mueller MB, Tuan RS. Anabolic/catabolic balance in patho-genesis of osteoarthritis: identifying molecular targets. *PM R*. 2011;6(suppl 1):S3–11.

97. Van Beuningen HM, van der Kraan PM, Arntz OJ, et al. In vivo protection against interleukin-1-induced articular cartilage damage by transforming growth factor-beta 1: age-related differences. *Ann Rheum Dis*. 1994;53(9):593–600.

98. Van Beuningen HM, van der Kraan PM, Arntz OJ, et al. Transforming growth factor-beta 1 stimulates articular chon-drocyte proteoglycan synthesis and induces osteophyte forma-tion in the murine knee joint. *Lab Invest*. 1994;71(2):279–290.

99. Ekenstedt KJ, Sonntag WE, Loeser RF, et al. Effects of chronic growth hormone and insulin-like growth factor 1 deficiency on osteoarthritis severity in rat knee joints. *Arthritis Rheum*. 2006;54(12):3850–3858.

100. Brama PAJ, TeKoppele JM, Bank RA, et al. Development of biochemical heterogeneity of articular cartilage: influences of age and exercise. *Equine Vet J*. 2002;34(3):265–269.

101. Albro MB, Cigan AD, Nims RJ, et al. Shearing of synovial fluid activates latent TGF-β. *Osteoarthr Cart*. 2012;20(11):1374–1382.

102. Wilsman NJ. Cilia of adult canine articular chondrocytes. *J Ultrastruct Res*. 1978;64(3):270–281.

103. Muhammad H, Rais Y, Miosge N, et al. The primary cilium as a dual sensor of mechanochemical signals in chondrocytes. *Cell Mol Life Sci*. 2012;69(13):2101–2107.

104. Mouw JK, Imler SM, Levenston ME. Ion-channel regulation of chondrocyte matrix synthesis in 3D culture under static and dynamic compression. *Biomech Model Mechanobiol*. 2007;6(1-2):33–41.

105. Walker PS, Dowson D, Longfield MD, et al. "Boosted lubrica-tion" in synovial joints by fluid entrapment and enrichment. *Ann Rheum Dis*. 1968;27(6):512–520.

106. Hui AY, McCarty WJ, Koichi M, et al. A systems biology approach to synovial joint lubrication in health, injury, and disease. *Wiley Interdiscip Rev Syst Biol Med*. 2012;4(1):15–37.

107. Radin EL, Paul IL, Swann DA, et al. Lubrication of synovial membrane. *Ann Rheum Dis*. 1971;30(3):322–325.

108. Elsaid KA, Jay GD, Warman ML, et al. Association of articular cartilage degradation and loss of boundary-lubricating ability of synovial fluid following injury and inflammatory arthritis. *Arthritis Rheum*. 2005;52(6):1746–1755.

109. Antonacci JM, Schmidt TA, Serventi LA, et al. Effects of equine joint injury on boundary lubrication of articular car-tilage by synovial fluid: role of hyaluronan. *Arthritis Rheum*. 2012;64(9):2917–2926.

110. Safari M, Bjelle A, Gudmundsson M, et al. Clinical assess-ment of rheumatic diseases using viscoelastic parameters for synovial fluid. *Biorheology*. 1990;27(5):659–674.

111. Holliday CM, Ridgely RC, Sedlmayr JC, et al. Cartilagi-nous epiphyses in extant archosaurs and their implications for reconstructing limb function in dinosaurs. *PLoS One*. 2010;5(9):e13120.

112. Herzog W, Federico S. Considerations on joint and articular cartilage mechanics. *Biomech Mod Mechanobiol*. 2006;5(2-3):64–81.

113. Brama PAJ, TeKoppele JM, Bank RA, et al. Topographical mapping of biochemical properties of articular cartilage in the equine fetlock joint. *Equine Vet J*. 2000;32(1):19–26.

114. Brama PAJ, Karssenberg D, Barneveld A, et al. Contact areas and pressure distribution on the proximal articular surface of the proximal phalanx under sagittal plane loading. *Equine Vet J*. 2001;33(1):26–32.

115. Brommer H, Brama PAJ, Laasanen MS, et al. Functional adaptation of articular cartilage from birth to maturity under the influence of loading: a biomechanical analysis. *Equine Vet J*. 2005;37(2):148–154.

116. Niissalo S, Hukkanen M, Imai S, et al. Neuropeptides in experimental and degenerative arthritis. *Ann N Y Acad Sci*. 2002;966:s384–s399.

117. Haegerstrand A, Dalsgaard CJ, Jonzon B, et al. Calcitonin gene-related peptide stimulates proliferation of human endothelial cells. *Proc Natl Acad Sci U S A*. 1990;87(9):1299–1303.

118. Schuelert N, McDougall JJ. Electrophysiological evidence that the vasoactive intestinal peptide receptor antagonist VIP6-28 reduces nociception in an animal model of osteoarthritis. *Osteoarthr Cart.* 2006;14(11):1155–1162.

119. Goldring SR, Goldring MB. The role of cytokines in cartilage matrix degradation in osteoarthritis. *Clin Orthop Relat Res.* 2004;427(suppl):S27–36.

120. Goldring MB, Goldring SR. Osteoarthritis. *J Cell Physiol.* 2007;213(3):626–634.

121. Pettipher ER. Pathogenesis and treatment of chronic arthritis. *Sci Prog.* 1989;73(292):521–534.

122. De Grauw JC, van de Lest CHA, van Weeren PR, et al. Arthrogenic lameness of the fetlock: synovial fluid markers of inflammation and cartilage turnover in relation to clinical joint pain. *Equine Vet J.* 2006;38(4):305–311.

123. Guerrero AT, Verri WA, Cunha TM, et al. Involvement of LTB4 in zymosan induced joint nociception in mice: participation of neutrophils and PGE_2. *J Leukoc Biol.* 2008;83(1):122–130.

124. De Grauw JC, Brama PAJ, Wiemer P, et al. Cartilage-derived biomarkers and lipid mediators of inflammation in horses with osteochondritis dissecans of the distal intermediate ridge of the tibia. *Am J Vet Res.* 2006;67(7):1156–1162.

125. Bouloux GF. Temporomandibular joint pain and synovial fluid analysis: a review of the literature. *J Oral Maxillofac Surg.* 2009;67(11):2497–2504.

126. Suzuki T, Segami N, Nishimura M, et al. Bradykinin expression in synovial tissues and synovial fluids obtained from patients with internal derangement of the temporomandibular joint. *Cranio.* 2003;22(4):265–270.

127. Kirker-Head CA, Chandna VK, Agarwal RK, et al. Concentrations of substance P and prostaglandin E_2 in synovial fluid of normal and abnormal joints of horses. *Am J Vet Res.* 2000;61(6):714–718.

128. Miller RJ, Jung H, Bhangoo SK, et al. Cytokine and chemokine regulation of sensory neuron function. *Handb Exp Pharmacol.* 2009;194:417–449.

129. Van Loon JPAM, de Grauw JC, van Dierendonck M, et al. Intra-articular opioid analgesia is effective in reducing pain and inflammation in an equine LPS induced synovitis model. *Equine Vet J.* 2010;42(5):412–419.

130. Knoop J, Dekker J, van der Leeden M, et al. Knee joint stabilization therapy in patients with osteoarthritis of the knee: a randomized, controlled trial. *Osteoarthr Cart.* 2013;21(8):1025–1034.

131. Stubbs NC, Riggs CM, Hodges PW, et al. Osseous spinal pathology and epaxial muscle ultrasonography in thoroughbred racehorses. *Equine Vet J.* 2010;42(suppl 38):654–661.

132. Mohammadi F, Roozdar A. Effects of fatigue due to contraction of evertor muscles on the ankle joint position sense in male soccer players. *Am J Sports Med.* 2010;38(4):824–828.

133. Zhuo QY, Yang W, Chen J, et al. Metabolic syndrome meets osteoarthritis. *Nat Rev Rheumatol.* 2012;8(12):729–737.

134. Lötvall J, Rajendran L, Gho YS, et al. The launch of Journal of Extracellular Vesicles (JEV), the official journal of the International Society for Extracellular Vesicles – about microvesicles, exosomes, ectosomes and other extracellular vesicles. *J Extracell Vesicles, Apr 16.* 2012;1. http://dx.doi.org/10.3402/jev.v1i0.18514.

135. Boere J, van de Lest CHA, Nolte-'t Hoen EN, et al. Extracellular vesicles isolated from equine synovial fluid are internalized and processed by chondrocytes and synoviocytes in vitro. *Congr Int Soc for Extracellular Vesicles.* 2014. Rotterdam, the Netherlands, April 30-May 3, 2014.

Biomechanics in Joints

Christopher E. Kawcak

Although the field of biomechanics is complex and often outside the minds of clinicians, a basic understanding of the biomechanics of the equine limb and axial skeleton and how abnormalities in the mechanical forces throughout the body can lead to disease may improve not only the understanding of the pathologic processes that occur, but also the effectiveness of diagnostics and therapeutics. The complex mechanisms that lead to pathologic changes in the joint are numerous; however, with the advent of newer therapies that target specific pathologic processes, an understanding of the basic mechanisms that lead to disease can enhance understanding and justification for the use of certain diagnostic methods and therapies. The goal of this chapter is to discuss basic biomechanical principles that play a role in normal and diseased joints. The influence of these biomechanics on normal joint homeostasis will be characterized, as will the acute and chronic effects of abnormal biomechanical forces on joint tissues. The known pathologic mechanisms that occur within joints will be discussed and examples will be given for specific joints.

BIOMECHANICAL CONSIDERATIONS THAT INFLUENCE JOINT DISEASE

Types of Joints Relevant to Equine

Joints are best characterized by their primary plane of motion. Hinge-type joints typically move in only the sagittal plane, although other types of joints such as the ball-and-socket joint can move in the sagittal, frontal, and transverse planes. These movements are restricted based on a complex organization of joint shape and extraarticular soft tissue support, namely ligaments. Joints below the shoulder and stifle typically move in the sagittal plane; however, out-of-plane motion such as in the frontal and transverse planes, albeit small in magnitude, may be of significance. Joints such as the shoulder, stifle, and hip have complex three-dimensional motions that are difficult to characterize. The joints of the axial skeleton have not been thoroughly characterized and are influenced not only by the periarticular ligaments but also by the large muscle and tendon masses as well as the intervertebral discs. The contributions of these large muscle masses are not entirely understood, but they are assumed to contribute significantly to back pain, both as a primary pathologic entity and as a

compensatory component.[1] An understanding of normal articulation is necessary to understand the normal changes that can occur within the joints in response to growth, exercise, and disease.

Ground Reaction Forces

The limbs of the horse undergo a tremendous amount of stress. This is most influential in the joints during the weight-bearing phase of stride between when the heel touches the ground and the toe lifts off.[2-7] Ground reaction force is defined as the force placed on the limb by the ground during contact. This force is dissipated as it moves proximally through the limb because of the coordinated efforts of soft tissues, subchondral bone, and articular cartilage. Therefore, the influence of ground reaction force on each joint is dependent on its location, its congruity, and the material properties of the tissues in that area (Figure 2-1). Abnormal tissue characteristics, such as occur with disease, can also influence the dissipation of ground reaction force and its transmission up the limb. Therefore, damage to any supporting tissue within a limb can have an effect on other joints and tissues because of its change in ability to dissipate or transfer forces.

Ground reaction force can be assessed several ways in the horse. The most accurate method is by kinetic measurement, which can be done with the use of a force plate, pressure film, or a force shoe.[8] Each of these methods is cumbersome, and all require time and expertise to ensure that data are accurate. Stationary force plates require dedicated space and equipment, and measurement is limited to a specific stationary site for assessment, thereby taking the horse out of its natural working environment. In addition, the force plate can often be sensed by the horse, whether by handler cues or change in ground characteristics, often leading to abnormal movement. Data acquired from a stationary force plate can often have considerable statistical variability, leading to inaccuracy in detecting disease or response to therapy. Pressure film has also been used to assess limb use and has been commercially packaged as easy to use.[9] However, pressure film systems require continuous calibration and can suffer from degradation of signal over time. Force shoes have recently been developed to allow the horse to be assessed in its natural working environment.[10] These shoes and associated wiring are cumbersome, which can affect the horse's natural gait. However, the data are thought to represent a more accurate picture of limb use compared with other techniques, especially at higher speeds.

The ground reaction force that is transmitted through the limb is also influenced by the limb conformation. Although force through the limb is needed to maintain proper

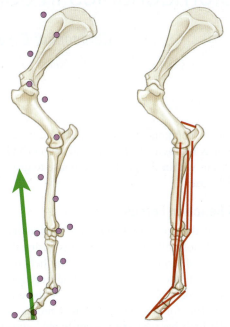

FIGURE 2-1 Ground reaction force (green arrow) is demonstrated moving from the ground, through the limb. This force is translated through the joints, in addition to the muscle forces imposed at each site. (Redrawn from Harrison S.M., Whitton R.C., Kawcak C.E., et al. (2014). Evaluation of a subject-specific finite-element model of the equine metacarpophalangeal joint under physiological load. J Biomech, 47(1), 65-73.)

metabolism and turnover of the musculoskeletal tissues, abnormal distribution of these forces can lead to pathologic manifestations. An understanding of this principle is necessary to influence these conformational abnormalities at a young age and to provide expectations to owners for horses with conformational abnormalities.

Extraarticular Forces

Ground reaction force is not the only force that influences the joints. A large magnitude of force is transmitted by the muscles through the tendons across the joints.[2-6] In addition, tendons can store energy during the loading phase of stride, which can influence the joints as well.[6] Ligaments can contribute to the force generation mechanism, and they restrict joints within certain planes, which can significantly influence the force distribution across the joint (Figure 2-2).

Calculation of both the ground reaction forces and the extraarticular forces can be used to characterize more objectively the stresses seen within the joint. Finite element modeling, in which these forces are characterized and optimized with the patient's bone and joint shape, is commonly used to characterize the forces across the joint at various gaits.[6] Abnormalities within conformation, muscle activation and timing, shoeing, and disease within various tissues can be programmed into the finite element model and the resultant joint stresses characterized. With the development of volumetric imaging techniques, such as magnetic resonance imaging and computed tomography, these modeling techniques may have a clinical use in the future.

Tissue Biomechanics
Soft Tissues

Muscle force influences joint stress based on the muscle's cross-sectional area, muscle fiber composition, and timing of

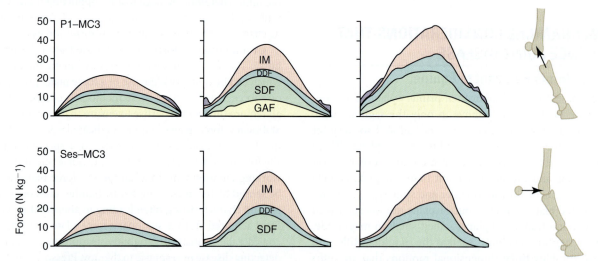

FIGURE 2-2 The graphs demonstrate the contribution of force of each muscle, tendon, and ligament to the MC3-P1 articulation (top) and the MC3-Ses articulation (bottom). Note the significant contribution of soft tissues to the overall force through each articulation. On the vertical axes are force and on the horizontal axes is stance (%). *DDF,* Deep digital flexor tendon; *GAF,* ground reaction force; *IM,* intraosseous muscle (proximal suspensory ligament); *SDF,* superficial digital flexor tendon. (Redrawn from Harrison S.M., Whitton R.C., Kawcak C.E., et al. (2014). Evaluation of a subject-specific finite-element model of the equine metacarpophalangeal joint under physiological load. J Biomech, 47(1), 65-73.)

firing.[3,4] Consequently, any change to a muscle caused by primary damage, physiologic abnormalities, or neuromuscular timing can indirectly influence the magnitude and timing of individual muscles and also the timing of activation among the different muscles that may influence a joint.

On a tissue level, ligaments, tendons, and the fibrous joint capsule are structurally and biomechanically similar. Each of these tissues is sparsely cellular but contains an abundant extracellular matrix composed of predominantly types I and III collagen, elastin, proteoglycan, glycosaminoglycans, and water. Although tendons are considered to be passive in their influence on limb and joint forces, they are a source of energy storage.[5] Consequently, damage to a tendon can reduce its energy storage capacity, which may lead to increased magnitude and direction of force on the limb.

The collagen of ligaments is arranged in nearly parallel bundles oriented to maximize resistance against tensile forces. The elastin of ligaments permits a small degree of elongation with tension, and this protects the bony insertion points of the proximal and distal ends of the ligament. The slightly random configuration of collagen bundles in ligaments enables the ligament to withstand small tensile forces in other directions besides the plane in which they lie. Therefore, although the lateral and medial collateral ligaments of the carpus and fetlock can resist medial-to-lateral movement, these are less effective against bending (in the dorsopalmar or plantar plane) or rotational forces applied to the joints. These forces must be countered or dissipated by other ligaments, such as the intercarpal ligaments (against rotational loads) that are positioned in a different plane, or by the flexor retinaculum (carpal extension). In the fetlock, the suspensory ligament and distal sesamoidean ligaments support the joint in a dorsopalmar (or plantar) plane during fetlock extension.[11]

Unlike ligament collagen, tendon collagen exhibits a highly ordered parallel arrangement with a characteristic wave and periodicity appearance. This is biomechanically important because tendons must resist high uniaxial loads during activity as they transmit the load from muscle to bone to produce motion.

The joint capsule inserts within bone around the periphery of the joint margin, providing stability to the joint surface, but it is also a significant source of nerve endings that can play a role in joint pain. Ligaments, tendons, muscles, the joint capsule, and the geometric shape of the articulating bones provide support to the joint.[12]

The proteoglycan-glycosaminoglycan component in the matrix of ligaments, tendons, and the fibrous joint capsule attracts and holds water. This imparts a gel-like quality to the matrix, which not only adds structure to the matrix but also helps support the collagen arrangement. Proteoglycans have long been recognized for their ability to resist compressive forces within the articular cartilage matrix, but this function is not as important in ligaments, tendons, and the fibrous joint capsule since they are designed to resist tensile forces.[12] However, changes in proteoglycan concentration and/or composition as a result of training, injury, or immobilization can alter the mechanical capability of the collagen by changing

the electrostatic interactions between the glycosaminoglycans and collagen.[13-15] The effect may be to change the site of tissue failure. The change in the composition of the soft tissues of the joint in response to loading has been considered an extension of Wolff's law, implying that the soft tissue of the joint adapts to an applied stress as seen in bone.[14]

The biomechanical structural behavior of isolated ligaments, tendons, and joint capsule is qualitatively identical, with differences existing in the amount of force the tissue is able to withstand and in the slope of the stress-strain curve (i.e., tissue modulus).[12,14] Tissue differences are related to the elastin/collagen ratio and to collagen arrangement (previously described). The elastin/collagen ratio of tendon (1:50) is much lower than that of ligament (1:4).[12] Initially, as force is applied, all three tissues exhibit a nonlinear toe region that curves upward (Figure 2-3). This toe region corresponds to the straightening of the collagen and/or elastin fibril wave and permits a large displacement or elongation of the tissue without placing any significant tension on the insertion site. As a result, ligaments, which contain a higher content of elastin compared with tendons, function at the lower portion of the physiologic strain range. With further tension, collagen fibers are increasingly recruited until tension develops against the insertion site. The load increases sharply into the linear region of the curve. The organization and quantity of collagen and elastin fibers determine the length and shape of the toe region and the slope of the linear region. Extremity ligaments typically have a shortened toe region compared with the fibrous joint capsule, in which the collagen is randomly organized, and compared with tendons, which have a longer wave periodicity.[12,13,16] Since the collagen of the tissue matrix stores the applied stress as energy, the quantity of collagen and its association with matrix glycosaminoglycans determine the strength and stiffness of the tissue.[11]

The linear region of the load-elongation curve represents the recruitment of all collagen fibers, which increase in tension as more displacement is applied until the tissue fails

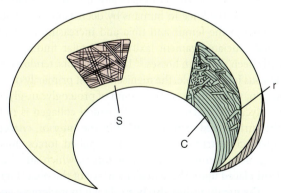

FIGURE 2-3 Collagen ultrastructure of the menisci. Notice the radial arrangement (r) of collagen fibrils on the surface (S) of the menisci that becomes circumferential (C) in the deep zone of the menisci in order to attenuate and dissipate the force applied to the tibial articular cartilage. (From Fithian D.C., Kelly M.A., Mow V.C. (1990). Material properties and structure-function relationships in the menisci. Clin Orthop, 252, 19-31.)

either at the insertion point or within the tissue. Because tendons and ligaments are generally subjected to loads well below those required for abrupt failure, injury to tendons and ligaments is generally viewed as a cumulative failure of individual collagen fibers, which eventually results in tissue failure under the applied load. However, it is reasonable to hypothesize that even failure of a few collagen fibers may subtly alter the stability of the joint during loading and result in excessive stretching of the joint capsule and synovial lining, which in turn may predispose intraarticular joint ligaments to injury through the release of inflammatory mediators.

Ligaments, tendons, and the fibrous joint capsule, just like the articular cartilage and subchondral bone, all exhibit viscoelastic behavior (i.e., their mechanical behavior is a function of the rate of the load application), which influences the mechanism of failure of the tissue.[17] Like bone and cartilage, ligaments and tendons are stiffer (i.e., the linear portion of the load-elongation curve becomes steeper) at higher strain rates.[12] As demonstrated in a study in rabbits, bone is the most strain-rate-sensitive tissue when compared with tendon and ligament.[16] In the same study, tendon was more strain-rate-sensitive than ligament. In addition, the mechanism of failure is altered as the strain rate is increased. In mature animals, failure occurs within the ligament at both low and high strain rates since the ligament is strongly attached to the bone, and at high strain rates bone is stronger than the ligament.[17] If the same holds true for equine joint tissues, it is reasonable to hypothesize that some trauma to the limb joints during racing may occur in the ligaments, destabilizing the joint and putting further strain on tendons, articular cartilage, and subchondral bone. In the equine distal limb joints (i.e., fetlock, carpus), this effect may be compounded by the anatomic lack of muscle, and therefore the importance of minor ligament tissue failure to joint stability may be exaggerated.

In the stifle, the menisci also play an important role in stabilizing the femorotibial joint during movement and in increasing joint congruency.[18,19] Once thought of as a fairly innocuous procedure, partial and/or total meniscectomy has been repeatedly shown to dramatically alter the normal biomechanics of the knee in humans by decreasing the contact area between the femur and tibia and increasing joint capsule and cruciate ligament laxity.[19-21] Similar findings have recently been shown in horses.[22] Like ligaments, tendons, and the fibrous joint capsule, the menisci consist primarily of type I collagen, water, and a small amount of proteoglycan-glycosaminoglycan. The arrangement of menisci collagen is radial on the surface and circumferential in the interior, enabling the menisci to transfer compressive applied forces during loading into circumferential tensile forces, which attenuates the load placed upon the articular surface of the tibia (Figure 2-4).[21] The meniscus has also been shown to undergo a good deal of cranial-caudal translation during flexion and extension, which puts increased stress on the cranial ligament of the medial meniscus.[23,24]

Alterations in the macromolecular composition of the soft tissues of the joint associated with training and inflammation may also affect the normal function or failure of the joint.[25,26]

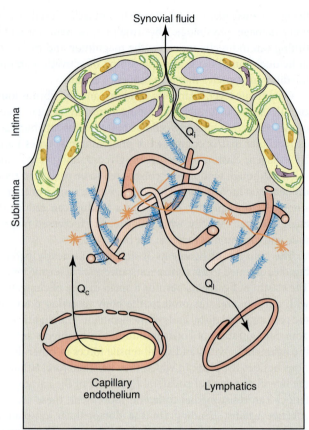

FIGURE 2-4 The organization of the synovial membrane allows the movement of the capillary filtrate through the interstitial fluid into the synovial cavity. The movement of the filtrate through the endothelium (Q_c) is controlled by the capillary hydrostatic pressure and the colloid osmotic pressure of the plasma. Movement through the interstitium (Q_i) is controlled by the interstitial hydrostatic pressure and the colloid osmotic pressure of the interstitial fluid. Excess synovial fluid is drained from the joint by valved lymphatic vessels.

Training increases the tensile stiffness and strength of ligaments, tendons, fibrous joint capsule, and their interfaces by increasing the number and type of collagen cross-links and diameter of the collagen fibril.[27,28] Therefore, an appropriate training regimen should further stabilize the joint and protect against injury originating from a soft tissue disturbance.

Synovial Fluid

There are many theories as to how the joint remains lubricated under various loading conditions (Table 2-1).[29] The synovial fluid viscosity and lubrication are imparted by hyaluronic acid and lubricin.[30-34] Boundary lubrication functions to resist shearing stresses between two cartilage surfaces and between the articular cartilage and synovial membrane, and it may also play a role in opposing articular surface tracking, possibly contributing to overall joint stability.[35] Boundary lubrication occurs because of the function of synovial fluid components that have an influence on articular and synovial surfaces. These components include hyaluronan, proteoglycan-4, and surface active phospholipids.[36] Changes in the joint environment can influence these synovial fluid

TABLE 2-1	Proposed Mechanisms of Joint Lubrication
Lubrication	**Mechanism of Action**
Fluid film Hydrodynamic Self-generating Squeeze film	A converging layer of synovial fluid is dragged between surfaces at continuous high-speed motion. This motion rarely occurs and therefore is not a primary lubrication mechanism. Fluid exudes from tissues at the leading and trailing edges of loading, resulting in a continuous supply of lubricant. Loading creates viscous resistance as fluid is squeezed.
Self-pressurized hydrostatic (weeping lubrication)	Tissue compression leads to self-pressurization of interstitial fluid
Boosted	Compression forces water into the articular cartilage and hyaluronic acid remains at the surface since it is too large to move through the pores.
Boundary	Multiple components such as lubricin and surface active phospholipid remain at the surface.

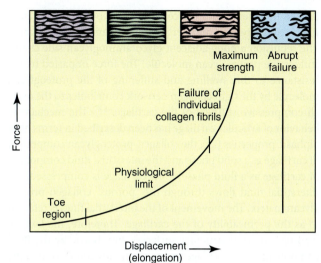

FIGURE 2-5 Idealized load-elongation curve of ligament, tendon, and joint capsule. At the initiation of tension, the toe region of the load-elongation curve corresponds to a straightening of the collagen-elastin fibril wave pattern, permitting a large displacement without significant tension being placed on the tissue. With increasing tension, collagen fibers are recruited and the load increases sharply into the linear portion of the curve. Further increases in tension result in individual collagen fiber rupture. Ultimate failure occurs when the tissue fails at the insertion site or midbody.

components, thereby negatively affecting the boundary lubrication of the joint. As an example, Antonacci et al. have shown that in acute joint disease in the horse, the boundary lubrication properties of the synovial fluid were considered poor and correlated with diminished hyaluronan concentration and molecular weight.[36] In addition, synovial fluid from acutely injured joints had higher proteoglycan-4 and surface active phospholipid concentrations. Therefore, the change in these biochemical parameters negatively influenced the ability of synovial fluid to perform as a boundary lubricant. In this study, the significant decrease in hyaluronic acid concentration and size appeared to outweigh the increases in proteoglycan-4 and surface active phospholipids. Furthermore, application of exogenous hyaluronic acid improved the boundary lubrication function of synovial fluid. Under high-speed situations, however, boundary lubrication is less effective, and the load is thought to be supported primarily through fluid-film lubrication, which appears to function by forcing fluid into the joint from tissues and creating a physical area of fluid pressure that resists loading.[37,38] Another theory of joint lubrication termed "natural lubrication" refers to the simultaneous movement of synovial fluid into and out of the articular cartilage as the joint surfaces slide across each other during articulation.[39,40]

Overall there have been several theories concerning lubrication in the joint, many of which have been contentious and some disproven. It is likely most accurate to summarize joint lubrication as the interaction of interstitial fluid pressure, boundary lubrication, and fluid film lubrication. These mechanisms probably work together to maintain low friction, movement, and lack of wear in the tissues.

Synovium

The synovial lining of the joint capsule is a thin structure, a 1- to 3-cell-thick layer that lines all articular surfaces except the articular cartilage. The synovial lining itself serves no known biomechanical function but like any soft tissue is capable of responding to mechanical stress through an increase in collagen production, alterations in transsynovial diffusion, and/or changes in synoviocyte metabolism (Figure 2-5).[41-43] Joint inflammation can be produced by stretching of the synovial lining through repeated hyperextension. The release of enzymes from the synovial membrane can affect all tissues within the joint including intraarticular ligaments and articular cartilage.[44,45] These changes are probably very subtle but may slightly alter the ability of the joint to respond appropriately to loading during motion. Disturbances in the arrangement of ligament or fibrous joint capsule collagen have been shown to result in increased ligamentous extensibility, decreased stiffness, reduced energy absorption, and less flexible joint capsules.[13] Even subtly, these changes in a joint of a performing animal may greatly predispose the overall joint to injury.

Articular Cartilage

The compressive stiffness of cartilage is related to the presence of negatively charged side chains of aggrecan, which are closely packed together within the collagen fibers of the extracellular matrix and repel one another and attract fluid into the matrix. The repulsion among adjacent glycosaminoglycan side chains stiffens the proteoglycan molecule. The force imparted by the resistance to this swelling and stiffening of the proteoglycan molecule by the tight collagen network contributes to the overall compressive stiffness of the cartilage.[46,47] The mechanical behavior of articular cartilage has been described in terms of its biphasic properties (i.e., the collagen-proteoglycan component of cartilage as a solid phase and the interstitial fluid component of cartilage as a fluid phase).[48] As cartilage is compressed, the interstitial fluid flows through the "porous" collagen-proteoglycan matrix. The movement of the interstitial fluid is referred to as the permeability of the cartilage. Therefore, the bulk of load placed on an articular surface is first borne by the fluid component of the cartilage and subsequently transferred to the solid component of the cartilage after all the fluid is squeezed out of the compressed region.[11,39,49] This property is characteristic of all viscoelastic materials.

The tissue material property of articular cartilage varies through its thickness. In the superficial layer of the cartilage, the collagen content and cross-link density is the highest. Combined with the parallel orientation of the collagen to the articular surface, this imparts a great tensile stiffness and strength to the cartilage surface.[49] Matrix molecule composition and orientation changes throughout the depth of the cartilage and as a result each area has a different inherent biomechanical capability.

The material properties of articular cartilage are also dependent on its loading history. Several studies of canine stifle joints have demonstrated that the biomechanical and biochemical response of articular cartilage is extremely dependent upon the level of activity experienced by the joint.[50-56] The results of these studies have established that there exists a critical level after which the beneficial effect of exercise is overwhelmed by the potential consequences of articular damage associated with loading. In the horse, investigations of the equine carpus have demonstrated that the response to load is both location-dependent and activity-dependent.[57-59] This has also been shown to occur in the metacarpophalangeal joint.[60] This may be functionally important in the adaptation of the articular cartilage to enhance the congruency of the joint and protect the cartilage from damage associated with exercise.

Subchondral Bone

Subchondral bone is highly responsive to loading and consequently can respond quickly to training and injury. Bone, like cartilage, is a biphasic material but is composed of an inorganic component of mineral salts [hydroxyapatite crystals $Ca_{10}(PO_4)_6(OH)_2$] and an organic component of predominantly type I collagen, proteoglycan, glycosaminoglycans, and water. The inorganic phase imparts a hardness and rigidity to the subchondral bone; whereas, the organic phase provides flexibility and resiliency.

Early mechanical studies clearly demonstrated the ability of the subchondral bone to attenuate axial loads and spare the overlying articular cartilage from damage.[61-66] The

transition zone between the uncalcified articular cartilage and the stiff subchondral bone is the calcified cartilage. The interface between these two mechanically dissimilar tissues (articular cartilage and subchondral bone) assists in minimizing the shear stresses via the calcified cartilage's intermediate mechanical properties and characteristic undulating insertions into the subchondral layer.[67] These undulations further dissipate mechanical stresses over a larger surface area. Articular cartilage is supported by the calcified cartilage, which is supported by the subchondral bone plate, which in turn is supported by the subchondral trabecular bone and ultimately the cortical bone. Increased trabecular bone compliance allows a degree of deformation on joint loading to absorb the load and dissipate energy and probably to assist in joint congruency. Morphometric analysis, radiographic analysis, and bone scintigraphy have demonstrated that repeated loading to the joint results in subchondral bone thickening and sclerosis, which may be amplified by trabecular microfractures and subsequent subchondral bone healing.[66,68-73] Consequently, subchondral bone thickening results in increased transverse stress at the base of the cartilage and the appearance of horizontal clefts in the deep zone of the cartilage, which may progress to the articular surface.[27,73-78]

REFERENCES

1. Greve L, Dyson SJ. The interrelationship of lameness, saddle slip and back shape in the general sports horse population. *Equine Vet J.* 2013;46(6):687–694.
2. Brown NA, Pandy MG, Buford WL, et al. Moment arms about the carpal and metacarpophalangeal joints for flexor and extensor muscles in equine forelimbs. *Am J Vet Res.* 2003;64(3):351–357.
3. Brown NA, Pandy MG, Kawcak CE, et al. Force- and moment-generating capacities of muscles in the distal forelimb of the horse. *J Anat.* 2003;203(1):101–113.
4. Brown NA, Kawcak CE, McIlwraith CW, et al. Architectural properties of distal forelimb muscles in horses, Equus caballus. *J Morphol.* 2003;258(1):106–114.
5. Harrison SM, Whitton RC, Kawcak CE, et al. Relationship between muscle forces, joint loading and utilization of elastic strain energy in equine locomotion. *J Exp Biol.* 2010;213(part 23):3998–4009.
6. Harrison SM, Whitton RC, King M, et al. Forelimb muscle activity during equine locomotion. *J Exp Biol.* 2012;215(part 17):2980–2991.
7. Harrison SM, Whitton RC, Kawcak CE, et al. Evaluation of a subject-specific finite-element model of the equine metacarpophalangeal joint under physiological load. *J Biomech.* 2014;47(1):65–73.
8. Keegan KG. Objective assessment of lameness. In: Baxter GM, ed. *Adams and Stashak's lameness in horses.* 6th ed. Wiley-Blackwell; 2011:154–172.
9. Perino VV. *Comparing pressure measurement systems and a force platform as tools for equine gait analysis.* PhD Dissertation: Colorado State University; 2007.
10. Roland ES, Hull ML, Stover SM. Design and demonstration of a dynamometric horseshoe for measuring ground reaction loads of horses during racing conditions. *J Biomech.* 2005;38(10):2102–2112.

11. Palmer JL, Bertone AL. Joint biomechanics in the pathogenesis of traumatic arthritis. In: McIlwraith CW, Trotter GW, eds. *Joint disease in the horse*. Philadelphia, PA: Saunders; 1996:104–119.

12. Carlstedt CA, Nordin M. Biomechanics of tendons and ligaments. In: Nordin E, Frankel VH, eds. *Basic biomechanics of the musculo-skeletal system*. Philadelphia, PA: Lea & Febiger; 1989:59–74.

13. Akeson WH, Amiel D, Abel MF, et al. Effects of immobilization on joints. *Clin Orthop*. 1987;219:28–37.

14. Akeson WH, Garfin S, Amiel D, et al. Para-articular connective tissue in osteoarthritis. *Semin Arthritis Rheum*. 1989;18(4 suppl 2):41–50.

15. Egan JM. A constitutive model for mechanical behavior of soft connective tissues. *J Biomech*. 1987;20(7):681–692.

16. Danto MI, Woo SLY. The mechanical properties of skeletally mature rabbit anterior cruciate ligament and patellar tendon over a range of strain rates. *J Orthop Res*. 1993;11(1):58–67.

17. Woo SLY, Peterson RH, Ohland KJ, et al. The effects of strain rate on the properties of the medial collateral ligament is skeletally immature and mature rabbits: a biomechanical and histological study. *J Orthop Res*. 1990;8(5):712–721.

18. Ghosh P, Taylor TFK. The knee joint meniscus: a fibrocartilage of some distinction. *Clin Orthop*. 1987;224:52–63.

19. McBride ID, Reid JG. Biomechanical considerations of the menisci of the knee. *Can J Sport Sci*. 1988;13(4):175–187.

20. Maistrelli G, Gerundini M, Bombelli R. The inclination of the weight bearing surface in the hip joint: the clinical significance of abnormal force. *Orthop Rev*. 1986;15(5):23–31.

21. Fithian DC, Kelly MA, Mow VC. Material properties and structure-function relationships in the menisci. *Clin Orthop*. 1990;252:19–31.

22. Fowlie J, Arnoczky S, Lavagnino M, et al. Resection of grade III cranial horn tears of the equine medial meniscus alter the contact forces on medial tibial condyle at full extension: an in-vitro cadaveric study. *Vet Surg*. 2011;40(8):957–965.

23. Fowlie JG, Arnoczky SP, Stick JA, et al. Meniscal translocation and deformation throughout the range of motion of the equine stifle joint: an in vitro cadaveric study. *Equine Vet J*. 2011;43(3):259–264.

24. Fowlie JG, Arnoczky SP, Lavagnino M, et al. Stifle extension results in differential tensile forces developing between abaxial and axial components of the cranial meniscotibial ligament of the equine medial meniscus: a mechanistic explanation for meniscal tear patterns. *Equine Vet J*. 2012;44(5):554–558.

25. Kim W, Kawcak CE, McIlwraith CW, et al. Influence of early conditioning exercise on the development of gross cartilage defects and swelling behavior of cartilage extracellular matrix in the equine midcarpal joint. *Am J Vet Res*. 2009;70(5):589–598.

26. Kim W, Kawcak CE, McIlwraith CW, et al. Histologic and histomorphometric evaluation of midcarpal joint defects in Thoroughbreds raised with and without early conditioning exercise. *Am J Vet Res*. 2012;73(4):498–507.

27. Vener MJ, Thompson RC, Lewis JL, et al. Subchondral damage after acute transarticular loading: an in vitro model of joint injury. *J Orthop Res*. 1992;10(6):759–765.

28. Firth EC. The response of bone, articular cartilage and tendon to exercise in the horse. *J Anat*. 2006;208(4):513–526.

29. Ateshian GA, Mow VC. Friction, lubrication and wear of articular cartilage and diarthrodial joints. In: Mow VC, Huiskes R, eds. *Basic orthopaedic biomechanics and mechano-biology*. 3rd ed. Philadelphia, PA: Lippincott Williams & Wilkins; 2005:447–494.

30. Chappuis J, Sherman IA, Neumann AW. Surface tension of animal cartilage as it relates to friction in joints. *Ann Biomed Eng*. 1983;11(5):435–449.

31. Hills BA. Oligolamellar lubrication of joints by surface active phospholipid. *J Rheumatol*. 1989;16(1):82–91.

32. Linn FC, Radin EL. Lubrication of animal joints: III. The effect of certain chemical alterations of the cartilage and lubricant. *Arthritis Rheum*. 1968;11(5):674–682.

33. Orford CR, Gardner DL. Ultrastructural histochemistry of the surface lamina of normal articular cartilage. *Histochem J*. 1985;17(2):223–233.

34. Swann DA, Silver FH, Slayter HS, et al. The molecular structure and lubricating activity of lubricin isolated from bovine and human synovial fluids. *Biochem J*. 1985;225(1):195–201.

35. Simkin PA. Biology and function of synovium. In: Finerman GAM, Noyes FR, eds. *Biology and biomechanics of the traumatized synovial joint: the knee as a model*. Rosemont, IL: Am Acad Orthop Surg; 1992:5–16.

36. Antonacci JM, Schmidt TA, Serventi LA, et al. Effects of equine joint injury on boundary lubrication of articular cartilage by synovial fluid. *Arthritis Rheum*. 2012. 2012;64(9):2917–2926.

37. Hou JS, Mow VC, Lai WM, et al. An analysis of the squeeze-film lubrication mechanism for articular cartilage. *J Biomech*. 1992;25(3):247–259.

38. Jin ZM, Dowson D, Fisher J. The effect of porosity of articular cartilage on the lubrication of a normal human hip joint. *Proc Inst Mech Eng*. 1992;206(3):117–124.

39. Mansour JM, Mow VC. The permeability of articular cartilage under compressive strain and at high pressure. *J Bone Joint Surg*. 1976;58(4):509–516.

40. O'Hara B, Urban J, Maroudas A. Influence of cyclic loading on the nutrition of articular cartilage. *Ann Rheum Dis*. 1990;49(7):536–539.

41. Barlow Y, Willoughby J. Pathophysiology of soft tissue repair. *Br Med Bull*. 1992;48(3):698–711.

42. Walker ER, Boyd RD, Wu DD, et al. Morphologic and morphometric changes in synovial membrane associated with mechanically induced osteoarthritis. *Arthritis Rheum*. 1991;34(5):515–524.

43. Dulin JA, Drost WT, Phelps MA, et al. Influence of exercise on the distribution of technetium Tc 99m medronate following intra-articular injection in horses. *Am J Vet Res*. 2012;73(3):418–425.

44. Frost L, Ghosh P. Microinjury to the synovial membrane may cause disaggregation of proteoglycans in rabbit knee joint articular cartilage. *J Orthop Res*. 1984;2(3):207–220.

45. McIlwraith CW, Frisbie DD, Kawcak CE, et al. The OARSI histopathology initiative - recommendations for histological assessments of osteoarthritis in the horse. *Osteoarthritis Cartilage*. 2010;18(suppl 3):S93–105.

46. Broom ND. Further insights into the structural principles governing the function of articular cartilage. *J Anat*. 1984;139(part 2):275–294.

47. Broom ND, Marra DL. New structural concepts of articular cartilage demonstrated with a physical model. *Connect Tissue Res*. 1985;14(1):1–8.

48. Mow VC, Gibbs MC, Zhu WB, et al. Biphasic indentation of articular cartilage: II. A numerical algorithm and an experimental study. *J Biomech*. 1989;22(8-9):853–861.

49. Setton LA, Zhu W, Mow VC. The biphasic poro-viscoelastic behavior of articular cartilage: role of the surface zone in governing the compressive behavior. *J Biomech*. 1993;26(4-5):581–592.

50. Jurvelin J, Kiviranta I, Tammi M, et al. Softening of canine articular cartilage after immobilization of the knee joint. *Clin Orthop.* 1989;207:246–252.

51. Jurvelin J, Kiviranta I, Saamanen AM, et al. Indentation stiffness of young canine knee articular cartilage – influence of strenuous joint loading. *J Biomech.* 1990;23(12):1239–1246.

52. Kiviranta I, Tammi M, Jurvelin J, et al. Moderate running exercise augments glycosaminoglycans and thickness of articular cartilage in the knee joint of young beagle dogs. *J Orthop Res.* 1988;6(2):188–195.

53. Kiviranta I, Tammi M, Jurvelin J, et al. Articular cartilage thickness and glycosaminoglycan distribution in the canine knee joint after strenuous running exercise. *Clin Orthop.* 1992;283:302–308.

54. Lammi MJ, Hakkinen TP, Parkkinen JJ, et al. Effects of long-term running exercise on canine femoral head articular cartilage. *Agents Actions.* 1993;39(suppl):95–99.

55. Oettmeier R, Arokoski J, Roth AJ, et al. Quantitative study of articular cartilage and subchondral bone remodeling in the knee joints of dogs after strenuous running training. *J Bone Miner Res.* 1992;7(suppl 2):419–424.

56. Parkkinen JJ, Lammi MJ, Karjalainen S, et al. A mechanical apparatus with microprocessor controlled stress profile for cyclic compression of cultured articular cartilage explants. *J Biomech.* 1989;22(11-12):1285–1291.

57. Palmer JL, Bertone AL, Mansour J. *Site specific indentation characteristics of third carpal articular cartilage in exercised versus non-exercised horses.* San Francisco, CA: Proceedings 39th Annual Meeting of the Orthopaedic Research Society; 1993. 184.

58. Murray RC, Birch HL, Lakhani K, et al. Biochemical composition of equine carpal articular cartilage is influenced by short-term exercise in a site-specific manner. *Osteoarthritis Cartilage.* 2001;9(7):625–632.

59. Murray RC, Smith RK, Henson FM, et al. The distribution of cartilage oligomeric matrix protein (COMP) in equine carpal articular cartilage and its variation with exercise and cartilage deterioration. *Vet J.* 2001;162(2):121–128.

60. Brama PA, Holopainen J, van Weeren PR, et al. Influence of exercise and joint topography on depth-related spatial distribution of proteoglycan and collagen content in immature equine articular cartilage. *Equine Vet J.* 2009;41(6):557–563.

61. Hoshino A, Wallace WA. Impact-absorbing properties of the human knee. *J Bone Joint Surg.* 1987;69(5):807–811.

62. Radin EL, Paul IL. Does cartilage compliance reduce skeletal impact load? The relative force-attenuating properties of articular cartilage, synovial fluid, periarticular soft tissues and bone. *Arthritis Rheum.* 1970;13(2):139–144.

63. Radin EL, Paul IL. Response of joints to impact loading: I. In vitro wear. *Arthritis Rheum.* 1971;14(3):356–362.

64. Radin EL, Paul IL. Importance of bone in sparing articular cartilage from impact. *Clin Orthop.* 1971;78:342–344.

65. Radin EL, Paul IL, Lowy M. A comparison of the dynamic force transmitting properties of subchondral bone and articular cartilage. *J Bone Joint Surg.* 1970;52(3):444–456.

66. Radin EL, Parker HG, Pugh JW, et al. Response of joints to impact loading: III. Relationship between trabecular microfractures and cartilage degeneration. *J Biomech.* 1973;6(1):51–57.

67. Radin EL, Rose RM. Role of subchondral bone in the initiation and progression of cartilage damage. *Clin Orthop.* 1986;213:34–40.

68. Christensen SB. Osteoarthritis; changes of bone, cartilage and synovial membrane in relation to bone scintigraphy. *Acta Orthop Scand.* 1985;214:1–43.

69. Noble J, Alexander K. Studies of tibial subchondral bone density and its significance. *J Bone Joint Surg Am,* Feb: 1985;67(2):295–302.

70. Radin EL, Martin RB, Burr DB, et al. Effects of mechanical loading on the tissues of the rabbit knee. *J Orthop Res.* 1984;2:221–234.

71. Young DR, Richardson DW, Markel MD, et al. Mechanical and morphometric analysis of the third carpal bone of thoroughbreds. *Am J Vet Res.* 1991;52(3):402–409.

72. Kawcak CE, McIlwraith CW, Norrdin RW, et al. The role of subchondral bone in joint disease: a review. *Equine Vet J.* 2001;33(2):120–126.

73. Kawcak CE, McIlwraith CW, Norrdin RW, et al. Clinical effects of exercise on subchondral bone of carpal and metacarpophalangeal joints in horses. *Am J Vet Res.* 2000;61(10):1252–1258.

74. Radin EL. The relationship between biological and mechanical factors in the etiology of osteoarthritis. *J Rheumatol.* 1983;10(suppl 9):20–21.

75. Radin EL, Burr DB, Caterson B, et al. Mechanical determinants of osteoarthritis. *Semin Arthritis Rheum.* 1991;21(3, suppl 2):12–21.

76. Thompson RC, Oegema TR, Lewis JL, et al. Osteoarthritis changes after transarticular load. *J Bone Joint Surg.* 1991;73(7):990–1001.

77. Norrdin RW, Kawcak CE, Capwell BA, et al. Subchondral bone failure in an equine model of overload arthrosis. *Bone.* 1998;22(2):133–139.

78. Norrdin RW, Kawcak CE, Capwell BA, et al. Calcified cartilage morphometry and its relation to subchondral bone remodeling in equine arthrosis. *Bone.* 1999;24(2):109–114.

Traumatic Arthritis and Posttraumatic Osteoarthritis in the Horse

C. Wayne McIlwraith

TRAUMATIC ARTHRITIS

In its broader sense, "traumatic arthritis" includes a diverse collection of pathologic and clinical states that develop after single or repetitive episodes of trauma. It may include one or all of the following:

1. Synovitis (inflammation of the synovial membrane)
2. Capsulitis (inflammation of the fibrous joint capsule)
3. Sprain (injury of specific ligaments associated with the joint)
4. Intraarticular fractures
5. Meniscal tears (femorotibial joints)
6. Osteoarthritis (OA) (when degradative changes have occurred in the articular cartilage)

Any one of the first five conditions above can potentially progress to OA. To facilitate discussion of pathobiology it is convenient to divide articular trauma into three entities:

Type I: Traumatic synovitis and capsulitis without obvious disturbance of the cartilage or destruction of major supporting structures. This includes acute synovitis and most sprains.

Type II: Disruptive trauma with damage to the articular cartilage or complete rupture of a major supporting structure. This includes severe sprains, meniscal tears, and intraarticular fractures.

Type III: Posttraumatic OA. This may be considered as a group of disorders characterized by a common end-stage in which progressive deterioration of the articular cartilage is accompanied by changes in the bone and soft tissues of the joint. It is inevitably the result of severe trauma to the joint or ineffective treatment of any of the predisposing conditions.

The joint is an organ and all tissues of this organ can be injured. There are a number of ways in which traumatic damage occurs to the joint organ, ultimately resulting in degradation of articular cartilage (Figure 3-1). Interestingly, this figure was initially developed by the author in 1996 and emphasized inflammation of the soft tissues (traumatic synovitis and capsulitis) as well as subchondral bone disease as important contributors to the osteoarthritic process. A review of human OA by two prominent researchers in 2007 noted that "current knowledge segregates the risk factors for development of OA into two fundamental mechanisms related either to the adverse effects of 'abnormal' loading on normal cartilage or of 'normal' loading on abnormal cartilage."[1] In the equine athlete, cyclic trauma to synovial membrane and fibrous joint capsule results in synovitis and capsulitis, and it is a common entity in the equine athlete. Direct trauma can occur to the articular cartilage and subchondral bone, whereas inflammatory mediators resulting from synovitis can cause biochemical damage. Intraarticular and extraarticular ligaments of the joint can be injured, as can the menisci in the stifle, resulting in tearing.

The reaction in the various joint-associated tissues should not be considered in isolation, as evidenced by the example of the carpus of a racehorse. Considerable damage may be inflicted directly to the articular cartilage and bone, resulting in cartilage ulceration and intraarticular fractures of the carpus that cause varying degrees of articular cartilage loss. However, cyclic fatigue damage to the collagen network could be an important step in the pathogenesis of a more insidious osteoarthritic entity, exposing chondrocytes to deleterious physical forces and inducing injury and metabolic changes. Primary damage to the subchondral bone other than fracture also may occur (subchondral bone disease) and lead to secondary damage to the articular cartilage, either from loss of support or secondarily from release of cytokines. Subchondral sclerosis may also lead to further physical damage to the articular cartilage because of decreased shock absorption. Acute synovitis and capsulitis are common problems in these same joints and may also contribute to the degenerative process by the release of deleterious mediators.[2]

In summary, when considering a traumatically injured joint, two basic pathobiologic processes should be considered: inflammation of the synovial membrane and fibrous joint capsule (synovitis and capsulitis), and physical and/or biochemical damage to the articular cartilage and bone.[2] Acute synovitis and capsulitis can cause significant clinical compromise and may also contribute to the posttraumatic degradative process by releasing enzymes, inflammatory mediators, and cytokines. These processes are outlined in Figures 3-1 and 3-2.

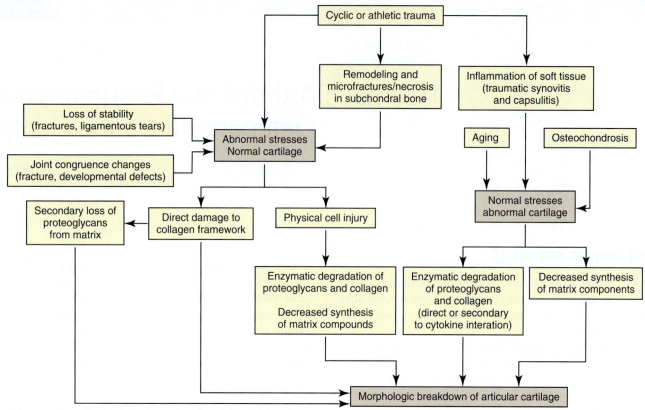

FIGURE 3-1 Possible pathways for degradation of articular cartilage secondary to joint trauma in the horse. (Reproduced with permission from McIlwraith C.W. (2005). Frank Milne lecture: from arthroscopy to gene therapy – 30 years of looking in joints. In: Proc Am Assoc Equine Pract, 51, 65-113.)

Osteoarthritis in the Horse

Spontaneous joint disease is a common clinical problem in the horse.[3] Surveys estimate that up to 60% of lameness is related to OA.[4] Koch and Betts have observed[5] that human OA is not a well-defined entity, in that pathologists define OA on a structural basis[6] and epidemiologists define OA based on pain.[7] The situation is similar in horses, where the clinical importance has been emphasized by a large U.S. Department of Agriculture survey of lameness in the horse (defined as an abnormality of gait such that the horse cannot be used for its intended purpose or could only be used if intervention [such as medication, corrective shoeing, or rest] was employed), which found that lameness was because of a joint problem in approximately 15% of cases.[8] On the structural side, however, a number of pathologic studies in the metacarpophalangeal joint (an important high-motion joint) of the horse have been published[9-11] and objective parameters of macroscopic and microscopic examination of clinical OA as well as experimental OA have been defined.[12]

Equine degenerative arthritis was first reported in 1938 and the pathological changes were compared with human OA.[13] Although examination of osteoarthritic joints was initially limited to morphologic observations,[13-17] equine OA received its first clinical attention by the American Association of Equine Practitioners in 1966, and its relationship with lameness and "use trauma" became a central etiologic concept.[18,19] By 1975 articular cartilage lesions were considered the indispensable criteria of OA, but it was also recognized that they may not be the centrally important cause of clinical disease. Today equine OA may be considered as a group of disorders characterized by a common end stage: progressive deterioration of the articular cartilage accompanied by changes in the bone and soft tissues of the joint.[19] This definition is simpler but comparable with one created for human OA at a workshop sponsored by the American Academy of Orthopaedic Surgeons, the National Institute of Arthritis, Musculoskeletal, and Skin Diseases, the National Institute on Aging, the Arthritis Foundation and the Orthopaedic Research and Education Foundation, where OA was redefined as "a group of overlapping distinct diseases which may have different etiologies, but with similar biologic, morphologic, and clinical outcomes."[20]

The OA disease processes do not only affect the articular cartilage but also involve the entire joint, including the subchondral bone, ligaments, capsule, synovial membrane, and periarticular tissues. Ultimately the articular cartilage degenerates with fibrillation, fissures, ulceration, and full thickness loss of the joint surface.[21,22] It has now been recognized that the equine OA disease process can start with disease in synovial membrane, fibrous joint capsule, subchondral bone, and ligaments as well as articular cartilage or a combination of the above.[19]

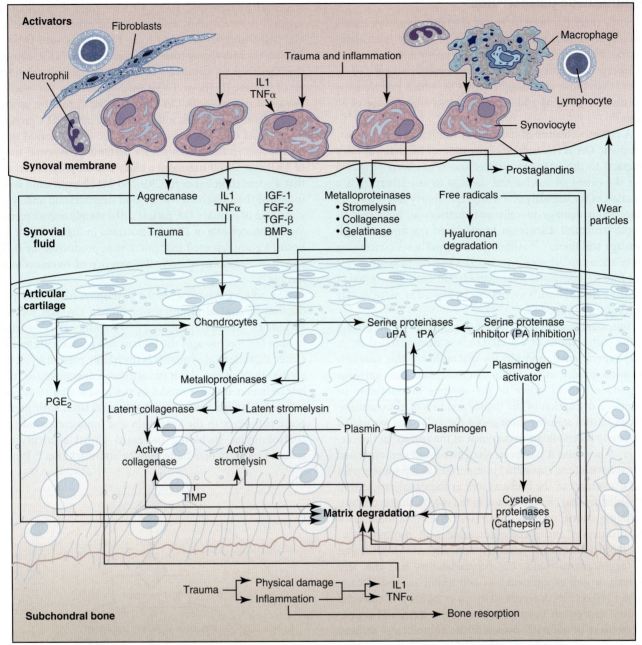

FIGURE 3-2 The factors involved in enzymatic degradation of articular cartilage matrix. Dotted lines indicate factors that may inhibit degradation. *BMPs*, bone morphogenetic proteins; *FGF-2*, fibroblast growth factor-2; *IGF-1*, insulin-like growth factor-1; *IL1*, interleukin-1; *TGF-β*, transforming growth factor-β; *PA*, plasminogen activator; *PG*, prostaglandin; *PLA₂*, phospholipase A2; *PGE₂*, prostaglandin E(2); *TIMP*, tissue inhibitor of metalloproteinases; *TNFα*, tumor necrosis factor-α; *tPA*, tissue plasminogen activator; *uPA*, urokinase plasminogen activator. (Reproduced with permission from McIlwraith CW (2005). Frank Milne lecture: from arthroscopy to gene therapy – 30 years of looking in joints. In: Proc Am Assoc Equine Pract, 51, 65-113.)

The metacarpophalangeal (MCP) joint is the most common joint for spontaneous OA in the racehorse, followed by the carpal joints. Both joints have close fitting articular surfaces that can quickly develop linear erosions and wear lines in association with osteochondral fragmentation. In the last 10 to 15 years, improvements in arthroscopic techniques and a higher competitive standard in Western performance equestrian events have resulted in recognition of a new spectrum of femorotibial traumatic disease and OA, which has much analogy to human OA of the knee. OA can occur early in equine athletes or later in older horses.[23-25] Arthroscopic grading systems have been used for osteochondral disease in high motion joints[26,27] and biomarkers related to macroscopic and histological cartilage lesions have been evaluated.[28,29]

Posttraumatic Osteoarthritis

Recently there has been increased attention to posttraumatic osteoarthritis (PTOA) in humans.[20,30,31] It has been demonstrated that early onset of OA can occur within 10 years of injury.[32] Patients with PTOA are much younger (18-44 years) than those with degenerative OA, which prevalence is increased with aging and is more evident after the age of 50 years.[30]

A common feature of joint injury leading to human posttraumatic OA is the sudden application of mechanical force (impact) to the articular surface, and it has been proposed that the extent of mechanical damage to any structure is a function of the intensity of the impact.[20] Injury and responses range from damage to cells and matrices without macroscopic structural disruption to displaced fractures through cartilage and bone.[33-35] Although the hypotheses concerning the relationship between joint injuries and the biologic events that lead to progressive joint degradation cannot be tested in human patients,[20] such events can be looked at more closely with equine OA models.

The significance of synovial membrane inflammation in the pathogenesis of equine OA was demonstrated in an early experimental model by the first author.[36] This induced-synovitis model using filipin demonstrated that cartilage degradation could occur in the absence of instability or traumatic disruption of the tissues and loss of glycosaminoglycan (GAG) staining throughout the ECM was associated with early morphologic breakdown of the surface of the cartilage. Since then it has been recognized and demonstrated that synovitis (and capsulitis) is important as it produces pain and discomfort in the horse as well as increased production of mediators that can contribute to the osteoarthritic process, including matrix metalloproteinases (MMPs), a member of the disintegrin and metalloproteinase with thrombospondin motif (ADAMTS) family, specifically ADAMTS-4 and -5 (aggrecanase-1 and -2), prostaglandins E2, and free radicals as well as interleukin-1 and tumor necrosis factor-alpha (TNFα).[37-44] A recent study on cytokine and catabolic enzyme expression in synovium, synovial fluid, and articular cartilage of naturally osteoarthritic equine carpi showed that TNFα was abundantly expressed in synovial membrane and cartilage, compared with interleukin-1beta (IL-1β) being overexpressed in OA cartilage but not to a significant extent in synovium.[45] Expression of ADAMTS-5 and MMP-13 was also significantly increased in synovial tissue and ADAMTS-4 and MMP-13 also were significantly expressed in OA cartilage. In summary acute synovitis and capsulitis is the most common problem in high-motion joints of the equine athlete and may contribute to the degradative process in articular cartilage by release of enzymes, inflammatory mediators, and cytokines (Figure 3-2).

The role of equine IL-1 in producing OA in the equine carpus was well demonstrated by total inhibition of OA production by gene therapy with interleukin-1 receptor antagonist (IL-1ra).[41,46] Interleukin-1beta (IL-1β) has also been called the master cytokine in human OA,[47] and although TNFα is thought to be the most prominent cytokine in the acute stages of human OA, IL-1β remains high throughout all stages.[48] A recent study evaluating gene expression in synovial tissue samples obtained from 12 patients with OA and 32 patients undergoing total knee replacement (TKR) showed that there was no significant difference in the expression levels of MMPs, IL-1β, or TNFα mRNA between the synovial tissues of patients with OA and TKR but C reactive protein (CRP) level was significantly increased in the OA group.[49] The authors concluded that because the study showed similar changes in the inflammatory patterns of synovial tissue of TKR and OA, it suggested a likely disease progression and that a correlation between CRP and MMP expression levels indicated their essential role in joint degeneration and synovial tissue of primary OA patients. The simple overall picture for the master role of IL-1 is illustrated in Figure 3-3. It has been recently reported that low innate production of IL-1β and IL-6 is associated with the absence of human OA in old age.[50]

The role of synovitis in the pathophysiology and production of clinical symptoms of human OA was recently reviewed.[51] Gradual emergence of recognition of synovitis in human OA has brought the human and equine entities into closer alignment as synovitis is invariably present in all OA entities in the horse.[19,44] It has also been demonstrated in an intraarticular fracture model in the mouse that increasing intraarticular fracture severity was associated with greater acute pathology in the synovium and bone compared with control limbs, including increased global synovitis and reduced periarticular bone density and thickness.[52] Proper

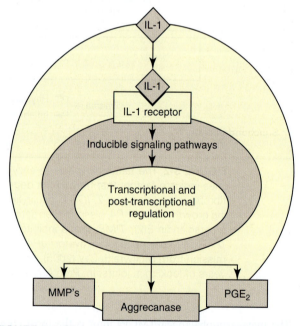

FIGURE 3-3 Diagram of interleukin-1 (IL-1) activating matrix metalloproteinases (MMPs), aggrecanase and prostaglandin E2 (PGE2) release acting through IL-1 receptors on the cell membrane. (Reproduced with permission from McIlwraith C.W. (2005). Frank Milne lecture: from arthroscopy to gene therapy – 30 years of looking in joints. In: Proc Am Assoc Equine Pract, 51, 65-113.)

balance of anabolic and catabolic activities is crucial for the maintenance of cartilage integrity and for the repair of molecular damage sustained during daily use[19,53] (Figure 3-4). Recognition that the balance of anabolic and catabolic activities is compromised in OA has led to various therapeutic efforts to promote anabolism and inhibit catabolism. Although the anticatabolic effects of equine IL-1ra gene therapy[46,41] has clearly demonstrated its ability to prevent or decrease the development of equine OA, another study also demonstrated that repair of articular defects could be enhanced by the combination of IL-1ra and IGF-1 gene therapy.[54]

Athletic Activity Potentially Leading to a Pathologic Process

It is well accepted that equine athletes carry an increased risk for development of OA. It should be noted that intact articular cartilage possesses optimal load-bearing characteristics that adjust to the level of activity. Increasing weight-bearing activity in athletes and adolescents has been shown to improve the volume and thickness of articular cartilage[55] and increased cartilage glycosaminoglycan content in the human knee.[56] In the healthy human athlete, a positive linear dose response relationship apparently exists for repetitive loading activities and articular cartilage function.[57] However, studies also indicate that the dose-response curve reaches a threshold and activity beyond this threshold can result in maladjustment and injury of articular cartilage.[58]

High-impact joint loading above this threshold has been shown to decrease cartilage proteoglycan content, increase levels of degradative enzymes, and cause chondrocyte apoptosis.[59,60] If the integrity of the functional weight-bearing unit is lost, either through acute injury or chronic trauma in the high-impact athlete, a chondropenic response is initiated that can include loss of articular cartilage volume and stiffness, elevation of contact pressures, and development or progression of articular cartilage defects.[57] It has been proposed that concomitant factors such as ligamentous instability, malalignment, meniscal injury, or deficiency can further

support progression of the chondropenic cascade and that without intervention chondropenia leads to progressive deterioration of articular cartilage function and may ultimately progress to OA.

Evidence has accumulated with regard to various inflammatory mediators having an impact on matrix homeostasis of articular chondrocytes by altering their metabolism.[61] A recent study on inflammatory factors involved in human OA cited evidence that points to the proinflammatory cytokine IL-1β as the most important factor responsible for the catabolism in OA.[61] However, the authors pointed out that new members of the IL-1 super family have recently been identified (ILF-5, ILF-10), some of which may be of interest for arthritic disease, and that other proinflammatory cytokines such as TNFα-6 and other interleukins can be contributing factors. They also noted that the exact role and importance of each within the OA process is not yet clearly identified. In addition to cytokines, other inflammatory mediators that may play a major role in the OA process include nitric oxide (NO), eicosanoids (prostaglandins and leukotrienes), and a newly identified cell membrane receptor family, the proteases-activated receptors (PARs).

Discussion of mediators for equine traumatic joint disease and OA in this chapter focuses on mediators that have been shown to be increased in equine joint disease and/or of which inhibition can ameliorate progression of OA.

When considering a traumatically injured joint, two basic pathobiologic processes should be considered: inflammation of the synovial membrane and fibrous joint capsule (synovitis and capsulitis), and physical or biochemical damage to the articular cartilage and bone. Acute synovitis and capsulitis can cause significant clinical compromise and may also contribute to the degenerative process by releasing enzymes, inflammatory mediators, and cytokines.[19] These processes are outlined in Figures 3-1 and 3-2.

Anabolic/Catabolic Balance and Pathogenesis of Osteoarthritis

In healthy cartilage there is a low turnover of extracellular matrix molecules, and proper balance of anabolic and catabolic activities is crucial for maintenance of cartilage tissue integrity and for the repair of molecular damages sustained during daily usage (Figure 3-4). In OA this balance is compromised and degradation predominates over the capacity for repair. It has been proposed that effects of abnormal mechanical loading in synovial inflammation likely contribute to dysregulation of chondrocyte function favoring disequilibrium between the catabolic and anabolic activities of the chondrocyte in remodeling the cartilage extracellular matrix.[1] Local loss of proteoglycans and cleavage of type II collagen occur initially at the cartilage surface where there has been a compensatory increase in type II collagen synthesis in deeper regions of the articular cartilage, signifying increased changes in both anabolism and catabolism.[1] Various anabolic and catabolic factors have been reviewed in identifying molecular targets for therapy.[53] Details of these various factors as they apply to the horse are reviewed below.

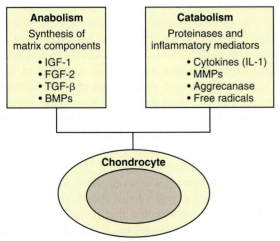

FIGURE 3-4 Homeostasis in articular cartilage related to balance between catabolic and anabolic factors.

The Importance of Synovitis

Synovitis (and capsulitis) is important to the horse because it produces pain, the increased synovial effusion is uncomfortable, it eliminates the normal small negative pressure within the joint (therefore promoting micro-instability), and it produces products that are deleterious to joint health as a whole and articular cartilage in particular. The mediators currently considered to be of significance in equine joint disease include metalloproteinases and aggrecanases, prostaglandins, free radicals, cytokines, IL-1, and possibly TNFα (Figure 3-2). As mentioned previously, human OA was long considered a "wear and tear" disease leading to loss of cartilage and previously OA was considered the sole consequence of any process leading to increased pressure on a joint (e.g., overload or anatomical joint in congruency) or fragility of cartilage matrix (genetic alterations of matrix components).[62] Apparently this paradigm was based on the observation that chondrocytes had low metabolic activity and no ability to repair cartilage and once damaged could not respond by the usual inflammatory response. This paradigm has been modified by molecular biology and the discovery that many soluble mediators such as cytokines and prostaglandins can increase the production of MMPs by chondrocytes, leading to the first steps of an "inflammatory" theory. It was noted in 2013 that it took a decade before synovitis was accepted as a critical feature of OA and more recently some studies have enhanced the idea of synovitis being a driver of the OA process (this has been considered an important process for a long time in the horse). In addition, more recent experimental data have shown that subchondral bone has a substantial role in the OA process as a mechanical damper as well as a source of inflammatory mediators implicated in the OA process and in the degradation of the deeper layers of cartilage.[62] Human OA is now considered a more complex disease with inflammatory mediators released by cartilage, bone, and synovium and the source and types of inflammatory mediators may also differ by OA phenotype.[63] Most recently, it has been proposed that OA has a considerable hereditary component and that genetic mutations associated with OA can be placed on a continuum.[64] It is proposed that early-onset OA is caused by mutations in matrix molecules often associated with chondrodysplasias; whereas, less destructive abnormalities or mutations confer increased susceptibility to injury or malalignment that can result in middle age onset. Finally, mutations in molecules that regulate subtle aspects of joint development and structure lead to late-onset OA.[64]

Matrix Metalloproteinases and Aggrecanases

MMPs are a group of zinc-dependent endopeptidate enzymes involved in extracellular matrix degradation and collectively are able to degrade all components of extracellular matrix. Though expression of MMPs contributes to tissue remodeling and turnover in healthy articular cartilage, in the development of OA proinflammatory cytokines such as IL-1β bind their respective cell receptors in chondrocytes and activate signaling pathways that involve the transcription factors NF-κB and activating protein-1 (AP-1) resulting in the upregulation of the expression of MMPs.[53] Three collagenases have been identified and they are interstitial or tissue collagenase (also called MMP-1), polymorphonuclear cells (PMN) collagenase (or MMP-8), and collagenase 3 (also known as MMP-13). Based on evidence in both human and equine studies it appears that the primary collagenase involved in the degradation of type II collagen of articular cartilage is collagenase 3 (MMP-13).[65,66] Caron et al.[65] found that MMP-13 is produced by equine chondrocytes and that MMP-13 expression is significantly stimulated by rhIL-1.

It is now generally accepted that loss of aggrecan from articular cartilage is a proteolytic process driven predominantly by aggrecanases-1 and -2 (also known as ADAMTS-4 and -5).[67-69] It has been demonstrated in mice that blocking aggrecanase cleavage in the aggrecan interglobular domain aggravates cartilage erosion and promotes cartilage repair.[68] In human OA it is still not clear whether ADAMTS-4 or -5 has the major aggrecanase-degrading activity, and differences between species have been noted.[67] MMP-3 has a wide variety of substrates, including proteoglycans (aggrecan, decorin, fibromodulin, link protein) and type IV, V, VII, IX, and XI collagen. It also cleaves type II collagen in nonhelical sites.[70] An in vitro study of IL-1-induced cartilage degeneration has revealed evidence of collagen degradation that could be attributed to MMP-3 in addition to that attributed to collagenase.[71] Molecular cloning and cartilage gene expression of equine stromelysin 1 (MMP-3) have been described.[37] MMP-3 cleaves the protein backbone of cartilage proteoglycans at the asparagine 341-phenylalanine 342 bond. Cleavage caused by aggrecanase has been classically reported as occurring at the GLU373-ALA374 bond and the ITEGE[37] neoepitope has been used to confirm this location. However, ADAMTS-4 and -5 have been shown to preferentially cleave aggrecan in the CS-2 domain, but blocking of cleavage at the 373-374 location not only diminished aggrecan loss and cartilage erosion in surgically induced OA but also appeared to stimulate cartilage repair following acute inflammation.[68]

Based on preliminary work in the horse using markers that differentiate these two cleavage sites, it appears that aggrecanase is the principal enzyme degrading aggrecan in equine joint disease (Little & McIlwraith, unpublished data, 2004). The relative roles of ADAMTS-4 and -5 in equine cartilage degradation are still open. Knockdown of gene expression of both ADAMTS-4 and ADAMTS-5 in human cartilage explants results in reduction of aggrecan depletion, indicating that both enzymes are involved in the loss of extracellular matrix in degenerative cartilage diseases.[69] Regulation of both ADAMTS-4 and ADAMTS-5 in human cartilage after IL-1 stimulation has also been reported.[72] In human OA both ADAMTS-4 and -5 are expressed and ADAMTS-4 is regulated by IL-1 and TNFα.[73] Studies also suggest that in human synovial cells both ADAMTS-4 and -5 are constitutively expressed and that IL-1 does not regulate ADAMTS-5 expression but that IL-1, TNFα and TGF-β regulate ADAMTS-4 expression.[53] Besides inhibition of MMP activity TIMP-3 is a potent inhibitor of ADAMTS-4 and -5 activity[74].

Equine MMPs 2 and 9 are two gelatinases that have been characterized in the horse.[38,39] It is known that the one-fourth and three-fourths fragments generated by cleavage of fibrin or collagens by collagenases can unwind and are then susceptible to further cleavage by MMP-2 and MMP-9. MMPs 2 and 9 are produced by a variety of equine cell types, and these enzymes have been demonstrated in elevated levels in synovial fluids from horses with joint disease.[38,39]

The metalloproteinases are inhibited by two tissue inhibitors of metalloproteinase and these are known commonly as TIMP (TIMP-1 and TIMP-2).[75,76] TIMP is found in many connective tissues and may be the most important inhibitor found in articular cartilage. The current belief is that the balance between MMPs and TIMP is important to prevent progression of articular cartilage degradation.

In summary, MMPs are considered to play a major role in articular cartilage degradation. They are secreted as latent proenzymes and activated extracellularly by serine proteinases. Plasmin may activate stromelysin, which in turn is an important activator of collagenase. Upregulation of these enzymes in synovial membrane and articular cartilage samples from traumatic equine joint disease has been demonstrated.[44] It is also known that the production of MMPs is upregulated by IL-1.

Studies of the ability of generalized inhibition of MMPs with MMP inhibitors have shown mediocre results and side effects. The identification of new aggrecanase inhibitors has been reviewed elsewhere.[77]

Prostaglandins

Prostaglandins (primarily E group) are produced in inflamed joints and can cause a decrease in the proteoglycan content of the cartilage matrix.[43] The presence of prostaglandin E2 (PGE2) in synovial fluid from inflamed joints has been demonstrated in the horse. Prostaglandin E2 is considered one of the main mediators of inflammation and pain in OA.[78] The production of PGE2 requires two enzymes, cycloogenase-2 (COX-2) and prostaglandin E synthase, both of which are induced by IL-1β.

Interestingly, blocking PGE2 potentiates the antianabolic effect of IL-1β.[1,79] Nonsteroidal antiinflammatory drugs (NSAIDs) act by inhibiting COX-2, and this action would relieve pain but is not considered to ameliorate cartilage loss in persons with OA.[53] It is therefore unclear whether suppression of prostaglandin synthesis by COX inhibition is beneficial to humans, but there is some evidence in the horse that topical NSAIDs can improve the status of articular cartilage.[80] In the author's laboratory at Colorado State University, PGE2 measurements are used as an objective index of the level of synovitis.[42,81] Actions of PGE2 in joints include vasodilation, enhancement of pain perception, and proteoglycan depletion from cartilage (by both degradation and inhibition of synthesis), bone demineralization, and promotion of plasminogen activator secretion. PGE2 is released from chondrocytes on stimulation of these cells by IL-1 and TNFα.

Oxygen-Derived Free Radicals

Oxygen-derived free radicals, including superoxide anion, hydroxyl radicals, and hydrogen peroxide, may be released from injured joint tissues. Studies have demonstrated cleavage of hyaluronic acid by free radicals.[82,83] There is also evidence that superoxide can degrade the alpha chains of collagen based on the finding that superoxide treatment inhibits its gelatin.[84] Proteoglycans may be cleaved by free radicals.[84] Increased free radicals in the synovial fluid of cases of equine joint disease have also been demonstrated.[40] Mechanical injury has been associated with an increase in production of reactive oxygen species (ROS) and decreased antioxidant capacity. NO upregulates the NF-κB pathway. Excessive free radical production has been reported in human patients with posttraumatic arthritis.[85]

More recently, nitric oxide, another free radical, has been shown to be produced by osteoarthritic chondrocytes[86] and that overexpression of inducible nitric oxide synthase (iNOS) in osteoarthritic chondrocytes results in an excess of NO.[87] iNOS is induced by both mechanical factors and inflammatory cytokines such as IL-1β and TNFα and inhibition of IL-1β can reduce NO production.[53] In addition, NO is an inductor of chondrocyte apoptosis and excess amounts produce both chondrocyte death and matrix degradation.[30]

Cytokines and Articular Cartilage Degradation

Cytokines are soluble peptides produced by one cell affecting the activity of other cell types. Early studies of cytokines in joint tissues suggest that IL-1 and TNFα modulate the synthesis of metalloproteinases by both chondrocytes and synovial cells[88-90] and are therefore important mediators in joint disease. Normal turnover of the extracellular matrix of the articular cartilage is likely regulated by the chondrocytes under the control and influence of cytokines and mechanical stimuli. Articular cartilage degradation in association with disease represents an exacerbation of these normal processes. It is widely accepted that the cytokine IL-1 induces proteoglycan depletion in articular cartilage by either increasing the rate of degradation or decreasing synthesis in association with the release of MMPs, aggrecanases and PGE2 from chondrocytes (Figure 3-3). The IL-1 system consists of the two agonist members, IL-1α and IL-1β, and these evoke signal production in response to binding IL-1R transmembrane receptors to induce downstream effects (see Figure 3-3). The presence of IL-1 in equine osteoarthritic joints was first reported by Morris et al.[91] An equine IL-1-containing extract was produced by May and colleagues in 1990.[92]

The significant role of equine IL-1 has been further consolidated, starting with construction of the cDNA sequences for IL-1α and IL-1β.[92] After generation of these DNA sequences, the IL-1α and IL-1β recombinant proteins were purified. Before that, only human recombinant IL-1 protein was available. Using equine articular cartilage explants, significant proteoglycan release was induced by both rEq-IL-1α and rEq-IL-1β at concentrations greater than or equal to 0.01 ng/mL with 38% to 76% and 88% to 90% of total glycosaminoglycan released by 4 and 6 days, respectively.[43] Significant inhibition of proteoglycan synthesis (42% to 64%) was observed at IL-1 concentrations greater than or equal to 0.01 ng/mL at 2 and 4 days. Increased PGE2 concentrations were observed at IL-1 concentrations greater than or equal to 1.0 ng/mL at 2 and 4 days. This work showed that the much lower concentrations of equine IL-1 could cause these effects compared with previously reported studies using human recombinant IL-1.[43] The significant role of IL-1 in the pathogenesis of cartilage degradation in the horse was best demonstrated by Frisbie et al. (2002)[41] with IL-1ra using gene therapy. This study demonstrated that if IL-1 can be inhibited, articular cartilage degradation in experimental OA can essentially be stopped. As mentioned previously, the simple overall picture for the master role of IL-1 is illustrated in Figure 3-3.

The role of TNFα in equine OA is less certain. Induction of intraarticular TNF was first demonstrated as part of an acute inflammatory response in equine arthritis.[93] It appears that IL-1 is the principal cytokine responsible for articular cartilage degradation and that TNFα contributes more to clinical morbidity and pain. IL-1 and TNFα have been demonstrated using RT-PCR in the synovial membrane of inflamed equine joints,[44] and increased serum concentrations of soluble TNF receptors (S TNF-r) have been detected in human patients with RA and OA in comparison to healthy controls.[94] A minireview of the role of cytokines as inflammatory mediators in OA concluded that it is generally accepted that IL-1 is the pivotal cytokine in early and late stages of OA, although TNFα is involved primarily in the onset of arthritis.[79] Both receptors of TNF have been identified in synovial tissue, with greater numbers seen in joints affected by RA in comparison to OA.[95]

Growth Factors

Transforming Growth Factor Beta

Transforming growth factor beta (TGF-β) promotes the expression of collagen type II and aggrecan and downregulates matrix-degradating enzymes, thus counteracting IL-β-induced cartilage matrix degradation.[53] The effect of TGF-β is reduced with aging and may be responsible for the higher level of cartilage degradation in aged cartilage in humans. Bone morphogenetic proteins (BMPs) are members of the TFG-β super family of signaling proteins and are involved in many developmental and physiologic properties. BMP-2 is upregulated in OA chondrocytes by the inflammatory cytokines IL-1β and TNFα, but BMP-7 is downregulated in osteoarthritic chondrocytes and has a positive effect on matrix biosynthesis. Experimental evidence in the horse suggests that BMP-7 has stronger antidegradative effects than BMP-2.[96] The activities in vivo are regulated by BMP antagonists and expression of the BMP antagonists gremlin and follistatin is regulated during OA reflecting a complex control system.[53] Insulin-like growth factor 1 (IGF-1) has a crucial role in cartilage homeostasis, stimulating extracellular matrix production and inhibiting matrix degradation. The anabolic effects of IGF-1 are likely involved in the response of osteoarthritic chondrocytes to inflammatory signals and there is evidence that IGF-1 protects cartilage against IL-1β-induced catabolic effects by upregulation of the IL-1 decoy receptor IL-1RII.[97]

Basic fibroblast growth factor (bFGF), also referred to as FGF-2, and FGF-18 have been studied in OA. The effects of FGF-2 are mixed but FGF-18 has demonstrated distinct anabolic effects on extracellular matrix biosynthesis.[62] A possible mechanism to explain the differential effects of FGF-2 and FGF-18 is the suppression of the BMP antagonist noggin by FGF-18.[98]

Transcription Factors and Regulatory Pathways

NF-κB signaling has been mentioned previously and plays a central role in the catabolic processes in articular cartilage. NF-κB is activated by both IL-1β and TNFα in chondrocytes and suppresses SOX9 expression, thus downregulating cartilage extracellular matrix protein such as type II collagen. Most MMPs are regulated transcriptionally and contain AP-1 binding sites. AP-1 is a transcription factor that is activated by growth factors and cytokines. NF-κB is also a positive regulator of the expression of proinflammatory cytokines such as TNFα, IL-1β, and IL-6. The growth factors IGF-1 and TGF-β act, at least in part, by induction of SOX-9.[53] SOX-9 is a key regulator of a mesenchymal chondrogenesis during embryonic development and enhances expression of cartilage-specific genes collagen type II and aggrecan.

The actions of the various regulatory factors in cartilage homeostasis are further complicated by the interactive signaling pathways and must be considered when evaluating therapeutic targets as untoward side effects could result. BMP-7 counteracts IL-1β-induced MMP-13 expression, but BMP-2 cannot counteract the negative effects of IL-1β.[53] TGF-β counteracts IL-1β-induced suppression of proteoglycan biosynthesis in chondrocytes and IGF-1 upregulates IL-1 decoy receptor IL-RII that binds IL-1β and therefore inhibits this signaling pathway. IGF-1 also inhibits IL-1β-induced MMP-13 expression.

Primary Disease of Subchondral Bone

In addition to synovial mediated degradation of articular cartilage and direct mechanical damage, the subchondral bone can play a primary role in disease development (Figure 3-5).[99]

Among possible pathways for mechanical destruction of articular cartilage in human OA, it has been suggested that early subchondral bone sclerosis causes a reduction in the joint's shock-absorbing ability and thereby places cartilage at risk of shear-induced tensile failure of cartilage cross-links, particularly under repetitive impulsive loading conditions.[100] However, further work on the relationship between bone and cartilage has revealed complex and sometimes contradictory changes in subchondral bone associated with OA in humans and experimental models.[101] Work in the author's laboratory[102] has demonstrated that when horses are subjected to athletic exercise on the treadmill, microdamage in the subchondral bone can develop early. On postmortem examination of racehorse joints (euthanized for catastrophic injuries in another limb), the range of microdamage includes not only microfractures but also primary osteocyte death. It is thought that not only is the mechanical support of the articular cartilage lost when subchondral bone microdamage progresses

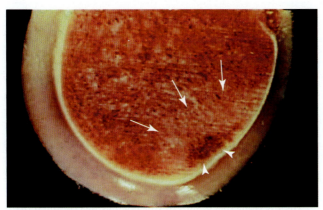

FIGURE 3-5 Postmortem sample of a distal metacarpus from the leg opposite to that suffering a catastrophic injury in a racehorse. Although there is intact articular cartilage, subchondral bone necrosis (arrowheads) and sclerosis (arrows) can be seen. (Reproduced with permission from Norrdin R.W., Kawcak C.E., Capwell B.A., et al. (1998). Subchondral bone failure in an equine model of overload arthrosis. Bone, 22(2), 133-139.)

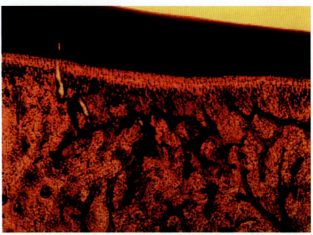

FIGURE 3-6 Histologic view of a section of articular cartilage and subchondral bone bulk-stained with basic fuchsin depicting microdamage with microcrack formation in the subchondral bone. (Reproduced from C.E. Kawcak with permission from McIlwraith C.W. (2005). Frank Milne lecture: from arthroscopy to gene therapy – 30 years of looking in joints. In: Proc Am Assoc Equine Pract, 51, 65-113.)

to macrodamage, but that cytokine release from the bone can also potentially influence the state of the articular cartilage.[23,99,102] Figure 3-5 illustrates a specimen from a horse euthanized because of catastrophic injury in the other limb. An incidental finding at postmortem was the presence of subchondral bone necrosis, with a peripheral area of sclerosis and intact cartilage in the distal palmar area of the metacarpus. Figure 3-6 shows microdamage that can occur quite early in association with exercise.

Gross examination of metacarpo/metatarsophalangeal joints from racehorses revealed defects on the condylar surface that ranged from cartilage fibrillation and erosion to focal cartilage indentation and cavitation in subchondral bone. These lesions represented a spectrum of mechanically induced arthrosis in which microdamage is thought to play a role.[99] Lesions in the subchondral bone ranged from thickening of subchondral bone and underlying trabeculae, advancing sclerosis with increasing amounts of osteocyte necrosis, vascular channels with plugs of matrix debris, and osteoclastic remodeling. Apparent fragmentation lines in the subchondral bone suggested increased matrix fragility. Trabecular microfractures developed at a depth of a few millimeters, with increased vascularity with hemorrhage, fibrin, and fibroplasia seen in the marrow spaces at the more advanced stage. The articular cartilage in most of these instances was variously indented but remained largely viable, with degeneration and erosion limited to the superficial layers. Focally, breaks in the calcified layer appeared to lead to collages and cartilage in-folding. In metacarpal condyles from experimental horses run on a treadmill,[23] the change in the metacarpal condyles was milder. The significance of osteochondral injury in joint disease has also been previously reviewed by Riggs.[103]

In addition to its role in contributing to OA, the presence of subchondral bone injury contributing to complete failure of the subchondral bone and fractures is important.[104] "Impact

fracture" is a term that has been used recently to describe a pathologic fracture that shows up as an area of lucency in the bone.[105] Pathologic change in the distal condyles of the third metacarpal and third metatarsal bones of the horse as a predisposing factor for condylar fractures was first investigated in detail by Riggs et al.[25,106,107] Recognition of this change potentially leading to fractures has led to investigations of imaging techniques to diagnose this at an early stage.[9]

Lubrication and Changes with Traumatic Joint Disease—Significance?

In synovial joints, articular cartilage bears load and moves relative to opposing tissue surfaces, with friction and wear reduced through various mechanisms, including boundary lubrication. In healthy joints synovial fluid (SF) is present between articulating cartilage surfaces, functioning as effective boundary lubrication.[108] During cartilage articulation, both interstitial fluid pressurization and boundary mode lubrication may ameliorate friction between articulating surfaces. In boundary lubrication, load is supported by surface-to-surface contact and friction between articular surfaces is thus dictated by bound surface lubricant molecules, which may become increasingly important with prolonged loading as interstitial fluid pressure diminishes.[109] Lubrication of articular cartilage is mediated by SF components and normal SF contains the molecules hyaluronan (HA), proteoglycan 4 (PRG4) (also known as lubricin, superficial zone protein, and megakaryocyte-stimulating factor) and surface-active phospholipids.[110]

Previous studies have shown that alteration of the friction-lowering function of SF may contribute to the deterioration of articular cartilage in joint disease and after joint injury in the horse.[108,110] In studies looking at the kinetic friction coefficient ($\mu_{kinetic}$) of equine SF from joints with acute injury, chronic injury, and controls, SF from joints with acute injury had higher $\mu_{kinetic}$ (39%) compared with normal equine SF; they also had a lower HA concentration (approximately 30%), higher PRG4 concentrations (+38%), and higher surface-active phospholipid (SAPL) concentrations. Equine SF from joints with chronic injury had $\mu_{kinetic}$, PRG4, and SAPL characteristics intermediate to those of equine SF from joints with acute injury and normal equine SF.[110] Regression analysis revealed that the $\mu_{kinetic}$ value decreased with increasing HA concentration. The addition of high-molecular-weight HA to equine SF from joints with acute injury reduced the $\mu_{kinetic}$ to a value near that of normal SF, which supports that a lubrication deficiency after acute injury could be a factor in the pathogenesis of articular cartilage disease. In the later chronic stage after injury, the boundary lubrication function of SF appears to be partially recovered, possibly caused by restoration and normalization of HA, PRG4, and SAPL concentrations and articular cartilage may be vulnerable when boundary lubrication is deficient in the acute stage of injury and during this time, addition of lubricant molecules to SF may restore its lubrication and function. Further in vivo work is needed to clarify this role.

The Pathways to Morphologic Breakdown of Articular Cartilage—the Critical Manifestation of OA

Trauma can cause an immediate physical defect or initiate a degradative process by direct damage to chondrocytes, causing release of enzymes as well as cytokine-initiated release of MMPs, aggrecanases, and PGE2 from chondrocytes in response to IL-1. As outlined in Figure 3-1, any instability in a joint can lead to damage of normal cartilage. On the other hand, cartilage compromised by loss of aggrecan (and component glycosaminoglycans) or collagen is vulnerable to normal forces. As has been previously discussed, as cartilage is compressed, the collapse of the collagen network is countered by the resistance offered by the proteoglycan gel. The precise nature of the forces exerted through the network are complex and related both to mechanical entrapment and chemical bonding effects between the fibers and the proteoglycans.[111] The same author has addressed the general problem of abnormal softening in articular cartilage with simultaneous micromechanical testing, interference-light microscopy, and transmission electron microscopy. A model has been developed in which this abnormal softening in articular cartilage is related to the presence of collagen fibers strongly aligned in a radial direction and this structure, having lost its three-dimensional character, would have limited ability to contain the swelling proteoglycan aggregates remaining in the tissue and would therefore reflect a state of softening in articular cartilage.[111]

The most common reason for degradation of articular cartilage and the development of OA is generally synovitis and capsulitis (but as discussed previously, pathologic processes in other soft tissues and subchondral bone are important contributors). With synovitis and capsulitis, there is a progression beginning with acute synovitis, when biochemical change can take place in the articular cartilage, but there is

no morphologic change. With critical loss of matrical components, however, morphologic damage ensues, going through a cycle of chondromalacia with softening of the cartilage and swelling caused by loss of GAG and absorption of water, followed by superficial fibrillation, fibrillation down to the middle zone of cartilage, and lastly fibrillation progressing through the deeper layer of cartilage, which then allows for loss of articular cartilage components and full-thickness erosion. Figure 3-7 illustrates four stages of OA in which there is a progression from acute to chronic synovitis and capsulitis and corresponding progressive change in articular cartilage degradation and loss.

The previous discussion in this chapter has outlined principal pathobiologic processes that are known to occur with traumatic arthritis and traumatic OA in the horse. This leads to identification of a number of targets, and treatments addressing some or all of these targets will be presented in Chapters 7 through 14, covering the principal treatment options, and Chapters 15 through 21, where specific therapies based on region will be detailed.

Articular Cartilage Repair

This chapter has focused on the pathobiology of OA and targets for therapeutic intervention to counteract OA development. When the severity of the disease or lack of response to treatment has resulted in full-thickness articular cartilage defects, however, a new therapeutic challenge is presented: repairing these defects. This section summarizes factors known to play a role in normal cartilage repair.

Healing refers to restoration of the structural integrity and function of the tissue after injury or disease, but repair usually has a more restricted meaning.[112] Repair refers to the replacement of damaged or lost cells and matrix with new cells and matrix, a process that does not necessarily restore the original structure or function of a tissue. Regeneration may be considered a special form of repair in which the cells replace lost or damaged tissue with a tissue identical to the original. It has been suggested that with the exception of bone fractures, most injuries and diseases of the musculoskeletal tissues do not stimulate regeneration of the original tissue.[112]

The limited potential of articular cartilage for regeneration and healing has been appreciated for more than 2 centuries. In 1743, Hunter stated, "If we consult the standard Chirurgical. Writers from *Hippocrates* down to the present Age, we shall find, that an ulcerated Cartilage is universally allowed to be a very troublesome Disease; that it admits of a Cure with more Difficulty than a carious Bone; and that, when destroyed, it is not recovered."[113] (Figure 3-8.) There is a limited response of cartilage to tissue damage and an inability of natural repair responses from adjacent tissues to produce tissue with the morphologic, biochemical, and biomechanical properties of articular cartilage.

The major limiting factor in the successful rehabilitation of any joint after injury or disease is the failure of osteochondral defects to heal.[114] Three mechanisms have been recognized as possible contributors to articular cartilage repair. Intrinsic

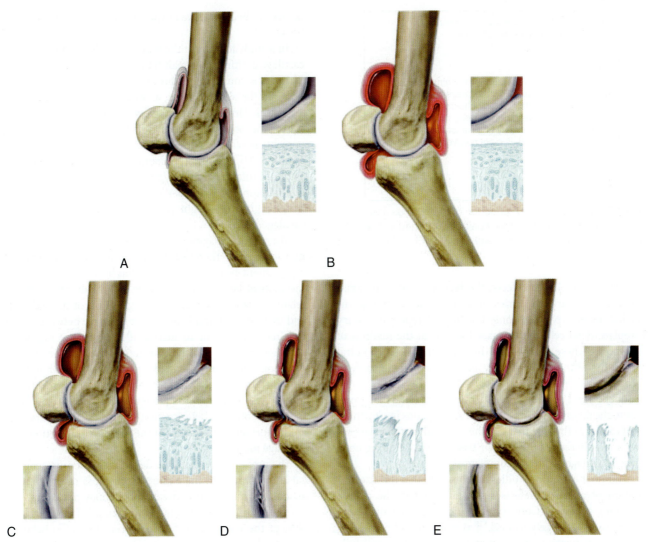

A   B

C   D   E

FIGURE 3-7 Diagrammatic series of development of osteoarthritis in a fetlock joint associated with cyclic trauma and traumatic synovitis and capsulitis. **A,** Diagram of a normal joint, as well as macroscopic and microscopic views of articular cartilage. **B,** Stage 1 acute synovitis without morphologic change in the articular cartilage. **C,** Stage 2 with synovitis persisting and early development of superficial fibrillation in the articular cartilage. **D,** Stage 3 synovitis and capsulitis becoming chronic, and articular cartilage fibrillation down into the deep zone of articular cartilage. **E,** Stage 4 development of full-thickness erosions in the articular cartilage that are visible macroscopically and microscopically. Joint capsule change is chronic with fibrosis, but some degree of active synovitis is still present. (Reproduced with permission from McIlwraith CW (2011). Joint injuries and disease and osteoarthritis. In: Baxter GM (Ed). Adams and Stashak's lameness in horses (6th ed) pp. 871-889. Wiley.)

repair (from within the cartilage) relies on the limited mitotic capability of the chondrocyte and a somewhat ineffective increase in collagen and proteoglycan production. Extrinsic repair comes from mesenchymal elements from the subchondral bone participating in the formation of new connective tissue that may undergo some metaplastic change to form cartilage elements. The third phenomenon, known as matrix flow, may contribute to equine articular cartilage repair by forming lips of cartilage from the perimeter of the lesion that migrate toward the center of the defect.[115,116]

The depth of the injury (full or partial thickness), size of defect, location and relation to weight-bearing or non-weight-bearing areas, and age of the animal influence the repair and remodeling of an injured joint surface.[117-119]

With a partial-thickness defect, some repair occurs with increased GAG synthesis and increased collagen synthesis.[119] However, the repair process is never completely effective. In humans, complete repair of chondromalacia of the patella has been reported to occur if matrical depletion and surface breakdown is minimal.[120] However, more recent work with arthroscopic débridement of partial-thickness defects in humans questions any actual regeneration.[121] In addition, superficial defects are not necessarily progressive and do not necessarily compromise joint function.

> *On the Structure and Diseases of Articulating Cartilages, by William Hunter, Surgeon.*
>
> If we consult the standard Chirurgical Writers from *Hippocrates* down to the present Age, we shall find, that an ulcerated Cartilage is universally allowed to be a very troublesome Disease; that it admits of a Cure with more Difficulty than a carious Bone; and that, when destroyed, it is not recovered.
>
> Read June 2.
> 1743.

FIGURE 3-8 Facsimile reproduction of the famous statement by William Hunter on cartilage repair as published in the Philosophical Transactions of the Royal Society of London in 1743.

With full-thickness defects, the response from the adjacent articular cartilage varies little from that after superficial lesions and provides only the limited repair necessary to replace dead cells and damaged matrix at the margins of the wound. These defects heal by ingrowth of subchondral fibrous tissue that may or may not undergo metaplasia to fibrocartilage.[116,118,122-125]

Subchondral bone defects either heal with bone that grows up into the defect or fill in with fibrocartilaginous ingrowth.[125] Duplication of the tide mark in the calcified cartilage layer is rare, and adherence of the repair tissue to surrounding non-injured cartilage is often incomplete.[122,123]

A number of equine studies demonstrate that the size and location of articular defects significantly affect the degree of healing achieved. Convery et al. first reported that large defects were less likely to heal.[118] A more recent study distinguished between large (15 mm^2) and small (5 mm^2) full-thickness lesions in weight-bearing and non-weight-bearing areas of the antebrachiocarpal (radiocarpal), middle carpal (intercarpal), and femoropatellar joints.[116] At 1 month, small defects were filled with poorly organized fibrovascular repair tissue; by 4 months, repair was limited to an increase in the amount of organization of this fibrous tissue, and by 5 months, small radiocarpal and femoropatellar lesions were hardly detectable because of combinations of matrix flow and extrinsic repair mechanisms. Large lesions showed good initial repair, but at 5 months, perilesional and intralesional subchondral clefts developed.

The repair tissue that forms after full-thickness injury to hyaline cartilage or as a natural repair process in joints with OA is primarily comprised of type I rather than type II collagen, at least at 4 months.[117,126] Identification of type II collagen is the critical biochemical factor distinguishing hyaline cartilage from repaired fibrous tissue and fibrocartilage. It is thought that the presence of an abnormal subchondral bone plate and the absence of a tide mark reforming may create a stiffness gradient and that shear stresses of the junction of the repair tissue and underlying bone develop. The propagation of such shear stresses would lead to the degradation of repair fibrocartilage and exposure of the bone. This mechanical

failure has been observed experimentally and clinically in the horse.[27,116]

In a study looking at the long-term effectiveness of sternal cartilage grafting, the repair tissue in the nongrafted defects at 12 months consisted of fibrocartilaginous tissue with fibrous tissue in the surface layers, as was seen in control defects at 4 months. However, on biochemical analysis, the repair tissue of the nongrafted defects had a mean type II collagen percentage of 79%, compared with being nondetectable at 4 months.[126,127] On the other hand, the GAG content expressed as mg of total hexosamine/g of dried tissue was 20.6 ± 1.85 mg/g, compared with 26.4 ± 3.1 mg/g at 4 months and 41.8 ± 4.3 mg/g dry weight (DW) in normal equine articular cartilage.[126,127]

The fibrocartilaginous repair seen in normal full-thickness defects is therefore biomechanically unsuitable as a replacement-bearing surface and has been shown to undergo mechanical failure with use. The lack of durability may be related to faulty biochemical composition of the old matrix and incomplete remodeling of the interface between old and repaired cartilage or to increased stress in the regenerated cartilage because of abnormal remodeling of the subchondral bone plate and calcified cartilage layer. Although earlier work implied that it may be possible to reconstitute the normal collagen type in equine articular cartilage,[126] clearly there is continued deterioration of GAG content, and these are important components in the overall composition of the cartilage matrix.

The presence of a cartilage defect may not represent clinical compromise. In the equine carpus, loss of up to 30% of articular surface of an individual bone may not compromise the successful return of a horse to racing.[27] However, loss of 50% of the articular surface or severe loss of subchondral bone leads to a significantly worse prognosis.

The inadequate healing response may not necessarily apply to immature animals or to non-weight-bearing defects. An example is the young horse after surgery for osteochondritis dissecans that shows impressive or at least functional healing responses. This may be related to increased chondrocytic capacity for mitosis and matrix synthesis and the presence of intracartilaginous vascularity. Complete restoration of the ultrastructure and surface configuration in a hinge-like gliding joint surface such as the femoropatellar joint may be unnecessary for clinical soundness, compared with the more severe loading on an osteochondral defect located on the weight-bearing portion of the medial condyle of the femur or the midcarpal joint.

Increasing age may affect the response of cartilage to injury in humans because the ability of the chondrocytes to synthesize and assemble matrix micromolecules could decline with age.[112] Buckwalter cites a study of transplanted chondrocytes, suggesting that older chondrocytes produce a more poorly organized matrix than younger chondrocytes,[112] and other studies demonstrate that the proteoglycan synthesized by the chondrocytes changes with age.[128,129] Much research is being done to develop better methods of cartilage repair and these have been reviewed elsewhere.[19,130]

REFERENCES

1. Goldring MB, Goldring SR. Osteoarthritis. *J Cell Physiol.* 2007;213(3):626–634.
2. McIlwraith CW. Joint injuries and disease and osteoarthritis. In: Baxter GM, ed. *Adams and Stashak's lameness in horses.* 6th ed. Wiley; 2011:871–889.
3. Caron JP. Osteoarthritis. In: Ross MW, Dyson SJ, eds. *Diagnosis and management of lameness in the horse.* 2nd ed. Elsevier Saunders; 2011:655–668.
4. Caron JP, Genovese RL. Principles and practices of joint disease treatment. In: Ross MW, Dyson SJ, eds. *Diagnosis and management of lameness in the horse.* Philadelphia, PA: Elsevier; 2003.
5. Koch TG, Betts DH. Stem cell therapy for joint problems using the horse as a clinically relevant animal model. *Expert Opin Biol Ther.* 2007;7(11):1621–1626.
6. Pritzker KP, Gay S, Jimenez SA, et al. Osteoarthritis cartilage histopathology: grading and staging. *Osteoarthritis Cartilage.* 2006;14(1):13–29.
7. Dray A, Read SJ. Arthritis and pain. Future targets to control osteoarthritis pain. *Arthritis Res Ther.* 2007;9(3):212–226.
8. USDA lameness and laminitis in U.S. horses. *USDA: APHIS: VS CEAH.* Fort Collins, CO: National Animal Health Monitoring System; 2000. N318.0400.
9. Drum MG, Kawcak CE, Norrdin RW, et al. Comparison of gross and histopathologic findings with quantitative computed tomographic bone density in the distal third metacarpal bone of racehorses. *Vet Radiol Ultrasound.* 2007;48(6):518–527.
10. Neundorf RH, Lowerison MB, Cruz AM, et al. Determination of the prevalence and severity of metacarpophalangeal joint osteoarthritis in Thoroughbred racehorses via quantitative macroscopic evaluation. *Am J Vet Res.* 2010;71(11):1284–1293.
11. Norrdin RW, Stover SM. Subchondral bone failure in overload arthrosis: a scanning electron microscopic study in horses. *J Musculoskelet Neuronal Interact.* 2006;6(3):251–257.
12. McIlwraith CW, Frisbie DD, Kawcak CE, et al. The OARSI histopathology initiative: recommendations for histological assessments of osteoarthritis in the horse. *Osteoarthritis Cartilage.* 2010;18(supply 3):S93–S105.
13. Callender GR, Kelser RA. Degenerative arthritis: a comparison of the pathological changes in man and equines. *Am J Pathol.* 1938;14(3):253–272.
14. Mackay-Smith MP. Pathogenesis and pathology of equine osteoarthritis. *J Am Med Vet Assoc.* 1962;141:1246–1252.
15. Nilsson G, Olsson SC. Radiologic and patho-anatomical changes in the distal joints and phalanges of the Standardbred horse. *Acta Vet Scand.* 1973;44(suppl 1):1.
16. Raker CW, Baker RH, Wheat JD. Pathophysiology of equine degenerative joint disease and lameness. In:. *Proc Am Assoc Equine Pract.* 1966;12:229–241.
17. Rooney JR. *Biomechanics of lameness in horses.* Baltimore, MD: Williams & Wilkins; 1969.
18. McIlwraith CW. General pathobiology of the joint and response to injury. In: McIlwraith CW, Trotter GW, eds. *Joint disease in the horse.* Philadelphia, PA: Saunders; 1996:40–70.
19. McIlwraith CW. Frank Milne lecture: from arthroscopy to gene therapy – 30 years of looking in joints. In:. *Proc Am Assoc Equine Pract.* 2005;51:65–113.
20. Anderson DD, Chubinskaya S, Guilak F, et al. Posttraumatic osteoarthritis: improving understanding and opportunities for early intervention. *J Orthop Res.* 2011;29(6):802–809.
21. Brandt KD, Dieppe P, Radin E. Etiopathogenesis of osteoarthritis. *Med Clin North Am.* 2008;34(3):531–559.
22. McIlwraith CW. Diseases of joints, tendons and related structures. In: Stashak TS, ed. *Adams' lameness in horses.* 5th ed. Philadelphia, PA: Lippincott, Williams & Wilkins; 2002:457–644.
23. Kawcak CE, McIlwraith CW, Norrdin RW, et al. The role of subchondral bone in joint disease: a review. *Equine Vet J.* 2001;33(2):120–126.
24. McIlwraith CW. Current concepts in equine degenerative joint disease. *J Am Vet Med Assoc.* 1982;180(3):239–250.
25. Riggs CM, Whitehouse CH, Boyde A. Pathology of the distal condyles of the third metacarpal and third metatarsal bones of the horse. *Equine Vet J.* 1999;31(2):140–148.
26. Kawcak CE, McIlwraith CW. Proximodorsal first phalanx osteochondral chip fragmentation in 336 horses. *Equine Vet J.* 1994;26(5):392–396.
27. McIlwraith CW, Yovich JV, Martin GS. Arthroscopic surgery for the treatment of osteochondral chip fractures in the equine carpus. *J Am Vet Med Assoc.* 1987;191(5):531–540.
28. Frisbie DD, Ray CS, Ionescu M, et al. Measurement of synovial fluid and serum concentrations of the 846 epitope of chondroitin sulfate and of carboxy propeptides of type II procollagen for diagnosis of osteochondral fragmentation in horses. *Am J Vet Res.* 1999;60(3):306–309.
29. Fuller CJ, Barr AR, Sharif M, et al. Cross-sectional comparison of synovial fluid biochemical markers in equine osteoarthritis and the correlation of these markers with articular cartilage damage. *Osteoarthritis Cartilage.* 2001;9(1):49–55.
30. Chubinskaya S, Wimmer MA. Key pathways to prevent posttraumatic arthritis for future molecule-based therapy. *Cartilage.* 2013;4(suppl 3):13S–21S.
31. Lotz MK. Posttraumatic osteoarthritis: pathogenesis and pharmacological treatment options. *Arthritis Res Ther.* 2010;12:211–219.
32. Roos H, Adalberth T, Dahlberg L, et al. Osteoarthritis of the knee after injury to the anterior cruciate ligament or meniscus: the influence of time and age. *Osteoarthritis Cartilage.* 1995;3(4):267–268.
33. Buckwalter JA. Articular cartilage injuries. *Clin Orthop Relat Res.* 2002;402:21–37.
34. Buckwalter JA, Brown TD. Joint injury, repair, and remodelling: roles in posttraumatic osteoarthritis. *Clin Orthop Relat Res.* 2004;423:7–16.
35. Olson SA, Guilak F. From articular fracture to posttraumatic arthritis: a black box that needs to be opened. *J Orthop Trauma.* 2006;20(10):661–662.
36. McIlwraith CW, Van Sickle DC. Experimentally induced arthritis of the equine carpus: histologic and histochemical changes in the articular cartilage. *Am J Vet Res.* 1981;42(2):209–217.
37. Balkman CE, Nixon AJ. Molecular cloning and cartilage gene expression of equine stromelysin 1 (matrix metalloproteinase 3). *Am J Vet Res.* 1998;59(1):30–36.
38. Clegg PD, Burke RM, Coughlan AR, et al. Characterisation of equine matrix metalloproteinase 2 and 9; and identification of the cellular sources of these enzymes in joints. Equine Vet J, 29(5), 335–342.

39. Clegg PD, Coughlan AR, Riggs CM, et al. Matrix metalloproteinases 2 and 9 in equine synovial fluids. *Equine Vet J.* 1997;29(5):343–348.

40. Dimock AN, Siciliano PD, McIlwraith CW. Evidence supporting an increased presence of reactive oxygen species in the diseased equine joint. *Equine Vet J.* 2000;32(5):439–443.

41. Frisbie DD, Ghivizzani SC, Robbins PD, et al. Treatment of experimental equine osteoarthritis by in vivo delivery of the equine interleukin-1 receptor antagonist gene. *Gene Ther.* 2002;9(1):12–20.

42. Kawcak CE, Frisbie DD, Trotter GW, et al. Effects of intravenous administration of sodium hyaluronate on carpal joints in exercising horses after arthroscopic surgery and osteochondral fragmentation. *Am J Vet Res.* 1997;58(10):1132–1140.

43. Takafuji VA, McIlwraith CW, Howard RD. Effects of recombinant equine interleukin-1 alpha and interleukin-1 beta on proteoglycan metabolism and prostaglandin E2 synthesis in equine articular cartilage explants. *Am J Vet Res.* 2002;63(4):551–558.

44. Trumble TN, Trotter GW, Oxford JR, et al. Synovial fluid gelatinase concentrations and matrix metalloproteinase and cytokine expression in naturally occurring joint disease in horses. *Am J Vet Res.* 2001;62(9):1467–1477.

45. Kamm JL, Nixon AJ, Witte TH. Cytokine and catabolic enzyme expression in synovium, synovial fluid and articular cartilage of naturally osteoarthritic equine carpi. *Equine Vet J.* 2010;42(8):693–699.

46. Frisbie DD, McIlwraith CW. Gene therapy: future therapies in osteoarthritis. *Vet Clin North Am Equine Pract.* 2001;17(2):233–243.

47. Berenbaum F. The quest for the Holy Grail: a disease-modifying osteoarthritis drug. *Arthritis Res Ther.* 2007;9(6):111.

48. Toncheva A, Remichkova M, Ikonomova K, et al. Inflammatory response in patients with active and inactive osteoarthritis. *Rheumatol Int.* 2009;29(10):1197–1203.

49. Wassilew GI, Lehnigk U, Duda GN, et al. The expression of proinflammatory cytokines and matrix metalloproteinases in the synovial membranes of patients with osteoarthritis compared with traumatic knee disorders. *Arthroscopy.* 2010;26(8):1096–1104.

50. Goekoop RJ, Kloppenburg M, Kroon HM, et al. Low innate production of interleukin-1beta and interleukin-6 is associated with the absence of osteoarthritis in old age. *Osteoarthritis Cartilage.* 2010;18(7):942–947.

51. Sellam J, Bernbaum F. The role of synovitis in pathophysiology and clinical symptoms of osteoarthritis. *Nature Rev Rheum.* 2010;6(11):625–635.

52. Lewis JS, Hembree WC, Furman BD, et al. Acute joint pathology in synovial inflammation is associated with increased intraarticular fracture severity in the mouse knee. *Osteoarthritis Cartilage.* 2011;19(7):864–873.

53. Mueller MB, Tuan RS. Anabolic/catabolic balance in pathogenesis of osteoarthritis: identifying molecular targets. *PM R.* 2011;3(6 suppl 1):S3–S11.

54. Morisset S, Frisbie DD, Robbins PD, et al. IL-1ra/IGF-1 gene therapy modulates repair of microfractured chondral defects. *Clin Orthop Relat Res.* 2007;462:221–228.

55. Jones DL, Barber SM, Doige CE. Synovial fluid and clinical changes after arthroscopic partial synovectomy of the equine middle carpal joint. *Vet Surg.* 1993;22(6):524–530.

56. Roos EM, Dahlberg L. Positive effects of moderate exercise on glycosaminoglycan content in knee cartilage. *Arthritis Rheum.* 2005;52(11):3507–3514.

57. McAdams TR, Mandelbaum BR. Articular cartilage regeneration in the knee. *Curr Orthop Pract.* 2008;19:140–146.

58. Kiviranta I, Tammi M, Jurvelin J, et al. Articular cartilage thickness and glycosaminoglycan distribution in the canine knee joint after strenuous exercise. *Clin Orthop.* 1992; 283:302–308.

59. Arokoski J, Kiviranta I, Jurvelin J, et al. Long-distance running causes site-dependent decrease of cartilage glycosaminoglycan content in the knee joint. *Arthritis Rheum.* 1993;36(10):1451–1459.

60. Lohmander LS, Roos H, Dahlberg L, et al. Temporal patterns of stromelysin, tissue inhibitor and proteoglycan fragments in synovial fluid after injury to the knee, cruciate ligament or meniscus. *J Orthop Res.* 1994;12(1):21–28.

61. Martel-Pelletier P, Pelletier J-P. Inflammatory factors involved in osteoarthritis. In: Buckwalter JA, Lotz M, Stoltz J-F, eds. *Osteoarthritis, inflammation and degradation: a continuum.* Amsterdam: IOS Press; 2007:3–13.

62. Berenbaum F. Osteoarthritis is an inflammatory disease (osteoarthritis is not osteoarthrosis!). *Osteoarthritis Cartilage.* 2013;21(1):16–21.

63. Kapoor M, Martel-Pelletier J, Lajeunesse D, et al. Role of proinflammatory cytokines in the pathophysiology of osteoarthritis. *Nat Rev Rheumatol.* 2011;7(1):33–42.

64. Sandell LJ. Etiology of osteoarthritis: genetics and synovial joint development. *Nat Rev Rheumatol.* 2012;8(2):77–89.

65. Caron JP, Tardif G, Martel-Pelletier J, et al. Modulation of matrix metalloproteinase 13 (collagenase III) gene expression in equine chondrocytes by equine interleukin-1 and corticosteroids. *Am J Vet Res.* 1996;57(11):1631–1634.

66. Moldovan F, Pelletier JP, Hambor J, et al. Collagenase-3 (matrix metalloproteinase 13) is preferentially localized in the deep layer of human articular cartilage in situ. In vitro mimicking effect by transforming growth factor beta. *Arthritis Rheum.* 1997;40(9):1653–1661.

67. Fosang HA, Rodgerson FM. Identifying the human aggrecanase. *Osteoarthritis Cartilage.* 2010;18(9):1109–1116.

68. Little CB, Meeker CT, Golub SB, et al. Blocking aggrecanase cleavage in the aggrecan interglobular domain aggregates cartilage erosion and promotes cartilage repair. *J Clin Invest.* 2007;117(6):1627–1636.

69. Song RH, Tortorella MD, Malfait AM, et al. Aggrecan degradation in human articular cartilage explants is mediated by both ADAMTS-4 and ADAMTS-5. *Arthritis Rheum.* 2007;56(2):576–585.

70. Wu J-J, Lark M, Eyre DR. Sites of stromelysin cleavage in collagens type II, IX, X, and XI of cartilage. *J Biol Chem.* 1991;266(9):5625–5628.

71. Dodge GR, Poole AR. Immunohistochemical detection and immunochemical analysis of type II collagen degradation in human normal, rheumatoid, and osteoarthritic articular cartilage and in explants of bovine articular cartilage cultured with interleukin 1. *J Clin Invest.* 1989;83(2): 647–661.

72. Little CB, Hughes CE, Curtis CL, et al. Cyclosporin A inhibition of aggrecanase-mediated proteoglycan catabolism in articular cartilage. *Arthritis Rheum.* 2002;46(1): 124–129.

73. Bondeson J, Wainwright SD, Lauder S, et al. The role of synovial macrophages in macrophage-produced cytokines in driving aggrecanases, matrix metalloproteinases, and other destructive and inflammatory responses in osteoarthritis. *Arthritis Res Ther.* 2006;8(6):R187.

74. Kashiwagi M, Tortorella M, Nagase H, et al. TIMP-3 is a potent inhibitor of aggrecanase 1 (ADAMTS-4) and aggrecanase 2 (ADAMTS-5). *J Biol Chem.* 2001;276(16):12501–12504.

75. Nagase H, Woessner Jr JF. Role of endogenous proteinases in the degradation of cartilage matrix. In: Woessner Jr JF, Howell DS, eds. *Joint cartilage degradation: basic and clinical aspects.* New York, NY: Marcel-Dekker; 1993:159–185.

76. Slether-Stevenson WG, Krutsch HC, Liotta.LA. Tissue inhibitor of metalloproteinase (TIMP-2). A new member of the metalloproteinase family. *J Biol Chem.* 1989;264(29):17374–17378.

77. De Rienzo F, Saxena P, Filomia F, et al. Progress towards identification of new aggrecanase inhibitors. *Curr Med Chem.* 2009;16(19):2395–2415.

78. Park JY, Pillinger MH, Abramson SB. Prostaglandin E2 synthesis and secretion. The role of PGE2 synthases. *Clin Immunol.* 2006;119(3):229–240.

79. Goldring MB. The role of cytokines as inflammatory mediators in osteoarthritis: lessons from animal models. Mini review. *Overseas Publishers Assoc.* 1999:1–11.

80. Frisbie DD, McIlwraith CW, Kawcak CE, et al. Evaluation of topically administered diclofenac liposomal cream for treatment of horses with experimentally induced osteoarthritis. *Am J Vet Res.* 2009;70(2):210–215.

81. Frisbie DD, Kawcak CE, McIlwraith CW, et al. Effects of 6α-methylprednisolone acetate on an in vivo equine osteochondral fragment exercise model. *Am J Vet Res.* 1998;59:1619–1628.

82. Greenwald R, Moy W. Effect of oxygen-derived free radicals on hyaluronic acid. *Arthritis Rheum.* 1980;23(4):455–463.

83. Wong S, Halliwell B, Richmond R, et al. The role of superoxide and hydroxyl radicals in the degradation of hyaluronic acid induced by metal ions and by ascorbic acid. *J Inorg Biochem.* 1981;14(2):127–134.

84. Greenwald R, Moy W. Inhibition of collagen gelatin by actions of the superoxide radical. *Arthritis Rheum.* 1979;22:251–259.

85. Ostalowska A, Kasperczyk S, Kasperczyk A, et al. Oxidant and anti-oxidant systems of synovial fluid from patients with knee posttraumatic arthritis. *J Orthop Res.* 2007;25(6):804–812.

86. Abramason SB. Osteoarthritis and nitric oxide. *Osteoarthritis Cartilage.* 2008;16(suppl 2):S15–S20.

87. Melchiorri C, Meliconi R, Frizziero L, et al. Enhanced and coordinated in vivo expression of inflammatory cytokines and nitric oxide synthase by chondrocytes from patients with osteoarthritis. *Arthritis Rheum.* 1998;41(12):2165–2174.

88. Dayer J-M, Beutler B, Serami A. Cachectin/tumor necrosis factor stimulates collagenase and prostaglandin E2 production by human synovial cells and dermal fibroblasts. *J Exp Med.* 1985;162(6):2163–2168.

89. Dayer J-M, de Rochemonteix B, Burrus B, et al. Human recombinant interleukin-1 stimulates collagenase and prostaglandin E2 production by human synovial cells. *J Clin Invest.* 1986;77(2):645–648.

90. Wood DD, Ihrie EJ, Hamerman D. Release of interleukin-1 from human synovial tissue in vitro. *Arthritis Rheum.* 1985;28(8):853–862.

91. Morris EA, McDonald BS, Webb AC, et al. Identification of interleukin-1 in equine osteoarthritic joint effusion. *Am J Vet Res.* 1990;51(1):59–64.

92. Howard RD, McIlwraith CW, Trotter GW, et al. Cloning of equine interleukin-1 alpha and equine interleukin-1 beta and determination of their full length cDNA sequences. *Am J Vet Res.* 1998;59(6):704–711.

93. Billinghurst RC, Fretz PB, Gordon JR. Induction of intraarticular tumor necrosis factor in acute inflammatory responses in equine arthritis. *Equine Vet J.* 1995;27(3):208–216.

94. Cope AP, Gibbons D, Brennan FM, et al. Increased levels of soluble tumor necrosis factor receptors in the sera and synovial fluid of patients with rheumatic diseases. *Arthritis Rheum.* 1992;35:1160–1169.

95. Deleuran BW, Chu CQ, Field M, et al. Localization of tumor necrosis factor receptors in the synovial tissue and cartilage/pannus junction in patients with rheumatoid arthritis. *Arthritis Rheum.* 1992;35(10):1170–1178.

96. Carpenter RS, Goodrich LR, Frisbie DD, et al. Osteoblastic differentiation of human and equine adult bone marrow-derived mesenchymal stem cells when BMP-2 or BMP-7 homodimer genetic modification is compared to BMP-2/7 heterodimer genetic modification in the presence and absence of dexamethasone. *J Orthop Res.* 2010;28(10):1330–1337.

97. Wang J, Elewau TD, Veys EM, et al. Insulin-like growth factor 1-induced interleukin-1 receptor II overrides the activity of interleukin-1 and controls the homeostasis of the extracellular matrix of cartilage. *Arthritis Rheum.* 2003;48(5):1281–1291.

98. Reinhold MI, Abe M, Kapadia RM, et al. FGF18 represses noggin expression and is induced by calcineurin. *J Biol Chem.* 2004;279(37):38209–38219.

99. Norrdin RW, Kawcak CE, Capwell BA, et al. Subchondral bone failure in an equine model of overload arthrosis. *Bone.* 1998;22(2):133–139.

100. Radin EL, Rose RN. The role of subchondral bone in the initiation and progression of cartilage damage. *Clin Orthop Rel Res.* 1986;213:34–40.

101. Goldring MB, Goldring SR. Bone and cartilage in osteoarthritis: is what's best for one good or bad for the other? *Arthritis Res Ther.* 2010;12(5):143–144.

102. Kawcak CE, McIlwraith CW, Norrdin RW, et al. Clinical effects of exercise on subchondral bone of carpal and metacarpophalangeal joints in horses. *Am J Vet Res.* 2000;61(10):1252–1258.

103. Riggs CM. Osteochondral injury and joint disease in the athletic horse. *Equine Vet Educ.* 2006;18(2):100–112.

104. Martinelli MJ. Subchondral bone and injury. Clinical commentary. *Equine Vet Educ.* 2009;21(5):253–256.

105. Cullimore AM, Finney JW, Marmion WJ, et al. Severe lameness associated with impact fracture of the proximal phalanx in a filly. *Equine Vet Educ.* 2009;21(5):247–251.

106. Riggs CM. Multidisciplinary investigation of the aetiopathogenesis of parasagittal fractures of the distal metacarpal and third metatarsal bone–review of the literature. *Equine Vet J.* 1999;31:116–120.

107. Riggs CM, Whitehouse CH, Boyde A. Structural variations of the distal condyles of the third metacarpal and third metatarsal bones of the horse. *Equine Vet J.* 1999;31(2):130–139.

108. Wong BL, Kim SHC, Antonacci JM, et al. Cartilage shear dynamics during tibio-femoral articulation: effect of acute joint injury in tribosupplementation on synovial fluid lubrication. *Osteoarthritis Cartilage.* 2010;18(3):464–471.

109. Armstrong CG, Lai WM, Mow VC. An analysis of the unconfined compression of articular cartilage. *J Biomech Eng.* 1984;106(2):165–173.

110. Antonacci JM, Schmidt TA, Serventi LA, et al. Effects of equine joint injury on boundary lubrication of articular cartilage by synovial fluid: role of hyaluronan. *Arthritis Rheum.* 2012;64(9):2917–2926.

111. Broom ND. Abnormal softening in articular cartilage. Its relationship to the collagen framework. *Arthritis Rheum.* 1982;25(10):1209.

112. Buckwalter JA, Mau DC. Cartilage repair in osteoarthritis. In: Moskowitz RW, Howell DS, Goldberg VM, et al., eds. *Diagnosis and medical/surgical management.* 2nd ed. Philadelphia, PA: Saunders; 1992:71–107.

113. Hunter W. Of the structure and diseases of articulating cartilage. *Phil Trans R Soc London 9, 514-521.* 1743. [Reprinted in: Clin Orthop Relat Res (1995) 317, 3–6.].

114. McIlwraith CW, Vachon AM. Review of pathogenesis and treatment of degenerative joint disease. *Equine Vet J.* 1988;S6:3–11.

115. Hurtig MB. Experimental use of small osteochondral grafts for resurfacing the equine third carpal bone. *Equine Vet J.* 1988;S6:23–27.

116. Hurtig MB, Fretz PB, Doige CE, et al. Effect of lesion size and location on equine articular cartilage repair. *Can J Vet Res.* 1988;52(1):137–146.

117. Calandruccio RA, Gilmer S. Proliferation, regeneration and repair of articular cartilage of immature animals. *J Bone Joint Surg Am.* 1962;44(3):431–455.

118. Convery FR, Akeson WH, Keown GH. Repair of large osteochondral defects – an experimental study in horses. *Clin Orthop Relat Res.* 1972;82:253.

119. Meachim G. The effect of scarification on articular cartilage in the rabbit. *J Bone Joint Surg Br.* 1963;45(1):150–161.

120. Bentley G. Articular cartilage changes in chondromalacia patellae. *J Bone Joint Surg Br.* 1985;67(5):769–774.

121. Schmid A, Schmid F. Ultrastructural studies after arthroscopic cartilage shaving. *Arthroscopy.* 1987;3:137.

122. Grant BD. Repair mechanisms of osteochondral defects in Equidae: a comparative study of untreated and x-irradiated defects. In:. *Proc Am Assoc Equine Pract.* 1975;21:95–114.

123. Mankin HJ. The reactions of articular cartilage to injury and osteoarthritis. *N Engl J Med.* 1974;291(24):1285–1292.

124. Riddle WE. Healing of articular cartilage in the horse. *J Am Vet Med Assoc.* 1970;157(11):1471.

125. Vachon AM, McIlwraith CW, Trotter GW, et al. Morphologic study of repair of induced osteochondral defects of the distal portion of the radial carpal bone in horses by use of glued periosteal autografts. *Am J Vet Res.* 1991;52(2):317–327.

126. Vachon AM, McIlwraith CW, Powers BE, et al. Morphologic and biochemical study of sternal cartilage autografts for resurfacing induced osteochondral defects in horses. *Am J Vet Res.* 1992;53(6):1038–1047.

127. Vachon AM, Keeley FW, McIlwraith CW, et al. Biochemical analysis of normal articular cartilage in horses. *Am J Vet Res.* 1990;51(2):1905–1911.

128. Bennett GA, Bauer W. Joint changes resulting from patellar displacement and their relation to degenerative joint disease. *J Bone Joint Surg.* 1937;19(3):667–682.

129. Repo RB, Mitchell N. Collagen synthesis in mature articular cartilage of the rabbit. *J Bone Joint Surg Br.* 1971;53(3):541–548.

130. McIlwraith CW, Nixon AJ, Wright IM. *Diagnostic and surgical arthroscopy in the horse.* 4th ed. Elsevier; 2014.

4

Pathologic Manifestations of Joint Disease

Christopher E. Kawcak

PATHOGENESIS OF JOINT DISEASE

Over the last 50 years there have been numerous studies to characterize the gross and histologic appearance of joint injuries, and with the development and use of volumetric imaging techniques such as computed tomography (CT) and magnetic resonance imaging (MRI), it is becoming evident that most joint injuries, although acute in clinical appearance, are the end result of a chronic pathologic process. Humane euthanasia of young racehorses is an unfortunate event in the equine industry, but by examining postmortem materials from young, actively training horses, a pathologic sequence of events has emerged leading to the documentation of chronic fatigue injury as a common problem in athletic horses. Pool first presented this hypothesis over 20 years ago through his observation of postmortem samples.[1] These observations were later confirmed by other investigators,[2-4] and additional support was gained from CT and MRI.[5] These findings have improved our understanding of injuries and allowed for earlier diagnosis of joint disease. The purpose of this chapter is to provide an overview of the pathologic mechanisms that lead to joint disease in the equine athlete.

BIOMECHANICAL INFLUENCES ON JOINT DISEASE

Acute Injury

The fact that a horse may become acutely lame does not necessarily mean that the injury itself is acute in nature. We are beginning to understand that true acute traumatic injuries, although common to the horse industry, are a relatively uncommon cause of injury in the equine athlete. Acute traumatic forces can result in osteochondral damage (fracture, fragmentation, and contusion), primary articular cartilage damage, intraarticular and extraarticular ligament injury, joint capsule injury, meniscal injury, and synovitis (Figure 4-1). Acute injuries are typically unusual in nature in the sense that they occur in areas of the joint that are not commonly injured, and pathologic examination of these lesions show that the injury usually occurs through normal tissue. Acute lesions typically lack any sign of healing/adaptive responses that are characteristic of chronic fatigue injuries.

Subchondral bone is composed of a subchondral bone plate and underlying trabecular bone, which together act to dampen forces that are transmitted through the joint.[2] Acute fracture or fragmentation of subchondral bone does occur but is rare as a cause of lameness in equine athletes. Most biomechanical mechanisms and pathologic sequence of events that describe acute cortical bone fracture also play a role in acute subchondral bone fracture. It is highly likely that shear, torsional, and compressive forces lead to acute subchondral bone fracture, and it is unlikely that bending and tensile forces play a role. These forces can result in either a complete fracture through the bone (involving two joint surfaces) or fragmentation in which the edge of the bone fractures into either the joint or joint capsule (Figure 4-2). Microdamage in the form of microfractures occur within the subchondral and trabecular bone layers. These microfractures can coalesce into gross fractures (this occurs with chronic fatigue fractures) or may stimulate an adaptive/healing response within the bone. The bone can respond by the formation of a contusion (an area of microscopic damage and bruising) or edema.[6] This can occur within the immediate subchondral bone plate, the deeper trabecular bone, or at sites of soft tissue attachment (such as joint capsule or ligamentous insertions) (Figure 4-3). The consequences of bone contusion and edema are difficult to identify in the horse. In humans, bone contusion can lead to an ischemic event in the proximal femur leading to osteonecrosis and osteoarthritis (OA).[7] One place where acute subchondral bone injury can occur is in the recovery stall, in which a poor recovery can lead to osteochondral fracture/fragmentation in the caudal aspect of the joint (see Figure 4-1). These injuries are difficult to prognosticate because of their low incidence and unusual configuration, which is typical of most acute injuries. If a subchondral bone fracture can be realigned and there is minimal articular cartilage damage, the prognosis for repair is typically good.

Similar to subchondral bone, primary articular cartilage injury can occur anywhere in the joint and the damage can lie somewhere between the biochemical and gross levels. Subtle injury can lead to biochemical changes in the articular cartilage matrix, leading to progressive degradation of the collagen and aggrecan components, which may impart either no significant lesion or only subtle clinical signs, usually in the

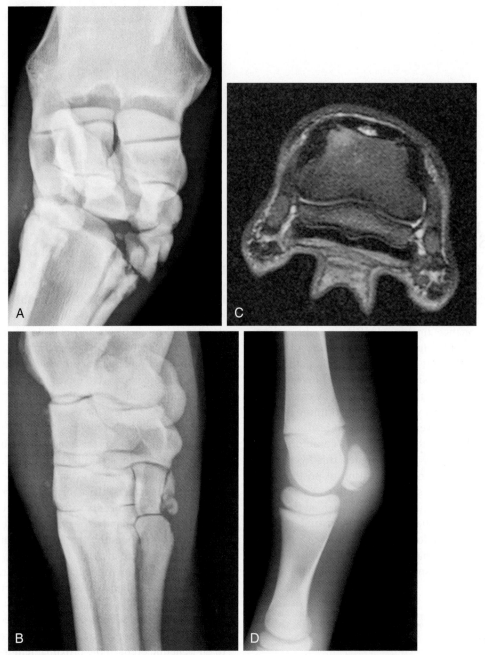

FIGURE 4-1 Examples of acute injuries that occurred through normal tissue. **A,** An acute joint fracture and luxation in the carpus without any signs of chronic fatigue. **B,** Acute osteochondral fracture of the palmar aspect of the second carpal bone detected after recovery from anesthesia for an unrelated problem. **C,** An MRI of a bone contusion of the distal second phalanx, which may be acute in nature. **D,** A fracture of the basal aspect of the proximal sesamoid bone in a foal with no signs of chronic disease.

form of synovitis. True acute damage, however, usually results in gross articular cartilage damage, often with an associated subchondral bone reaction and soft tissue damage, which sometimes leads to instability and progression of damage.[7] In these cases, synovitis and usually some form of capsulitis are seen as well. Articular cartilage fibrillation, partial thickness erosion or full thickness erosion can result. Damage can also occur at the calcified cartilage level which can lead to osteoarthritis.[8,9]

Acute injury can also occur in either the intraarticular or extraarticular ligaments. Intraarticular ligament injury is rare in the horse, but has become better characterized because of volumetric imaging.[10,11] Complete characterization of injury to the cruciate ligaments in the stifle, however, is limited by the ability to image the area.[12] Only a few MRI units can accommodate the stifle of an adult horse, and only horses with specific body types can fit within the machine. Contrast-enhanced CT has been used and can provide valuable

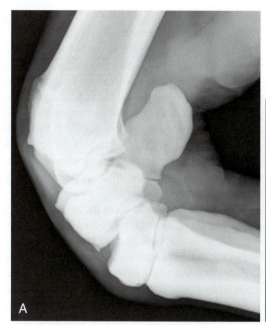
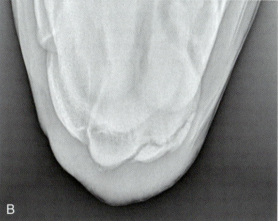

FIGURE 4-2 Examples of fragmentation and complete fracture. **A,** An osteochondral fragment that has broken out of the dorsal aspect of the distal radial carpal bone. **B,** A third carpal slab fracture that has spanned both the proximal and distal edges of the bone to involve two joints.

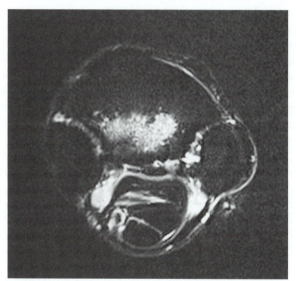

FIGURE 4-3 MRI showing bone edema within the ligamentous insertion site of the proximal third metatarsal bone.

information as long as the injury is such that it allows the inflow of contrast to the lesion.[10,11] A lesion that only involves the center of the ligaments without surface damage may be missed using this technique. In other species, there is emerging evidence that cruciate ligament disease may be chronic in its development, but such a pathologic mechanism has not been established in the horse.[13] Injury to the intersesamoidean ligaments, intercarpal ligaments, and collateral ligaments has been reported and the prognosis is variable depending on the severity of injury. These injuries can be characterized with volumetric imaging techniques, which have helped to optimize treatment.

Injury to the joint capsule is difficult to diagnose and treat. Without MRI in the acute stages, the injury may go unrecognized. The horse may have no other findings and may respond well to intraarticular treatment. Only later can an enthesophyte be seen on subsequent radiographs. In some instances of primary joint disease, such as with osteochondral fracture or fragmentation, there may be no signs of joint capsule injury, again only to show up later on radiographs. Many of these subsequent changes can be incidental if the primary disease is treated, but some may be indicative of a persistent problem in the joint capsule that leads to pain. Synovial membrane can repair after acute injury[14]; however, if disease is persistent then a fibrotic response can result.

Meniscal injury in the horse is becoming more commonly recognized because of the development of advanced imaging techniques. The meniscus, meniscal ligaments and bone attachments can be involved in an acute event. Multiple imaging techniques are needed to fully characterize the extent of meniscal injury in horses.[12] Unlike in other species, the full extent of the meniscus cannot be visualized arthroscopically in the horse. In addition, few MRI units can accommodate the stifle of the horse, and contrast-enhanced CT is of some help for characterizing the disease.[10]

Chronic Fatigue Injury

We are beginning to learn that chronic fatigue injury commonly occurs in the equine athlete. This term is used to characterize the pathologic processes that start at the molecular and biochemical levels, leading to histologic evidence of tissue damage and ultimately tissue failure that results in clinical signs. These injuries can be termed pathologic injuries but should not be confused with injuries that occur through tissues compromised by other diseases such as cancer. Chronic fatigue injuries result from cyclic loading of tissues below the biomechanical threshold of tissue failure. The progression of damage can occur by (1) microdamage formation within the tissues, resulting in molecular and biochemical processes that either repair the injury or result in its progression; (2) microdamage may be absent, but the biochemical and tissue responses to cyclic loading can create an area of weakness in the tissues, thus predisposing it to damage; or (3) adaptive tissue responses that fatigue the tissues, resulting in chronic progressive changes to its material properties, leading ultimately to injury.

The clinical manifestations of chronic fatigue injuries are consistent in nature, but can differ by breed, use, and age. In particular, the locations of the disease processes that lead to clinical signs are consistent and the pathologic appearances (both grossly and histologically) are consistent in character.[3] It is now understood that chronic fatigue injury consistently occurs in subchondral bone in the equine athlete, and there is some evidence to suggest that it occurs in the articular cartilage and is likely worsened by degradation process associated with synovitis.[1,2,14-16] Although clinical impressions lead some individuals to believe that chronic fatigue injury can occur in areas such as suspensory ligaments and tendons, the evidence supporting those processes is weak. It becomes obvious that conformational abnormalities in the limb can lead to chronic fatigue stress to any of the tissues in the musculoskeletal system and consequently disease. The difficulty in characterizing chronic fatigue processes is that the tissues will typically remodel abnormally to the stresses that occur within that area. This must be discerned from the normal adaptive response that occurs in so many tissues.[2] As an example, the palmar aspect of the third metacarpal condyles normally becomes sclerotic in response to training in young Thoroughbred racehorses. The difficulty lies in discerning when that response becomes pathologic (Figure 4-4). Consequently, the horse rarely demonstrates clinical

signs until the pathologic process lead to subchondral bone pain or gross damage within the joint.[17]

Chronic fatigue injury in subchondral bone was first described by Pool based on gross and histologic appearances of tissues from equine athletes that became injured.[1,14] Multiple studies then supported these findings by characterizing gross, histologic, and material properties of subchondral bone tissues in postmortem specimens.[3,8,18-22] Volumetric imaging of postmortem and clinical samples confirmed the presence of a normal adaptive process in subchondral bone at specific sites, but also divergence in the appearance of those tissues when they become diseased.[5,23]

Bone has tremendous capacity to change shape, strength, and immediacy of response based on age, exercise intensity and duration, and gait in the face of normal growth. Growth at the proximal and distal ends of the bones occurs by endochondral ossification, in which a cartilage template is replaced by bone. This bone is then remodeled into a secondary spongiosa. Remodeling of bone occurs when packets of bone are resorbed and new bone is formed. The reformation phase of bone remodeling is temporarily slow compared with the resorption phase, leaving the athlete prone to fracture through weak bone.[15] In normal bone remodeling, bone does reform in the areas of resorption. However, in some diseased states such as overstressed bone (which can occur with excessive training), resorption and formation can become uncoupled leaving the bone prone to damage.[15] Bone modeling also occurs during growth and response to stress.[2,15] Bone resorption and formation are uncoupled normally, allowing for separate areas of bone resorption and formation to occur. This allows for bone sclerosis to occur and also allows for bone "drift" to occur, changing the shape of the bone in response to stress.

Several factors can influence bone response to athletic endeavors. Microdamage is known to occur in most tissues, but has been classically described in bone.[24] Microdamage can take the form of microfracture or microcracks

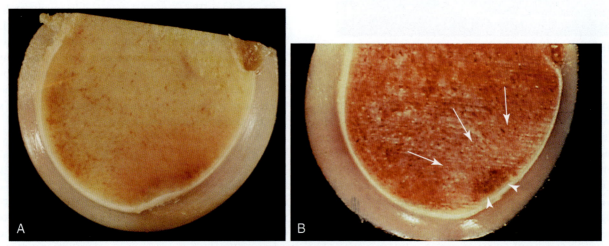

FIGURE 4-4 Sclerosis of the distal third metacarpal condyles associated with adaptation (**A**) and osteonecrosis (**B**). In B, arrows show areas of intense sclerosis, and arrowheads show areas of necrosis.

in the bone tissue. These are small cracks that take up basic fuchsin stain when applied in a bulk-staining technique.[21] Diffuse microdamage can also occur in bone tissue and is identified as a darkly stained area in bone. These areas have been shown to contain microcracks at the ultrastructural level. Microdamage occurs in normal remodeling and modeling bone, and is likely a stimulus to initiate bone turnover, to optimize bone strength.[15] However, with continued loading (exercise) there is a chance that the microdamage could coalesce and create a gross fracture. Pathologic bone formation can also occur, in which the resorptive phase can outpace the formative phase of bone remodeling and modeling, creating a weakened structure because of the intense bone resorption from continued training. For trabecular bone, excessive bone tissue formation may create a sclerotic response that could become damaging to the tissues. In cortical bone, excess bone formation can be seen to expand the size of the bone. However, in subchondral bone, expanding the size of the trabeculae reduces bone marrow spaces, leading some to believe that an ischemic state can occur.[14] In addition, as the formative phase of bone remodeling and modeling becomes more rapid, the mineral characteristics of the new bone can change, leading to a crystalline structure that has poor material properties compared with normal bone.[25] Finally, during bone modeling, newly formed bone likely has different material properties compared with the old bone tissues. When the new bone is formed on top of the old bone, a disparity in material properties can create poor integration between the tissues, thus causing an area of weakness and fracture.[25] All of these factors are likely responsive to various levels of work intensity and duration.

Chronic fatigue damage can also occur in the calcified cartilage area,[19] leading to osteochondral fracture, osteochondral necrosis, or articular cartilage thinning (indicative of OA). These changes have been best characterized in the third metacarpal condyles and third carpal bones of racehorses. Recent work has demonstrated that the calcified cartilage area of the parasagittal groove of yearling Thoroughbred horses has areas of apparent weakness. These areas in the calcified cartilage show poor material properties and often form into gross lesions.[26] The correlation between these findings in young horses and subsequent fracture has not been established but merits further study. Advancement of the tidemark into and through the noncalcified cartilage is commonly seen in the third metacarpal condyles of horses with joint disease.[8] In fact, it is not uncommon to see the subchondral bone front invade into and through the calcified cartilage layer and into and through the noncalcified cartilage layer in joints with OA. The initiating factors and the cause of the overwhelming response are unknown. It is also common to see fracture and necrosis of the calcified cartilage in areas of damage, especially in those areas classified as undergoing palmar necrosis (palmar osteochondral disease). In these cases, the subchondral bone and calcified cartilage become necrotic, which later induces massive resorption and ultimately articular cartilage collapse and osteoarthritis. The

cause of necrosis is unknown but can be caused by either overadaptation and an ischemic response or bone insufficiency. This cascade of events has led some investigators to conclude that ischemia must be an initiating factor. Recent work has shown that vascular perfusion of the palmar aspect of the condyles decreases with loading, lending more evidence to that theory.[27]

The presence of fatigue injury in articular cartilage is difficult to characterize, but likely occurs in those cases that demonstrate articular cartilage erosion over time. As part of the pathologic process of OA, it has been well established that the tidemark regularly duplicates in many species, and that the osseous front invades both calcified and noncalcified cartilage.[2] This process likely places abnormal forces upon the articular cartilage, leading to progressive damage and erosion. However, in the horse, duplication of the tidemark is a common finding in nondiseased sites, likely reflecting the magnitude of loading on the joints. However, it is not uncommon to see advancement of the tidemark into noncalcified articular cartilage in areas of disease (Figure 4-5).

Chronic fatigue injury likely occurs in the soft tissues of the joint but, as with articular cartilage fatigue injury, can be difficult to verify. Acute injuries are known to occur, but the role of chronic fatigue injury on development of soft tissue injury and pain is now starting to emerge. As mentioned above, synovial membrane can reform after an acute, single injury. However, with chronic, repetitive injury or chronic inflammation, synovial intima can become modified and the subintima fibrotic.[14] Joint capsule can heal by granulation tissue formation and become fibrotic in an unpredictable fashion, likely changing the joint mechanics and making it difficult to give an accurate prognosis for soundness.[14] A classic example of this is in the dorsal aspect of the fetlock joint, where the synovial membrane and joint capsule can become edematous and fibroplastic, with associated articular cartilage damage around that area.[14]

Although these high-speed injuries are best characterized in the fetlock and carpal joints, similar pathologic mechanisms likely occur in the coffin and stifle joints. For instance, in the medial femorotibial joint, there is evidence that the changes seen in the articular cartilage, subchondral bone, and soft tissues could be caused by fatigue injury.[28] In the coffin joint, synovitis is common, and subchondral bone changes are becoming more apparent from volumetric imaging studies. This area is complicated because of the navicular bone and soft tissues, which often appear to be prone to injury.

Chronic changes also appear to occur in the meniscus. Postmortem samples of meniscal tissues in Western performance horses have demonstrated abnormal shape and consistency in some cases (Figure 4-6), likely indicating a chronic change in tissues. It is likely, based on our understanding of musculoskeletal tissues, that normal tissue adaptation and the pathologic mechanisms (closely related to the adaptive process) that lead to chronic fatigue injury occur in all tissues.

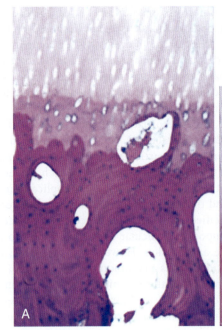
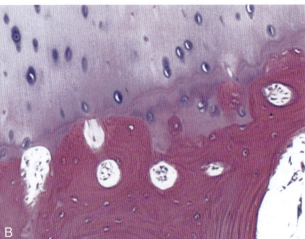
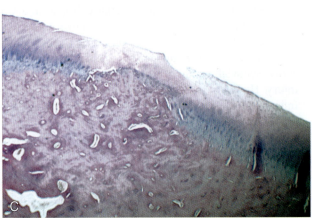
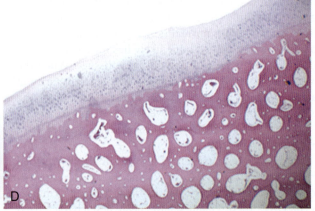

FIGURE 4-5 Histologic sections through the third metacarpal condyles of horses with various levels of disease. **A,** Osteoclastic invasion into the calcified cartilage layer. **B,** Mineralization through the calcified cartilage layer. **C,** Mineralization into the noncalcified articular cartilage layer. **D,** An osteochondral section demonstrating various degrees of mineralization through the calcified cartilage layer.

Developmental orthopedic disease (DOD) is described in Chapters 5 and 6. Similar to chronic fatigue injury, the pathologic mechanisms that occur are often subclinical and it is only when the tissues become unstable that the clinical manifestations occur. Whether or not the subtle changes seen in the palmar metacarpal calcified cartilage and subchondral bone in the parasagittal groove are manifestations of DOD remains to be seen.

Biochemical Influences on Joint Disease

Although biomechanical forces typically lead to synovitis, the disease process continues even after the abnormal biomechanical forces have been mitigated. As described in Chapter 3, synovitis typically results in the release of biochemical mediators that influence all cells within all tissues of the joint. This includes the synoviocytes, inflammatory cells, and chondrocytes which induces a chronic, progressive, vicious cycle of amplified biochemical mediator production and release within the joint. It is also likely that progressive articular cartilage damage is caused by a combined effect of biochemical and biomechanical factors. One example of a true biochemical pathologic manifestation is septic arthritis, in which bacterial stimulation of the joint and the immune system results in significant localization of white blood cells to the joint and release of inflammatory mediators. This is clinically demonstrated by the intense pain that occurs within the joint caused by infection, and the significant pain relief that occurs when the joint is lavaged of those inflammatory mediators and cells.

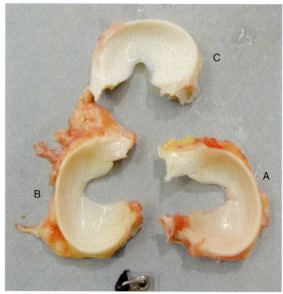

FIGURE 4-6 Gross images of the menisci from a horse with chronic stifle pain. Note the elongated shape to the damaged meniscus (**A**) as well as the meniscus from the contralateral side (**B**). This horse was a high-level Western performance athlete. (**C**) A meniscus from a similar-sized horse of the same age as in **A** but that was not an athlete.

SUMMARY

The biomechanical influences on joint tissues are complex and difficult to measure; however, as measurement techniques become more user friendly, the equine industry will begin to commercialize methods that are promoted as lameness/disease monitors. These techniques should be closely scrutinized through objective experimental and clinical studies. In addition, as the pathologic mechanisms that lead to disease are better understood, the neuromuscular influence on joint disease needs to be further studied to better understand and modify the individual animal's response to injury. There is concern that once injured, an animal's individual pain threshold and associated response to the injury can worsen the primary disease.

REFERENCES

1. Pool RR, Meagher DM. Pathologic findings and pathogenesis of racetrack injuries. *Vet Clin North Am Equine Pract.* 1990;6(1):1–30.
2. Kawcak CE, McIlwraith CW, Norrdin RW, et al. The role of subchondral bone in joint disease: a review. *Equine Vet J.* 2001;33(2):120–126.
3. Martig S, Chen W, Lee PVS, et al. Bone fatigue and its implications for injuries in racehorses. *Equine Vet J.* 2014;46(4):408–415.
4. McIlwraith CW, Frisbie DD, Kawcak CE, et al. The OARSI histopathology initiative – recommendation for histological assessments of osteoarthritis in the horse. *Osteoarthritis Cartilage.* 2010;18(suppl 3):S95–S105.
5. Powell SE. Low-field standing magnetic resonance imaging findings of the metacarpo/metatarsophalangeal joint of racing Thoroughbreds with lameness localised to the region: a retrospective study of 131 horses. *Equine Vet J.* 2012;44(2):169–177.
6. Roemer FW, Frobal R, Hunter DJ, et al. MRI detected subchondral bone marrow signal alterations of the knee joint: terminology, imaging appearance, relevance and radiological differential diagnosis. *Osteoarthritis Cartilage.* 2009;17(9):1115–1131.
7. Schenker ML, Mauck RL, Ahn J, et al. Pathogenesis and prevention of posttraumatic osteoarthritis after intraarticular fracture. *J Am Acad Orthop Surg.* 2014;22(1):20–28.
8. Drum MG, Kawcak CE, Norrdin RW, et al. Comparison of gross and histopathologic findings with quantitative computed tomographic bone density in the distal third metacarpal bone of racehorses. *Vet Radiol Ultrasound.* 2007;48(6):518–527.
9. Thompson Jr RC, Oegma Jr TR, Lewis JL, et al. Osteoarthrotic changes after acute transarticular load. An animal model. *J Bone Joint Surg Am.* 1991;73(7):990–1001.
10. Vekens EV, Bergman EH, Vanderperren K, et al. Computed tomographic anatomy of the equine stifle joint. *Am J Vet Res.* 2011;72(4):512–521.
11. Crijns CP, Gielen IMVL, van Bree HJJ, et al. The use of CT and CT arthrography in diagnosing equine stifle injury in a Rheinlander gelding. *Equine Vet J.* 2010;42(4):367–371.
12. Barrett MF, Frisbie DD, McIlwraith CW, et al. The arthroscopic and ultrasonographic boundaries of the equine femorotibial joints. *Equine Vet J.* 2012;44(1):57–63.
13. Comeford EJ, Smith K, Hayashi K. Update on the aetiopathogenesis of canine cranial cruciate ligament disease. *Vet Comp Orthop Traumatol.* 2011;24(2):91–98.
14. Pool RR. Pathological manifestations of joint disease in the athletic horse. In: McIlwraith CW, Trotter GW, eds. *Joint disease in the horse.* Philadelphia, PA: Saunders; 1996:98–99.
15. Frost HM. Joint anatomy, design and arthroses: insights of the Utah paradigm. *Anat Rec.* 1999;255(2):162–174.
16. Silver FH, Bradica G, Tria A. Viscoelastic behavior of osteoarthritic cartilage. *Connect Tissue Res.* 2001;42(3):223–233.
17. Tull TM, Bramlage LR. Racing prognosis after cumulative stress-induced injury of the distal portion of the third metacarpal and third metatarsal bones in Thoroughbred racehorses: 55 cases (2000-2009). *J Am Vet Med Assoc.* 2011;238(10):1316–1322.
18. Norrdin RW, Kawcak CE, Capwell BA, et al. Subchondral bone failure in an equine model of overload arthrosis. *Bone.* 1998;22(2):133–139.
19. Norrdin RW, Kawcak CE, Capwell BA, et al. Calcified cartilage morphometry and its relation to subchondral bone remodeling in equine arthrosis. *Bone.* 1999;24(2):109–114.
20. Kawcak CE, McIlwraith CW, Firth EC. Effects of early exercise on metacarpophalangeal joints in horses. *Am J Vet Res.* 2010;71(4):405–411.
21. Kawcak CE, McIlwraith CW, Norrdin RW, et al. Clinical effects of exercise on subchondral bone of carpal and metacarpophalangeal joints in horses. *Am J Vet Res.* 2000;61(10):1252–1258.
22. Turley SM, Thambyah A, Riggs CM, et al. Microstructure changes in cartilage and bone related to repetitive overloading in an equine athlete model. *J Anat.* 2014;224(6):647–658.
23. Kawcak CE, Frisbie DD, Werpy NM, et al. Effects of exercise vs experimental osteoarthritis on imaging outcomes. *Osteoarthritis Cartilage.* 2008;16(12):1519–1525.

24. Carter DR, Hayes WC. Compact bone fatigue damage: a microscopic examination. *Clin Orthop Relat Res*. 1997;127:265–274.

25. Boyde A. The real response of bone to exercise. *J Anat*. 2003;203(2):173–189.

26. Firth EC, Doube M, Boyde A. Changes in mineralised tissue at the site of origin of condylar fracture are present before athletic training in Thoroughbred horses. *N Z Vet J*. 2009;57(5):278–283.

27. Alber MT, Brown MP, Merritt KA, et al. Vascular perfusion of the dorsal and palmar condyles of the equine third metacarpal bone. *Equine Vet J*. 2014;46(3):370–374.

28. Walker WT, Kawcak CE, Hill AE. Medial femoral condyle morphometrics and subchondral bone density patterns in Thoroughbred racehorses. *Am J Vet Res*. 2013;74(5):691–699.

5

Osteochondritis Dissecans

P. René van Weeren

HISTORY AND TERMINOLOGY

The surgical removal of fragments from a joint was reportedly performed for the first time in 1558 by the famous French surgeon Ambroise Paré (1510-1592), who is generally regarded as the father of modern surgery, based on the immense expertise he gained on many battlefields.[1] However, nothing is known of the nature of the fragments removed by Paré, which may well have been traumatic in origin. The term "osteochondritis dissecans" (Latin for inflammation of bone and cartilage resulting in the formation of loose fragments) was first used by the German surgeon Franz König (1832-1910). In his study on loose bodies in joints he discussed three possible causes. First, severe trauma that would lead to breaking off of fragments through direct mechanical impact. Second, lesser trauma causing necrosis of subchondral bone that would at a later stage result in separation of fragments. Third, fragments formed without any substantial trauma but because of some (unidentified) underlying lesion.[2] Evidence for the existence and nature of such underlying lesions came 50 years after König's publication when Ribling (cited by Barrie, 1987[3]) published his radiologic studies on disturbances of the process of endochondral ossification.

In human literature the term "osteochondritis dissecans" (OCD) has from the start led to much confusion, as the term is used for articular fragmentation of many different causes.[3] In the equine veterinary literature the term is almost exclusively used for König's third category (i.e., for fragmentation based on disturbances of endochondral ossification). In 1986 Poulos[4] defined the terms "osteochondrosis," "osteochondrosis dissecans," and "osteochondritis dissecans," which are often incorrectly used as synonyms, as follows: osteochondrosis is the disorder itself, osteochondritis is the inflammatory response to it, and in OCD an area of cartilaginous or osteochondral separation is present. These are very good working definitions. This does not mean, by the way, that the terminology in the equine literature has been always unambiguous. Far from that. After the recognition in the 1970s and early 1980s that foals, especially those from fast growing breeds, may exhibit a wide variety of orthopedic growth disturbances, there has been a tendency to group these all together as manifestations of a single syndrome. The term "metabolic bone disease" to cover this syndrome was first used and stood for some time.[5] However, this was not the best choice, as the term is commonly used in human medicine in cases of mineral loss of bone caused by osteoporosis,[6] which is a disease of elderly people rather than a developmental disorder. In 1986 the term "developmental orthopedic disease" (DOD) was coined by a panel of specialists.[7] This term encompasses virtually all noninfectious orthopedic faulty developments of growing, young horses of which OC is the most common, but which includes also cervical vertebral malformation (Wobbler disease), collapse of cuboidal bones, angular and flexural limb deformities, bone cysts, and physitis.

The term "osteochondrosis" has withstood many attempts at being replaced by other names that were deemed more appropriate, such as "dyschondroplasia" or "chondrodysplasia."[8] These latter terms may reflect better the developmental background of the diseases and the pathologic changes in cartilage formation that are characteristic of OC, but they have the disadvantage of already being used for certain hereditary growth disturbances causing short stature and/or vertebral or limb deformities in humans and animals.[9] Further, the terms do not recognize the extensive involvement of (subchondral) bone in OC.

Recently, a consensus paper was published that introduced a new term, juvenile osteochondral conditions (JOCCs), for those developmental orthopedic disorders that are related to the immature joint or growth plate.[10] The term includes OC(D), cuboidal bone disease, and various other forms of failure of the immature skeleton such as formation of (articular) juvenile bone cysts, osteochondral collapse, or avulsion at insertion sites and physitis. The term does not include Wobbler disease, flexural limb deformities, or angular limb deformities unrelated to developmental skeletal disorders. With the terms DOD for the wide panel of orthopedic disorders related to disturbances in musculoskeletal development, JOCC for the subset of lesions representing the different types of epiphyseal/metaphyseal developmental disorders, and OC(D) for the specific disturbance of endochondral ossification of the articular-epiphyseal complex, semantics now seem well covered with a maximum of clarity in an area that has long been confusing.

THE PROCESS OF ENDOCHONDRAL OSSIFICATION

In all mammals the primordial skeleton is laid down first as a cartilaginous structure that already during the fetal stage starts to transform into bone, a process that continues until well after birth. During this entire period there are thus two processes simultaneously going on: growth and ossification (Figure 5-1). Unlike mature articular cartilage, these fetal cartilaginous structures are well vascularized by vessels running through so-called cartilage canals. Ossification of the primary centers of ossification in the diaphyses of the long bones starts early in fetal life, and at the time of birth, all diaphyses are bony structures. However, many secondary centers of ossification located in the epiphyses of the long bones and in other sites such as apophyses and cuboidal bones in complex joints are still partly cartilaginous at the time of birth.

Longitudinal growth of long bones is effectuated by the growth plates or physes. In these structures from a germinal layer of cells (resting cells), chondrocytes proliferate and lay down a scaffold of extracellular matrix. These cells subsequently hypertrophy and later go into apoptosis. The scaffold forms the basis for the apposition of primary bone by osteoblasts that originate from the metaphysis (Figure 5-2). The primary spongiosa that is formed will undergo continuous remodeling under the influence of biomechanical loading according to Wolff's law during the entire growth period of the foal. In the mature animal, the process of remodeling of the bone will continue when loading changes, for instance, when the skeleton is exposed to athletic challenges, providing

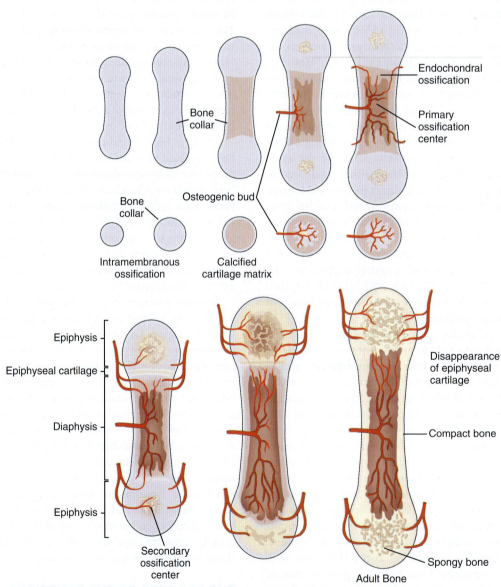

FIGURE 5-1 Semischematic drawing of the ossification process of the long bones in mammals. After closing of the growth plates, the only cartilage left is the articular cartilage. Note the rich vascularization of the cartilaginous precursor of the long bone and the absence of vascularization of mature articular cartilage. (From: Van Weeren P.R. (2006). Etiology, diagnosis and treatment of OC(D). Clin Techn Equine Pract, 5(4), 248-258.)[238]

the animal with the ability to adapt to changes in biomechanical challenges.[11] This entire process of cartilage remodeling, followed by calcification of cartilage, deposition of primary bone, and successive remodeling into bony trabeculae as occurring in the young, growing animal, is known as endochondral ossification.[12]

Transversal growth (increase in diameter) of the long bone is the product of a different but simultaneous and coordinated process and is realized by appositional growth from the periosteum. This results in the formation of compact cortical bone around the Haversian canals.

In the epiphyses of the long bones a similar growth process takes place, but is less advanced than in the diaphyses at birth. Initially there is a complete ring of cartilage around the ossification center that is located in the center of the epiphysis, connecting the cartilage at the articular side with the growth plate. Ossification of this cartilage ring takes place first at the border of the physis and at the perimeter of the epiphysis. The thick cartilage mass at the articular side of the epiphysis functions as a type of growth plate with simultaneously occurring processes of growth, remodeling, and ossification. It is at this level that the characteristic lesions of equine osteochondrosis develop. After cessation of growth a considerably thinner layer of articular cartilage remains in the mature animal. Whereas the thick layer of epiphyseal growth cartilage seems a homogeneous mass at macroscopic inspection and plain microscopy, in fact the epiphyseal growth cartilage that will eventually turn into bone and the articular cartilage that will remain are distinct tissues that can be discerned already during early gestation. In a benchmark study on the early development of articular cartilage a research group from Québec investigated very early changes in epiphyseal growth cartilage and articular cartilage (and the relationship between the two) in both fetuses (6 to 11 months gestation length) and neonates (0 to 8 days). Using picrosirius red staining and polarized light microscopy, they could clearly identify the future layer of articular cartilage and differentiate this in fetuses of 6- to 8-month gestation time from the epiphyseal growth cartilage that would become (subchondral) bone[13] (Figure 5-3). Modern imaging technology facilitates in vivo monitoring of the process of endochondral ossification and lesion formation/resolution,[14] and further progress in basic knowledge about this process can be expected.

CLINICAL PRESENTATION OF OC

The typical OC patient is a yearling that presents with effusion of the tarsocrural or femoropatellar joint. The horse usually is not lame, and radiographic examination may show a fragment at the cranial end of the distal intermediate ridge of the tibia (Figure 5-4) or irregularities at the lateral trochlear ridge of the distal femur (Figure 5-5).

However, many variations on this theme are possible. Age at which the disease becomes manifest can vary from young foals (which may sometimes present with large lesions in the femoropatellar joints causing severe lameness) to horses over 10 years old. However, in this last category lesions must have been present in a clinically silent form from foal age, as OC(D) is a disorder of endochondral ossification and no new lesions can possibly form after cessation of this process. OC often becomes manifest at the age the animals are put into training and the joints become biomechanically challenged by athletic activity. The age at which this occurs varies with the equestrian discipline and is hence also breed-related. Warmblood horses typically start athletic activities at about 3 years of age or older and racing Thoroughbreds and Standardbreds start work at about 18 months. Histopathologic signs of synovial inflammation have been shown to be associated with effusion but not with other clinical signs, including lameness.[15] Radiographic signs may also be less severe than the presence of fragments and may show as minor irregularities in the articular contour of the subchondral bone or as only a flattening of this contour. Further, other joints may be affected. Most common are the metacarpophalangeal and metatarsophalangeal joints, but OC has been diagnosed in virtually all diarthrodial joints. Osteochondrosis in cervical facet joints is quite common and has long been related to cervical stenotic myelopathy, being a cause of the "wobbler syndrome" in young horses.[16] However, the relationship does not seem to be straightforward, although common pathogenetic pathways may exist.[17] Sufficiently powered epidemiologic studies linking cervical facet joint OC (Figure 5-6) at juvenile age with the occurrence of ataxia in older animals are still lacking at present.

Radiography has long been and still is the gold standard for diagnosing OC. Minor radiographic aberrations can be reliably classified as OC by an experienced radiologist. In one study, there was a correlation of 0.87 ($P < 0.001$) between radiographic classification of OC of the distal intermediate

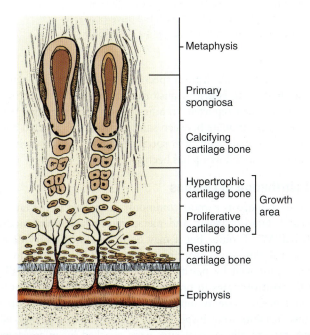

FIGURE 5-2 Schematic representation of the process of growth and ossification of long bones that takes place at the level of the physis. (From: Van Weeren P.R. (2012). Osteochondrosis. In: Auer J.A., Stick J.A. (Eds.) Equine surgery (4th ed.) (pp. 1239-1255). St. Louis, MO: Elsevier-Saunders.)

Metaphysis

Primary spongiosa

Calcifying cartilage bone

Hypertrophic cartilage bone

Growth area

Proliferative cartilage bone

Resting cartilage bone

Epiphysis

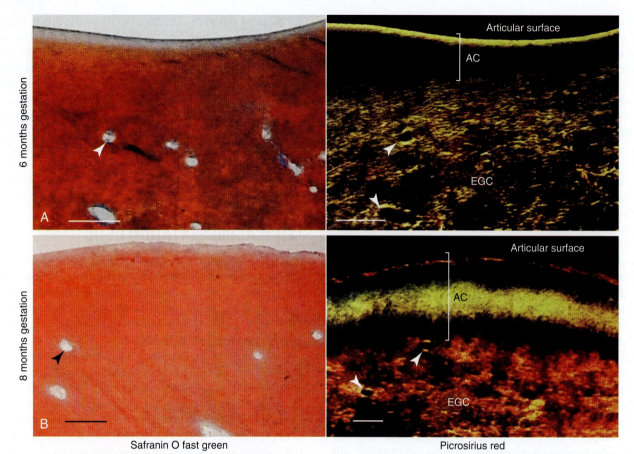

FIGURE 5-3 Equine fetal cartilage (**A**) 6-month-old fetus; (**B**) 8-month-old fetus stained with safranin O fast green and picrosirius red. In the picrosirius red-stained sections viewed under polarized light microscopy, the future articular cartilage can be clearly distinguished; this is not possible in the safranin O fast green-stained sections. *AC,* Articular cartilage; *EGC,* epiphyseal growth cartilage. Arrowheads: cartilage canals in the EGC, not present in the AC. Scale bars = 500 μm. (From: Lecocq M., Girard C.A., Fogarty U., et al (2008). Cartilage matrix changes in the developing epiphysis: early events on the pathway to equine osteochondrosis? Equine Vet J, 40, 442-454.)

ridge of the tibia on a 0 to 4 scale[18] and histology.[19] However, this diagnostic modality has several drawbacks: lesions limited to the cartilage layer may be more severe than radiographic appearance suggests, or cartilaginous lesions may be present without changes in the subchondral bone and hence not detectable. Subtle bony lesions may also be easily missed because of superposition with other structures. In very young animals the low mineralization grade of the subchondral bone may preclude diagnosis of all but the larger lesions. All in all, specificity of radiography for the detection of OC lesions is quite good, but sensitivity is not very high. More advanced diagnostic modalities such as CT and MRI perform better.[20] High-field MRI is a useful tool to image the layer of articular cartilage, but this technique remains expensive and its availability is limited. Ultrasonography has become increasingly used to image the integrity of joint surfaces and has proven to be a very useful, widely available and relatively inexpensive tool to diagnose OC that outperforms radiography on those joint surfaces that can be imaged using this modality.[21,22] Also, other approaches using a variety of biochemical and molecular markers have been tried with varying success. Further, the

use of infrared absorption spectral characterization of synovial fluid using Fourier-transform infrared (FTIR) spectroscopy has been reported. In a first report this technique was able to discriminate between samples from OC-affected and normal animals with 50% specificity and 73% sensitivity.[23] However, no follow-up has been given since.

Distribution of Lesions

Osteochondrosis is most commonly diagnosed in the tarsocrural, femoropatellar, and metacarpo/metatarsophalangeal (MCP/MTP) joints, but it may occur in almost every diarthrodial joint. In an experimental study, 43 Warmblood foals were produced by pairing OC-positive sires with partially OC-positive mares to produce offspring with a high prevalence of OC. Twenty-four foals were sacrificed at 5 months and all joints were inspected at necropsy. Subsequently, all macroscopically suspect sites were checked by microscopy to confirm the diagnosis of OC.[24] Lesions were found to be most numerous in the tarsocrural joint (average of two lesions per animal), followed by the femoropatellar and the cervical intervertebral (facet) joints (one lesion per animal),

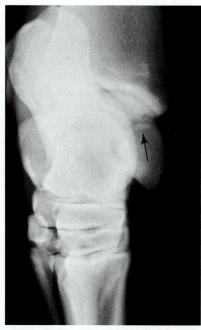

FIGURE 5-4 Radiograph showing a typical osteochondritic lesion of the dorsal aspect of the distal intermediate ridge of the tibia (arrow). (Courtesy Dr. AJM van den Belt, University of Utrecht, Netherlands. IN Auer JA, Stick JA: Equine Surgery, 4th edition, St. Louis, 2012, Elsevier Saunders.)

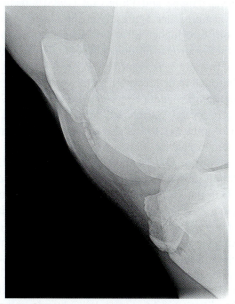

FIGURE 5-5 Oblique radiographic view showing osteochondrotic fragmentation at the lateral trochlear ridge of the distal femur. (Courtesy AJM van den Belt, Utrecht University. IN Van Weeren PR: Etiology, diagnosis and treatment of OC(D). Clin. Techn. Equine Pract. 5, 248-258, 2006.)

MTP joint (0.6), MCP and carpal joints (0.4), humeroradial joint (0.2), and scapulohumeral joint (0.04).[19] The prevalence of OC in this study was artificially high and not representative for the overall population, but the relative distribution is in agreement with clinical experience in the Warmblood. There are breed differences with regard to lesion distribution

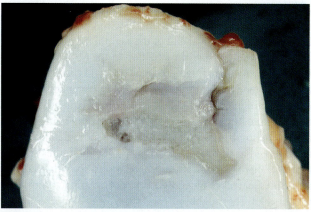

FIGURE 5-6 Osteochondrotic lesion on the articular surface of the caudal intervertebral process of the sixth vertebra. (From: Van Weeren P.R., Barneveld A. (1999). The effect of exercise on the distribution and manifestation of osteochondrotic lesions in the Warmblood foal. Equine Vet J, 31(Suppl 31):16-25.)

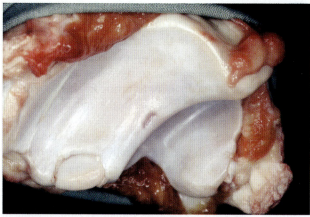

FIGURE 5-7 Typical osteochondrotic lesion of the distal intermediate ridge of the tibia at necropsy. The thin cartilage area in the center of the intermediate ridge is a synovial groove, which is a physiological phenomenon in non-weight bearing areas common to many diarthrodial joints. (From: Van Weeren P.R. (2012). Osteochondrosis. In: Auer J.A., Stick J.A. (Eds.) Equine surgery (4th ed.) (pp. 1239-1255). St. Louis, MO: Elsevier-Saunders.)

and relative clinical importance. In Warmbloods and Standardbreds, tarsocrural OC is most frequent,[25-29] but in racing Thoroughbreds femoropatellar OC is the predominant manifestation.[30]

Lesions of OC almost always occur at certain predilection sites within a joint. In the tarsocrural joint, the most common site is the cranial end of the distal intermediate ridge of the tibia (Figures 5-4 and 5-7), followed by the distal end of the lateral trochlea of the talus and the medial malleolus of the tibia.[31] In the femoropatellar joint, the lateral trochlear ridge of the femur is most commonly affected. Less common sites here are the medial trochlear ridge of the femur, the trochlear groove, and the distal end of the patella.[32] Subchondral cysts in the medial femoral condyle are not uncommon and a manifestation of osteochondrosis as well. These are discussed in depth in the following chapter. In the shoulder joint, osteochondrosis is commonly located on the glenoid and the humeral head.[33] The predilection site in the MCP/MTP joints is the dorsal end of the sagittal ridge of the metacarpus and metatarsus. The situation in the MCP/MTP joints is complex, as many fragments may occur in these joints that are not osteochondrotic in origin. Palmar or plantar osteochondral fragments (so-called POFs) are frequently seen in these joints. They were originally reported as being part of the osteochondrosis complex,[34] but after more detailed studies emerged as traumatic in origin.[35,36] Later studies showed that POF had a significant linear relationship with grades of wear lines, cartilage ulceration, and dorsal impact injuries in a cohort of Thoroughbred racehorses, and hence could be classified as a manifestation of traumatic overload arthrosis.[37] A histologic study on POFs harvested from mature (average age 6 years) horses made clear that, even in long-present intraarticular fragments, histology may give an indication about the original etiology; there were more indications of osteoarthritis (higher Mankin score) in fragments than of osteochondrosis.[38] The different pathogenetic events that are going on in joints with OC-based fragments and traumatic fragments are reflected in the markers of collagen metabolism that can be detected in the synovial fluid. In joints with osteochondrotic fragments the collagen degradation marker C2C was increased and in joints featuring fragments on traumatic basis there was an increase in the collagen synthesis marker CPII.[39]

Lesions are often encountered bilaterally in the tarsocrural and femoropatellar joints and bilaterally or even quadrilaterally in the MCP/MTP joints.[40] Bilateral presence, however, often with unilateral clinical manifestation, can occur in the tarsocrural and femoropatellar joints in more than 50% of clinical cases.[32] In horses with unilateral clinical signs in one of these joints it is therefore advisable to examine the contralateral joint radiographically as well. Concomitant occurrence in other joints or joint pairs is much less common, which probably has to do with the differences in time windows during which OC lesions develop in different joints (discussed later). In a study of 225 horses with OC in the tarsocrural joint, lesions were found in other joints in not more than eight cases.[40] For this reason, there is generally no need to examine joints other than the contralateral, unless clinical signs exist.

PREVALENCE AND EVOLUTION OF OSTEOCHONDROSIS

An Emerging Disease

The first report on what is retrospectively judged to have been OC appeared in 1947 when Nilsson described fragments in the femoropatellar joints of Ardenner horses.[41] In the following decades some reports described intraarticular fragments that might have been osteochondrotic[42] and even the term osteochondrosis was used,[43] but the real history of OC starts with the classic publication by Birkeland and Haakenstad in 1968.[44] The authors described a series of seven cases of OC of the distal ridge of the tibia, but still did not use the term.

From the early 1970s onwards more publications started to appear,[45,46] but the breakthrough came in the mid-1970s when a comprehensive study on osteochondrosis in a multitude of species was published.[47-51]

Osteochondrosis is a very common disorder, at least radiographically. It has been estimated that annually 20,000 to 25,000 foals are born in northwestern Europe that will develop some degree of OC.[24] The prevalence is high in many breeds and the disease is frequently diagnosed radiographically in the racing breeds. Many of the initial surveys have been carried out in Scandinavian countries. In Swedish Standardbreds, a prevalence of 10.5% was reported in the tarsal joints,[28] which is comparable to the 12% found by others[26] but considerably less than the figure of 26% reported in earlier work on Scandinavian Standardbreds.[52] A high prevalence of 35% in Standardbreds in a Canadian population was reported in the femoropatellar and MCP/MTP joints combined.[53] There are fewer studies in Thoroughbreds, but the prevalence in that breed is reportedly relatively high as well.[33,54,55] Low figures of 4% OC in the tarsocrural joint and 3% in the femoropatellar joint are mentioned in a study on New Zealand Thoroughbreds. However, the study was based on the evaluation of repository films taken at yearling sales, which means that the population was strongly preselected and the figures are thus of limited value.[56]

The first data on the Warmblood horse also come from Scandinavia. Hoppe and Philipsson (1985)[52] mentioned a 15% prevalence. Later figures from the Dutch Warmblood population were higher (25% in the tarsocrural joint and 15% in the femoropatellar joint).[18] A study on 1180 horses in France (mainly Selle Français and Anglo-Arabs, a minority of Thoroughbreds), reported a prevalence of 13.3% in the tarsocrural joint,[29] and a large-scale field study in Germany focusing on several Warmblood breeds noted 19.5% for the MCP/MTP joints, 11.1% for the tarsocrural joint, and 7.2% for the femoropatellar joint.[57] In a study almost a decade later in almost 10,000 Hanoverian Warmbloods, Hilla and Distl[58] found substantially smaller figures: 5.4% of the horses had OCD in the MCP/MTP joints, the tarsocrural joint was affected in 6.9% and 2.6% had OC in the femoropatellar joint. In a nonpreselected population from a single breeder and comprising views of the distal and proximal interphalangeal, metacarpophalangeal and metatarsophalangeal, tarsocrural, and femoropatellar joints, radiographic evidence of OC(D) was found in not less than 44.3% of clinically sound Dutch Warmblood horses.[59] In general, Warmbloods are at higher risk to develop OC than Thoroughbreds.[60] Recent work in Norwegian Trotters found a prevalence of tarsocrural OC/OCD of 19.3%. The prevalence of OC/OCD in MCP joints was not more than 3.6%.[61]

Not all types and breeds of horses suffer from OC to the same degree. Osteochondrotic lesions are only rarely encountered in ponies.[62] It is interesting to note that in feral horses the disease is not nonexistent, but the prevalence is low. In a survey of 80 feral horses, an extremely low prevalence of 2.5% was found in the tarsocrural joint and no signs of OC were seen in the femoropatellar joint.[63] Because osteochondrosis is a disease that has been described only relatively recently and of which the incidence has soared from the 1970s onwards, these observations strongly implicate breeding policies and possibly management aspects as key factors in this disease.

Age-dependent Spontaneous Repair: the Dynamic Character of Osteochondrosis

Osteochondrosis was originally seen as a largely static condition, but this concept gradually changed. Strömberg (1979)[64] reported changes in the radiographic appearance of femoropatellar OC after repeated radiographic examinations. Other researchers observed, after taking sequential radiographs of foals, that osteochondrotic lesions of the distal femur could progress until the age of 9 months.[65] In the same year, another group published a study in which they followed a cohort of 77 horses by sequential radiographing and found that no major new osteochondrotic lesions developed after the age of 8 months in the tarsocrural joint. Interestingly, the regression of a number of minor lesions before the age of 8 months was also observed. These lesions had been first detected between ages 1 and 3 months.[27]

In a large experimental study focusing on the influence of exercise at early age on the development of osteochondrosis, the EXOC study (for exercise and osteochondrosis),[24] the tarsocrural and femoropatellar joints of 43 foals were radiographed on a monthly basis from the age of 1 month until age

5 months and in 19 of these until age 11 months. That study showed that not only minor lesions but also radiographically visible larger fragments could repair spontaneously[18] (Figure 5-8). The predominant ages at which lesions originated and at which most of them had spontaneously healed varied for each joint (Figure 5-9A-C). In the tarsocrural joint, most of the lesions at the distal intermediate ridge of the tibia and at the distal aspect of the lateral trochlear ridge of the talus that had been detected within the first few months of life had repaired spontaneously, and hence become undetectable on radiographs, before the age of 5 months. After that age no major changes occurred and lesions still existing at that moment remained visible. In the femoropatellar joint, of which the epiphyseal maturation is known to be late compared with other joints,[13,66] lesions originated later and peaked at approximately 6 months before declining in number until about 8 months, after which the situation remained stable[18] (Figure 5-9C).

This highly dynamic character of OC, in which multiple lesions are formed at early age—the majority of which will, however, resolve without leaving traces in the following months—was confirmed in later longitudinal studies. In a study focusing on the influence of nutrition on OC in the French Saddlebred[67] that also featured sequential radiographic examinations, a similar pattern emerged. In the BOSAC (Breeding, Osteochondral Status, and Athletic Career) study, a large field study on JOCCs conducted in

1 month
Large concavity/fragmentation

2 months
Fading fragment

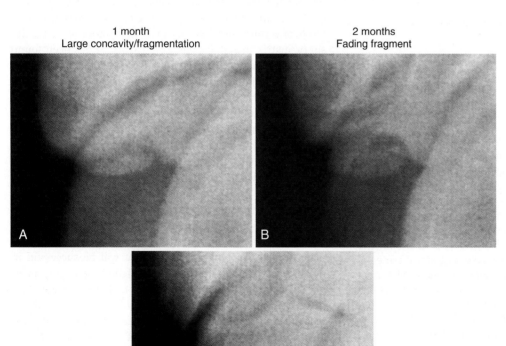

3 months
Normal

FIGURE 5-8 Complete resolution of a lesion at the intermediate ridge of the distal tibia. At 1 month there is a large concavity with fragmentation, at 2 months the fragments fade, and the lesion has resolved at age 3 months. (From: Dik K.J., Enzerink E.E., van Weeren P.R. (1999). Radiographic development of osteochondral abnormalities, in the hock and stifle of Dutch Warmblood foals, from age 1 to 11 months. Equine Vet J, 31(Suppl 31), 9-15.)

France on 400 foals born in 2002, 2003, or 2004,[68,69] 85.7% of the osteochondrotic lesions in the femoropatellar joint were found to regress (disappear or improve) between 6 and 18 months. In the tarsocrural joint, 53.1% of OCD lesions of the intermediate ridge of the tibial cochlea remained stable, confirming the differences in progression-regression patterns

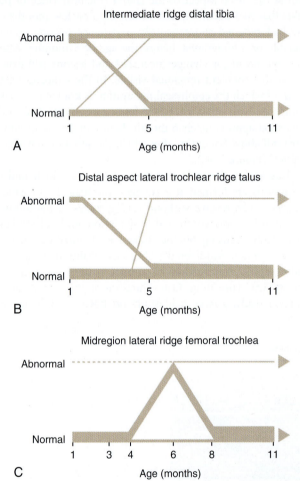

A, Schematic diagram of the early development

FIGURE 5-9 A, Schematic diagram of the early development of osteochondral lesions at the distal intermediate ridge of the tibia. At age 1 month several lesions are already detectable. Most of these will heal (thick arrow, pointing down). Only a few lesions originate after the age of 1 month (thin arrow pointing upwards) and from the age of 5 month the situation remains stable. **B,** Comparable diagram of the early development of osteochondral lesions at the distal aspect of the lateral trochlear ridge of the talus. The same general pattern exists as in (A), but the healing potential is better. **C,** Diagram of the early development of osteochondral lesions of the lateral ridge of the femoral trochlea. The pattern is clearly distinct here, probably because the development of the femoropatellar joint lags behind in comparison to most other joints of the limbs. Lesions develop only after the age of 3 months, peak at about 6 months, and for the most part have resolved at the age of 8 months, although some may remain. (From: Dik K.J., Enzerink E.E., van Weeren P.R. (1999). Radiographic development of osteochondral abnormalities, in the hock and stifle of Dutch Warmblood foals, from age 1 to 11 months. Equine Vet J, 31(Suppl 31), 9-15.)

per joint.[70] There may be breed differences. In an interesting study in Lusitano foals, Baccarin et al (2012)[71] confirmed the dynamic character of OC and the general pattern established by earlier studies, but found more lesions in the femoropatellar joint at the early age of 1 month than in the original study by Dik et al. (1999).[18] Also, they established the "age of no return" at 12 months, rather than the originally proposed 5 months for the tarsocrural joint and 8 months for the femorotibial joint. Indeed, in most cases a stable situation has been reached at age 12 months and it seems most safe and practical to stick to that age for the entire animal. After that age no major OC lesions will be formed anymore, nor will existing large lesions resolve. Minor changes are still possible, however, as was confirmed in a study in which Warmblood foals were followed for 24 months.[72] In that study, very little change in radiographic appearance was noted from 12 to 24 months.

The dynamic character of OC in which lesions appear and apparently heal (and thus may disappear) during the first months of life can be explained by the interaction of several etiologic factors (see later) and the specific characteristics of articular cartilage metabolism in young, growing horses.

Whereas the metabolic activity of mature articular cartilage is reputedly low with reported half-life times for articular collagen of more than 100 years,[73] the situation is essentially different in the young, growing individual where continuous remodeling and formation of cartilage takes place. The huge difference in metabolism is reflected well by synovial fluid levels of certain proteinases. The concentration of stromelysin or matrix metalloproteinase-3 (MMP-3) has been found to be increased 80-fold in samples from fetal joints compared with levels in joints from mature individuals. At young age (5 to 11 months) MMP-3 levels had fallen dramatically, but were still two-fold to three-fold higher than in mature joints.[74] This pattern is exemplary for the change in cartilage metabolism over time with extremely high levels of turnover at the fetal and neonatal stage that decrease rapidly after birth, but still remain significantly higher up to at least 1 year of age (see also Chapters 1 and 8). It is in this period of initially turbulent remodeling that the process of endochondral ossification, in itself a feature of growth and development, takes place. Lesion formation is incited by etiologic factors (see later) and immediately triggers a repair response that will be successful in most cases thanks to the large remodeling capacity of juvenile articular cartilage. However, the metabolic activity and hence the capacity for repair reduces sharply after birth, so that with increasing age lesions will heal with more difficulty. The gradual closing of the window of repair—that will preclude the repair of either lesions that have originated late or that are too large—differs per joint. The femoropatellar joint lags considerably behind the tarsocrural joint, which explains the difference in time course of the evolution of lesions in different joints (Figure 5-9A-C). Lesions that remain after the window for repair has closed in a certain joint may become clinically manifest, either when the joint is challenged because of increased loading (e.g., when training starts), or earlier.

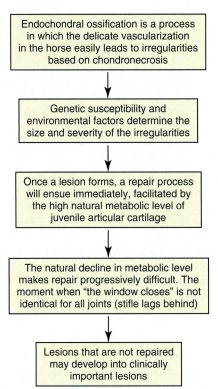

```
┌─────────────────────────────────────┐
│  Endochondral ossification is a       │
│  process in which the delicate        │
│  vascularization in the horse easily  │
│  leads to irregularities based on     │
│  chondronecrosis                      │
└─────────────────────────────────────┘
                  │
                  ▼
┌─────────────────────────────────────┐
│  Genetic susceptibility and           │
│  environmental factors determine the  │
│  size and severity of the irregularities │
└─────────────────────────────────────┘
                  │
                  ▼
┌─────────────────────────────────────┐
│  Once a lesion forms, a repair process│
│  will ensue immediately, facilitated  │
│  by the high natural metabolic level  │
│  of juvenile articular cartilage      │
└─────────────────────────────────────┘
                  │
                  ▼
┌─────────────────────────────────────┐
│  The natural decline in metabolic     │
│  level makes repair progressively     │
│  difficult. The moment when "the      │
│  window closes" is not identical for  │
│  all joints (stifle lags behind)      │
└─────────────────────────────────────┘
                  │
                  ▼
┌─────────────────────────────────────┐
│  Lesions that are not repaired        │
│  may develop into clinically          │
│  important lesions                    │
└─────────────────────────────────────┘
```

FIGURE 5-10 Flow chart of events over time in OC, emphasizing the dynamic character of the disorder in which many of the lesions that originate will repair, depending on the age of the animal. (From: Van Weeren P.R. (2012). Osteochondrosis. In: Auer J.A., Stick J.A. (Eds.) Equine surgery (4th ed.) (pp. 1239-1255). St. Louis, MO: Elsevier-Saunders.)

Figure 5-10 presents a flow chart for the putative sequence of events in OC based on this concept. The fact that clinical OC can be considered as the final outcome of at least two complex, but probably unrelated, processes (the initiation of lesions by specific etiologic factors and the ensuing probably largely unspecific repair process,[75,76]) makes OC into a very complex disorder.

The Relative Value of Figures for the Incidence or Prevalence of Osteochondrosis

Given the dynamic character of OC as explained previously, figures on the incidence or prevalence of OC should be considered with utmost caution. The age at which a population is screened is important and any survey performed at ages younger than approximately 12 months cannot be considered to be representative of a stable situation. However, the common ages for screening by studbooks (3 or 4 years) is also far from ideal, as any form of preselection by breeders (which is common) will affect prevalence figures as well. The effects of these factors may be dramatic. In a study on 811 yearlings that had not been preselected, a staggering 67.5% prevalence was reported in Dutch Warmbloods, when combining results from tarsocrural, femoropatellar, MCP, and MTP joints.[77] When measured at the age of 3 years, the mean figure for this breed is approximately 30%. A similarly high prevalence for tarsocrural and MCP/MTP OC (61.7%) was found in a population of South German Coldbloods that contained many young animals.[78] It can be stated that all surveys conducted at the conventional ages of 3 or 4 years yield severe underestimations of the real prevalence of OC. Further, even surveys conducted in populations that have not been preselected will not identify animals that have had (radiographically detectable) OC lesions in one or more joints at foal age and that have resolved spontaneously afterwards. Studies such as the above-mentioned EXOC study, in which the development of lesions in foals was followed, suggest that the percentage of animals that have had lesions at foal age but are clean when radiographed at adult age may be considerable. This is of great importance for the definition of nonsufferers in genetic studies and may be one of the reasons why genetic research into OC (see later) has yielded relatively little conclusive data thus far. A last important point when considering epidemiologic OC data is the fact that OC has been described in almost every diarthrodial joint, but screenings are normally restricted to a few joints only. These factors and the differences in experimental design between many surveys make comparisons between these studies a very hazardous undertaking and may explain the large range of percentages that have been reported.

THE PATHOPHYSIOLOGIC MECHANISM BEHIND OSTEOCHONDROSIS

Although there has always been consensus in the veterinary literature that OC is a disturbance of the process of endochondral ossification of the articular epiphyseal complex, there has been ample controversy about the etiopathogenesis. Despite many attempts to do so, no single causative factor, environmental or genetic, could be pinpointed, and the disease is now generally acknowledged to be multifactorial. The pathogenetic mechanism was long thought to be of primary biomechanical nature, but excellent and original work in pigs and horses by Scandinavian groups has now provided convincing evidence for a predominantly vascular pathogenetic mechanism. A large problem in the research in this field is that samples were often taken from long-existing lesions that had undergone extensive secondary processes, which had long effaced any possible traces of primary events.[79] This problem is much larger still in human medicine where it is virtually impossible to get hold of material from very early (and almost invariably asymptomatic) patients.[80] In almost all studies using clinical material it is unfortunately not possible to say whether any abnormalities are primary or the expression of a secondary response, as it is known that the reactive repair process starts immediately after the initial lesion formation. The evidence for a vascular pathogenetic mechanism for OC comes from experimental studies.

Vascular Events in Early OC

The thick layer of epiphyseal cartilage of the growing joint that is destined to change into bone via the process of endochondral ossification is irrigated by vessels running through so-called cartilage canals. These canals were described as early as 1933 by Wheeler Haines, who stated that *"the primary function of cartilage canals is the nutrition of cartilage too large to be supplied by diffusion of nutriments through their substance."*[81] The author also described the gradual process of obliteration of these canals, called chondrification, which precedes ossification. This last process is time-dependent and varies per joint, as not all joints mature simultaneously, which is exemplified by the sometimes large differences in closure times of physes.[82] In a study on chondrification of cartilage canals in the distal end of the proximal phalanx, the distal end of the tibia, and the medial femoral condyle, patent cartilage canals were not seen in the proximal phalanx after age 3 weeks, but in the femoral condyle they were still present at 4.5 months (which had all disappeared at age 7 months). The distal tibia was in between.[83]

The initial studies on the vascularization of juvenile cartilage, the physiologic process of regression of cartilage canals, and the disturbances thereof as possible causes for OC have mostly been conducted in the pig, a species in which OC is common and a cause of important economic losses. The regression of cartilage canals is a highly predictable process that follows an age-dependent pattern, as revealed by a study on femoral condyles of pigs.[84] It had been shown earlier in this species that areas of chondronecrosis related to obliterated cartilage canals can be found, which are much larger in commercial pig breeds than in miniature pigs of wild hog ancestry.[85] Artificial devascularization can create islands of cartilage without vascular supply, which may develop into OC-like lesions.[86] These observations led to the hypothesis that premature interruption of the vascular supply of the growth cartilage of the articular epiphyseal complex may lead to necrotic areas in the cartilage layer, which can subsequently become engulfed in the ossification front and result in the typical irregularities and cartilage islands seen in OC.[87] In a follow-up study in which only a limited number of cartilage canals was sectioned, OC-like lesions could also be produced,[88] suggesting that OC is caused by local biomechanical damage to cartilage canals, especially to the anastomosing branches that run through the ossification front from the bone marrow.[89] The initial chondronecrotic areas that do not give rise to clinical symptoms are not visible macroscopically or with help of standard imaging methods and are called *osteochondrosis latens*. Depending on environmental factors and the efficacy of the repair process, these lesions may resolve or become clinically apparent, in which case they are designated as *osteochondrosis manifesta*.[90] Recent genetic work has provided further indirect support for the involvement of vascular disturbances in the pathogenesis of OC. In a genome-wide association study in pigs, an SNP in the gene encoding T-box transcription factor 5 (TBX5), a transcription factor interacting with two genes involved in vascularization, was significantly associated with OC lesion scores.[91]

The process of endochondral ossification is similar in mammalian species and OC is common in many of them. Therefore a similar early pathogenesis as in the pig would presumably occur in the young foal. In a cross-sectional study in random source foals (ranging from 191 days gestation to

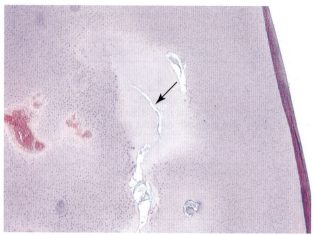

FIGURE 5-11 Microphotograph of a femur of a 114-day-old foal. The arrow indicates a necrotic cartilage vessel, surrounded by an area of necrotic matrix. (From: Olstad K., Ytrehus B., Ekman S., et al. (2011). Early lesions of articular osteochondrosis in the distal femur of foals. Vet Pathol, 48(6), 1165-1175.)

153 days old), lesions resembling those in pigs, that is, characterized by chondrocyte necrosis and apparently caused by cartilage canal failure, were present in the distal tibia of 9 out of 100 animals[92] (Figure 5-11). Interestingly, in all but the two youngest individuals (aged 12 and 18 days) an ongoing repair process was also noted. A follow-up experimental study of the development of the vascularization of the tarsus in seven very young foals (0 to 7 days old) used a special technique in postmortem specimens to clear the tissues surrounding the vessels to obtain a good view of the vascular structure. It elegantly showed how the advancing ossification front induces a change in the arterial supply of the cartilage canals. Whereas the cartilage canals are initially supplied by arteries from perichondral origin, the advancing ossification front engulfs the midportion of the vessels in the canal. Subsequently, a shift occurs such that vessels in the distal terminus come to use subchondral, rather than perichondral, vessels as their arterial source. At the site where these vessels traverse the ossification front, they are supposed to be more vulnerable to mechanical influences (Figure 5-12). In this study the authors found 12 lesions, characterized by areas of chondronecrosis, in these seven foals (that were genetically more susceptible to the development of OC). All lesions were located where vessels crossed the ossification front to supply cartilage canals.[93] In a similar study focusing on the distal femur, another predilection site of osteochondrosis, the same authors found in principle similar changes in vascularization, but the regression of blood vessels was much less extensive at this early age than in the tarsus and no lesions could be found.[94] This agrees with the fact that the femoropatellar joint lags behind in its development[13,66] and that the peak of osteochondrotic lesion development is later than in most other joints.[18] In a later study, lesions were found in 7 of 30 foals. Again, the lesions were located in regions where cartilage canal vessels traversed the chondro-osseous junction. Lesions were found in animals from 31 to 336 days old (mean 148 days).[95] In the MCP/MTP

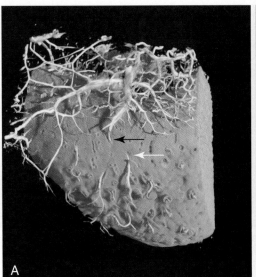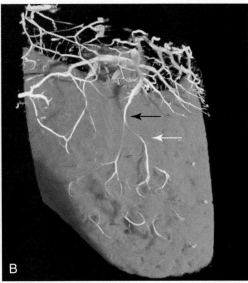

FIGURE 5-12 Images of three-dimensional volume-rendered models of micro-CT scans of a tissue block (measuring approximately 2 cm in all directions) from the cranial part of the distal intermediate ridge of the tibia of a 3-week old foal. The block contained a permanent barium angiogram, and only the grayscale segments representing barium and bone are shown. **A,** A vessel originating from the perichondrial plexus on the cranial aspect of the distal tibia courses into the subchondral bone towards the cranial apex of the distal intermediate ridge (black arrow). Distal and caudal to this, towards the distal articular surface of the intermediate ridge, vessels emerge into the growth cartilage directly from subchondral bone (white arrow). **B,** The greyscale segment for bone has been rendered less opaque/more translucent than in (**A**), illustrating how the midsection of cartilage canal vessels is incorporated into the advancing ossification front during growth. This traversing of junctions between tissues of different qualities such as bone and cartilage is believed to render vessels particularly vulnerable to failure. (Images courtesy of Dr. K. Olstad, Norwegian School of Veterinary Science. IN Auer JA, Stick JA: Equine Surgery, 4th edition, St. Louis, 2012, Elsevier Saunders.)

joint, again the pattern of changes in vascularization was similar; in this case one ("latens") lesion was found.[96] A very interesting observation made by microcomputed tomography of the early lesions was that the secondary repair process follows almost immediately after formation of the lesion[97] (Figure 5-13). The final proof for the role of vascular disturbances in the pathogenetic mechanism of OC in the horse was provided by an experimental study in which at the age of 13 to 15 days two vessels supplying the epiphyseal growth cartilage of the lateral trochlear ridge of the left distal femur were transected in 10 pony foals. The animals were one by one sacrificed at 1, 4, 7, 10, 14, 21, 28, 35, 42, and 49 days after surgery, respectively. It appeared that transection of blood vessels running in epiphyseal cartilage canals resulted in ischemic chondronecrosis that was associated with a focal delay in endochondral ossification (OC) in foals examined 21 days or more after transection. In one foal a pathological cartilage fracture (OCD) was observed 42 days after transection.[98]

Thus failure of vascularization through occlusion of cartilage canals plays a crucial mechanistic role in the early pathogenesis of OC in the horse, which is contradictory to a suggestion in earlier work on cartilage canals in the horse where it was speculated that cartilage canal retention rather than premature closure was related to dyschondroplasia.[99] Many features of equine OC, such as the joint-specific time windows (related to joint-specific patterns in the progress

of the ossification front and subsequent vascular rearrangements), and the frequent bilateral occurrence can be easily explained in this way. However, it should be realized that the complex vascular rearrangements that take place during the process of endochondral ossification and that create a window of vulnerability are common to all individuals of a species and not only to those developing osteochondrotic lesions. Therefore, there are other, etiologic factors that incite lesion formation during this vulnerable period. Biomechanical loading is a very obvious candidate here, but other factors, such as differences in the biochemical and/or biomechanical characteristics of key tissue components, may play a role, too. These factors may be either genetically or environmentally determined and may be heavily influenced by the management of the young horse. These factors, which are dealt with in the paragraph on etiologic factors, will determine in the end why a given horse will develop OC and another will not.

Molecular Events in OC

Many studies have focused on changes in the events at cellular and molecular level in OC-affected tissue compared with normal tissue. However, here a caveat should be made; given the strong interaction of lesion formation and the repair process as signaled earlier, it is hardly ever possible in observational studies to determine with certainty which and to what extent observations can be ascribed to the primary pathogenesis of

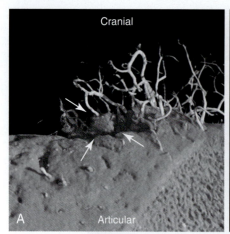
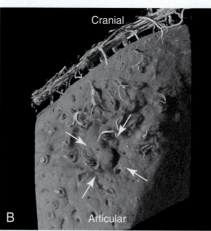
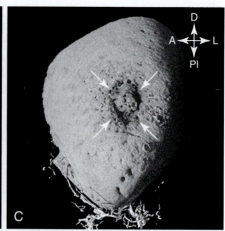

FIGURE 5-13 Lesions of osteochondrosis associated with ongoing ossification. The figure shows images of three-dimensional volume-rendered models of blocks containing permanent barium angiograms; only the grayscale segment representing bone and barium is shown. *A*, Axial; *D*, dorsal; *L*, lateral; *Pl*, plantar. **A**, 2-week-old foal, distal intermediate ridge of tibia, oblique distal view: A perfused vessel descended on the cranial aspect of the process to terminate within the growth cartilage immediately superficial to a triangular indented defect in the subchondral bone plate. The vessel terminus was surrounded by a spherical bone opacity (arrows). This appearance was compatible with a separate center of ossification, seen as an early manifestation of the repair process. **B**, 3-week-old foal, intermediate coronoid process, distal view: There was a circular indented defect in the subchondral bone plate (arrows). The defect was partially filled by a hemispherical bone opacity. In cross-section, endochondral ossification appeared to be progressing within the hemisphere. **C**, 7-week-old foal, lateral trochlear ridge, distal view. There was a circular indented defect in the subchondral bone plate (arrows) that was partially filled by a hemispherical bone opacity, representing the repair process. (From Olstad K, Cnudde V: Masscahele B, et al. Micro-computed tomography of early blood supply of osteochondrosis in the tarsus of foals, Bone 43(3):574-583, 2008.)

OC lesions and which are secondary. The borderline between the OC lesion itself and repair tissue is vague, probably because the onset of repair is almost immediate after formation of a lesion and because events are taking place in juvenile cartilage that still has considerable regenerative capacity. When comparing OC tissue with tissue from healing, surgically created osteochondrotic fragments, the two could not be discerned. Both resembled an anabolic, reparative process when compared with age-matched controls. However, the OC tissue bed stained positive for chondroitin sulfate and collagen type II, and the fracture bed did not.[66]

The Chondrocyte in OC

Chondrocytes freshly harvested from fetal growth cartilage undergo hypertrophy and subsequently apoptosis when cultured in either the commonly used fetal calf serum, or horse serum, in a situation that strongly resembles the natural process of endochondral ossification. Chondrocytes from animals older than 5 months old did, however, not undergo hypertrophy and chondrocytes from neonates (7 days) showed intermediate behavior.[100] This study once more stresses the importance of age when studying OC.

Chondrocytes harvested from early osteochondrotic lesions have a higher metabolic level (in terms of proteoglycan synthesis measured as ^{35}S-incorporation), but cannot be stimulated to an overall higher level than chondrocytes from normal

cartilage by addition of serum. Interestingly, when harvested from longer-existing lesions, their native metabolic rate is lower than in normal cells and stimulation is hardly possible anymore.[101] This phenomenon may indicate a reactive up-scaling of metabolic activity in response to lesion formation, which, when repair is unsuccessful, may develop into some stage of exhaustion and loss of vitality of the chondrocytes. Given the sequence of events, this is almost certainly a secondary phenomenon that can explain why OC lesions in arthroscopically removed fragments had significantly lower quantity of uronic acid, total GAG, and CS, compared with normal cartilage.[102]

Failure to undergo hypertrophy has been suggested as a main cause for OC.[103,104] However, this was disproved in a study in which OC was induced in 3- to 6-month-old foals by a high-energy diet and in which the expression of hypertrophy-related genes such as collagen I, II and X, matrix metalloproteinase-13 (MMP-13), and the transcription factor Runx2 (known to induce hypertrophy and expression of type X collagen and of MMP-13), was investigated. The higher expression of collagen X and MMP-13 (the main matrix metalloproteinase involved in collagen degradation) indicated that failure of chondrocytes to undergo hypertrophy is not the cause of OC.[105]

Hormonal Factors

Parathyroid hormone-related protein (PTHrP) and Indian hedgehog (Ihh) have a well-known role in controlling cartilage differentiation and hypertrophy in the growth plate.[106] Bone morphogenic proteins serve as signaling peptides. The hypothesis that these molecules would have a similar role in cartilage differentiation in the equine articular-epiphyseal complex and hence could be implicated in the pathogenesis of OC was tested by measuring parathyroid hormone-related peptide and Indian hedgehog expression patterns in samples from naturally acquired equine osteochondrosis. Indeed, elevated PTH-rP protein and mRNA expression were identified in the deeper layers of affected articular cartilage and there was a trend in Ihh.[107] However, expression of bone morphogenic proteins 6 and 2 was not changed.[108] Also, expression of transcription factors Gli1 and Gli3 was not increased, suggesting either a different transcription factor in osteochondrotic tissue, a dysfunction in local receptor activation, or elevations in Ihh inhibitors. It should be noted that these investigations were performed on samples from horses aged 6 to18 months, which makes their outcome likely to be representative for early repair rather than for the pathogenesis of lesions.[104] In a more recent study animals aged 1 to 6 months were used. Equine-specific Ihh, PTH-rP, vascular endothelial growth factor (VEGF), platelet-derived growth factor (PDGF)-A, MMP-13, and MMP-3 mRNA expression levels were evaluated by real-time (RT)-PCR. In full-thickness cartilage samples, there was significantly increased Ihh, MMP-3, and MMP-13 gene expression in OC samples, suggesting alteration of pathways involving cartilage maturation and ossification in early OC.[109]

Collagen

Much work has been done comparing normal and abnormal (dyschondroplastic) cartilage with respect to the expression of the various collagen types present in the extracellular cartilage matrix (collagen types II, VI, and X), and with respect to the expression of the major growth factors (TGF-β, IGF-I, IGF-II) known to play a role in the development and maturation of cartilage.[110-114] Not unexpectedly, there are distinct differences in expression with high levels of activity around the chondrocyte clusters or chondrones in early cases of OC, in line with the overall increase in chondrocyte metabolism mentioned earlier, which most likely represents an attempt at repair[115] and hence is secondary. In agreement with the higher metabolic activity is the increase in activity of gelatinases (MMP-2 and MMP-9) in osteochondrotic cartilage.[116] Also, levels of matrix metalloproteinases (MMPs) were found to be elevated in copper-deficient horses with clinical OC lesions.[117] However, expression of membrane-type matrix metalloproteinase-3 (MT3-MMP) is not significantly altered in osteochondrotic cartilage.[118] The distribution of cathepsins B, D, and L in normal and abnormal cartilage has been studied by the group from Cambridge. They found physiologic differences in distribution,[119-121] but also a strong increase in cathepsin B activity in chondrocyte clonal clusters in OC,[122] which observation was later confirmed in a study on the effect of copper supplementation.[123]

Gene Expression

The different signature of osteochondrotic cartilage with respect to proteoglycan and collagen metabolism was further detailed by a study on expression patterns and chondrogenic potential of osteochondrotic cartilage (from mature animals) versus normal cartilage (from age-matched controls). In this study OC cartilage showed increased expression of collagen types I, II, III, and X and of MMP-13, ADAMTS-4, and TIMP-1 and decreased expression of TIMP-2 and TIMP-3.[124] Additional evidence for the crucial role of collagen was provided by studies demonstrating differences in posttranslational modifications of collagen type II in samples from early lesions.[125] Pellet cultures produced from OC tissues contained significantly less GAGs,[124] which is in agreement with earlier work like that of van den Hoogen et al.[101]

Subchondral Bone

Relatively little work has been done on the subchondral bone underlying the cartilage defects, but changes in bone morphogenic enzymes and in membrane lipid composition of the cellular components of the subchondral bone have been demonstrated.[126] Interestingly, there is a strong correlation between serum osteocalcin levels in synovial fluid as early as at 2 weeks of age with radiographically scored OC at 5.5 and 11 months and postmortem scores at 11 months (i.e., when lesions had become virtually immutable),[127] indicating the implication of bone in the early events in OC. In another study where serum from foals aged 1 to 49 days was used no such correlation was found,[128] which may indicate that osteocalcin is reflecting very early events indeed and osteocalcin might therefore be a potential marker for the susceptibility of individual animals to develop OC.

ETIOLOGIC FACTORS

Whereas there now is strong evidence for a single, uniform early pathogenetic mechanism of OC in the form of damage to the vessels in the cartilage canals with ensuing chondronecrosis, the etiologic factors that trigger this pathogenetic chain of events are multiple. They include, as in many disorders, genetic and environmental components. In both fields much progress has been made in recent years. The rapidly developing molecular genetic techniques have facilitated an intensive quest for genes that could be associated with OC and related genetic markers. The first large field study on juvenile osteochondral conditions,[10] a subset of the group of DOD[129] of which OC is the most important, has yielded many interesting results with respect to the influence of a number of management factors.[69] These consist of two main groups: those related to biomechanical loading of the joint, such as exercise regimen and roughness of terrain, and those related to nutrition. There are, therefore, three main categories of etiologic factors: genetics, biomechanical factors, and nutritional factors.

Genetics

There are large differences in the incidence of OC between wild animals and their domesticated counterparts of the same species and between breeds of animals. Osteochondrosis seems to be nonexistent in wild boars, but has a very high incidence in many breeds of domesticated pigs.[87] As mentioned earlier, in a population of feral horses (that stem from domesticated horses but have not undergone artificial selection for a long time) the prevalence of OC was very low[63] and in ponies osteochondrotic lesions have been reported, but are very rare.[62] These are all strong indications for an important role of genetics in OC.

Many studies have been performed to determine heritability estimates (h^2) for OC. However, this area is far from straightforward. Because of the dynamic and complex character of OC, any genetic study is heavily dependent on the definition of the phenotype. In all heritability studies with regard to OC, the phenotype is determined radiographically. This means that the phenotype is dependent on the radiographic protocol with less extensive protocols featuring limited numbers of views such as used for large-scale field studies[130] being more likely to detect fewer lesions than the very extensive protocols used for repository films at sales.[56] Although having a large variety of number of views is very important in the clinical setting, to judge the value of individual animals at sales and give well-founded advice to the owner, the lesions that are missed when using field protocols are of less impact on large epidemiologic field studies that aim at establishing the prevalence of OC in a population. For those studies the impact of preselection (owners screening their animals beforehand and not presenting them at selection events when affected, thus biasing the outcome of prevalence studies) is more important. Another confounding factor is that in some studies all osteochondral fragments are counted as OC lesions whereas others discriminate between fragments likely to be osteochondrotic in nature and those known to be of other origin, such as the POFs alluded to earlier. The outcome of genetic studies will also depend on whether OC is defined at the animal level or at the joint level and, given the highly dynamic character of the disorder, on the age at which phenotypic measurements are performed. Lastly, not all studies use the same methodology. Sire models only account for paternal half-sib relationships. Animal models use information on all relatives of an animal without reduction to specific structures of relatives. Osteochondrosis is virtually always a categorical variable and in those cases a threshold model or a transformation to the underlying distribution has to be applied to avoid underestimation of the heritability.[131] All these factors together make genetic studies on OC somewhat hazardous and may explain why the reported heritabilities vary widely.

Reported values for heritability of OC in the tarsocrural joint range from 0.04 (in South German Coldbloods[132]) to 0.52 (in Standardbred Trotters[133]), but most values are around 0.30.[26,134-138] For the metacarpophalangeal/metatarsophalangeal joints these figures are lower at approximately 0.15,[132,137,139] but occasionally higher values are mentioned.[135,140,141] Ricard et al. (2013)[141] reported an h^2 of 0.29, but this figure relates to all juvenile osteochondral conditions, of which OC is a subset. Data on the femoropatellar joint are scarce, but reported heritabilities are substantially lower than for other joints, staying consistently under 0.10[135,139] with values as low as 0.05 for OC and 0.02 for OCD in the Dutch Warmblood.[137] The last study consistently discriminated between OC without (OC) and with (OCD) fragmentation and discovered that heritabilities were distinct; within all joints OC was to a larger degree heritable than OCD. For a detailed overview see the review by Distl (2013).[131]

A heritability is a population measure that is specific to the population and environment under scrutiny. It measures the proportion of the phenotypic variance that is the result of genetic factors. The higher the heritability, the quicker progress can be made. The heritabilities that were found for OC were deemed by several studbooks to be high enough to warrant some kind of selection and many studbooks have implemented such programs. However, any progress has been slow. The Royal Dutch Warmblood Studbook (KWPN) has long followed a strict selection program. They started rejecting any candidate sire with any sign of tarsocrural OC in 1984 and of femoropatellar OC in 1992, but no substantial decrease in incidence had been realized in the mid-2010s. This in contrast to the conditions of navicular disease and bone spavin, where a similar selection policy had been followed and where a substantial decrease in incidence had been realized.[142] There are various explanations for this that relate to the confounding factors for heritability studies referred to earlier. First, both population genetic studies and molecular genetic investigations (see later) have now made clear that different genes are involved in different joints. This translates to different heritabilities for different joints. The study by van Grevenhof et al. (2009)[137] even suggests that different manifestations of OC (fragmentation versus flattening of the joint) may represent different traits. A second complicating factor for the genetic approach of OC is its dynamic nature. Many animals are radiographically free of lesions at age 3 or 4 years when they enter the stallion selection process and are subject to routine radiographic screening, yet they will have had evidence of the disease as a foal. Hence, these foals are genetically predisposed to OC and will pass this trait on. A third and not unimportant factor is that some traits that are known to be implicated in OC (such as a high growth rate) are seen as desirable and actively selected for. The complexity of the genetic background of OC (and the pressure from breeders, who saw approximately 30% of their products with often promising performance potential eliminated each year because of often tiny OC lesions) has urged certain studbooks to change their breeding policies. The KWPN now uses a more differentiated approach, classifying lesions on an A-E scale with A being normal and E showing large lesions. Animals with limited number of B-C lesions may now still pass. It is up to the breeders to decide whether or not to mate their mares with such a stallion. This decision may depend on the OC status of the mare and the balance between the higher risk of OC and the expected positive effects of such a mating. Further, approval is temporary and data from the first crops of offspring are now included in the selection procedure and used to calculate breeding values. If a provisionally approved sire produces a high prevalence of OC in its offspring, it may still be eliminated.

Advances in molecular genetics have been tremendous in the past decades. The genome of the horse was published in 2009[143] and in 2008 the first equine microarray containing more than 54,000 single nucleotide polymorphism markers (SNPs) came on the market, allowing genome-wide association studies.[130] Osteochondrosis was among the first disorders to be investigated by quantitative molecular genetic techniques. The outcome of those studies gave further evidence for the complexity of OC. Linkage and association analyses and genome-wide association studies identified regions of the genome that were associated with some phenotypic manifestation of OC on not less than 22 of the 33 chromosomes of the horse.[130,140,144-155] Most of these quantitative trait loci (QTL) were breed specific, and there is little overlap between metacarpophalangeal and metatarsophalangeal OC and tarsal OC, suggesting a different genetic background.[130,137] Based on these molecular genetic studies, several candidate genes that are potentially implicated in OC have been identified (Table 5-1). Many of these genes cannot be directly related to cartilage or bone turnover, but have more general roles. The equine gene for collagen IX that is located on chromosome 2 harboring a QTL for osteochondrosis has been characterized, but no significant association with OC could be made.[156] An interesting QTL has been identified on chromosome 18, located very closely to the parathyroid hormone 2 receptor gene.[151] This PTH2R gene has earlier been implicated in familial early-onset osteoarthritis (OA) in humans.[157] As mentioned earlier, in the pig the gene encoding T-box transcription factor 5 (TBX5) has been identified as being associated with OC,[91] which is potentially very interesting as this transcription factor is involved in vascularization. No data on the horse exist thus far.

Another molecular genetic approach was taken by a group that compared gene expression profiles of leucocytes from horses affected by OC and normal controls. They identified dysregulation of a number of pathways, among others Wnt, Ihh, and TGF-β signaling, in OC-affected animals.[158] Ihh is an interesting target, given its role together with parathyroid hormone-releasing peptide (PTHrp) in the feedback loop involved in chondrogenesis.[107] However, the problem with this approach, as with the earlier described genome-wide scans, is that material from horses with established OC is used so that no discrimination can be made between primary and secondary processes. In a study on genetic polymorphism of the Ihh gene no relation with OC could be demonstrated in Polish Halfbreds.[159] Scientifically, the work performed on very young foals from the experimental study by Olstad et al. (2008)[93] on vascular changes in the growth cartilage is more interesting. In that study the Tousler-like kinase 2 gene (TLK2) and an unknown gene were found to be upregulated in foals predisposed to OC.[160]

Clearly, the genetic background of OC is complex and not very easy to unravel. An important limiting factor in genetic OC research is the lack of homogeneity in the definition of the phenotype, which inevitably leads to differences in outcome. Another point is that there is now mounting evidence that the genetic background is very complex indeed with large differences between breeds, joints, and even manifestations of OC (fragmentation or not). When trying to confirm in Thoroughbreds a number of QTLs found to be associated with OC in Hanoverian Warmbloods only 2 of 24 showed agreement.[144] The phenotypic and genotypic association between OC in the tarsocrural joint and in the MCP/MTP joints has been reported to be very low in various studies.[61,77,137] Hence, there is no doubt that OC is partially genetically determined,

TABLE 5-1   Candidate Genes Potentially Involved in Equine Osteochondrosis as Identified by Quantitative Molecular Genetic Investigations

Abbreviation	Gene Name	#	Phenotypic Trait	Breed	Reference
NCDN	Nerochondrin	2	OC(D) TC; MCP/MTP	HW	Dierks et al. 2010[147]
HECW1	HECT, C2 and WW domain containing E3 ubiquitin protein ligase 1	4	OC TC; MCP/MTP	HW	Dierks et al. 2010[148] (Cited by Distl, 2013)[131]
AOAH	Acycloxyacyl hydrolase	4	OCD MCP/MTP	SGC	Wittwer et al. 2008[236]
CLCA4	Chloride channel, calcium activated, family member 4	5	OC(D) TC; MCP/MTP	NT	Lykkjen et al. 2010[153]
COL24A1	Collagen type XXIV, alpha 1	5	OC(D) TC OC(D) TC; MCP/MTP	HW NT	Lampe et al. 2009[150] Lykkjen et al. 2010[153]
LOC100073151	Protein-coding gene similar to serum/glucocorticoid-regulated kinase	10	OC(D) TC; MCP/MTP		Lykkjen et al. 2010[153]
XIRP2	Xin actin-binding repeat containing 2	18	OC TC; OC(D) MCP/MTP	SGC	Wittwer et al. 2009[237]
PTH2R	Parathyroid hormone 2 receptor	18	OC(D) TC; MCP/MTP	HW	Lampe et al. 2009[151]
FBXO25	F-box protein 25	27	OC(D) TC; MCP/MTP	NT	Lykkjen et al. 2010[153]
TBC1D22A	TBC1 domain family, member 22A	28	OC(D) TC; MCP/MTP	NT	Lykkjen et al. 2010[153]

HW, Hanovarian Warmblood; *MCP/MTP*, metacarpophalangeal/metatarsophalangeal joint; *#*, number of chromosome; *NT*, Norwegian Trotter; *OC(D)*, osteochondrosis (osteochondritis dissecans); *SGC*, South German Coldblood; *TC*, tarsocrural joint.

but this genetic contribution is far from straightforward. It is therefore highly unlikely that OC can ever be selected against using a simple genetic test that detects one or two culprit genes. This does not mean that there may not be a place for genomic selection in the horse in the future.[161] The big advantage of genomic selection is the reduction of the generation interval. However, the large reference populations that are necessary to develop genomic selection strategies are difficult to establish in the equine species.[137] The large differences between the reported heritabilities per joint further show that the relative contribution of genetics to the total variance in the population is variable, with OC in the femoropatellar joint being much more influenced by environmental conditions than other joints. It is clear anyhow that environmental factors contribute relatively more to the manifestation of OC than genetics.

Environmental Factors

There are two major groups of environmental factors that have been identified as playing a role in equine osteochondrosis: biomechanical loading and nutritional factors. Within these wider groups several more specific environmental factors can be discerned. Biomechanical loading is mainly determined by the exercise regimen of the foals or yearlings, but also roughness of the terrain or conformation may be contributing factors. Nutrition will influence growth rate (which in itself is also partially genetically determined), but will, depending on the composition of the ration, also influence hormonal balances, especially with respect to glucose metabolism. Nutritional imbalances may also affect the mineral and trace element status of animals with possible effects on the process of endochondral ossification.

Biomechanical Influences

There is little doubt that biomechanical loading plays an important role in the pathogenesis of OC. The well-defined and consistent predilection sites within joints strongly point in this direction. In fact, biomechanical factors are thought to play a prominent role in the occurrence of the entire group of JOCCs, of which OC is one.[10] It is probable that the dramatic changes in biomechanical loading that take place after birth are an important trigger factor for initiating lesions. In a pathologic study of the femoropatellar and tarsocrural joints of 9 fetuses and 10 foals aged 0 to 35 days, in only one 3-day-old foal and in none of the fetuses was an osteochondrotic lesion detected.[50] Tiny areas of chondronecrosis were found in all 21 fetuses studied by another group, but these were seen as a feature of normal development and not as osteochondrotic lesions, as no specific changes in the collagen matrix compatible with early OC were encountered in any of them.[13] A triggering role for biomechanical forces fits very well with the vascular early pathogenetic mechanism discussed earlier.[80,89] Biomechanical forces—acting on the vessels running in the cartilage canals during the time window when these are especially vulnerable because of progression of the ossification front and related changes in their sources—may well

induce the areas of chondronecrosis that are commonly seen as early lesions of OC. Also the areas in the growth cartilage, notably between the proliferative and hypertrophic zones near the ossification front where a dramatic change in collagen fiber organization has been shown,[13] may be very prone to biomechanically induced trauma. Whether or not a lesion will develop will be determined by the combination of the biomechanical insult (magnitude, direction of force, repetition) and the "quality" of the tissue at that particular moment in time. The latter factor may be influenced by genetics, but also by nutritional and related hormonal imbalances (see next section).

Biomechanical (over)loading of joints may be caused by a variety of causes. In the pig, rough transport has been shown to be an important causative factor of OC.[162] In the horse, the joints are principally challenged by the exercise regimen the animals are subjected to. There is now compelling evidence that in the horse (as probably in most other mammalian species including humans) physical exercise in the juvenile period has a crucial role in the conditioning of the entire musculoskeletal system with consequences for injury resistance and proneness for the development of chronic degenerative joint disorders later in life[163,164] (see Chapter 8 for a more exhaustive discussion). It is exactly in this early juvenile period of rapid growth and development that osteochondrotic lesions develop and these processes are therefore intricately linked.[75] Hence, exercise can be expected to be an important factor in the development of OC, and it seems likely that an optimum should exist between lack of exercise, known to affect cartilage composition in a permanent fashion,[164] and biomechanical overloading caused by excessive exercise. Experimental data indicate that this indeed seems to be the case.

In a preliminary study, in which controlled exercise was given to foals from 3 to 24 months of age using a high-speed horse walker, the incidence of OC was found to be 6% in the high-exercise group and 20% in the low-exercise group. These results seemed to point at an important protective effect of exercise, but unfortunately the results were flawed because of a concurrently running nutritional study employing different energy levels that were not consistently provided.[165,166] The large EXOC study mentioned earlier did not yield conclusive results, although there was a tendency toward a decrease in severity of OC lesions in the exercised groups.[19] In a large field study, one researcher found fewer OC lesions on the distal sagittal ridge of the metacarpus and metatarsus in the MCP and MTP joints of foals that got more exercise during the first months of life. There was, however, no effect on the incidence of OC in the tarsocrural joint.[167] The other large field study mentioned earlier, the so-called BOSAC study, was more conclusive. It showed there were associations of both the prevalence and the severity of osteochondrotic lesions with irregular access to pasture, as well as with keeping animals in very large plots.[60,168] From the same study it became clear that "mixed housing" (stabling overnight and pasture access during the daytime, as opposed to continuous housing in either stables or at pasture) and rough and slippery grazing grounds were risk factors as well.[169] These results are in line with another study on the relationship between breeding management and OC in which it was shown that foals housed exclusively at pasture until 1 year of age are significantly less affected by OC than foals exclusively housed in box or, alternatively, in box and at pasture.[170]

It can be concluded that, apart from direct blunt trauma that will cause an osteochondral fracture, biomechanical forces are considered a necessary additive factor rather than a sole cause of OC. Exercise is certainly a factor codetermining the final appearance of osteochondrotic lesions, but does not seem to be of primary pathogenetic importance. A balanced exercise regimen, in which at least a minimal basic level of exercise is given to allow for the proper development of the musculoskeletal system in general and articular cartilage in particular and characterized by regularity and devoid of high peak loading, is most protective against osteochondrotic lesions.

Nutrition: Growth Rate, Energy Intake, and Mineral Imbalances

Nutritional factors have been extensively studied as possible causes for OC. In this research, attention has focused on two distinct areas: imbalances in mineral and trace element supply and excesses in energy intake, the latter with concomitant hormonal disturbances. Research into high-energy intake was prompted by the observation in many species that OC seemed to be principally a disorder of large-framed, rapidly growing individuals or breeds.[47,64] However, the situation turned out to be less simple than that. Several studies found no relation to growth rate,[25,171,172] but others reported a larger prevalence in horses taller at the withers[26,60] or in horses having a higher average daily weight gain.[173] Sometimes this was only true for a limited period of development.[174,175] In the French BOSAC study a poor osteoarticular status (including other disorders than OC alone) was associated with a number of growth variables (overall increase in height from 0 to 6 months, height at the withers, and girth perimeter at 30 days of age), but there was no significant association with feeding practices.[168] However, no accurate estimate of roughage intake was available in this study. The fact that in some studies no direct relationship with absolute body weight is found although there is a relationship between the occurrence of lesions with growth rate in a specific time window, may well be related to the known windows in time when certain joints are more vulnerable to develop osteochondrotic lesions. In a study where a normal level of nutrition was compared with an increase of 120% to 150% in all components of the diet, a fast growth rate was associated with a higher amount of osteochondrotic lesions, regardless whether the fast growth rate was determined by a higher nutritional level or by genetic predisposition.[67] A similar lack of effect of feeding level in foals was seen in a study in 223 foals in Belgium. However, the feeding practice of the mare had an influence in this study in the sense that mares not fed any concentrates during pregnancy were less likely to produce offspring with OC than mares that did receive some quantity of concentrates.[170]

There is now ample evidence to state that a high growth rate, at least a high growth rate during certain periods of time, most likely those coinciding with the various windows of vulnerability of specific joints, is a factor that is associated with more or more severe OC lesions. Mechanistically it is possible that a high growth rate just puts the physiologic process of endochondral ossification under excessive pressure, resulting in larger than normal irregularities and a higher vulnerability of the tissues. However, when the high growth rate is caused by the use of high-energy diets, hormonal imbalances may occur that may have a negative effect on the process of endochondral ossification.

Excessive levels of energy, especially when fed in the form of easily digestible carbohydrates,[176,177] result in a strong postprandial hyperinsulinemia. This response is not the same in all horses and may explain some of the (genetically determined) variation in OC susceptibility, as horses with OC have been shown to have higher postprandial glucose and insulin responses to feeding with high-grain ratios than did normal horses.[178] Insulin and its derivatives insulin-like growth factor (IGF)-I and IGF-II have a direct effect on the process of endochondral ossification. These growth factors act as mitogens for chondrocytes and stimulate chondrocyte survival or suppress apoptosis.[179] Many of today's horses live under strongly changed conditions when compared with their ancestors only a couple of decades ago, because of the changes in societal role of the horse and the related, rather dramatic changes in the keepers of horses. These changes have increased the risk for OC.[180] Many horses are fed excessively and have low activity levels. As in humans, these conditions may lead to obesity and insulin resistance. The latter condition has been related to many pathologic conditions, including laminitis and osteochondrosis.[181,182]

Insulin also stimulates a rapid removal from the circulation of the thyroid hormones T3 and T4,[183] which are involved in the final stages of chondrocyte differentiation and in the invasion of growth cartilage by blood vessels before its conversion to bone.[103] In fact, OC-positive foals have significantly lower IGF-I activity than OC-negative foals.[184] In this way, high carbohydrate levels would induce a transient relative hypothyroidism and hence a retardation of the maturation of growth cartilage. The clinical syndrome of hypothyroidism in horses has indeed been shown to produce skeletal lesions, although they are not equivalent to those seen in OC.[185] It is interesting to note that the effect of carbohydrates on thyroid hormone levels can be demonstrated in weanlings, but is not present in yearlings,[186] which may be a factor in the determination of the specific time windows for OC.

Experimentally, it has been possible to induce cartilaginous lesions by administering diets with high levels of digestible energy.[187,188] A field study in Kentucky on the influence of the season on the occurrence of OC has yielded further circumstantial evidence for the importance of carbohydrate levels in the feed. Early foals appeared to have a significantly higher incidence of OC in the tarsocrural joints, but late foals had a higher incidence in the femoropatellar joints. This seemingly contradictory effect of the season could be explained by the different windows of vulnerability of these joints, which appeared to coincide with the spring and autumn peaks in the energy value of the famous Kentucky bluegrass.[55]

There is hardly any doubt that the nutrition-related hormonal imbalances play a role in the development of equine OC and it may well be that these imbalances increase the vulnerability of the tissues that undergo the complex process of endochondral ossification for early vascular damage as outlined above. However, it is highly unlikely that it is the sole etiological factor, as OC lesions can also be found in horses eating perfectly normal diets without any indication of abnormalities in their insulin metabolism. Further, many lesions provoked by the administration of high-carbohydrate diets were similar but not always identical to clinical OC lesions. Lastly, many lesions were seen in the growth plate.[172] In contrast to other species, clinical OC is rarely, if ever, seen in the growth plate in the horse.

Imbalances in trace elements, especially copper, have been incriminated as possible causes of OC from the early days of OC research. A report on the relationship between low copper levels in serum, ceruloplasmin, and OC raised interest here.[189] Studies were initiated on the effect of low-copper diets[190] and the possible role of zinc in inducing a relative copper deficiency.[191] The mechanism was thought to act via the enzyme lysyl oxidase, a copper-dependent enzyme that is essential for the formation of collagen cross-links. Zinc, as well as cadmium, is a copper antagonist by displacing it from the sulfhydryl binding sites on metallothionein.[192] It was indeed possible to provoke osteochondral lesions resembling those seen in natural OC, but copper or zinc levels had to be excessively low or excessively high, respectively and the lesions were in general more severe than those seen in clinical disease. Nevertheless, epidemiologic studies on the relationship between dietary mineral and trace element levels and the incidence of DOD (DOD in a wider sense than OC alone) in Ohio and Kentucky seemed to give further evidence for a key role of copper.[5]

The original National Research Council (NRC) recommendation[193] of 10 ppm copper in dry matter, based on a study with only four (!) foals,[194] was questioned, and supplementation studies were started to confirm the crucial role of copper. These studies yielded positive results to some extent,[117,195,196] but they certainly were not conclusive enough to incriminate copper deficiency as the sole or even the major cause of OC.[197] Higher dietary copper levels of 20 to 25 ppm[117] or 50 ppm[198] were recommended. The validity of those recommendations was later questioned when it was shown that the low natural copper level of 4.3 to 8.6 ppm in grass in New Zealand, a country with a low incidence of OC and where many horses are kept year round on grass only, was sufficient for a healthy development of bone and cartilage.[199] The evidence on the effect of copper supplementation to pregnant mares is equivocal. Foals are, as many mammalian species, born with a large stock of copper in the liver that declines gradually to normal levels when they eat enough grass to ensure sufficient daily intake.[200] In Thoroughbreds mean liver copper concentrations have been reported to

decline from 374 mg/kg DM at birth to 21 mg/kg DM at 160 days.[201] One supplementation study showed an increase of liver copper concentration in newborn foals after prenatal supplementation of mares during late pregnancy[202] and noted a (minor) reduction in articular cartilage lesions at age 5 months.[199] However, another study conducted in the same country (New Zealand) failed to demonstrate both effects.[203] In both studies lesions were minimal, however, and no clinical OC was seen. Therefore, if any effect on the initiation of lesions exists, it will be minor. However, copper supplementation of pregnant mares or newborn foals, which may also raise liver copper content,[204] may still have clinical benefit. A relationship has been shown between neonatal liver copper concentration and the resolution of lesions, leading to the conclusion that copper had a positive effect on the repair of osteochondrotic lesions but not on their pathogenesis.[205] This will have a positive effect on final outcome as would have any decreasing effect on initiation of lesions. This influence on lesion resolution may explain many of the somewhat contradictory and inconclusive earlier findings.

Mechanistically, the effect of copper via lysyl oxidase has been challenged,[206] but in vitro research yielded additional information on possible mechanisms, as copper appeared to have a chondroprotective effect through reduction of the activity of the proteinases cathepsin B and cathepsin D.[207]

The calcium/phosphorus ratio is important for bone metabolism and (severe) aberrations are well-known to cause various bone disorders. With respect to OC, high calcium levels were shown to have no influence on the incidence in foals, but high levels (four times the NRC recommendation) of phosphorus resulted in significantly more lesions.[208] The mechanism was supposed to act via the induction of secondary hyperparathyroidism, which would lead to increased osteoporosis and subsequent weakening of the subchondral bone. The study is interesting because foals were studied in the period from 2.5 to 6.5 months of age, an age interval that much later was identified as a period when the dynamic process of OC is very active and animals are very susceptible to the disorder.

TREATMENT

Osteochondrosis may manifest as joint effusion without lameness, joint effusion with lameness of varying degrees, or abnormalities only on imaging with no clinical signs. The need and reasons for treatment may vary accordingly. The presence of lameness makes intervention necessary to obtain functional recovery, joint effusion may be treated for esthetic reasons and interventions on asymptomatic joints are often urged by the wish to present "clean" animals at sales and are hence principally economically driven. The (relatively weak, see later) effect of asymptomatic OC on long-term performance may be another reason to treat.

The basic treatment options are conservative treatment and surgical intervention; the latter is the option of choice in the vast majority of cases.

Conservative Treatment

Nonsurgical treatment consists principally of rest and controlled exercise. Systemic NSAIDs and intraarticular medication (corticosteroids to enhance resolution of joint effusion and certain disease-modifying osteoarthritic drugs such as hyaluronan, chondroitin sulfate, or pentosan sulfate) may be administered, but they are not seen as of great value in OC.[209] There may even be some risk associated with medication, as there are anecdotal reports of horses treated with intraarticular corticosteroids to reduce effusion before going to sales that developed acute lameness and suffered from acute stripping of cartilage.[210]

Conservative treatment is the first advised treatment in a limited number of conditions. Theoretically, nonsurgical management can only be expected to be successful in either very young animals, where there is still good capacity for regeneration, or in very mild cases. Small femoral lesions are known to resolve until the age of at least 11 months[18] and can be treated conservatively. Indeed, several animals in three crops of Thoroughbred foals that were longitudinally followed without intervention showed improvement and repair of a variety of stifle lesions.[30] Healing with conservative treatment is deemed likely when lesions are less than 2 cm long and less than 5 mm deep without radiographic fragmentation being present.[210] Also in those cases of OC of the sagittal ridge of the metacarpus or metatarsus where only flattening and no fragments are visible (so-called type I OC), initial conservative treatment is advised.[210] Conservative treatment of OC in the scapulohumeral joint had been qualified as having a very poor prognosis,[211] but recent data suggest that it may be a worthwhile option in mild cases where the glenoidal cavity is involved.[210] Opinions on the treatment of tarsocrural OC differ to a certain extent. Some advise surgical intervention in all cases with clinical signs and when an athletic career has been planned.[210] One group described a favorable outcome of nonsurgical treatment of tarsocrural OC in a group of Standardbreds, half of which were treated nonsurgically and half surgically. The authors noted, however, that these results were biased, because the more severe cases tended to be treated surgically.[212] In racing Standardbreds, single, small, radiographically obvious OC lesions in the tarsocrural joint without effusion did not influence performance, in contrast to joints where there was significant effusion.[134]

Surgical Management

Surgical management is the treatment of choice in most cases.[210,213,214] Since the introduction of arthroscopy in equine surgery in the early 1980s,[215] arthroscopy has taken the place of arthrotomy for almost every possible indication. The advantages of arthroscopic surgery over arthrotomy are numerous: soft-tissue trauma is less, the convalescent period is considerably shorter, and functional and cosmetic recovery is better. Further, a more comprehensive examination of the joint is possible.[32] A direct comparison of arthroscopy with arthrotomy showed that hospitalization time after arthroscopy was almost one fifth of that after arthrotomy. Not unimportantly, horses returned significantly more often to their intended use.[216]

Arthroscopic surgery is widely used on a routine basis in all joints where OC is frequently encountered. Standard approaches and some variations thereof have been described for every relevant joint.[217] The approach is relatively straightforward for the majority of joints where OC is encountered (tarsocrural, femoropatellar, metacarpophalangeal/metatarsophalangeal joints), but is much more difficult in the scapulohumeral joint.[33] After extensive inspection and careful probing of the cartilage to detect loose flaps or hidden cysts, loose fragments and/or loose cartilage flaps are removed and the remaining surrounding tissue débrided (Figure 5-14A-C). Bare subchondral bone should not be débrided too aggressively in young animals, as this tissue is often still relatively soft in them.[210] A relatively recently introduced surgical technique in which polydioxanone pins are used to fix large flaps[218] seems to yield encouraging results. Long-term follow-up in 26 horses with reattached flaps showed a 95% success rate in those horses (n=20) for which long-term performance data were available.[219]

PROGNOSIS

The prognosis after surgical intervention varies by joint and depends on the amount and extent of the lesion. Whereas the very extensive lesions in the femoropatellar joint occasionally encountered in foals are inoperable and carry a poor prognosis, prognosis after surgery is much better for most other manifestations of OC. Nevertheless, the prognosis also depends on the definition of "favorable outcome." In most racing Thoroughbreds and Standardbreds, a favorable outcome means a sound horse that can compete at its maximal athletic capacity. The possible presence of some effusion is of less importance here. In many show horses the biomechanical challenges may be less, but cosmetic appearance is important as well. In horses meant for sale, the only goal of surgical intervention is often to make them look "clean" on the radiographs. In general, prognosis for a return to athletic activity is fair to good for the majority of joints involved.

For the femoropatellar joint a 64% success rate was reported in a mixed population of racehorses and nonracehorses.[220] Horses with smaller lesions (grade I, <2 cm in length) were more successful than horses with larger lesions (grade II, 2 to 4 cm and grade III, >4 cm). The overall figure might be too pessimistic because the study included many horses operated on at a young age before their first performance. Therefore, it included a number of horses that would never have raced anyhow because attrition rates in Thoroughbred training are high and many young horses will never race. Jockey Club records indicate that only about 60% of all Thoroughbreds intended for racing ever reach the starting gate in the United States. In another study that compared arthroscopy with arthrotomy, 19 of 25 arthroscopically treated horses (76%) were able to perform their intended use.[216] A more recent study that analyzed the outcome of arthroscopic treatment of OC lesions of the lateral femoral trochlear ridge in sport horses showed

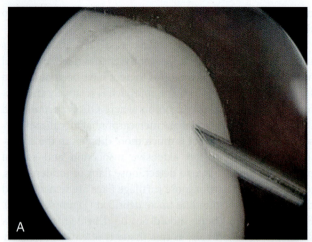

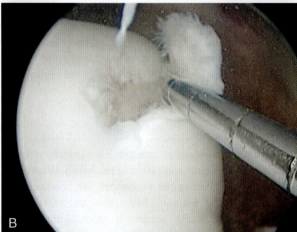

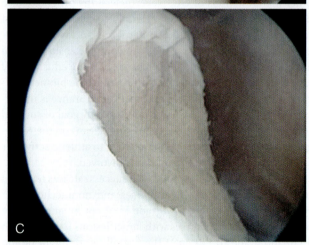

FIGURE 5-14 Arthroscopic views of OCD of the lateral trochlear ridge of the femur before probing (A), during elevation of OCD flap (B), and after débridement of osteochondrotic tissue (C). (From McIlwraith CW: Lameness in the young horse: Osteochondrosis, Chapter 11e. IN Baxter GM (ed): Adams and Stashak's lameness in horses, 6/e, Wiley Blackwell 2011.)

that 29 of 37 horses did not have any complications after surgery. Long-term follow-up was available for 29 horses; of these 19 (65%) were functioning in a fully satisfactory way, 5 performed below the expected level, and 5 could not be used. The depth of the lesion was significantly associated with

short-term complications (effusion and lameness) but not with the long-term outcome. However, involvement of structures other than the lateral trochlear ridge (patella, medial trochlear ridge) was associated with a worse prognosis.[221]

In a large survey of 183 horses operated for tarsocrural OC one group reported success rates of 73% and 83% in racehorses and nonracehorses, respectively. Synovial effusion resolved in 89% of racehorses and 74% of nonracehorses.[31] In a study on 64 Thoroughbreds and 45 Standardbred horses that had been treated for OC by arthroscopic intervention before the age of 2 years and were compared with unaffected (and hence untreated) siblings, less horses raced as 2-year-olds, but a similar proportion raced as 3-year-olds. This indicated that surgery had affected the start of their career but not their overall potential to race.[222] This outcome was in line with another study showing that horses treated surgically for OCD of the distal intermediate ridge of the tibia performed equally well as matched control horses.[212] The overall good prognosis of the surgical removal of OC fragments in the tarsocrural joint was confirmed in a later study in a mixed population of Standardbreds and Warmblood horses in which joint effusion, reaction to the flexion test, and lameness were longitudinally monitored over a period of up to 20 months. Score reductions for lameness and reaction to the flexion test were 80% to 90% and around 50% for resolution of joint effusion.[223]

In the MCP and MTP joints the most frequently seen location of OC is the sagittal ridge of the metacarpus/metatarsus. A discrimination is made between lesions type I (flattening only), type II (flattening with fragmentation), and type III (flattening with or without fragmentation at the lesion site and a loose body present). Whereas type I is treated conservatively, advised treatment for types II and III is surgical. In one study a successful outcome was reported in 57% of cases after surgery. This figure is negatively biased because 18% of the cases were classified as unsuccessful for other reasons that made the horse unsuitable for use.[224] A more recent source mentions a 90% return to athletic activity rate if the lesion is located in the more proximal part of the sagittal ridge but an unspecified lower rate for lesions in weight-bearing areas.[225] A frequently encountered problem with the more severe lesions when treated at a late stage is the quick development of osteoarthritis.[210]

The other OC site in the MCP/MTP joints is the proximal margin of the first phalanx. Clinical signs, if present, are often mild (joint effusion rather than lameness). Often the fragments are found when the horses are radiographed for sales and fragments are removed for economical rather than clinical reasons. Treatment is surgical and no studies exist on the specific prognosis of these lesions, but the clinical impression is that it is good.

Of all joints regularly affected by OC, prognosis is least favorable in the shoulder joint. The arthroscopic approach of this joint is difficult and not all locations within the joint can be reached.[211] Whereas in one study a favorable outcome of only 15% was found after surgery in racehorses (but higher in nonracehorses) suffering from shoulder OC, irrespective if treatment was surgical or nonsurgical,[226] other preliminary data suggest successful outcome in approximately 50% of cases.[210] The same study mentions the clinical impression that conservative treatment of early recognized lesions may be relatively successful. This could well be related with the specific window of time for the development and regression of OC lesions in the shoulder joint, which has not been determined thus far.

ECONOMIC AND WELFARE IMPACT OF OSTEOCHONDROSIS

Osteochondrosis is obviously not a life-threatening disease, but its impact on both the economics of the equine industry and equine welfare is large because of the high prevalence of the disorder.

Effects on Performance

In the cases where lameness is the main clinical sign the effect on performance is evident, but in the majority of cases in which clinical signs are mild or even absent, the situation is less straightforward. In most studies performed until now some impact of OC on performance could be demonstrated, but in many cases differences with unaffected animals are not very large. Trotters with lesions in the tarsocrural joint had a significantly lower number of starts and somewhat lower earnings compared with controls.[227] In a retrospective cohort study on racing performance of Trotters related to abnormal radiographic findings (including OCD, but not limited to this condition) no significant association between the presence or type of radiologic abnormalities and the subsequent performance and longevity could be found, but horses with multiple lesions had a tendency to lower earnings and poorer survival than horses with single lesions.[228] Racing performance in Thoroughbreds treated for OC in the femoropatellar joint was not different from that in unaffected siblings, but fewer horses raced as 2-year-olds and earnings were less, both at 2 and 3 years of age.[229] Also, 2-year-old Thoroughbreds and Standardbreds that were operated on for osteochondrotic lesions in the tarsocrural joint were less likely to race, compared with unaffected siblings at 2 years of age, but findings were not different between groups at 3 years of age.[222] The differences might have been mainly the result of the delay in training caused by the surgery. In a recent study in racing Thoroughbreds (flat and hurdle racing) that took into account all radiographic findings related to juvenile osteochondral conditions (hence including more than OC only) it was shown that fewer horses with radiographic findings raced as 2-year-olds and fewer won prizes as 3-year-olds compared with horses without radiographic anomalies.[230] It was further shown that there was no association between the presence of radiographic findings and earnings, but the total radiographic score, calculated as the sum of all weighted findings,[231] was well correlated with performance. The results of this study largely confirmed the findings of an earlier study in racing Standardbreds in which osteoarticular lesions appeared to be directly responsible for nonqualification in 31%, leading to the conclusion that most radiographic findings are compatible with beginning a racing career, but that severe or multiple abnormalities significantly compromise future racing career.[232]

In nonrace horses studies are scarce. In Show Jumpers no significant difference was found between horses with lesions of the tarsocrural joint and controls. However, horses with osteochondrosis of the lateral trochlear ridge of the femur had both significantly lower performance scores and numbers of performances compared with controls and a significantly lower number of performances was recorded for horses with metacarpo/metatarsophalangeal OCD.[233]

Other Economic Effects and Impact on Welfare

Even if the effect on performance is limited, OC has a huge effect on the economics of the equine industry, mainly because of the high prevalence. Apart from the direct losses of the cases where lesions are too large to be treated, tens of thousands of horses have to be operated on each year, causing significant costs for the equine sector. Further, horses that show signs of OC on radiographs or are clean but still show signs of surgical intervention have an economic value that is considerably less than if that were not the case, even if the chance that their eventual performance will be affected is minimal. Not unimportantly, the fact that so many horses each year are forced to undergo a major surgical procedure means there is an important welfare issue associated with OC(D).

Effects on Breeding

Apart from the direct economic loss, there is an even larger indirect cost of the disease, because many studbooks will not approve horses with (major or minor, depending on studbook policy) evidence of OC. Taking into account the high incidence of the disease, this means that a large proportion (in some cases up to 30%) of potentially good breeding stock is excluded from stallion selection procedures. This of course directly affects breeders, but it also means elimination of a significant part of the gene pool. It was this aspect of OC that led the KWPN to change its very strict selection policy, as mentioned earlier.

CONCLUSION AND POINTERS FOR FURTHER RESEARCH

Osteochondrosis is a multifactorial and complex disorder that, despite its nonlethal and relatively little invalidating character, has a huge impact on the equine industry. Much progress has been made since it became a focus of research in the late 1980s and early 1990s when there were many aspects of OC that were identified as pointers for future research.[8] We now know that OC, as a developmental disorder, can only be understood in the wider framework of the developing musculoskeletal system in the juvenile horse and the genetic and environmental factors acting thereon[234] (Chapter 8 of this book). There is still much conflicting data on incidence and heritability, but we now know why this is so. We have good insight in the early pathogenetic mechanisms, although the knowledge of the exact way of triggering these mechanisms by the numerous etiologic factors is still incomplete. The (surgical) treatment has evolved well and generally carries a fair to good prognosis, but better prevention would be much more desirable for economic and welfare reasons.

From all our current knowledge it is clear that no simple "cure" for OC exists and that we shall not be able to eliminate the disorder if we stick to current breeding goals regarding performance and aesthetics and to current management conditions.[235] However, the disease can become better manageable through further research. Progress can be expected from detailed studies at the molecular level by which it might be possible to discriminate between events related to the normal process of endochondral ossification, those related to the primary etiopathogenesis, and those reflecting the secondary repair process. Further, more epidemiologic studies in which a more refined discrimination is made between lesions of various types and at different locations (which are now known to have a different genetic background) may help to develop better selection strategies and result in more differentiated prognostication.

REFERENCES

1. Malgaigne J-F. *Oeuvres complètes d'Ambroise Paré, revues et collationnées sur toutes les éditions, avec les variantes; ornées de 217 planches et du portrait de l'auteur; accompagnées de notes historiques et critiques et précédées d'une introduction sur l'origine et les progrès de la chirurgie en Occident du sixième siècle au seizième siècle et sur la vie et les ouvrages d'Ambroise Paré.* Paris: J-B. Baillière; 1841.
2. König F. Über freie Körper in den Gelenken. *Dtsch Z Klin Chir.* 1887;27:90–109.
3. Barrie HJ. Osteochondritis dissecans 1887–1987. A centennial look at König's memorable phrase. *J Bone Joint Surg.* 1987; 69-B(5):693–695.
4. Poulos P. Radiologic manifestations of developmental problems. In: McIlwraith CW, ed. *American quarter horse developmental orthopedic diseases symposium.* Amarillo, TX: American Quarter Horse Association; 1986:1–2.
5. Knight DA, Gabel AA, Reed SM, et al. Correlation of dietary mineral to incidence and severity of metabolic bone disease in Ohio and Kentucky. *Proc Am Assoc Equine Pract.* 1985;31:445–460.
6. Mankin HJ, Mankin CJ. Metabolic bone disease: a review and update. *Instr Course Lect.* 2008;57:575–593.
7. Beeman GM, McIlwraith CW. Summary of panel findings. In: McIlwraith CW, ed. *AQHA developmental orthopedic disease symposium.* Amarillo, TX: American Quarter Horse Association; 1986:55–63.
8. Jeffcott LB. Problems and pointers in equine osteochondrosis. *Equine Vet J.* 1993;25(S16):1–3.
9. Parnell SE, Phillips GS. Neonatal skeletal dysplasias. *Pediatr Radiol.* 2012;42(suppl 1):S150–S157.
10. Denoix J-M, Jeffcott LB, McIlwraith CW, et al. A review of terminology for equine juvenile osteochondral conditions (JOCC) based on anatomical and functional considerations. *Vet J.* 2013;197(1):29–35.
11. Wolff J. *Das Gesetz der Transformation der Knochen.* Berlin: Hirschwald; 1892.
12. Hurtig MB, Pool RR. Pathogenesis of equine osteochondrosis. In: McIlwraith CW, Trotter GW, eds. *Joint disease in the horse.* 1st ed. Philadelphia, PA: Saunders; 1996:335.
13. Lecocq M, Girard CA, Fogarty U, et al. Cartilage matrix changes in the developing epiphysis: early events on the pathway to equine osteochondrosis? *Equine Vet J.* 2008;40(5): 442–454.
14. Tóth F, Nissi MJ, Zhang J, et al. Histological confirmation and biological significance of cartilage canals demonstrated using high field MRI in swine at predilection sites of osteochondrosis. *J Orthop Res.* 2013;31(12):2006–2012.
15. Brink P, Skydsgaard M, Teige J, et al. Association between clinical signs and histopathologic changes in the synovium of the tarsocrural joint of horses with osteochondritis dissecans of the tibia. *Am J Vet Res.* 2010;71(1):47–54.
16. Alitalo I, Kärkkäinen M. Osteochondrotic changes in the vertebrae of four ataxic horses suffering from cervical vertebral malformation. *Nord Vet Med.* 1983;35(12):468–474.
17. Nout YS, Reed SM. Cervical vertebral stenotic myelopathy. *Equine Vet Educ.* 2003;15(4):212–223.
18. Dik KJ, Enzerink EE, van Weeren PR. Radiographic development of osteochondral abnormalities, in the hock and stifle of Dutch Warmblood foals, from age 1 to 11 months. *Equine Vet J.* 1999;31(suppl 31):9–15.
19. Van Weeren PR, Barneveld A. The effect of exercise on the distribution and manifestation of osteochondrotic lesions in the Warmblood foal. *Equine Vet J.* 1999;31(suppl 31):16–25.
20. Fontaine P, Blond L, Alexander K, et al. Computed tomography and magnetic resonance imaging in the study of joint development in the equine pelvic limb. *Vet J.* 2013;197(1): 103–111.
21. Relave F, Meulyzer M, Alexander K, et al. Comparison of radiography and ultrasonography to detect osteochondrosis lesions in the tarsocrural joint: a prospective study. *Equine Vet J.* 2009;41(1):34–40.
22. Beccati F, Chalmers HJ, Dante S, et al. Diagnostic sensitivity and interobserver agreement of radiography and ultrasonography for detecting trochlear ridge osteochondrosis lesions in the equine stifle. *Vet Radiol Ultrasound.* 2013;54(2):176–184.
23. Vijarnson M, Riley CB, Ryan DA, et al. Identification of infrared spectral characteristics of synovial fluid of horses with osteochondrosis of the tarsocrural joint. *Am J Vet Res.* 2007;68(5):517–523.
24. Van Weeren PR, Barneveld A. Study design to evaluate the influence of exercise on the development of the musculoskeletal system of foals up to age 11 months. *Equine Vet J.* 1999;31(suppl 31):4–8.
25. Hoppe F. Radiological investigations of osteochondrosis dissecans in Standardbred trotters and Swedish Warmblood horses. *Equine Vet J.* 1984;16(5):425–429.
26. Schougaard H, Falk Rønne J, Philipsson J. A radiographic survey of tibiotarsal osteochondrosis in a selected population of trotting horses in Denmark and its possible genetic significance. *Equine Vet J.* 1990;22(4):288–289.
27. Carlsten J, Sandgren B, Dalín G. Development of osteochondrosis in the tarsocrural joint and osteochondral fragments in the fetlock joints of Standardbred trotters. I. A radiological survey. *Equine Vet J.* 1993;25(suppl 16):42–47.

28. Sandgren B, Dalin G, Carlsten J. Osteochondrosis in the tarsocrural joint and osteochondral fragments in the fetlock joints in Standardbred trotters. I. Epidemiology. *Equine Vet J.* 1993;25(Suppl 16):31–37.
29. Denoix JM, Valette JP. Pathologie ostéo-articulaire chez le jeune cheval (incidence, évaluation clinique, facteurs de risque et conséquences). *Proc Journée d'étude des Haras Nationaux.* 2001;27:101–113.
30. McIntosh SC, McIlwraith CW. Natural history of femoropatellar osteochondrosis in three crops of Thoroughbreds. *Equine Vet J.* 1993;25(suppl 1):54–61.
31. McIlwraith CW, Foerner JJ, Davis DM. Osteochondritis dissecans of the tarsocrural joint: results of treatment with arthroscopic surgery. *Equine Vet J.* 1991;23(3):155–162.
32. McIlwraith CW. Subchondral cystic lesions (osteochondrosis) in the horse. *Compend Contin Educ Pract Vet.* 1982;4:S282–S293.
33. McIlwraith CW. Clinical aspects of osteochondrosis dissecans. In: McIlwraith CW, Trotter GW, eds. *Joint disease in the horse.* 1st ed. Philadelphia, PA: Saunders; 1996:362.
34. Sønnichsen HV, Kristoffersen J, Falk-Rønne J. Joint mice in the fetlock joint-osteochondritis dissecans. *Nord Vet Med.* 1982;34(11):399–403.
35. Dalin G, Sandgren B, Carlsten J. Plantar osteochondral fragments in the metatarsophalangeal joints in Standardbred trotters: results of osteochondrosis or trauma? *Equine Vet J.* 1993;25(suppl 16):62–65.
36. Nixon AJ, Pool RR. Histologic appearance of axial osteochondral fragments from the proximoplantar/proximopalmar aspect of the proximal phalanx in horses. *J Am Vet Med Assoc.* 1995;207(8):1076–1080.
37. Barr ED, Pinchbeck GL, Clegg PD, et al. Post mortem evaluation of palmar osteochondral disease (traumatic osteochondrosis) of the metacarpo/metatarsophalangeal joint in Thoroughbred racehorses. *Equine Vet J.* 2009;41(4):366–371.
38. Theiss F, Hilbe M, Fürst A, et al. Histological evaluation of intraarticular osteochondral fragments. *Pferdeheilk.* 2010;26(4):541–552.
39. Lettry V, Sumie Y, Mitsuda K, et al. Divergent diagnosis from arthroscopic findings and identification of CPII and C2C for detection of cartilage degradation in horses. *Jpn J Vet Res.* 2010;57(4):197–206.
40. McIlwraith CW. Inferences from referred clinical cases of osteochondrosis dissecans. *Equine Vet J.* 1993;25(suppl 16):27–30.
41. Nilsson F. Hästens goniter. *Svensk Vetidn.* 1947;52:1–14.
42. Numans SR, Wintzer HJ. Einige neue Indikationen zur Knochen-und Gelenkchirurgie des Pferdes. *Berl Münchn Tierärztl Wschr.* 1961;74:205–210.
43. Baker RH. Osteochondrosis of the tibial tuberosity of the horse. *J Am Vet Med Assoc.* 1960;137: 354–345.
44. Birkeland R, Haakenstad LH. Intracapsular bony fragments of the distal tibia of the horse. *J Am Vet Med Assoc.* 1968;152(10):1526–1529.
45. Birkeland R. Chip fractures of the first phalanx in the metatarsophalangeal joint of the horse. *Acta Radiol.* 1972;(suppl 319):73–77.
46. De Moor A, Verschooten F, Desmet P, et al. Osteochondritis dissecans of the tibiotarsal joint of the horse. *Equine Vet J.* 1972;4(3):139–143.
47. Olsson SE, Reiland S. The nature of osteochondrosis in animals. *Acta Radiol.* 1978;(suppl 358):299–306.
48. Reiland S. Morphology of osteochondrosis and sequelae in pigs. *Acta Radiol.* 1978;(suppl 358):45–90.
49. Reiland S, Strömberg B, Olsson SE, et al. Osteochondrosis in growing bulls. Pathology, frequency and severity on different feedings. *Acta Radiol.* 1978;(Suppl 358):179–196.
50. Rejnö S, Strömberg B. Osteochondrosis in the horse: II. Pathology. *Acta Radiol.* 1978;(suppl 358):153–178.
51. Strömberg B, Rejnö S. Osteochondrosis in the horse I. A clinical and radiologic investigation of osteochondritis dissecans of the knee and hock joint. *Acta Radiol.* 1978;(suppl 358):139–152.
52. Hoppe F, Philipsson J. A genetic study of osteochondrosis dissecans in Swedish horses. *Equine Pract.* 1985;7:7–15.
53. Alvarado AF, Marcoux M, Breton L. The incidence of osteochondrosis in a Standardbred breeding farm in Quebec. *Proc Am Assoc Equine Pract.* 1989;35:295–307.
54. O'Donohue DD, Smith FH, Strickland KL. The incidence of abnormal limb development in the Irish Thoroughbred from birth to 18 months. *Equine Vet J.* 1992;24(4):305–309.
55. Paasch KM, Bramlage LR. Influence of birth month on location of osteochondrosis dissecans. *Proc Am Assoc Equine Pract.* Focus on Joints Meeting. 2004;50:17–18.
56. Oliver LJ, Baird DK, Baird AN, et al. Prevalence and distribution of radiographically evident lesions on repository films in the hock and stifle joints of yearling Thoroughbred horses in New Zealand. *N Z Vet J.* 2008;56(5):202–209.
57. Arnan P, Hertsch B-W. Röntgenologische Untersuchung zur Erfassung der Osteochondrosis dissecans im Fessel-, Sprung- und Kniegelenk im Vergleich vom Fohlen zum Zweijährigen. In: Bruns E, ed. *Göttinger Pferdetage 2004.* Warendorf, Germany: FN-Verlag; 2004:115–124.
58. Hilla D, Distl O. Prevalence of osteochondral fragments, osteochondrosis dissecans and palmar/plantar osteochondral fragments in Hanoverian Warmblood horses. *Berl Munch Tierarztl Wochenschr.* 2013;126(5-6):236–244.
59. Vos NJ. Incidence of osteochondrosis (dissecans) in Dutch Warmblood horses presented for pre-purchase examination. *Ir Vet J.* 2008;61(1):33–37.
60. Lepeule J, Bareille N, Robert C, et al. Association of growth, feeding practices and exercise conditions with the prevalence of developmental orthopaedic disease in limbs of French foals at weaning. *Prev Vet Med.* 2009;89(3-4):167–177.
61. Lykkjen S, Roed KH, Dolvik NI. Osteochondrosis and osteochondral fragments in Standardbred trotters: prevalence and relationships. *Equine Vet J.* 2012;44(3):332–338.
62. Voûte LC, Henson FM, Platt D, et al. Osteochondrosis lesions of the lateral trochlear ridge of the distal femur in four ponies. *Vet Rec.* 2011;168(10):265.
63. Valentino LW, Lillich JD, Gaughan EM, et al. Radiographic prevalence of osteochondrosis in yearling feral horses. *Vet Comp Orthop Traumatol.* 1999;12(3):56–60.
64. Strömberg B. A review of the salient features of osteochondrosis in the horse. *Equine Vet J.* 1979;11(4):211–214.
65. Dabareiner RM, Sullins KE, White II NA. Progression of femoropatellar osteochondrosis in nine young horses. Clinical, radiographic and arthroscopic findings. *Vet Surg.* 1993;22(6):515–523.
66. Bertone AL, Bramlage LR, McIlwraith CW, et al. Comparison of proteoglycan and collagen in articular cartilage of horses with naturally developing osteochondrosis and healing osteochondral fragments of experimentally induced fractures. *Am J Vet Res.* 2005;66(11):1881–1890.

67. Donabédian M, Fleurance G, Perona G, et al. Effect of maximal vs. moderate growth related to nutrients intake on developmental orthopaedic diseases in horses. *Anim Res.* 2006;55:471–486.

68. Robert C, Valette JP, Jacquet S, et al. Study design for the investigation of likely aetiological factors of juvenile osteochondral conditions (JOCC) in foals and yearlings. *Vet J.* 2013;197(1):36–43.

69. Van Weeren PR, Denoix J-M. The Normandy field study on juvenile osteochondral conditions: conclusions regarding the influence of genetics, environmental conditions and management, and the effect on performance. *Vet J.* 2013;197(1):90–95.

70. Jacquet S, Robert C, Valette JP, et al. Evolution of radiological findings detected in the limbs of 321 young horses between the ages of 6 and 18 months. *Vet J.* 2013;197(1):58–64.

71. Baccarin RY, Pereira MA, Roncati NV, et al. Development of osteochondrosis in Lusitano foals: a radiographic study. *Can Vet J.* 2012;53(10):1079–1084.

72. Enzerink E, Dik KJ, Knaap JH, et al. Radiographic development of lesions in hock and stifle in a group of Dutch Warmblood horses from 1-24 months of age. *Proc Congr Br Equine Vet Assoc.* 2000;39:195.

73. Verzijl N, DeGroot J, Thorpe SR, et al. Effect of collagen turnover on the accumulation of advanced glycation end products. *J Biol Chem.* 2000;275(50):39027–39031.

74. Brama PAJ, TeKoppele JM, Beekman B, et al. Influence of development and joint pathology on stromelysin enzyme activity in equine synovial fluid. *Ann Rheum Dis.* 2000;59(2):155–157.

75. Van Weeren PR, Brama PAJ. Equine joint disease in the light of new developments in articular cartilage research. *Pferdeheilk.* 2003;19:336–344.

76. Van Weeren PR. Osteochondrosis: developmental disorder or disorderly development? (OC seen in the general framework of articular development in young animals). *Proc Eur Coll Vet Surg.* 2004;13:164–175.

77. Van Grevenhof EM, Ducro BJ, van Weeren PR, et al. Prevalence of various radiographic manifestations of osteochondrosis and their correlations between and within joints in Dutch Warmblood horses. *Equine Vet J.* 2009;41(1):11–16.

78. Wittwer C, Hamann H, Rosenberger E, et al. Prevalence of osteochondrosis in the limb joints of South German Coldblood horses. *J Vet Med A Physiol Pathol Clin Med.* 2006;53(10):531–539.

79. Pool RR. Difficulties in definition of equine osteochondrosis: differentiation of developmental and acquired lesions. *Equine Vet J.* 1993;25(suppl 16):5–12.

80. McCoy AM, Toth F, Dolvik NI, et al. Articular osteochondrosis: a comparison of naturally-occurring human and animal disease. *Osteoarthr Cart.* 2013;21(11):1638–1647.

81. Wheeler Haines R. Cartilage canals. *J Anat.* 1933;68(Pt 1):45–64.

82. Butler JA, Colles CM, Dyson SJ, et al. *Clinical radiology of the horse.* 3rd ed. Chichester, UK: John Wiley and Sons; 2011.

83. Carlson CS, Cullins LD, Meuten JD. Osteochondrosis of the articular-epiphyseal cartilage complex in young horses: evidence for a defect in cartilage canal blood supply. *Vet Pathol.* 1995;32(6):641–647.

84. Ytrehus B, Carlson CS, Lundeheim N, et al. Vascularization and osteochondrosis of the epiphyseal growth cartilage of the distal femur in pigs—development with age, growth rate, weight and joint shape. *Bone.* 2004;34(3):454–465.

85. Ekman S, Rodriguez Martinez H, Plöen L. Morphology of normal and osteochondritic porcine articular-epiphyseal cartilage. A study in the domestic pig and minipig of wild hog ancestry. *Acta Anat.* 1990;139(3):239–253.

86. Carlson CS, Meuten DJ, Richardson DC. Ischemia of cartilage in spontaneous and experimental lesions of osteochondrosis. *J Orthop Res.* 1991;9(3):317–329.

87. Ekman S, Carlson CS. The pathophysiology of osteochondrosis. *Vet Clin North Am Small Anim Pract.* 1998;28(1):17–32.

88. Ytrehus B, Andreas Haga H, Mellum CN, et al. Experimental ischemia of porcine growth cartilage produces lesions of osteochondrosis. *J Orthop Res.* 2004;22(6):1201–1209.

89. Ytrehus B, Carlson CS, Ekman S. Etiology and pathogenesis of osteochondrosis. *Vet Pathol.* 2007;44(4):429–448.

90. Ekman S, Carlson CS, van Weeren PR. Workshop report. Third international workshop on equine osteochondrosis. Stockholm, 29-30th May 2008. *Equine Vet J.* 2009;41(5):504–507.

91. Rangkasenee N, Murani E, Brunner RM, et al. Genome-wide association identifies TBX5 as candidate gene for osteochondrosis providing a functional link to cartilage perfusion as initial factor. *Front Genet.* 2013;4:78.

92. Olstad K, Ytrehus B, Ekman S, et al. Early lesions of osteochondrosis in the distal tibia of foals. *J Orthop Res.* 2007;25(8):1094–1105.

93. Olstad K, Ytrehus B, Ekman S, et al. Epiphyseal cartilage canal blood supply to the tarsus of foals and relationship to osteochondrosis. *Equine Vet J.* 2008;40(1):30–39.

94. Olstad K, Ytrehus B, Ekman S, et al. Epiphyseal cartilage canal blood supply to the distal femur of foals. *Equine Vet J.* 2008;40(5):433–439.

95. Olstad K, Ytrehus B, Ekman S, et al. Early lesions of articular osteochondrosis in the distal femur of foals. *Vet Pathol.* 2011;48(6):1165–1175.

96. Olstad K, Ytrehus B, Ekman S, et al. Epiphyseal cartilage canal blood supply to the metatarsophalangeal joint of horses. *Equine Vet J.* 2009;41(9):865–871.

97. Olstad K, Cnudde V, Masschaele B, et al. Micro-computed tomography of early blood supply of osteochondrosis in the tarsus of foals. *Bone.* 2008;43(3):574–583.

98. Olstad K, Hendrickson EH, Carlson CS, et al. Transection of vessels in epiphyseal cartilage canals leads to osteochondrosis and osteochondrosis dissecans in the femoro-patellar joint of foals; a potential model of juvenile osteochondritis dissecans. *Osteoarthr Cart.* 2013;21(5):730–738.

99. Shingleton WD, Mackie EJ, Cawston TE, et al. Cartilage canals in equine articular/epiphyseal growth cartilage and a possible association with dyschondroplasia. *Equine Vet J.* 1997;29(5):360–364.

100. Ahmed YA, Tatarczuch L, Pagel CN, et al. Hypertrophy and physiological death of equine chondrocytes in vitro. *Equine Vet J.* 2007;39(6):546–552.

101. Van den Hoogen BM, van de Lest CHA, van Weeren PR. Changes in proteoglycan metabolism in osteochondrotic articular cartilage of growing foals. *Equine Vet J.* 1999;31(suppl 31):38–44.

102. Lillich JD, Bertone AL, Malemud CJ, et al. Biochemical, histochemical and immunohistochemical characterisation of distal tibial osteochondrosis in horses. *Am J Vet Res.* 1997;58(1):89–98.

103. Jeffcott LB, Henson FM. Studies on growth cartilage in the horse and their application to aetiopathogenesis of dyschondroplasia (osteochondrosis). *Vet J.* 1998;156(3):177–192.

104. Semevolos SA, Strassheim ML, Haupt JL, et al. Expression patterns of hedgehog signaling peptides in naturally acquired equine osteochondrosis. *J Orthop Res.* 2005;23(5):1152–1159.

105. Mirams M, Tatarczuch L, Ahmed YA, et al. Altered gene expression in early osteochondrosis lesions. *J Orthop Res.* 2009;27(4):452–457.

106. Kronenberg HM, Lee K, Lanske B, et al. Parathyroid hormone-related protein and Indian hedgehog control the pace of cartilage differentiation. *J Endocrinol.* 1997;154(suppl 3):S39–45.

107. Semevolos SA, Brower-Toland BD, Bent SJ, et al. Parathyroid hormone-related peptide and Indian hedgehog expression patterns in naturally acquired equine osteochondrosis. *J Orthop Res.* 2002;20(6):1290–1297.

108. Semevolos SA, Nixon AJ, Strassheim M. Expression of bone morphogenic protein-6 and -2 and a bone morphogenic protein antagonist in horses with naturally acquired osteochondrosis. *Am J Vet Res.* 2004;65:110–115.

109. Riddick TL, Duesterdieck-Zellmer K, Semevolos SA. Gene and protein expression of cartilage canal and osteochondral junction chondrocytes and full-thickness cartilage in early equine osteochondrosis. *Vet J.* 2012;194(3):319–325.

110. Henson FMD, Schofield PN, Jeffcott LB. Expression of transforming growth factor-β1 in normal and dyschondroplastic articular growth cartilage of the young horse. *Equine Vet J.* 1997;29(6):434–439.

111. Henson FMD, Davies ME, Skepper JN, et al. Localisation of alkaline phosphatase in equine growth cartilage. *J Anat.* 1995;187(Pt 1):151–159.

112. Henson FMD, Davies ME, Schofield PN, et al. Expression of types II, VI and X collagen in equine growth cartilage during development. *Equine Vet J.* 1996;28(3):189–198.

113. Semevolos SA, Nixon AJ, Brower-Toland MA. Changes in molecular expression of aggrecan and collagen types I, II, and X, insulin-like growth factor-I, and transforming growth factor-β1 in articular cartilage obtained from horses with naturally acquired osteochondrosis. *Am J Vet Res.* 2001;62:1088–1094.

114. Henson FMD, Davies ME, Jeffcott LB. Equine dyschondroplasia (osteochondrosis)—histological findings and type VI collagen localization. *Vet J.* 1997;154(1):53–62.

115. Muir H. The chondrocyte, architect of cartilage. Biomechanics, structure, function and molecular biology of cartilage matrix macromolecules. *Bio Essays.* 1995;17(2):1039–1045.

116. Al-Hizab F, Clegg PD, Thompson CC, et al. Microscopic localization of active gelatinases in equine osteochondritis dissecans (OCD) cartilage. *Osteoarthr Cart.* 2002;10(8):653–661.

117. Hurtig M, Green SL, Dobson H, et al. Correlative study of defective cartilage and bone growth in foals fed a low-copper diet. *Equine Vet J.* 1993;25(suppl 16):66–73.

118. Garvican ER, Vaughan-Thomas A, Redmond C, et al. MT3-MMP (MMP-16) is downregulated by in vitro cytokine stimulation of cartilage, but unaltered in naturally occurring equine osteoarthritis and osteochondrosis. *Connect Tissue Res.* 2008;49(2):62–67.

119. Hernandez-Vidal G, Davies ME, Jeffcott LB. Localization of cathepsins B and D in equine articular cartilage. *Pferdeheilkunde.* 1996;12:371–373.

120. Hernandez Vidal G, Jeffcott LB, Davies ME. Cellular heterogeneity in cathepsin D distribution in equine articular cartilage. *Equine Vet J.* 1997;29(4):267–273.

121. Gläser KE, Davies ME, Jeffcott LB. Differential distribution of cathepsins B and L in articular cartilage during skeletal development in the horse. *Equine Vet J.* 2003;35(1):42–47.

122. Hernandez-Vidal G, Jeffcott LB, Davies ME. Immunolocalization of cathepsin B in equine dyschondroplastic cartilage. *Vet J.* 1998;156(3):193–201.

123. Gee E, Davies M, Firth E, et al. Osteochondrosis and copper: histology of articular cartilage from foals out of copper supplemented and non-supplemented dams. *Vet J.* 2007;173(1):109–117.

124. Garvican ER, Vaughan-Thomas A, Redmond C, et al. Chondrocytes harvested from osteochondritis dissecans cartilage are able to undergo limited in vitro chondrogenesis despite having perturbations of cell phenotype in vivo. *J Orthop Res.* 2008;26(8):1133–1140.

125. Van de Lest CHA, Brama PAJ, DeGroot J, et al. Extracellular matrix changes in early osteochondrotic defects in foals: a key role for collagen? *BBA Mol Basis Dis.* 2004;1690(1):54–62.

126. Van de Lest CHA, van den Hoogen BM, van Weeren PR, et al. Changes in bone morphogenic enzymes and lipid composition of equine osteochondrotic subchondral bone. *Equine Vet J.* 1999;31(suppl 31):31–37.

127. Donabédian M, van Weeren R, Perona G, et al. Early changes in biomarkers of skeletal metabolism and their association to the occurrence of osteochondrosis (OC) in the horse. *Equine Vet J.* 2008;40(3):253–259.

128. Vervuert I, Winkelsett S, Christmann L, et al. Evaluation of the influences of exercise, birth date, and osteochondrosis in plasma bone marker concentrations in Hanoverian Warmblood foals. *Am J Vet Res.* 2007;68(12):1319–1323.

129. McIlwraith CW, ed. *American quarter horse developmental orthopedic diseases symposium*. Amarillo, TX: American Quarter Horse Association; 1986:1–77.

130. Denoix JM, Jacquet S, Lepeule J, et al. Radiographic findings of juvenile osteochondral conditions detected in 392 foals using a field radiographic protocol. *Vet J.* 2013;197(1):44–51.

131. Distl O. The genetics of equine osteochondrosis. *Vet J.* 2013;197(1):13–18.

132. Wittwer C, Hamann H, Rosenberger E, et al. Genetic parameters for the prevalence of osteochondrosis in the limb joints of South German Coldblood horses. *J Anim Breed Genet.* 2007;124(5):302–307.

133. Grøndahl AM, Dolvik NI. Heritability estimation of osteochondrosis in the tibiotarsal joint and of bony fragments in the palmar/plantar portion of the metacarpo- and metatarsophalangeal joints of horses. *J Am Vet Med Assoc.* 1993;203(1):101–104.

134. Brendov E. *Osteochondrosis in Standardbred Trotters: Heritability and Effects on Racing Performance. Thesis.* Uppsala: Swedish University of Agricultural Sciences; 1997.

135. Jönsson L, Dalin G, Egenvall A, et al. Equine hospital data as a source for study of prevalence and heritability of osteochondrosis and palmar/plantar osseous fragments of Swedish Warmblood horses. *Equine Vet J.* 2011;43(6):695–700.

136. Philipsson J, Andréasson E, Sandgren B, et al. Osteochondrosis in the tarsocrural joint and osteochondral fragments in the fetlock joints in Standardbred trotters. II. Heritability. *Equine Vet J.* 1993;25(suppl 16):38–41.

137. Van Grevenhof I, Schurink A, Ducro BJ, et al. Genetic variables of various manifestations of osteochondrosis and their correlations between and within joints of Dutch Warmblood horses. *J Anim Sci.* 2009;87(6):1906–1912.

138. Willms F, Röh R, Kalm E. Genetische Analyse von Merk-malskomplexen in der Reitpferdezucht unter Berücksichtigung von Gliedmaßenveränderungen. *Züchtungskunde.* 1999;71:330–345.

139. Pieramati C, Pepe M, Silvestrelli M, et al. Heritability estimation of osteochondrosis dissecans in Maremmano horses. *Livest Prod Sci.* 2003;79(2-3):249–255.

140. Teyssèdre S, Dupuis MC, Guérin G, et al. Genome-wide association studies for osteochondrosis in French Trotter horses. *J Anim Sci.* 2012;90(1):45–53.

141. Ricard A, Perrocheau M, Couroucé-Malblanc A, et al. Genetic parameters of juvenile osteochondral conditions (JOCC) in French Trotters. *Vet J, 2013.* 2013;197(1):77–82.

142. Van den Belt AJM. *Personal communication.* 2010.

143. Wade CM, Giulotto E, Sigurdsson S, et al. Genome sequence, comparative analysis, and population genetics of the domestic horse. *Science.* 2009;26(5954):865–867.

144. Corbin LJ, Blott SC, Swinburne JE, et al. A genome-wide association study of osteochondritis dissecans in the Thoroughbred. *Mamm Genome.* 2012;23(3-4):294–303.

145. Dierks C, Mömke S, Drögemüller C, et al. A high-resolution comparative radiation hybrid map of equine chromosome 4q12-q22. *Anim Genet.* 2006;37(5):513–517.

146. Dierks C, Löhring K, Lampe V, et al. Genome-wide search for markers associated with osteochondrosis in Hanoverian Warmblood horses. *Mamm Genome.* 2007;18(10):739–747.

147. Dierks C, Komm K, Lampe V, et al. Fine mapping of a quantitative trait locus for osteochondrosis on horse chromosome 2. *Anim Genet.* 2010;41(Suppl 2):87–90.

148. Dierks C. *Fine mapping of a quantitative trait locus for osteochondrosis on horse chromosome 4. Thesis.* Hanover: University of Veterinary Medicine; 2010 [Cited by Distl, 2013].

149. Felicetti M. *Mapping of quantitative trait locus on equine chromosome 21 responsible for osteochondrosis in hock joints of Hanoverian Warmblood horses. Thesis.* Hanover: University of Veterinary Medicine; 2009 [Cited by Distl, 2013].

150. Lampe V, Dierks C, Distl O. Refinement of a quantitative trait locus on equine chromosome 16 responsible for fetlock osteochondrosis in Hanoverian Warmblood horses. *Anim Genet.* 2009;40(4):553–555.

151. Lampe V, Dierks C, Komm K, et al. Identification of a new quantitative trait locus on equine chromosome 18 responsible for osteochondrosis in Hanoverian Warmblood horses. *J Anim Sci.* 2009;87(11):3477–3481.

152. Lampe V, Dierks C, Distl O. Refinement of a quantitative trait locus on equine chromosome 5 responsible for fetlock osteochondrosis in Hanoverian Warmblood horses. *Anim Genet.* 2009;40(4):553–555.

153. Lykkjen S, Dolvik NI, McCue ME, et al. Genome-wide association analysis of osteochondrosis of the tibiotarsal joint in Norwegian Standardbred trotters. *Anim Genet.* 2010;41(suppl 2):111–120.

154. Orr N, Hill EW, Gu J, et al. Genome-wide association study of osteochondrosis in the tarsocrural joint of Dutch Warmblood horses identifies susceptibility loci on chromosomes 3 and 10. *Anim Genet.* 2012;44(4):408–412.

155. Wittwer C, Löhring K, Drögemüller C, et al. Mapping quantitative trait loci for osteochondrosis in fetlock and hock joints and palmar/plantar osseous fragments in fetlock joints of South German Coldblood horses. *Anim Genet.* 2007;38(4):350–357.

156. Boneker C, Kuiper H, Drögemüller C, et al. Molecular characterization of the equine collagen, type IX, alpha 2 (COL9A2) gene on horse chromosome 2p16→p15. *Cytogenet Genome Res.* 2006;115(2):107–114.

157. Meulenbelt I, Min JL, van Duijn M, et al. Strong linkage on 2q33.3 to familial early-onset generalized osteoarthritis and a consideration of two positional candidate genes. *Eur J Hum Genet.* 2006;14(12):1280–1287.

158. Serteyn D, Piquemal D, Vanderheyden L, et al. Gene expression profiling from leukocytes of horses affected by osteochondrosis. *J Orthop Res.* 2010;28(7):965–970.

159. Zabek T, Golonka P, Fornal A, et al. IHH gene polymorphism among three horse breeds and its application for association test in horses with osteochondrosis. *Hereditas.* 2013;150(2-3):38–43.

160. Austbø L, Rø KH, Dolvik NI, et al. Identification of differentially expressed genes associated with osteochondrosis in standardbred horses using RNA arbitrarily primed PCR. *Anim Biotechnol.* 2010;21(2):135–139.

161. Haberland AM, König von Borstel U, Simianer H, et al. Integration of genomic information into sport horse breeding programs for optimization of accuracy of selection. *Animal.* 2012;6(9):1369–1376.

162. Nakano T, Aherne FX. Involvement of trauma in the pathogenesis of osteochondrosis dissecans in swine. *Can J Vet Res.* 1988;52(1):154–155.

163. Helminen HJ, Hyttinen MM, Lammi MJ, et al. Regular joint loading in youth assists in the establishment and strengthening of the collagen network of articular cartilage and contributes to the prevention of osteoarthrosis later in life: a hypothesis. *J Bone Miner Metab.* 2000;18(5):245–257.

164. Brama PAJ, TeKoppele JM, Bank RA, et al. Development of biochemical heterogeneity of articular cartilage: influences of age and exercise. *Equine Vet J.* 2002;34(3):265–269.

165. Bruin G, Creemers J. Het voorkómen van osteochondrose. In: Bruin G, ed. *Praktijkonderzoek paarden (p. 15).* Lelystad, the Netherlands: Proefstation voor de Rundveehouderij, Schapenhouderij en Paardenhouderij; 1994.

166. Jeffcott LB. Osteochondrosis in the horse–searching for the key to pathogenesis. *Equine Vet J.* 1991;23(5):331–338.

167. Wilke A. *Der Einfluss von Aufzucht und Haltung auf Osteochondrose. Thesis.* Hannover: Tierärztliche Hochschule; 2003.

168. Lepeule J, Bareille N, Robert C, et al. Association of growth, feeding practices and exercise conditions with the severity of the osteoarticular status of limbs in French foals. *Vet J.* 2013;197(1):65–71.

169. Praud A, Dufour B, Robert C, et al. Effects of management practices as risk factors for juvenile osteochondral conditions in 259 French yearlings. *Vet J.* 2013;197(1):72–76.

170. Vander Heyden L, Lejeune JP, Caudron I, et al. Association of breeding conditions with prevalence of osteochondrosis in foals. *Vet Rec.* 2013;172(3):68.

171. Glade MJ, Krook L, Schryver HF, et al. Growth inhibition by chronic dexamethasone treatment of foals. *J Equine Vet Sci.* 1981;1:198–201.

172. Glade MJ, Belling TH. Growth plate cartilage metabolism, morphology and biochemical composition in over- and underfed horses. *Growth.* 1984;48(4):473–482.

173. Sandgren B, Dalin G, Carlsten J, et al. Development of osteochondrosis in the tarsocrural joint and osteochondral fragments in the fetlock joints of Standardbred trotters. II. Body measurements and clinical findings. *Equine Vet J.* 1993;25(suppl 16):48–53.

174. Firth EC, van Weeren PR, Pfeiffer DU, et al. Effect of age, exercise and growth rate on bone mineral density (BMD) in third carpal bone and distal radius of Dutch Warmblood foals with osteochondrosis. *Equine Vet J.* 1999;31(suppl 31):74–78.

175. Van Weeren PR, Sloet van Oldruitenborgh-Oosterbaan MM, Barneveld A. The influence of birth weight, rate of weight gain and final achieved height and sex on the development of osteochondrotic lesions in a population of genetically predisposed Warmblood foals. *Equine Vet J.* 1999;31(suppl 31):26–30.

176. Glade MJ. The control of cartilage growth in osteochondrosis: a review. *J Eq Vet Sci.* 1986;6(4):175–187.

177. Glade MJ. The role of endocrine factors in equine developmental orthopedic disease. *Proc Am Assoc Equine Pract.* 1987;33:171–189.

178. Ralston SL. Hyperglycaemia/hyperinsulinaemia after feeding a meal of grain to young horses with osteochondrosis dissecans (OCD) lesions. *Pferdeheilk.* 1996;12(3):320–322.

179. Henson FMD, Davenport C, Butler L, et al. Effects of insulin and insulin-like growth factors I and II on the growth of equine fetal and neonatal chondrocytes. *Equine Vet J.* 1997;29(6):441–447.

180. Robert C. Further evidence for better prevention of equine osteochondrosis. *Vet Rec.* 2013;172:66–67.

181. Firshman AM, Valberg SJ. Factors affecting clinical assessment of insulin sensitivity in horses. *Equine Vet J.* 2007;39(6):567–575.

182. Johnson PJ, Wiedmeyer CE, Messer NT, et al. Medical implications of obesity in horses—lessons for human obesity. *J Diabetes Sci Technol.* 2009;3(1):163–174.

183. Glade MJ, Gupta S, Reimers TJ. Hormonal responses to high and low planes of nutrition in weanling thoroughbreds. *J Anim Sci.* 1984;59(3):658–665.

184. Sloet van Oldruitenborgh-Oosterbaan MM, Mol JA, Barneveld A. Hormones, growth factors and other plasma variables in relation to osteochondrosis. *Equine Vet J.* 1999;31(suppl 31):45–54.

185. Shavers JR, Fretz PB, Doige CE, et al. Skeletal manifestations of suspected hypothyroidism in two foals. *J Equine Med Surg.* 1979;3:269–275.

186. Glade MJ, Reimers TJ. Effects of dietary energy supply on serum thyroxine, tri-iodothyronine and insulin concentrations in young horses. *J Endocrinol.* 1985;104(1):93–98.

187. Savage CJ, McCarthy RN, Jeffcott LB. Effects of dietary energy and protein on induction of dyschondroplasia in foals. *Equine Vet J.* 1993a;25(suppl 16):74–79.

188. Glade MJ, Belling TH. A dietary etiology for osteochondrotic cartilage. *J Equine Vet Sci.* 1986;6(3):151–155.

189. Bridges CH, Womack JE, Harris ED, Scrutchfield WL. Considerations of copper metabolism in osteochondrosis of suckling foals. *J Am Vet Med Assoc.* 1984;185(2):173–178.

190. Bridges CH, Harris ED. Experimentally induced cartilaginous fractures (osteochondritis dissecans) in foals fed low-copper diets. *J Am Vet Med Assoc.* 1988;193(2):215–221.

191. Bridges CH, Moffitt PG. Influence of variable content of dietary zinc on copper metabolism of weanling foals. *Am J Vet Res.* 1990;51(2):275–280.

192. Gunson DE, Kowalczyk DF, Shoop CR, et al. Environmental zinc and cadmium pollution associated with generalized osteochondrosis, osteoporosis, and nephrocalcinosis in horses. *J Am Vet Med Assoc.* 1982;180(3):295–299.

193. NRC - Nutritional Research Council, Committee on Animal Nutrition. *The nutrient requirements of horses.* 5th ed. Washington, DC: National Academic Press; 1989.

194. Cupps PJ, Howell CE. The effects of feeding supplemental copper to growing foals. *J Anim Sci.* 1949;8(2):286–289.

195. Knight DA, Weisbrode SE, Schmall LM, et al. The effects of copper supplementation on the prevalence of cartilage lesions in foals. *Equine Vet J.* 1990;22(6):426–432.

196. Hurtig MB, Green SL, Dobson H, et al. Defective bone and cartilage in foals fed a low-copper diet. *Proc Am Assoc Equine Pract.* 1990;36:637–643.

197. Cymbaluk NF, Smart ME. A review of possible metabolic relationships of copper to equine bone disease. *Equine Vet J.* 1993;25(suppl 16):19–26.

198. Lewis LD. Minerals for horses. In: Lewis LD, ed. *Equine clinical nutrition: feeding and care.* Baltimore, MD: Williams & Wilkins; 1995:25.

199. Pearce SG, Grace ND, Wichtel JJ, et al. Effect of copper supplementation on copper status of pregnant mares and foals. *Equine Vet J.* 1998;30(3):200–203.

200. Egan DA, Murrin P. Copper concentration and distribution in the livers of equine fetuses, neonates and foals. *Res Vet Sci.* 1973;15(1):147–148.

201. Gee EK, Grace ND, Firth EC, et al. Changes in liver copper concentration of Thoroughbred foals from birth to 160 days of age and the effect of prenatal copper supplementation to their dams. *Aust Vet J.* 2000;78(5):347–353.

202. Pearce SG, Grace ND, Firth EC, et al. Effect of copper supplementation on the copper status of pasture-fed young Thoroughbreds. *Equine Vet J.* 1998;30(3):204–210.

203. Gee EK, Firth EC, Morel PCH, et al. Articular/epiphyseal osteochondrosis in Thoroughbred foals at 5 months of age: influences of growth of the foal and prenatal copper supplementation of the dam. *N Z Vet J.* 2005;53(6):448–456.

204. Pearce SG, Firth EC, Grace ND, et al. Effect of copper supplementation on the evidence of developmental orthopaedic disease in pasture-fed New Zealand Thoroughbreds. *Equine Vet J.* 1998;30(3):211–218.

205. Van Weeren PR, Knaap J, Firth EC. Influence of liver copper status of mare and newborn foal on the development of osteochondrotic lesions. *Equine Vet J.* 2003;35(1):67–71.

206. Jeffcott LB, Davies ME. Copper status and skeletal development in horses: still a long way to go. *Equine Vet J.* 1998;30(3):183–185.

207. Davies ME, Pasqualicchio M, Henson F, Hernandez-Vidal G. Effects of copper and zinc on chondrocyte behaviour and matrix turnover. *Pferdeheilkunde.* 1996;12(3):367–370.

208. Savage CJ, McCarthy RN, Jeffcott LB. Effects of dietary phosphorus and calcium on induction of dyschondroplasia in foals. *Equine Vet J.* 1993b;25(suppl 16):80–83.

209. Carmona JU, Argüelles D, Deulofeu R, et al. Effect of the administration of an oral hyaluronan formulation on clinical and biochemical parameters in young horses with osteochondrosis. *Vet Comp Orthop Traumatol.* 2009;22(6):455–459.

210. McIlwraith CW. Surgical versus conservative management of osteochondrosis. *Vet J.* 2013;197(1):19–28.

211. McIlwraith CW, Nixon AJ, Wright IM, et al. *Diagnosis and surgical arthroscopy of the horse*. 3rd ed. Edinburgh, UK: Mosby-Elsevier; 2006.

212. Laws EG, Richardson DW, Ross MW, et al. Racing performance of Standardbreds after conservative treatment and surgical treatment for tarsocrural osteochondrosis. *Equine Vet J*. 1993;25(3):199–202.

213. McIlwraith CW. Osteochondritis dissecans of the tibiotarsal (tarsocrural) joint. *Proc Am Assoc Equine Pract*. 1993;39:69–72.

214. McIlwraith CW. Osteochondritis dissecans of the femoropatellar joint. *Proc Am Assoc Equine Pract*. 1993;39:73–77.

215. McIlwraith CW, Fessler JF. Arthroscopy in the diagnosis of equine joint disease. *J Am Vet Med Assoc*. 1978;172(3):263–268.

216. Vatistas NJ, Wright IM, Dyson SJ. Comparison of arthroscopy and arthrotomy for the treatment of osteochondrotic lesions in the femoropatellar joint of horses. *Vet Rec*. 1995;137(25):629–632.

217. McIlwraith CW, Nixon AJ, Wright IM, et al. *Diagnosis and surgical arthroscopy of the horse*. 4th ed. Edinburgh, UK: Mosby-Elsevier; 2015.

218. Nixon AJ, Fortier LA, Goodrich LR, et al. Arthroscopic reattachment of select (OCD) lesions using resorbable polydioxanone pins. *Equine Vet J*. 2004;36(5):376–383.

219. Sparks HD, Nixon AJ, Fortier LA, et al. Arthroscopic reattachment of osteochondritis dissecans cartilage flaps of the femoropatellar joint: long-term results. *Equine Vet J*. 2011;43(6):650–659.

220. Foland JW, McIlwraith CW, Trotter GW. Arthroscopic surgery for osteochondritis dissecans of the femoropatellar joint of the horse. *Equine Vet J*. 1992;24(6):419–423.

221. UpRichard K, Elce YA, Piat P, et al. Outcome after arthroscopic treatment of lateral femoral trochlear ridge osteochondrosis in sport horses. A retrospective study of 37 horses. *Vet Comp Orthop Traumatol*. 2013;26(2):105–109.

222. Beard WL, Bramlage LR, Schneider RK, et al. Postoperative racing performance in Standardbreds and Thoroughbreds with osteochondrosis of the tarsocrural joint: 109 cases (1984-1990). *J Am Vet Med Assoc*. 1994;204(10):1655–1659.

223. Brink P, Dolvik NI, Tverdal A. Lameness and effusion of the tarsocrural joints after arthroscopy of osteochondritis dissecans in horses. *Vet Rec*. 2009;165(24):709–712.

224. McIlwraith CW, Vorhees M. Management of osteochondritis dissecans of the dorsal aspect of the distal metacarpus and metatarsus. *Proc Am Assoc Equine Pract*. 1990;36:547–550.

225. Richardson DW. Diagnosis and management of osteochondrosis and osseous cyst-like lesions. In: Ross MW, Dyson SJ, eds. *Diagnosis and management of lameness in the horse*. 2nd ed. Philadelphia, PA: Saunders; 2011:631–638.

226. Jenner F, Ross MW, Martin BB, et al. Scapulohumeral osteochondrosis. A retrospective study of 32 horses. *Vet Comp Orthop Traumatol*. 2008;21(5):406–412.

227. Grøndahl AM, Engeland A. Influence of radiographically detectable orthopedic changes on racing performance in Standardbred trotters. *J Am Vet Med Assoc*. 1995;206(7):1013–1017.

228. Jørgensen HS, Proschowsky H, Falk-Rønne J, et al. The significance of routine radiographic findings with respect to subsequent racing performance and longevity in standardbred trotters. *Equine Vet J*. 1997;29(1):55–59.

229. Hopper SA, Bramlage LR. Postoperative racing performance of Thoroughbred weanlings and yearlings surgically treated for femoropatellar joint osteochondrosis. *Proc Am Assoc Equine Pract*. 1996;42:168–169.

230. Robert C, Valette JP, Jacquet S, et al. Influence of juvenile osteochondral conditions on racing performance in Thoroughbreds born in Normandy. *Vet J*. 2013;197:83–89.

231. Lepeule J, Robert C, Bareille N, et al. A reliable severity scoring system for radiographic findings in the limbs of young horses. *Vet J*. 2013;197(1):52–57.

232. Robert C, Valette JP, Denoix JM. Correlation between routine radiographic findings and early racing career in French trotters. *Equine Vet J*. 2006;38(suppl 36):473–478.

233. Verwilghen DR, Janssens S, Busoni V, et al. Do developmental orthopaedic disorders influence future jumping performances in Warmblood stallions? *Equine Vet J*. 2013;45(5):578–581.

234. Barneveld A, van Weeren PR. Conclusions regarding the influence of exercise on the development of the equine musculoskeletal system with special reference to osteochondrosis. *Equine Vet J*. 1999;31(suppl 31):112–119.

235. Van Weeren PR, Jeffcott LB. Problems and pointers in osteochondrosis: twenty years on. *Vet J*. 2013;197(1):96–102.

236. Wittwer C, Dierks C, Harmann H, et al. Associations between candidate gene markers at a quantitative trait locus on equine chromosome 4 responsible for osteochondrosis dissecans in fetlock joints of South German Coldblood horses. *J Hered*. 2008;99(2):125–129.

237. Wittwer C, Hamann H, Distl O. The candidate gene XIRP2 at a quantitative gene locus on equine chromosome 18 associated with osteochondrosis in fetlock and hock joints of South German Coldblood horses. *J Hered*. 2009;100(4):481–486.

238. Van Weeren PR. Etiology, diagnosis and treatment of OC(D). *Clin Techn Equine Pract*. 2006;5(4):248–258.

6

Subchondral Cystic Lesions

C. Wayne McIlwraith

SUBCHONDRAL CYSTIC LESIONS

Subchondral cystic lesions (SCLs) and, in particular, their pathogenesis and consequent treatment methods still incite controversy.[1] The lesions were initially described as subchondral bone cysts. Later others described them as SCLs or osseous cystlike lesions to avoid the implication that they are a true cyst. However, when examined pathologically the author feels that they conform to most people's definition of a cyst in that they have a lining (Figure 6-1). They occur in a number of locations. Subchondral bone cysts were first reported as a clinical entity in 1968.[2] In that report there were 12 cases in the phalanges and one in the radial carpal bone. A series was reported in 1982 in the stifle and distal phalanx.[3] A third series of 69 cases with 64 horses was reported in 1970 under a modified name, osseous cystlike lesions.[4] In that series, there were 15 instances of cysts in the carpal bones, 10 in the third metacarpal bone, 3 in the radius, 5 in the proximal sesamoid, 6 in the proximal phalanx, 4 in the middle phalanx, 5 in the distal phalanx, 6 in the navicular bone, 12 in the femur, 2 in the tibia, and 3 in the tarsal bones. Since that time, the most common site of clinical cases reported has been the medial condyle of the femur.[5-12]

What Is a Subchondral Cystic Lesion and What Are We Treating?

This discussion will address SCLs of the medial femoral condyle (MFC) in the medial femorotibial joint of the stifle as this is the most common condition we deal with and studies on pathogenesis have been specific for this lesion.

In early literature, cases of SCLs had lameness, and radiographs usually showed an obvious lesion. Lameness is the usual reason that cases are presented to the veterinarian. Direct palpation of medial femorotibial joint effusion is uncommon, but it has been reported that approximately 60% of cases will have femoropatellar effusion.[5] This is presumably related to known communication (at least the potential) between the medial femorotibial joint and the femoropatellar joint. The condition is confirmed by radiographs (Figure 6-2). With the advent of digital radiographs and survey radiographs at yearling sales, more attention is now paid to subchondral defects and even flattening of the medial femoral condyle in addition to "traditional" SCLs. These cases are usually asymptomatic.

With regard to radiographic appearance and classification, there has been an evolution. Initially there were two types: Type I was a radiographically dome-shaped lucent area, which was confluent with a flattened joint surface, and type II had a circular lucent area within the condyle with a thinner radiographically lucent tract connecting the cysts to the articular surface of the condyle[12] (Figure 6-2). This early classification evolved into type I, 10 mm or less in depth; type II, more than 10 mm in depth; and type III, flattened or irregular contour of the subchondral bone.[5] More recently, five different types were described by Wallis et al. in 2008[13] (Figure 6-3).

Type 1 lesions were defined as being smaller than 10 mm in depth and were usually dome-shaped. Type 2A lesions were greater than 10 mm in depth and had a lollipop or mushroom shape with a narrow cloaca and a round cystic lucency. Type 2B lesions were greater than 10 mm in depth with a large dome shape extending down to a large articular surface defect. Type 3 lesions (noted incidentally on survey radiographs of yearlings) were defined as condylar flattening or small defects in the subchondral bone, usually noted in the limb contralateral to that of the clinically significant SCL. Type 4 lesions were defined as those that had lucency in the condyle with or without an articular defect, but had no radiographic evidence of a cloaca in the subchondral bone plate.

Digital radiographs and survey radiographs have led to increased scrutiny of radiographs. As part of a study to prospectively examine the significance of lesions in the medial femoral condyle of cutting horses, there was further definition of subchondral defects and flattening of MFCs.[14] In this study, to differentiate "lesions" that were being noted as potentially significant by some veterinarians, the MFC was classified as smooth and continuously convex in contour (grade 0); flattened without radiographic evidence of subchondral bone changes (grade 1); a small defect or change in, without extension through, the subchondral bone (grade 2); a shallow, crescent-shaped subchondral lucency that is wider than tall and confluent with the joint surface (grade 3); or a well-defined round or oval radiolucency in the middle of the MFC that communicated with the femorotibial joint (grade 4).[14] (In this classification grade 3 is equivalent to the type I of Wallis et al. (2008)[13] and grade 4 is equivalent to grade 2 without subdivision into a and b).

PATHOGENESIS

SCLs have been proposed as manifestations of osteochondrosis by a number of authors.[15,16] It is my opinion that with young horses and, particularly, in bilateral cases, this is the probable cause. On the other hand, there has been progressive recognition that subchondral bone cysts occur in older horses and some have been identified with an initial articular defect.[17,18] In an early study by Kold et al. (1986),[19] a

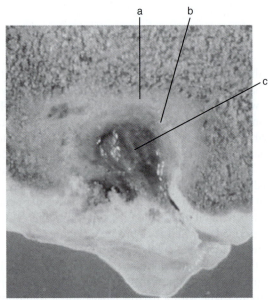

FIGURE 6-1 A gross sagittal section revealing the appearance of a subchondral cystic lesion. Sclerotic bone is present around the cyst (**a**), dense fibrous tissue lines the cyst (**b**), and the center is often filled with gelatinous material (**c**). (Reprinted from Wallis TW, Goodrich LR, McIlwraith CW, et al.: Arthroscopic injection of corticosteroids into the fibrous tissue of subchondral cystic lesions of the medial femoral condyle in horses: a retrospective study of 52 cases (2001-2006), Equine Vet J 40(5):461-7, 2008.)

subchondral bone cyst was produced experimentally in a pony by creating a linear cartilaginous defect in a central weight-bearing area of the medial femoral condyle. More recent work in our laboratory did not duplicate this finding but showed that a subchondral bone defect could induce an SCL. A full-thickness linear defect was created in the articular cartilage of the medial femoral condyle in six femorotibial joints in a group of exercised horses, and there was no formation of subchondral bone cysts.[20] However, in the same study, concurrent elliptical cartilaginous and subchondral bone defects (5 mm diameter and 3 mm deep) in the medial femoral condyle resulted in the development of cystic lesions in 5 of 6 horses. This experimental finding, as well as anecdotal clinical evidence, lends support to the theory that direct mechanical trauma to the subchondral bone plays a role in the development of subchondral bone cysts.

Some work from a collaborative study between the Orthopaedic Research Center at Colorado State University and the University of Zurich has demonstrated that the fibrous tissue contents of SCLs in horses produce prostaglandin E2 (PGE2) and nitric oxide (NO), as well as matrix metalloproteinases (MMPs). Of all the variables measured, PGE2 concentrations were the highest in cystic tissue of SCL compared with synovial membrane and articular cartilage from normal joints and joints with chip fractures, indicating that this mediator may play an important role in pathologic bone resorption associated with SCL. These findings were then supported by the observation that conditioned media of SCL tissue were capable of recruiting osteoclasts and increasing their activity.[21] Such active bone resorption may play a role in the pathogenesis of subchondral bone cysts and may also be significant in the continued enlargement of cystic lesions well after the cessation of endochondral ossification.[21] A second study investigated the potential association of interleukin-1beta (IL-1β) and interleukin-6 (IL-6) in SCLs in horses using in situ hybridization of paraffin sections of fibrous tissue of SCL and quantitative

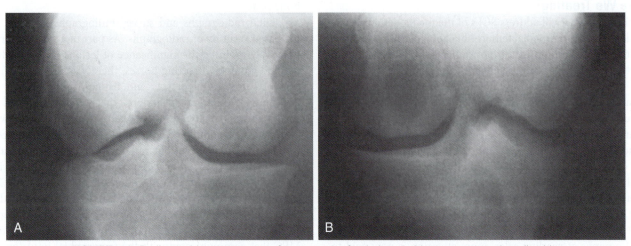

FIGURE 6-2 Radiographic appearance of two types of subchondral bone cysts as described by White K.K., McIlwraith C.W., Allen D. (1988). Curettage of subchondral bone cysts in medial femoral condyles of the horse. Equine Vet J, 20(Suppl s6),120-124. **A**, Type I dome-shaped lesion; **B**, Type II circular lucent defect.

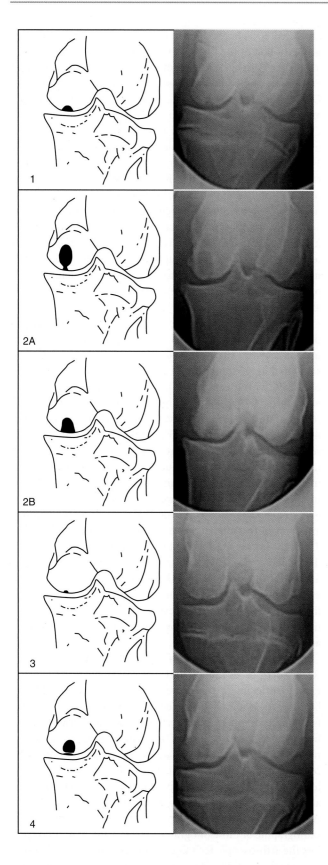

FIGURE 6-3 Classification of subchondral cystic lesions of the medial femoral condyle as described by Wallis T.W., Goodrich L.R., McIlwraith C.W., et al. (2008). Arthroscopic injection of corticosteroids into the fibrous tissue of subchondral cystic lesions of the medial femoral condyle in horses: a retrospective study of 52 cases (2001-2006). Equine Vet J 40(5), 461-467. Type 1 lesions were defined as being smaller than 10 mm in depth and were usually dome-shaped. Type 2A lesions were greater than 10 mm in depth and had a lollipop or mushroom shape with a narrow cloaca and a round cystic lucency. Type 2B lesions were greater than 10 mm in depth with a large dome shape extending down to a large articular surface defect. Type 3 lesions (noted incidentally on survey radiographs of yearlings) were defined as condylar flattening or small defects in the subchondral bone, usually noted in the contralateral limb to that of the clinically significant SCL. Type 4 lesions were defined as those that had lucency in the condyle with or without an articular defect, but had no radiographic evidence of a cloaca in the subchondral bone plate.

real-time PCR in fresh frozen tissue and undecalcified bone sections of SCL embedded in acrylic resin. Upregulation of mRNA of both cytokines could be demonstrated. Interestingly, mRNA of IL-1β was upregulated at the periphery of the cystic lesion adjacent to the normal bone; whereas, IL-6 mRNA was upregulated within the fibrous tissue found in the center of the SCL.[22] It was concluded that both cytokines are associated with the pathologic bone resorption observed in SCLs and in combination with increased production of PGE2 may be responsible for the slow healing, maintenance, or further expansion of the cystic lesions.

As an "intermediate" hypothesis, compressive forces encountered in normal weightbearing might encourage the formation of subchondral bone cysts by contributing to the deformation of thickened cartilage previously compromised by a disturbance in the endochondral ossification process.[23,24] Associated with this observation is the observation that subchondral bone cysts tend to occur at the location in a joint subjected to maximal weightbearing during the support phase of the stride.[17,25]

More recently a new treatment technique for SCLs has been developed using a cortical bone screw; the originator of the technique proposes that altering strain on the SCL will promote trabecular bone formation and remodeling (E.M. Santschi, unpublished data).

Treatment Based on Pathogenesis?

Treatment techniques have continued to be somewhat controversial, but initial success was reported with conservative therapy (rest and antiinflammatory agents).[6,11] However, older horses have a worse prognosis[11]; in the author's experience some horses progress to athletic activity (including racing) without surgery but most have persistent problems.

Some form of surgical intervention has generally been recommended when athletic activity is required. Criteria for "success" have varied and some horses with conservative treatment can go on to alternative and less demanding careers.

For instance, we have seen horses that are bred to race but end up being riding horses. The criterion for success, at least with athletes, is generally that the horse returns to the complete activity that it was undertaking before or for which the horse was bred and at the same level. Historically there have been a number of surgical treatments. From 1975 to 1978 the author attempted surgical treatment using an extraarticular approach and packed the defect with cancellous bone graft in similar fashion to the technique used in phalangeal cysts.[24] None of the initial six cases treated in this fashion achieved athletic soundness. This was attributed to inadequate curettage at the edge of the cyst and lack of penetration of the sclerotic bone, but of course this was based on the SCLs being considered inert structures that just required increase in healing without any awareness of progressive inflammation and osteolysis. Similarly, a periarticular approach with débridement and packing was considered successful.[26]

From 1979 to 1998 an intraarticular approach was used with arthrotomy into the medial femorotibial joint between the middle and medial patellar ligaments with the joint flexed.[9] Of 48 horses that did not have evidence of osteoarthritis before surgery, all improved and 35 were not lame when returned to athletic activity.[12] Of four with osteoarthritis signs before surgery, two remained lame and two improved. At that stage surgery was recommended for cases that had not responded to at least 3 months of rest; however, a long delay did not necessarily have detrimental effects because horses that had been lame for a year or more before surgery became sound after surgery.

Surgery using arthrotomy and packing of cancellous bone graft into the curetted cavity—with the rationale that this would improve healing—did not show any benefit of curettage alone.[7,27] Because curettage and leaving the cavity open had superior results, this was the technique adopted by most.[12]

In 1989 the author started using arthroscopic surgery as described by Lewis (1987)[8] to treat these lesions. Excellent visualization of the cystic lesion can be obtained, and a follow-up study reported on outcome for 41 horses with SCLs of the MFC treated by arthroscopic surgery.[5] There were 17 Quarter horses, 15 Arabians, 8 Thoroughbreds, and 1 Holsteiner; 28 (68%) of the horses were 1- to 3-years-old. For all horses the initial presentation was mild to moderate hindlimb lameness or altered gait. Bilateral radiographic abnormalities were detected in 27 horses and 19/27 horses had lesions identified at arthroscopic surgery. In addition to the SCL, 13 joints in 11 horses had an OCD lesion on the articular surface of the medial femoral condyle that extended from the opening of the SCL. Surgical débridement via arthroscopy was the only treatment for 37 lesions of 23 horses. Débridement followed by drilling of the defect bed was performed in 23 lesions of 18 horses. Complete follow-up information was obtained for 39 horses; 22 (56%) had a successful result and 17 (44%) had an unsuccessful result. However, in a separate analysis excluding horses with unsuccessful results because of factors not directly attributable to the SCL of the MFC (so-called censored analysis), 23/31 (74%) horses had a successful result

and 8/31 (26%) horses had an unsuccessful result. Within this group of horses the prognosis for a successful result was not associated with age, sex, size of lesion, unilateral versus bilateral lesions, whether the lesion was drilled, the presence of OCD associated with the SCL, or whether the lesion enlarged after surgery. Compared with Thoroughbreds and Arabians, Quarter horses had a poorer prognosis for success. Follow-up radiographs were available for 14 horses. In 9 of these 14 horses the SCL had enlarged after surgery. Postoperative cystic enlargement was significantly associated with drilling of the lesion bed at the time of surgery.[5] Subsequent to these findings, we ceased using subchondral bone drilling and also added the intralesional injection of 40 mg of methylprednisolone acetate (Depo-Medrol) to our regimen. The latter technique was based on extrapolation from the treatment of unicameral bone cysts in humans. Since commencing the use of corticosteroids at the time of curettage, we have not seen any cysts increase in size.

Other authors, reporting on results with arthroscopic débridement, have identified certain limitations. In a study in Kentucky of 150 cases, 70% of horses with a surface defect smaller than 15 mm started a race after surgery; whereas, only 54% with greater than 15 mm of surface defect diameter started a race after surgery.[28] In a UK study, 25/39 (64%) of horses aged 0 to 3 years of age returned to soundness; although only 16/46 (35%) of horses older than 3 years returned to soundness.[29] More recently, a retrospective study identified concurrent or sequential development of medial meniscal tears and SCLs within the medial femorotibial joint in horses.[30] In this study 21 horses (9.1% of all horses undergoing MFC arthroscopy during that period) were identified as having both a medial meniscal injury and SCL of the MFC. Thirteen horses had the abnormalities concurrently. Six developed a meniscal lesion subsequent to SCL débridement. This led to a hypothesis that the rim of a débrided SCL could cause damage to the medial meniscus or medial meniscotibial ligament. Two horses also developed an SCL subsequent to meniscal injury. Only 4/19 horses were classified as successful and returned to intended use.

During the time period of this study the findings of von Rechenberg et al. (2000, 2001)[21,22] led to development of a technique to inject corticosteroids directly into the fibrous lining of the cystic lesion under arthroscopic guidance.[13] This is a good example of laboratory bench research leading to an improved clinical technique. The rationale for intralesional injection of triamcinolone acetonide possibly improving results versus débridement included shorter convalescence, less articular disruption, less potential for cystic enlargement, and less potential for causing a subsequent meniscal lesion. Although the injection technique can be performed under radiographic or ultrasonographic monitoring, the author prefers the arthroscopic technique to débride any loose chondral or osteochondral flaps (as was seen early during arthroscopic débridement[5]). In a retrospective study on the results of arthroscopic injection of corticosteroids into the fibrous tissue of SCLs of the MFC in 52 cases, the inclusion criteria were lameness and radiographic evidence of an SCL. The results showed that 35/52 (67%) horses were successfully treated. An additional 5 horses, bringing the total to 40/52 (77%), were considered sound at veterinary recheck examination, but for various reasons were not performing their intended athletic discipline. When no other variable was considered other than the presence of an SCL, 56/73 SCLs (77%) treated by this procedure resulted in a sound leg. Of the SCLs from unilateral cases 28/31 (90%) were considered successful and of the bilateral SCLs, 28/42 (67%) were considered successful. This equated to 25/31 horses with unilateral SCLs (81%) classified as successful vs 10/21 horses with bilateral SCLs (48%) ($P = 0.01$). A change in radiographic size of SCLs was recorded in 22 SCLs that had pre- and postoperative radiographs available. In 7/9 (78%) SCLs there was a decrease in size and they were classified as successful. In 9/13 (69%) SCLs there was no change in size but they were still classified as successful. Only 1/22 SCLs had evidence of enlargement postoperatively and this was unsuccessful. There was no significant association between success and age when separated into age groups of up to 3 years and over 3 years of age. A total of 43/55 (78%) SCLs in horses aged 0 to 3 years old and 13/18 (72%) SCLs in horses aged more than 3 years old were classified as successful. This equated to 27/39 (69%) horses aged 0 to 3 years and 8/13 (62%) aged over 3 years old classified as successful. Radiographic findings of osteophytes were found on preoperative radiographs or listed in the radiograph report of 16/61 SCLs (26%). There was a significant association between absence of these osteophytes and success ($P = 0.04$), and 10/16 limbs (63%) with these radiographic signs were classified as successful versus 39/45 (87%) without any radiographic osteophytes being classified as successful.

SUMMARY

This chapter has presented thoughts on the pathobiology of SCLs with attention to targets and rationale for treatment. The focus has been on SCLs of the MFC in the medial femorotibial joint. SCLs occur elsewhere and these will be discussed in Section IV, Specifics of Anatomy, Clinical Diagnosis, Imaging Diagnosis, and Treatment by Region.

REFERENCES

1. McIlwraith CW. Subchondral bone cysts in the horse: aetiology, diagnosis and treatment options. *Equine Vet Educ*. 1998;10(6):313–317.
2. Pettersson H, Sevelius F. Subchondral bone cysts in the horse: a clinical study. *Equine Vet J*. 1968;1(2):75–80.
3. Verschooten F, DeMoor A. Subchondral cystic and related lesions affecting the equine pedal bone and stifle. *Equine Vet J*. 1982;14(1):47–54.
4. Reid CF. Radiographic diagnosis and appearance of osseous cyst-like lesions in horses previously reported as periarticular subchondral bone cysts. *Proc Am Assoc Equine Pract*. 1970;16:185–187.
5. Howard RD, McIlwraith CW, Trotter GW. Arthroscopic surgery for subchondral cystic lesions of the medial femoral condyle in horses. 41 cases (1988-1991). *J Am Vet Med Assoc*. 1995;206(6):842–850.
6. Jeffcott LB, Kold SE. Clinical and radiological aspects of stifle bone cysts in the horse. *Equine Vet J*. 1982;14(1):40–46.
7. Kold SE, Hickman J. Results of treatment of subchondral bone cysts in the medial condyle of the equine femur with an autogenous cancellous bone graft. *Comp Cont Educ Pract Vet*. 1984;4:S282–S294.
8. Lewis RD. A retrospective study of diagnostic and surgical arthroscopy of the equine femorotibial joint. *Proc Am Assoc Equine Pract*. 1987;23:887–893.
9. McIlwraith CW. Subchondral cystic lesions. *Vet Clinics North Am Large Anim Pract*. 1983;5:350–355.
10. McIlwraith CW. Subchondral cystic lesions in the horse – the indications, methods and results of surgery. *Equine Vet Educ*. 1990;2(2):75–80.
11. Stewart B, Reid CF. Osseous cyst-like lesions of the medial femoral condyle in the horse. *J Am Vet Med Assoc*. 1982;180(3):254–258.
12. White KK, McIlwraith CW, Allen D. Curettage of subchondral bone cysts in medial femoral condyles of the horse. *Equine Vet J*. 1988;20(Suppl s6):120–124.
13. Wallis TW, Goodrich LR, McIlwraith CW, et al. Arthroscopic injection of corticosteroids into the fibrous tissue of subchondral cystic lesions of the medial femoral condyle in horses: a retrospective study of 52 cases (2001-2006). *Equine Vet J*. 2008;40(5):461–467.
14. Contino EK, Park RD, McIlwraith CW. Prevalence of radiographic changes in yearling and 2-year-old Quarter Horses intended for cutting. *Equine Vet J*. 2012;44(2):185–195.
15. McIlwraith CW. Osteochondrosis. In: Stashak TS, ed. *Adams' lameness in horses (4*th *ed.)*. Philadelphia, PA: Lea & Febiger; 1987:396–410.
16. Stromberg J. A review of the salient features of osteochondrosis in the horse. *Equine Vet J*. 1979;11(4):211–214.
17. McIlwraith CW. What is developmental orthopedic disease, osteochondrosis, osteochondritis, metabolic bone disease? *Proc Am Assoc Equine Pract*. 1993;39:35–44.
18. Yovich JV, Stashak TS. Subchondral osseous cyst formation after an intra-articular fracture in a filly. *Equine Vet J*. 1989;21(1):72–74.
19. Kold SE, Hickman J, Melsen F. An experimental study of the healing process of equine chondral and osteochondral defects. *Equine Vet J*. 1986;18(1):18–24.
20. Ray CS, Baxter GM, McIlwraith CW, et al. Development of subchondral cystic lesions after articular cartilage and subchondral bone damage in young horses. *Equine Vet J*. 1996;28(3):225–232.
21. von Rechenberg B, Guenther H, McIlwraith CW, et al. Fibrous tissue of subchondral cystic lesions in horses produced local mediators and neutral metalloproteinases and caused bone resorption in vitro. *Vet Surg*. 2000;29(5):420–429.
22. von Rechenberg B, Leutenegger C, Zlinsky K, et al. Upregulation of mRNA of interleukin-1 and -6 are upregulated in equine subchondral cystic lesions of four horses. *Equine Vet J*. 2001;33(2):143–149.
23. Bramlage LR. Osteochondrosis related bone cysts. *Proc Am Assoc Equine Pract*. 1993;39:83.
24. Kold SE, Killingbeck M. The use of autogenous cancellous bone graft for treatment of subchondral bone cysts in the distal phalanges: 3 cases. *Equine Vet Educ*. 1998;10(6):307–312.
25. Nixon AJ. Osteochondrosis and osteochondritis dissecans of the equine fetlock. *Comp Cont Educ Pract Vet*. 1990;12:1463–1475.

26. White KK, Prades M. Grid assisted periarticular approach to subchondral cysts. *J Am Vet Med Assoc.* 1988;192:1762.

27. Kold SE, Hickman J. Use of an autogenous cancellous bone graft in the treatment of subchondral bone cysts in the medial femoral condyle of horses. *Equine Vet J.* 1983;15(4):312–316.

28. Sandler EA, Bramlage LR, Emberston RM, et al. Correlation of radiographic appearance, lesion size, and racing performance after arthroscopic surgical treatment of subchondral cystic lesions of the medial femoral condyle in Thoroughbreds: 150 cases. *Vet Surg.* 2002;31:495.

29. Smith MA, Walmsley JP, Phillips TJ, et al. Effect of age at presentation on outcome following arthroscopic debridement of subchondral cystic lesions of the medial femoral condyle: 85 horses (1993-2003). *Equine Vet J.* 2005;37(2):175–180.

30. Hendrix SM, Baxter GW, McIlwraith CW, et al. Concurrent or sequential development of medial meniscal or subchondral cystic lesions within the medial femorotibial joint in horses (1996-2006). *Equine Vet J.* 2010;42(1):5–9.

7

Septic Arthritis

P. René van Weeren

There is common agreement nowadays that virtually any joint disorder has an inflammatory component, including those earlier designated as "degenerative" only.[1] However, this inflammatory component is nowhere as present and as fulminant as in cases of joint infection. The condition is commonly called "septic arthritis," but has also been termed "infectious" or "infective" arthritis.[2] All of these terms are not entirely appropriate, as "infectious" might imply a transmittable disease, which is rarely the case; "septic" means pertaining to or causing sepsis (systemic infection), whereas joint infection is more often consequence than cause of sepsis; and "infective" is defined as "capable of causing infection" in the Churchill Livingstone Medical Dictionary,[3] which applies more to the causing agent than to the condition itself. The author has chosen to use the term "septic arthritis" throughout this chapter.

The primary cause may be either an abnormal exposure to pathogens or an abnormal weakness of the host defense, that is, in most cases some form of immunodeficiency. In equine septic arthritis the first mechanism commonly applies to cases in mature individuals, but in foals the second mechanism is common. This difference is important for treatment and prognosis, for which reason discrimination will be made between these two patient categories.

There are few conditions in equine medicine and surgery in which treatment and prognosis have changed so dramatically over the past few decades as with septic arthritis. The author can recall the early days of his career in the early 1980s when the prognosis of a horse with a septic arthritis because of trauma was poor, and many horses presented with this condition were euthanized because of this poor prognosis. Nowadays, there is common agreement that, if subjected to timely and aggressive treatment featuring arthroscopic lavage, the prognosis of most of these cases has become much better.[4]

This chapter will provide an overview of the pathophysiology (i.e., the effect on joint homeostasis), possible etiology and causative organisms, and prevalence, before embarking on clinical signs and diagnosis, followed by treatment and prognosis. The chapter concludes with a paragraph on the specific aspects of septic arthritis in foals.

PATHOPHYSIOLOGY

The body tends to respond vigorously to infection with microorganisms. The joint is no exception and in the majority of cases a fulminant inflammation will ensue, leading to severe clinical signs. This is not always the case, as both host conditions (immune response) and characteristics of the invading microorganism play a role. Joint infection may give rise to much less obvious and even subclinical signs under specific conditions and depending on the type of the microorganism involved.

After infection, the synovial membrane will respond with hyperemia. Increased vascular permeability will result in extravasation of fibrin, together with the efflux of macrophages. There will be joint effusion and severely increased hypersensitivity of the richly innervated articular capsule. A large number of inflammatory mediators will be released, including interleukin-1beta (IL-1β) and tumor necrosis factor alpha (TNF-α). These are the same mediators relevant in cases of much lower-grade inflammation occurring after joint trauma or in osteoarthritis (see Chapter 3 for a general overview), but they are released in much larger quantities.

In septic arthritis it is the balance between inflammatory and antiinflammatory mediators that is important. Research in other species has shown various factors that affect the response of the host. *Staphylococcus aureus* and other infectious agents produce a number of toxins and enzymes that trigger the inflammatory reaction by the host and exert negative effects on the tissues of the joint (Figure 7-1). These may be either extracellular virulence factors,[5] bacterial cell wall components such as staphylococcal protein A,[6] formylated peptides that mediate neutrophil recruitment and in this way contribute substantially to joint damage,[7] or even oligonucleotide sequences within bacterial DNA.[8] Some of these factors have been studied through the development of vaccinations against them. For instance, vaccinations against so-called adhesins (that facilitate *S. aureus* infection) were proven to be effective against intravenous challenging with this microorganism in mice.[9]

In samples of synovial fluid from infected joints, significant amounts of collagenase and caseinase activity were

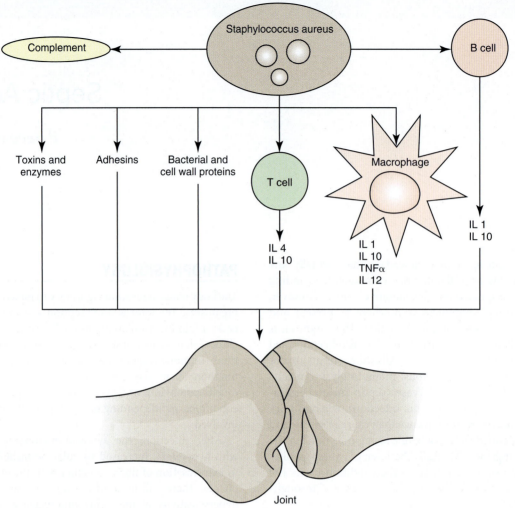

FIGURE 7-1 Pathogenesis of infection by *S. aureus* in humans. *IL*, Interleukin; *TNF-α*, tumor necrosis factor-alpha. (From: Mathews C.J., Weston V.C., Jones A., et al. (2010). Bacterial septic arthritis in adults. Lancet, 375(9717), 846-855.)

detected that were deemed to originate from both the synovial cells and neutrophils.[10] Further, synovial membrane infection increases the production of IL-1β and IL-6 by synoviocytes in an in vitro setting.[11] Medium that was collected from the infected cultures and subsequently filtered reduced proteoglycan synthesis and total glycosaminoglycan (GAG) content in cartilage explants; hyaluronic acid concentration was also lower with synovial infection. In vivo, the synovial membrane is thought to be an important element in septic arthritis, because hematogenous infection will enter the joint via the synovial membrane, but, above all, because microorganisms are known to colonize parts of the synovial membrane. This may make them hard to reach and eradicate with therapeutic interventions. Experimental work using a septic arthritis model in horses has largely been limited to therapy evaluation and has not focused on pathophysiologic aspects.[12-14] However, in a study in which septic synovitis was induced experimentally in one tarsocrural joint of six horses by intraarticular injection of Staphylococcus-saline suspension, the progression of the induced pfnectious arthritis was followed over a 9-day period by clinical examination

and classic clinical-chemical synovial fluid parameters (see the paragraph on diagnosis). Changes in synovial fluid were shown to be present before clinical signs of septic arthritis became manifest, with neutrophilia over 90% and pH under 6.9 as the most consistent findings in the infected synovia.[15]

If left untreated, septic arthritis will result in substantial joint damage. The initial proteoglycan loss from the extracellular matrix (ECM) is followed by damage to the collagen network, which will diminish biomechanical resistance and hence make the cartilage more susceptible to further damage.[16] In vitro work with infected cartilage cultures showed that up to 40% of glycosaminoglycans may be lost from the ECM within 48 hours.[17] In in vivo trials loss of collagen becomes significant between weeks 2 and 3 after infection and may reach up to 50% after 3 weeks in untreated animals.[16] In advanced cases substantial macroscopically visible damage to the articular cartilage may occur (Figure 7-2).

There are additional factors, apart from the primary infection, that play a role in the course of the disease after the initial stage. Large amounts of fibrin are often present in the joint cavity. These form niches for the microorganisms and severely

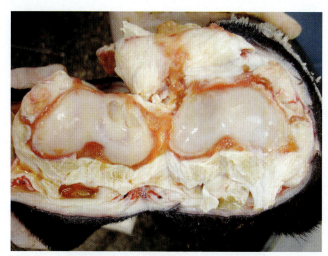

FIGURE 7-2 Severe cartilage damage in the interphalangeal joint of a horse with long-standing septic arthritis that was unresponsive to treatment. (Photo courtesy Dr. Harold Brommer.)

hamper reestablishment of joint homeostasis, because they also affect the normal flow of synovial fluid. Microorganisms within these fibrin aggregates will be difficult targets for medication that is administered systemically, by regional perfusion methods, or applied intraarticularly via through-and-through lavage, making drainage via arthrotomy or arthroscopy a critical part of treatment. The fibrin clots induce an increased synovial fibrinolytic activity, which has been measured in the horse as a significant increase in synovial D-dimer concentrations.[18] Both joint swelling and pain impede normal joint motion. The increased intraarticular pressure will affect blood flow to the synovial membrane, which may result in ischemia of that tissue and further damage and dysfunction. In a very advanced stage, signs may include pannus formation, erosion, and undermining of cartilage. Radiographic signs of subchondral osteolysis, erosions, and possible cyst formation may become evident. It is recognized in the horse that this very severe category would usually be grounds for humane euthanasia.

ETIOLOGY AND CAUSATIVE ORGANISMS

Classically, a microorganism may enter a joint via four routes:
1. The most common way in foals (and children) is *hematogenous* infection with the invading pathogens arriving via the vascularization of the synovial membrane. Although less common than in foals, the possibility of hematogenous infection should not immediately be discarded in mature animals. In a large retrospective study of 192 horses affected with septic arthritis or tenosynovitis, in 12/126 horses older than 6 months no etiology was found and the pathway of infection was probably hematogenous.[19]
2. A septic process in the neighborhood of a joint may also spread and invade the joint *(per continuitatem)*. This condition is not uncommon in cases of trauma followed by infection of the damaged tissue in which the joint was not involved in the primary lesion, but may become infected secondarily.

3. Perforating trauma is by far the most common etiology of joint infection in mature horses.
4. The development of arthritis after an intraarticular injection. This form is called *iatrogenic* and is in fact a specific variant of perforating trauma.

Numerous microorganisms have been implicated in septic arthritis in adult horses, partly depending on the origin of the infection and the patient population studied. Trauma is the most frequent cause and *Streptococcus spp.*, *Staphylococcus spp.*, *enterobacteriaceae*, among which *Escherichia coli* and *Salmonella spp.* are prominently present, and anaerobes are among the most frequently cultured pathogens.[2] Less common organisms, such as *Corynebacterium pseudotuberculosis* can be found occasionally.[20] In trauma patients it is not uncommon to find more than one organism.[19] *Staphylococcus aureus* is most commonly cultured in cases of iatrogenic infection. In one study concerning 15 cases of septic arthritis after intraarticular injections in Standardbreds, all isolates were Gram-positive *cocci*, of which 86% were *S. aureus*.[21] In another study, this percentage was 69%.[19] In that study, anaerobes were cultured in 12.3% of all cases and in 26.3% of the cases related to wounds. For common pathogens in foals, see the paragraph on septic arthritis in foals.

EPIDEMIOLOGY

Perforating trauma of a synovial cavity is a common and well-known complication of wounds in horses, especially those affecting the lower limbs where joints have virtually no layers of protective tissue. Wounds are common in these areas, which may explain why, in a large retrospective study,[19] the most frequently affected joint in all cases of septic arthritis was the tibiotarsal joint (34%), followed by the metacarpophalangeal/metatarsophalangeal (20%), carpus (18%), and femoropatellar joints (9%). Hematogenous infection is relatively rare in mature horses and no epidemiologic data exist, but several studies have addressed the incidence of septic arthritis after medical interventions, such as arthrocentesis and arthroscopy. In a recent study from Australia the risk of septic arthritis after intraarticular medication was calculated at 7.8 cases/10,000 injections, which is equivalent to one in 1249 joint injections. Risk factors were the treating veterinarian and the type of corticosteroid used with betamethasone having a lower risk than dexamethasone ($P = 0.024$).[22] The incidence of septic arthritis after elective arthroscopy without perioperative antimicrobial prophylaxis was 3 septic joints in 444 horses and 636 joints.[23] This is equal to an incidence of 0.5% per joint and 0.7% of cases. These figures are comparable with 0.9% of joints and 1.0% of horses in an earlier study concerning 932 joints in 682 horses.[24] These figures relate to the period of hospitalization. Of 461 horses for which follow-up information was available, none of the horses that had not developed septic arthritis during hospitalization developed the condition after dismissal. A difference between both studies was that the last one included horses with perforating trauma caused by a wound and the former only included elective patients. In that last study, breed (heavy breeds) and joint (tibiotarsal joint) were risk factors, but use of perioperative or intraarticular antimicrobials was not.

In an experimental study, joints inoculated with a subinfective dose of *S. aureus* were more likely to develop septic arthritis when injected simultaneously with PSGAGs than if injected with the microorganism alone.[25] A possible explanation in this case may be the antiinflammatory effect of PSGAGs, especially the inhibition of MMPs and the complement cascade.[26] However, predisposition to infection is presumably not just a result of antiinflammatory activity, as intraarticular application of corticosteroids did not significantly increase the risk of infection.[27]

CLINICAL SIGNS AND DIAGNOSIS

Clinical signs of septic arthritis alone include joint distension, periarticular swelling, often edematous in character, pain at palpation, reduced range of passive motion, and high-grade, often non-weight-bearing lameness. In many cases in which the primary cause of septic arthritis is a wound, these signs may be confounded or even obscured by clinical signs caused by the original trauma. In some of these cases it is not immediately evident if a joint is involved in a wound or not. Wounds may be contaminated, but they may drain well and therefore not be painful. In those cases arthrocentesis of the joint (in a place at a certain distance from the wound and not passing through possibly inflamed tissue) followed by the injection of a sterile fluid (after aspiration of a synovial fluid sample for analysis and culture) may be helpful to see whether there is a connection between the joint and the wound. When infusing saline remotely, it is a good idea to flex and extend the joint to see if the exit of fluid is position-dependent. Clinical signs typically develop over a couple of days. In an experimental study that used subinfective doses of the pathogen this period could be up to 10 days[25]; in another infection study this period was much shorter, but was prolonged if intraarticular corticosteroids were used.[27] Although the clinical signs will usually be sufficient to raise the suspicion of septic arthritis, the definitive diagnosis is normally based on synovial fluid analysis, imaging, and bacteriologic culture.

The aspect of synovial fluid (SF) from an infected joint differs markedly from normal SF. Normal SF is a lightly yellowish, clear, and very viscous liquid. The color of SF from septic joints may vary from normal to dark orange or red, it is often opaque or cloudy in appearance, and in most cases it has a more watery, that is, less viscous, aspect than normal SF (Figure 7-3). The most important laboratory analyses in suspected cases are total white blood cell count (WBC), differentiation of the cells in the SF, and determination of total protein content. In normal SF WBC is less than 500 cells/mm³; in septic joints this figure will rise to over 30,000 to 40,000 cells/mm³ and may easily reach values of over 100,000 cells/mm³. Although in normal SF monocytes and the odd macrophage are the predominant cell types, in septic SF polymorphonuclear leukocytes dominate and a persistent neutrophilia (>95% of WBC) is an important hallmark of a septic joint.[15] Total protein (TP) content is less than 2 g/dL in the normal joint, but will attain 4 to 5 g/dL in septic arthritis.[19,28] SF changes precede clinical

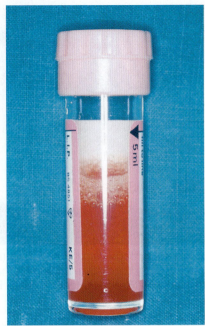

FIGURE 7-3 Hemorrhagic and turbid synovial fluid with reduced viscosity from a septic joint. This is only one manifestation of septic arthritis. Color of the fluid may vary from more or less normal to pink or red. Viscosity is usually reduced because of a lower content of hyaluronic acid, but the synovial fluid may contain flocculent material. (Photo courtesy Dr. Janny de Grauw.)

signs and were shown to occur within 24 hours after infection in experimental studies.[12,15] Apart from these long-proven laboratory analyses that are in routine use in every clinic, studies have been performed to identify other potential SF markers for septic arthritis. Serum amyloid A (SAA) concentrations in SF were significantly higher in septic or suspected septic joints than in normal SF, in which they were lower than the detection limit.[29] Because of the fact that SAA levels were not influenced by repeated arthrocentesis and because of the ease of detection, SAA was deemed a reliable marker for septic arthritis. In a follow-up study evaluating the effect of intraarticular amikacin, SAA concentration was not influenced by amikacin application although TP and WBC were. The authors concluded that SAA determination was more useful for the monitoring of a septic joint than TP or WBC.[30] In an interesting pilot study on cell viability in SF, the viability of neutrophils in SF from healthy joints or joints with OA was significantly less than in SF from septic joints; in addition, apoptosis was the predominant cell death type in the latter category versus necrosis in the former.[31]

Many inflammatory mediators and other molecules are known to be elevated in the SF of septic joints, and all are potential markers. Given the good sensitivity of the currently routinely used SF parameters, their ease of determination and low cost, and the relatively straightforward diagnosis of (suspected) septic arthritis, there is not much clinical need for more or better SF parameters, with a few possible exceptions for specific applications.

Sometimes, bacteria can be detected directly microscopically in synovial smears, which are then stained using haematoxylin and eosin (H&E) and Gram staining. In an experimental study and in a field study, approximately 25% of microorganisms could be detected in this way.[12,19] Bacterial culture is a more sensitive way to identify causative pathogens and should be performed in all cases of suspected septic arthritis. The procedure also provides the opportunity to determine the susceptibility of the causative agent for specific antimicrobials. Samples should be inoculated into vials containing blood culture medium or another enriched medium, which significantly improves the test sensitivity.[19,32,33] Culture is performed under both aerobic and anaerobic conditions. Success rate of bacteriologic culture varies; it is often more than 50%[28] and has been reported to be up to 70% when specific culture techniques are used.[2] Although samples for bacteriologic culture should ideally be taken before the onset of antimicrobial therapy, it is important to point out that valuable information can still be obtained after the onset of such therapy.[33] It has been suggested that culture of synovial membrane biopsies would be more effective than culture of SF, but this could not be substantiated.[28] Nevertheless, it is advisable to culture both if synovial membrane samples are available. In humans, real-time polymerase chain reaction (PCR) has been used successfully to identify the causative agents of septic arthritis. In a recent study in children, sensitivity and specificity for the diagnosis of septic arthritis were 0.47 and 1.00 for bacteriologic culture and 0.79 and 1.00 for real-time PCR, respectively.[34] PCR is also potentially applicable in horses.

Imaging is not the primary means to diagnose septic arthritis, but it may yield valuable additional information. In cases of septic arthritis related to wounds, radiography is routinely indicated. More sophisticated imaging techniques like computed tomography (CT) and magnetic resonance imaging (MRI) may be used, but they are expensive. In foals septic arthritis is often a sequel to or accompanied by septic physitis and osteomyelitis, and radiographic imaging is a must (see the paragraph on septic arthritis in foals). Ultrasonography may demonstrate the presence of flocculent material in synovial fluid and MRI will show soft tissue reactions in the joint capsule and around the joint. In a study in 14 horses with septic arthritis, MRI findings included diffuse hyperintensity within bone and extracapsular tissue on fat-suppressed images in all horses; there was further also joint effusion, synovial proliferation, capsular thickening, bone sclerosis, and evidence of cartilage and subchondral bone damage in most. Intravenous gadolinium administration helped in detecting fibrin deposition. It was concluded that MRI may allow earlier and more accurate diagnosis of septic arthritis compared with other imaging modalities.[35] Scintigraphy can be useful to localize lesions in the proximal parts of the limbs and in the axial skeleton. It should be noted that sites of infection may show on nuclear imaging as "cold" rather than "hot" spots, because of the presence of ischemia instead of inflammation-related hyperemia.[36,37] Contrast CT arteriographs may serve as well to document penetration into a synovial structure.[38]

TREATMENT

If there is any condition to which the millennia-old adage *ubi pus, ibi evacua* (where there is pus, it should be evacuated) applies, it may be septic arthritis. It is even found in the work of Hippocrates (460-370 BC). It was not until the absolute necessity of early physical cleaning by lavage or drainage by means of multiple-needle arthrocentesis, arthrotomy, or arthroscopy was recognized and universally applied that the prognosis of septic arthritis in immunocompetent horses improved dramatically. Nowadays arthroscopy is the treatment of choice. Cases of penetrating wounds of synovial structures and suspected septic arthritis will almost certainly be treated by emergency arthroscopic lavage with or without débridement of the synovial membrane. Additional to the surgical intervention and despite it being much less effective when used alone, antimicrobial treatment is indispensable and remains the other mainstay of the treatment of septic arthritis.

Antimicrobial Therapy

Ideally, every antimicrobial treatment should be guided by the causative organism(s) and its (or their) susceptibility to specific antibiotics. In practice, these data are not known when a patient suspected of septic arthritis is presented, but nevertheless treatment should start immediately. As the variety of possible causative organisms is large and may include both Gram-positive and Gram-negative species, the choice of a broad-spectrum antimicrobial therapy is justified. In many cases the combination of penicillin or another β-lactam antibiotic and an aminoglycoside, often amikacin or gentamicin, is chosen. The minimal inhibitory concentration (MIC) provides a guideline for the dosing of antibiotics. For gentamicin the MIC has been established at less than 2 μg/mL for most bacterial isolates, which can be achieved in synovial fluid after systemic application.[39] In cases where the presence of anaerobes is likely, for instance in certain heavily contaminated wounds, metronidazole may be added. It goes without saying that once bacteriologic and susceptibility data are available, the antibiotic regimen should be reconsidered.

Systemic administration of antibiotics has been the only way of antimicrobial therapy until recently, but current practice is to use additional local delivery systems wherever feasible. There are several reasons for this combined approach. Septic arthritis is normally, with the exception of polysynovitis in foals, a disorder of a single synovial cavity. Further, the effect of some classes of antibiotics, such as the aminoglycosides, is dose-dependent[40] and the use of extremely high doses can be warranted in cases of septic arthritis. Local application enables this, which is important as the therapeutic index of several antibiotics, including the aminoglycosides, is low. Another issue is the penetration into the synovial cavity after systemic application and the effect of the drug in that synovial cavity. Data from healthy horses are of little value, as joint homeostasis is severely disturbed in septic arthritis and changes in pH, vascular occlusion, and large amounts of fibrin, debris, and cells may affect the efficacy of medication one way or the other. For instance, in a study using the bacterial lipopolysaccharide (LPS) model for synovitis, after regional limb perfusion with amikacin sulfate the maximal attained intraarticular concentration was higher and time to maximal concentration shorter in inflamed joints versus controls.[41]

For all these reasons, there is currently much emphasis on local delivery of antibiotics in septic arthritis, in addition to systemic treatment. There are various ways to accomplish this.

Regional limb perfusion is now widely used as an adjunctive treatment. The principle is that a high dose of the antimicrobial is applied intravenously into a peripheral vessel close to the affected joint. The region is isolated from the systemic circulation by the placement of a tourniquet proximal to the joint. Both the classic rubber Esmarch tourniquet and pneumatic tourniquets can be used; the former was deemed more effective in preventing loss of amikacin from the infused region in a direct comparison and was less expensive.[42] In an earlier study comparing a pneumatic tourniquet and a narrow and a wider rubber tourniquet, the wider rubber and the pneumatic tourniquets came out as efficient, but the narrow tourniquet was ineffective.[43] Although regional limb perfusion was initially often performed under general anesthesia, this is not necessary in most cases. Discomfort to the horse can be alleviated by the use of regional anesthesia, which has been shown to have no effects on antibiotic concentrations.[44]

One of the first studies on regional perfusion investigated the effect of the technique on amikacin sulfate levels in the perfused joints (metacarpophalangeal/MCP, metatarsophalangeal/MTP, and distal interphalangeal/DIP) and on systemic concentrations after release of the tourniquet.[45] Injection of 125 mg of amikacin sulfate in 60 mL of balanced electrolyte solution resulted in concentrations in synovial fluid of over 200 μg/mL in the MCP/MTP joint and over 100 μg/mL in the DIP. The MIC for amikacin for sensitive organisms is about 4 μg/mL. High to very high concentrations remained detectable in the synovial fluid for at least 60 minutes after injection, which was 30 minutes after tourniquet removal. Serum levels did not pass 3 μg/mL after release of the tourniquet.[45] This study clearly illustrates the large impact of local delivery of antimicrobials on concentrations in SF. In later studies, safety and pharmacokinetics after regional intravenous perfusion of other drugs, including ceftiofur, vancomycin, enrofloxacin, and marbofloxacin, have been investigated.[46-49] All these antibiotics appeared safe for application via intravenous perfusion, and concentrations far above the MIC of the respective drugs were attained in all cases. However, not all combinations work. A combination of amikacin sulfate with ticarcillin/clavulanate during regional limb perfusion resulted in significantly lower amikacin synovial concentration and antimicrobial activity versus amikacin alone.[50] It is clear, however, that regional intravenous perfusion is a highly efficacious delivery route for many antimicrobial drugs in septic arthritis.

In most studies the palmar digital vein was used for delivery of the perfusion fluid, but the saphenous and cephalic veins were shown to be good alternatives in case access to the palmar digital vein is lost.[51] Loss of venous access may easily occur because of the need for repeated infusions and the often irritating character of the drug to be injected in high doses. To prevent vascular wall damage as much as possible, some authors recommend the use of a small-gauge butterfly catheter.[4] The concomitant use of a cream containing a nonsteroidal antiinflammatory drug (NSAID) during intravenous regional limb perfusion has been reported to be helpful in mitigating the inflammatory reaction at the sites used and hence may be useful to keep the vessel in good condition as long as possible.[52]

Alternatives for regional limb perfusion using venous access are intraarticular and intraosseous perfusion. In the first case an intraarticular catheter is used as an ingress portal, in the second cannulated screws are used. The intraosseous technique may have advantages in cases of concurrent osteomyelitis, but it is otherwise not a preferred option. In a case series of horses subjected to intravenous (n=155) and intraosseous (n=27) regional limb perfusion, the complication rate was found to be higher in horses treated with the latter (33%) versus the former technique (12%).[53] In a case report, intraosseous perfusion of gentamicin in a 10-year-old Warmblood treated for sepsis of the distal interphalangeal joint and the navicular bursa resulted in toxic osteonecrosis followed by pathologic fracture of the proximal phalanx that had been perfused.[54]

Implantation of antibiotic-impregnated materials, such as polymethylmethacrylate (PMMA) beads, is an alternative method to reach high local tissue concentrations of antibiotics. This approach obviates the need for repeated invasive and expensive perfusion sessions.[55] However, PMMA beads are inflexible and are not resorbed, making them unsuitable for high-motion joints. Flexible collagen sponges have been shown to be suitable for intraarticular use in the horse,[56] but have a release profile featuring a strong initial burst followed by a rapid decrease in synovial fluid concentrations of the active drug. Nevertheless, given the current interest in the development of controlled release platforms for intraarticular use in both humans and horses,[57] in most cases based on either hydrogel or microsphere technology, it can be anticipated that suitable platforms for safe prolonged intraarticular delivery of antibiotics will become available in the near future.

JOINT LAVAGE OR DRAINAGE

There are several reasons why cleaning of the joint space is of great importance in septic arthritis. The presence of purulent material may affect the potency of intraarticularly applied antimicrobials through protein binding. The drop in pH that is seen in septic joints reduces the activity of aminoglycosides, a group of antibiotics that is commonly used in septic arthritis. More importantly, cellular detritus and the myriad of inflammatory mediators and upregulated catabolic enzymes have a devastating effect on the cartilage extracellular matrix. Proteoglycan content is affected first. Proteoglycan loss is reversible, however, once the collagen network is severely affected, joint damage becomes irreversible (see previously). To prevent the infection from becoming established and for the immediate relief of pain and resulting better weight-bearing, intervention should take place as early as possible and horses suspected of septic arthritis should be treated as emergencies.

There are various ways to effect joint lavage. There is through-and-through lavage through a multineedle arthrocentesis system, arthrotomy, and arthroscopy. The first method is the least invasive and can often be performed without the need for general anesthesia,[12,13] especially in foals. A big disadvantage is that the joint cavity is not visualized. This may result in not noticing large fibrin clots, debris, or foreign material, the latter especially in cases of perforating trauma. In this technique, copious amounts (6 to 7 L on average) of a sterile fluid are used to flush the joint through at least two needles, but there may be more as several egress portals may be used for a single ingress portal. One of the pitfalls of the technique is that the fluid stream will take a fixed path within the joint, creating a "highway" and leaving large parts of the joint untouched. This can to a certain extent be counteracted by intermittently closing the egress portals and allowing the joint to distend while gently massaging it. Another frequent problem is clogging of the egress needles. A large bore needle (12 to 14 gauge) should be used as an egress portal, but the problem may still occur, requiring frequent reversal of flow. Some prefer to use a small stab incision as egress portal, because this will allow easy unplugging and even blind removal of fibrin clots through the incision by an experienced arthroscopist.[4] The joint anatomy must be taken into consideration during the procedure as all aspects of the joint (cranial and caudal in the tibiotarsal joint, for instance) must be lavaged. After the procedure the portal is left open and covered by a sterile bandage, or the skin is sutured in places where bandaging is impractical. A variant of the through-and-through lavage technique is the closed irrigation-suction system that has been reported to be effective in both humans and horses. In both species there is a success rate of approximately 80%.[58,59] With such a system, a flow reversal system using double tubing that prevents obstruction is necessary.[2]

Various fluids have been used for joint lavage. The basis is a sterile saline or Ringer solution. In a study using an equine septic arthritis model a balanced electrolyte solution containing 0.1% (weight/volume) of povidone iodine was not superior to the electrolyte solution alone.[13] When comparing solutions with 0.1%, 0.2%, and 0.5% of povidone iodine and a solution with 0.5% chlorhexidine with electrolyte solution alone, the two high concentrations of disinfectant caused severe lameness and induced synovitis.[2] In another study, even a 0.05% concentration of chlorhexidine caused synovial inflammation, ulceration, and fibrin accumulation[60] and is thus not advisable. Dimethylsulfoxide is a free radical scavenger that also has been used as an adjunct to fluids used for joint lavage. It does not seem to be harmful in both in vitro and in vivo work,[61,62] but any superiority to fluids alone has yet to be documented. There is general agreement that the use of antimicrobials in the lavage fluid is undesirable, based on the viewpoint to restrict use of antimicrobials in (veterinary) medicine to lessen development of resistance. However, after lavage, antimicrobials can be left in the joint (see the paragraph on antibiotic treatment). Outcome using multineedle lavage techniques is fair to good. In a study in 13 horses treated with a closed suction system, 10 returned to the previous level of exercise. In 11 of the horses arthroscopic lavage and débridement were also used, but they were not deemed essential by the authors.[59] A study using the through-and-through lavage technique reported an overall joint recovery rate of 81%. However, in some of the successful cases up to five lavages (performed every other day) were necessary.[63]

Both arthrotomy and arthroscopy offer the opportunity to inspect the joint cavity and remove large amounts of fibrin and debris and, in some cases of accidental wounds, to remove foreign material. Open drainage resulted in the elimination of infection in 26 horses with persistent or severe septic arthritis/tenosynovitis; 24 were discharged from the hospital.[64] In a study directly comparing both techniques in experimentally infected horses, arthrotomy was shown to eliminate joint infection earlier than arthroscopy with concurrent lessening of clinical signs, but arthrotomy was complicated by a higher rate of ascending infections.[65] In human medicine a direct comparison of open arthrotomy versus arthroscopy was performed in children with septic arthritis of the hip. Arthrotomy had excellent results in 7/10 children and good results in the other 3; with arthroscopy these figures were 9 and 1, respectively. This difference was not significant, but arthroscopically treated children had a significantly shorter hospitalization period.[66] Although in human medicine the jury still seems to be out with respect to the use of surgical intervention in cases of septic arthritis and the type of surgery needed,[67] in equine medicine there is now consensus that an aggressive approach, which includes early surgical intervention, is mandatory.[4] Thanks to the widespread availability of arthroscopic equipment, arthroscopy is the technique of choice in virtually all clinics where this type of patient is treated. Arthroscopy has the advantage of quicker recovery and the modern equipment that is available permits the handling of almost all conditions that can be encountered in the joint, including synovial resection with motorized equipment. Arthroscopy also reduces the risk of secondary infection, a risk that is substantially larger in equine than in human medicine. Nevertheless, it may be preferable to leave a small arthrotomy wound open and to implant a drain for flushing.[2] Further, in some cases of severely lacerated joints, open management of the joint is the only option.

Adjunctive Therapeutic Measures

Septic arthritis is a very painful condition and in the acute stage adjunctive therapy will virtually always include the oral application of NSAIDs. Phenylbutazone has for long been, and still is in the U.S. and many other places, the drug of choice. Phenylbutazone has proven to be very effective for musculoskeletal pain, but it has been banned in the European Union (EU) for use in food-producing animals. According to EU legislation, where the horse is considered a food-producing animal, treatment of horses with phenylbutazone must be recorded in their "horse passport," resulting in their definitive exclusion from slaughter for human consumption.[68] Although some EU member states permit the use of the drug in horses for the management of chronic bone and joint problems, for example, arthritis, under the above-mentioned conditions, others do not, severely limiting the use of phenylbutazone in those countries. Alternatives are more specific cyclooxygenase 2 (COX-2) inhibitors, such as firocoxib and meloxicam, that have been registered for use in the horse in large parts of the world. Oral application of meloxicam in horses with experimentally induced acute synovitis (by intraarticular injection of bacterial LPS) resulted in significant suppression of PGE_2 and of substance P release. It further decreased general MMP activity significantly versus placebo-treated controls and limited inflammation-induced cartilage catabolism.[69] In a recent study in horses using the LPS-induced synovitis model, phenylbutazone did not reduce MMP activity or substance P release and there was no reduction of cartilage catabolism, as with meloxicam. In contrast, concentration of the anabolic collagen marker CPII (see Chapter 10) was reduced, suggesting a transient reduction of collagen anabolism.[70] In rabbits, the NSAID naproxen was shown to have a chondroprotective effect in an experimental study of staphylococcal septic arthritis.[71]

Other adjunctive medical therapy that has been reported includes the intraarticular application of hyaluronic acid and of corticosteroids. In a study of six adult horses in which septic arthritis was experimentally induced by the injection of 1×10^4 colony-forming units of *S. aureus*, joints treated with sodium hyaluronate showed less signs of inflammation than the contralateral controls. Apart from injection with sodium hyaluronate or placebo, all horses were treated systemically with trimethoprim/sulfamethoxazole and phenylbutazone and all joints were lavaged with sterile Ringer solution 24 hours after inoculation. Glycosaminoglycan loss from the cartilage in treated joints was less than in control joints, but this difference was not significant.[72]

The use of corticosteroids in septic arthritis is controversial. In principle, corticosteroids are immunosuppressive and hence contraindicated in cases of acute infections in which the host defense system should be boosted rather than suppressed. Nevertheless, in a study in experimentally infected rabbits, the group treated with a combination of intraarticular corticosteroids and systemic antibiotics showed less histologic damage than the group treated with systemic antibiotics alone.[73] In the horse it is certainly not recommended to use corticosteroids in the acute phase of septic arthritis, owing to their immunosuppressive properties and also to their capacity to mask clinical signs for several days, as was shown in a study in artificially infected horses.[27] However, corticosteroids are potent antiinflammatory drugs and judicious use in a later phase of septic arthritis may be warranted, that is, in those cases in which the infection has been eliminated and clinical signs linger on because of a persistent, chronic inflammation. In these cases a single application of triamcinolone may have an immediate and lasting effect. The procedure is somewhat risky though and requires good clinical judgment, as it is difficult to be completely sure that the joint is entirely devoid of viable microorganisms.

Further adjunctive therapy includes restriction of motion (box confinement) in acute cases and the application and regular change of sterile bandages in case of open drainage wounds. If progress is good, physical therapy can be used to prevent stiffening of the periarticular area, which is a common sequel to septic arthritis, and a gradual rehabilitation regimen may be started. In some cases in which the damage to the joint is too extensive to allow for regaining acceptable joint function, ankylosis formation may still result in an acceptable outcome, depending on the joint involved (Figure 7-4), especially in animals of great genetic or emotional value. Ankylosis may occur spontaneously[74] or it can be facilitated surgically if degeneration occurs more rapidly than the horse can accommodate, to reestablish pain-free weight bearing on the affected limb for protection of the contralateral one.[75,76]

PROGNOSIS

A few decades ago the prognosis of septic arthritis in mature horses used to be poor or guarded at best. With the current more aggressive treatment practices prognosis has substantially improved, but septic arthritis in the horse is still a grave condition and outcomes can be disappointing.

In a large retrospective study that included 126 adult horses with septic arthritis or tenosynovitis because of various causes, 85% of the horses treated were released from the hospital. Success rate in tenosynovitis was higher than in arthritis, as all 14 horses diagnosed with tenosynovitis were discharged; success rate in septic joints was 74%.[19] In the study by Meijer et al.[63] using a multineedle lavage technique, 81% of the horses were discharged from the hospital. When using open drainage in combination with antibiotics, 24 of 26 horses (92%) were discharged.[64]

A more recent study investigated the influence of outcome of synovial fluid culture on short-term and long-term prognosis of horses with septic synovitis. The condition was defined as a nucleated cell count of more than 30,000 cells/mm³ or more than 90% neutrophils. Of the 67 horses in which bacteriologic culture was positive, 21% were euthanized because of persistent synovial sepsis versus only 1.5% of the animals (n=139) in which bacteriologic culture was negative. Successful long-term return to function was 50% in the first group and 71% in the second. However, this appeared to be related to the microorganism involved, as long-term outcome was favorable in not more than 30% of horses in which *S. aureus* was cultured and in 74% of horses in which other microbes were cultured (hence equivalent to the group with negative culture).[33]

In the quest for prognostic markers, the ratio between pro-MMP-9 and pro-MMP-2 was, besides WBC count, a good prognosticator for survival.[77] In that study no relationship between the interval from injury to referral for treatment and outcome was found, but average time between first clinical signs and referral was not more than 2.7 days with the upper limit of the range being 7 days. This is much less than in most other studies.

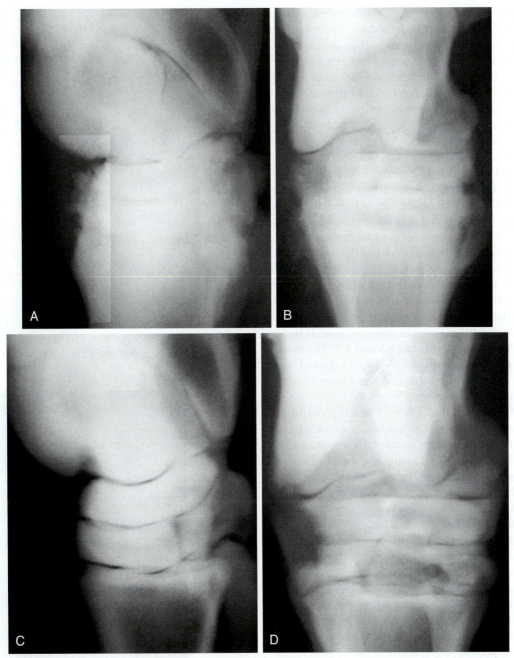

FIGURE 7-4 End stage of what started as septic arthritis of the tarsometatarsal joint 12 months earlier. Close-up lateral (**A**) and plantarodorsal (**B**) views show near-complete solidification of the lower half of the tarsus, making identification of joint spaces nearly impossible, especially distally. Lateral (**C**) and plantarodorsal (**D**) views of the normal opposite tarsus are provided for comparison. At this stage, this horse was only mildly lame, usually after prolonged exercise.

Overall, prognosis has improved with modern treatment methods and is on average about 80% for dismissal from the hospital and approximately 70% for full return to function. These are overall figures that may be different in more specific groups of patients.

SEPTIC ARTHRITIS IN FOALS

A very specific patient group is formed by (neonatal) foals. Septic arthritis is relatively common in newborn foals and often,

but not always, related to septicemia. In a large study of 2468 foals, of which 116 (4.7%) died, septicemia was the most common cause of death (30%) in foals aged less than 7 days. Septic arthritis was the cause of death in 12.5% of foals aged 8 to 30 days.[78] Umbilical infection is the classic source, but many other sources, such as pneumonia or enteritis, may be encountered. In a substantial number of cases there may be failure of passive transfer of antibodies, which makes these foals less immune competent and negatively influences prognosis. Because of the often hematogenous origin of septic arthritis in foals, the disease may often present as polyarthritis with more than one joint involved and arthritis may be secondary to primary foci of infection, often present as osteomyelitis. The combination of osteomyelitis and septic arthritis in foals is common. In a study of 118 Thoroughbred foals with osteomyelitis (mean age 39 days, range 1 to 180), 70% had concurrent septic arthritis.[79] Septic arthritis is a severe complication of septicemia, as odds for survival of septicemia are less when septic arthritis develops.[80]

Septic arthritis has been divided into four types: S, E, P, and T.[81] In S-type arthritis there is no bony involvement with only the synovial membrane and synovial fluid affected. In type E there is osteomyelitis of the epiphysis and concurrent septic arthritis of the adjacent joint, and in type P there is a focal infection in the physis that may result in septic arthritis as well, mostly via the attachment of the joint capsule. In type T the primary infection is located in one of the tarsal bones. The osteomyelitic lesions are located at predilection sites, often where the cartilage layer is thickest.[82] In very young foals transphyseal vessels exist, connecting the metaphyseal and epiphyseal blood supply and enabling the localization of bacteria in the synovial membrane and subchondral bone, hence leading to septic arthritis types S and E.[83] The transphyseal vessels close at approximately 7 to 10 days of age, restricting the infection to metaphyseal vessel loops in older foals and leading to P-type arthritis.[83]

Clinically, foals with arthritis types S and E present in a similar way: severe lameness, joint distension, which is painful at passive flexion, and often systemic illness because of septicemia. Total nucleated cell count is often in excess of 30,000 cells/mm^3 but may be lower, and percentage of neutrophils is typically 90% or more. Macroscopically, the synovial fluid may be turbid, with a color varying from normal to pink or red. In most cases the clinical picture, synovial fluid analysis, and regular radiography will be sufficient to make the diagnosis and to discriminate between types S and E (Figure 7-5). However, osseous lesions may be missed with this approach, as was shown in a study that evaluated the usefulness of MRI for the diagnosis of septic arthritis in foals. Of 19 lesions detected on MRI, only 4 were detected on digital radiography as well. The synovial fluid showed as a heterogeneous signal in most joints with septic arthritis, but in none of the foals with nonseptic arthritis.[84] There is thus a certain added value of MRI in the diagnosis of septic arthritis, but in most cases the diagnosis can be made without it. In P-type septic arthritis there is lameness too, but instead of synovial effusion there is marked periarticular swelling and foals often show pain upon palpation of the infected area. Here too, radiography (or MRI) is a helpful aid in making the diagnosis (Figure 7-6). A consistent laboratory finding in foals with osteomyelitis (E, P type) is hyperfibrinogenemia. Plasma fibrinogen level is greater than 900 mg/dL in the vast majority of affected foals. In a study in 17 foals with physeal or epiphyseal osteomyelitis, positive and negative predictive values for plasma fibrinogen concentrations between 900 and 1500 mg/dL were 84% and 98%, respectively. Foals with osteomyelitis also had greater total nucleated cell count gend neutrophil counts than foals with septic arthritis alone.[85]

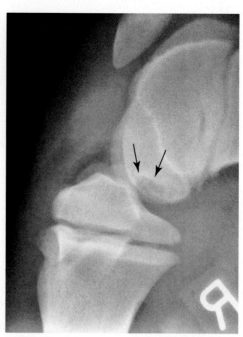

FIGURE 7-5 Radiograph of a foal with type-E septic arthritis showing involvement of the distal femoral epiphysis (arrows).

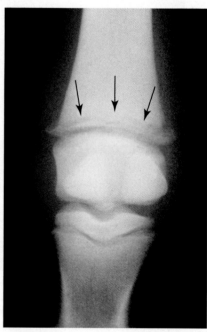

FIGURE 7-6 Radiograph of a foal with type-P septic arthritis showing involvement of the distal metacarpal physis (arrows). The soft tissues around the metacarpophalangeal joint are swollen. There are no radiographic alterations of the metacarpophalangeal joint itself.

The pathogens that can be involved in septic arthritis in foals are many. *Actinobacillus spp., Streptococcus spp.,* and *enterobacteriacea* such as *Salmonella spp.* and *Escherichia coli* are all regularly cultured.[4] Septic arthritis may also be a sequel to *Rhodococcus equi* infection.[86] Sometimes less common microorganisms are cultured. *Clostridium septicum* was cultured from the joints of three foals, two with polyarthritis and one with a single affected joint. All animals responded well to treatment consisting of joint lavage and benzyl penicillin.[87]

Treatment for septic arthritis in foals is not essentially different from that in mature horses. It was recently shown that, of a large amount of drugs used for the treatment of neonatal sepsis in foals, the MICs have increased significantly from 1979 to 2010.[88] Among these were the aminoglycosides of choice for septic arthritis, amikacin and gentamicin. Further, as in foals there is often septicemia and possibly immunosuppression, these conditions have to be treated with urgency as well. In cases of osteomyelitic foci, which are common in foals but rare in adult horses, surgical curettage is a good option. In a case series of 17 foals with septic physitis treated with surgical curettage, 15 were alive at 9-month follow-up. Apart from surgical curettage, these foals were all treated with systemic antibiotics, and some of them with intravenous regional perfusion and/or antibiotic-impregnated PMMA beads that were left at the surgical site. Eight of the foals had concurrent septic arthritis of the adjacent joint (hence a P-type septic arthritis), which did not affect outcome.[89] A case of septic osteomyelitis of the middle phalanx and septic arthritis of the proximal interphalangeal joint because of *Rhodococcus equi* infection was successfully treated with a combination of systemic antibiotic treatment, regional limb perfusion, and lavage and open drainage of the joint.[90]

The treatment of foals with septic arthritis and/or septicemia is expensive and outcome is uncertain at best. For commercially kept foals, such as in racing, the question is whether or not treatment is economically warranted. Many studies have focused on long-term prognosis for survival as well as for racing performance. In a retrospective study of 108 foals with osteomyelitis (of which 76 had concurrent septic arthritis), 79 survived long-term to reach racing age and 52 (48%) actually raced. Foals younger than 30 days, foals that were critically ill, and foals with multiple bone involvement were less likely to survive. Multiple septic joints were an unfavorable prognosticator for racing.[79] In another study of 423 bacteremic foals, 254 survived. Surviving foals did not differ from unaffected siblings regarding the percentage of starters, but had significantly less wins and earnings.[80] In a study focusing specifically on foals treated for septic arthritis (n=69), these foals had reduced likelihood of starting and they entered racing significantly later (1757 days versus 1273 days) than controls.[91] In an earlier study in 93 foals with septic arthritis, 73 survived to discharge and approximately a third raced. Presence of *Salmonella spp.* was associated with a lower chance of survival and multisystem disease with both a lower chance of survival and less chance to race.[92] It can be concluded that treatment for septic arthritis in foals has a less favorable prognosis than in adult horses, but prognosis is still fair to good for survival. After successful treatment, the foal may still develop into a top-level performance horse, but it should be realized that the odds for high-level athletic performance of survivors are lower than for foals that never suffered from the disorder. The choice of whether or not to treat may be based on the expectation value of the animal or on its emotional value.

CONCLUSION

Septic arthritis in horses is a severe condition that needs to be treated as an emergency. Although prognosis used to be rather poor in the days when the condition was treated with (systemic) antibiotics only, it has improved with the current, more aggressive approach consisting of immediate (arthroscopic) lavage and both systemic and local delivery of high doses of antibiotics using some kind of local perfusion technique. Early treatment is mandatory, as treatment of an established infection is more difficult and prognosis becomes much worse once substantial cartilage damage has occurred. In foals, the condition is seen relatively frequently as a consequence of septicemia and general illness, whether or not it is related to immune deficiency. In this category of patients, prognosis is not as good as it is in mature horses because of the concomitant disorders.

REFERENCES

1. Attur MG, Dave M, Akamatsu M, et al. Osteoarthritis or osteoarthrosis: the definition of inflammation becomes a semantic issue in the genomic era of molecular medicine. *Osteoarthritis Cartilage*. 2002;10(1):1–4.
2. McIlwraith CW. Specific diseases of joints: infective (septic) arthritis. In: Stashak TS, ed. *Adams' lameness in horses* 5th ed. Philadelphia, PA: Lippincott, Williams & Wilkins; 2002:577–588.
3. Brooker C. *Churchill Livingstone medical dictionary*. 16th ed. London: Churchill Livingstone; 2008.
4. Richardson DW, Ahern BJ. Synovial and osseous infections. In: Auer JA, Stick JA, eds. *Equine surgery* 4th ed. St. Louis, MO: Elsevier-Saunders; 2012:1189–1201.
5. Abdelnour A, Arvidson S, Bremell T, et al. The accessory gene regulator (agr) controls Staphylococcus aureus virulence in a murine arthritis model. *Infect Immun*. 1993;61(9): 3879–3885.
6. Palmqvist N, Silverman GJ, Josefsson E, et al. Bacterial cell wall-expressed protein A triggers supraclonal B-cell responses upon in vivo infection with Staphylococcus aureus. *Microbes Infect*. 2005;7(15):1501–1511.
7. Gjertsson I, Jonsson IM, Peschel A, et al. Formylated peptides are important virulence factors in Staphylococcus aureus arthritis in mice. *J Infect Dis*. 2012;205(2):305–311.
8. Deng GM, Tarkowski A. The features of arthritis induced by CpG motifs in bacterial DNA. *Arthritis Rheum*. 2000;43(2):356–364.
9. Nilsson IM, Patti JM, Bremell T, et al. Vaccination with a recombinant fragment of collagen adhesin provides protection against Staphylococcus aureus-mediated septic death. *J Clin Invest*. 1998;101(2):2640–2649.
10. Spiers S, May SA, Harrison LJ, et al. Proteolytic enzymes in equine joints with infectious arthritis. *Equine Vet J*. 1994;26(1):48–50.
11. Hardy J, Bertone AL, Malemud CJ. Effect of synovial membrane infection in vitro on equine synoviocytes and chondrocytes. *Am J Vet Res*. 1998;59(3):293–299.
12. Bertone AL, McIlwraith CW, Jones RL, et al. Comparison of various treatments for experimentally induced equine infectious arthritis. *Am J Vet Res*. 1987;48(3):519–529.

13. Bertone AL, McIlwraith CW, Jones RL, et al. Povidone-iodine lavage treatment of experimentally induced equine infectious arthritis. *Am J Vet Res.* 1987;48(4):712–715.

14. Bertone AL, Jones RL, McIlwraith CW. Serum and synovial fluid steady-state concentrations of trimethoprim and sulfadiazine in horses with experimentally induced infectious arthritis. *Am J Vet Res.* 1988;49(10):1681–1687.

15. Tulamo RM, Bramlage LR, Gabel AA. Sequential clinical and synovial fluid changes associated with acute infectious arthritis in the horse. *Equine Vet J.* 1989;21(5):325–331.

16. Smith RL, Schurman DJ. Comparison of cartilage destruction between infectious and adjuvant arthritis. *J Orthop Res.* 1983;1(2):136–143.

17. Smith RL, Schurman DJ. Bacterial arthritis. A staphylococcal proteoglycan-releasing factor. *Arthritis Rheum.* 1986;29(11):1378–1386.

18. Ribera T, Monreal L, Armengou L, et al. Synovial fluid D-dimer concentration in foals with septic joint disease. *J Vet Intern Med.* 2011;25(5):1113–1117.

19. Schneider RK, Bramlage LR, Moore RM, et al. A retrospective study of 192 horses affected with septic arthritis/tenosynovitis. *Equine Vet J.* 1992;24(6):436–442.

20. Nogradi N, Spier SJ, Toth B, et al. Musculoskeletal Corynebacterium pseudotuberculosis infection in horses: 35 cases (1999-2009). *J Am Vet Med Assoc.* 2012;241(6):771–777.

21. Lapointe JM, Laverty S, Lavoie JP. Septic arthritis in 15 Standardbred racehorses after intraarticular injection. *Equine Vet J.* 1992;24(6):430–434.

22. Steel CM, Pannirselvam RR, Anderson GA. Risk of septic arthritis after intraarticular medication: a study of 16,624 injections in Thoroughbred racehorses. *Aust Vet J.* 2013;91(7):268–273.

23. Borg H, Carmalt JL. Postoperative septic arthritis after elective equine arthroscopy without antimicrobial prophylaxis. *Vet Surg.* 2013;42(3):262–266.

24. Olds AM, Stewart AA, Freeman DE, et al. Evaluation of the rate of development of septic arthritis after elective arthroscopy in horses: 7 cases (1994-2003). *J Am Vet Med Assoc.* 2006;229(12):1949–1954.

25. Gustafson SB, McIlwraith CW, Jones RL. Comparison of the effect of polysulfated glycosaminoglycan, corticosteroids, and sodium hyaluronate in the potentiation of a subinfective dose of Staphylococcus aureus in the midcarpal joint of horses. *Am J Vet Res.* 1989;50(12):2014–2017.

26. Gustafson SB, McIlwraith CW, Jones RL, et al. Further investigations into the potentiation of infection by intraarticular injection of polysulfated glycosaminoglycan and the effect of filtration and intraarticular injection of amikacin. *Am J Vet Res.* 1989;50(12):2018–2022.

27. Tulamo RM, Bramlage LR, Gabel AA. The influence of corticosteroids on sequential clinical and synovial fluid parameters in joints with acute infectious arthritis in the horse. *Equine Vet J.* 1989;21(5):332–337.

28. Madison JB, Sommer M, Spencer PA. Relations among synovial membrane histopathologic findings, synovial fluid cytologic findings, and bacterial culture results in horses with suspected infectious arthritis: 64 cases (1979-1987). *J Am Vet Med Assoc.* 1991;198(9):1655–1661.

29. Jacobsen S, Thomsen MH, Nanni S. Concentrations of serum amyloid A in serum and synovial fluid from healthy horses and horses with joint disease. *Am J Vet Res.* 2006;67(10):1738–1742.

30. Sanchez Teran AF, Rubio-Martinez LM, Villarino NF, et al. Effects of repeated intraarticular administration of amikacin on serum amyloid A, total protein and nucleated cell count in synovial fluid from healthy horses. *Equine Vet J.* 2012;(Suppl 43):12–16.

31. Wauters J, Martens A, Pille F, et al. Viability and cell death of synovial fluid neutrophils as diagnostic biomarkers in equine infectious joint disease: a pilot study. *Res Vet Sci.* 2012;92(1):132–137.

32. Dumoulin M, Pille F, van den Abeele AM, et al. Use of blood culture medium enrichment for synovial fluid culture in horses: a comparison of different culture methods. *Equine Vet J.* 2010;42(6):541–546.

33. Taylor AH, Mair TS, Smith LJ, et al. Bacterial culture of septic synovial structures of horses: does a positive bacterial culture influence prognosis? *Equine Vet J.* 2010;42(3):213–218.

34. Choe H, Inaba Y, Kobayashi N, et al. Use of real-time polymerase chain reaction for the diagnosis of infection and differentiation between gram-positive and gram-negative septic arthritis in children. *J Pediatr Orthop.* 2013;33(3):e28–e33.

35. Easley JT, Brokken MT, Zubrod CJ, et al. Magnetic resonance imaging findings in horses with septic arthritis. *Vet Radiol Ultrasound.* 2011;52(4):402–408.

36. Levine DG, Ross BM, Ross MW, et al. Decreased radiopharmaceutical uptake (photopenia) in delayed phase scintigraphic images in three horses. *Vet Radiol Ultrasound.* 2007;48(5):467–470.

37. Uren RF, Howman-Giles R. The 'cold hip' sign on bone scan. A retrospective review. *Clin Nucl Med.* 1991;16(8):553–556.

38. Puchalski SM, Galuppo LD, Hornof WJ, et al. Intraarterial contrast-enhanced computed tomography of the equine distal extremity. *Vet Radiol Ultrasound.* 2007;48(1):21–29.

39. Bertone AL. Infectious arthritis. In: McIlwraith CW, Trotter GW, eds. *Joint disease in the horse.* 1st ed. Philadelphia, PA: WB Saunders; 1996:397–409.

40. Moore RD, Lietman PS, Smith CR. Clinical response to aminoglycoside therapy: importance of the ratio of peak concentration to minimal inhibitory concentration. *J Infect Dis.* 1987;155(1):93–99.

41. Beccar-Varela AM, Epstein KL, White CL. Effect of experimentally induced synovitis on amikacin concentrations after intravenous regional limb perfusion. *Vet Surg.* 2011;40(7):891–897.

42. Alkabes SB, Adams SB, Moore GE, et al. Comparison of two tourniquets and determination of amikacin sulfate concentrations after metacarpophalangeal joint lavage performed simultaneously with intravenous regional limb perfusion in horses. *Am J Vet Res.* 2011;72(5):613–619.

43. Levine DG, Epstein KL, Ahern BJ, et al. Efficacy of three tourniquet types for intravenous antimicrobial regional limb perfusion in standing horses. *Vet Surg.* 2010;39(8):1021–1024.

44. Mahne AT, Rioja E, Marais HJ, et al. Clinical and pharmacokinetic effects of regional or general anaesthesia on intravenous regional limb perfusion with amikacin in horses. *Equine Vet J.* 2014;46(3):375–379.

45. Murphey ED, Santschi EM, Papich MG. Regional intravenous perfusion of the distal limb of horses with amikacin sulfate. *J Vet Pharmacol Ther.* 1999;22(1):68–71.

46. Pille F, De Baere S, Ceelen L, et al. Synovial fluid and plasma concentrations of ceftiofur after regional intravenous perfusion in the horse. *Vet Surg.* 2005;34(6):610–617.

47. Rubio-Martínez LM, López-Sanromán J, Cruz AM, et al. Evaluation of safety and pharmacokinetics of vancomycin after intravenous regional limb perfusion in horses. *Am J Vet Res.* 2005;66(12):2107–2113.

48. Parra-Sanchez A, Lugo J, Boothe DM, et al. Pharmacokinetics and pharmacodynamics of enrofloxacin and a low dose of amikacin administered via regional intravenous limb perfusion in standing horses. *Am J Vet Res.* 2006;67(10):1687–1695.
49. Lallemand E, Trencart P, Tahier C, et al. Pharmacokinetics, pharmacodynamics and local tolerance at injection site of marbofloxacin administered by regional intravenous limb perfusion in standing horses. *Vet Surg.* 2013;42(6):649–657.
50. Zantingh AJ, Schwark WS, Fubini SL, et al. Accumulation of amikacin in synovial fluid after regional limb perfusion of amikacin sulfate alone and in combination with ticarcillin/clavulanate in horses. *Vet Surg.* 2014;43(3):282–288.
51. Kelmer G, Bell GC, Martin-Jimenez T, et al. Evaluation of regional limb perfusion with amikacin using the saphenous, cephalic, and palmar digital veins in standing horses. *J Vet Pharmacol Ther.* 2013;36(3):236–240.
52. Levine DG, Epstein KL, Neelis DA, et al. Effect of topical application of 1% diclofenac sodium liposomal cream on inflammation in healthy horses undergoing intravenous regional limb perfusion with amikacin sulfate. *Am J Vet Res.* 2009;70(11):1323–1325.
53. Rubio-Martínez LM, Elmas CR, Black B, et al. Clinical use of antimicrobial regional limb perfusion in horses: 174 cases (1999-2009). *J Am Vet Med Assoc.* 2012;241(12):1650–1658.
54. Parker RA, Bladon BM, McGovern K, et al. Osteomyelitis and osteonecrosis after intraosseous perfusion with gentamicin. *Vet Surg.* 2010;39(5):644–648.
55. Haerdi-Landerer MC, Habermacher J, Wenger B, et al. Slow release antibiotics for treatment of septic arthritis in large animals. *Vet J.* 2010;184(1):14–20.
56. Ivester KM, Adams SB, Moore GE, et al. Gentamicin concentrations in synovial fluid obtained from the tarsocrural joints of horses after implantation of gentamicin-impregnated collagen sponges. *Am J Vet Res.* 2006;67(9):1519–1526.
57. Petit A, Redout EM, van de Lest CH, et al. Sustained intraarticular release of celecoxib from in situ forming gels made of acetyl-capped PCLA-PEG-PCLA triblock copolymers in horses. *Biomaterials.* 2015;53:426–436.
58. Kawashima M, Torisu T, Kamo Y, et al. The treatment of pyogenic bone and joint infections by closed irrigation-suction. *Clin Orthop Relat Res.* 1980;148:240–244.
59. Ross MW, Orsini JA, Richardson D, et al. Closed suction drainage in the treatment of infectious arthritis of the equine tarsocrural joint. *Vet Surg.* 1991;20(1):21–29.
60. Wilson DG, Cooley AJ, MacWilliams PS, et al. Effects of 0.05% chlorhexidine lavage on the tarsocrural joints of horses. *Vet Surg.* 1994;23(6):442–447.
61. Adair HS, Goble DO, Vanhooser S, et al. Evaluation of use of dimethyl sulfoxide for intra-articular lavage in clinically normal horses. *Am J Vet Res.* 1991;52(2):333–336.
62. Smith CL, MacDonald MH, Tesch AM, et al. In vitro evaluation of the effect of dimethyl sulfoxide on equine articular cartilage matrix metabolism. *Vet Surg.* 2000;29(4):347–357.
63. Meijer MC, van Weeren PR, Rijkenhuizen AB. Clinical experiences of treating septic arthritis in the equine by repeated joint lavage: a series of 39 cases. *J Vet Med A Physiol Pathol Clin Med.* 2000;47(6):351–365.
64. Schneider RK, Bramlage LR, Mecklenburg LM, et al. Open drainage, intra-articular and systemic antibiotics in the treatment of septic arthritis/tenosynovitis in horses. *Equine Vet J.* 1992;24(6):443–449.
65. Bertone AL, Davis DM, Cox HU, et al. Arthrotomy versus arthroscopy and partial synovectomy for treatment of experimentally induced infectious arthritis in horses. *Am J Vet Res.* 1992;53(4):585–591.
66. El-Sayed AM. Treatment of early septic arthritis of the hip in children: comparison of results of open arthrotomy versus arthroscopic drainage. *J Child Orthop.* 2008;2(3):229–237.
67. Kang SN, Sanghera T, Mangwani J, et al. The management of septic arthritis in children: systematic review of the English language literature. *J Bone Joint Surg Br.* 2009;91(9):1127–1133.
68. European Food Safety Authority: FAQ on phenylbutazone in horsemeat (www.efsa.europa.eu/en/faqs/phenylbutazone.htm). Accessed January 2015.
69. De Grauw JC, van de Lest HA, Brama PAJ, et al. In vivo effects of meloxicam on inflammatory mediators, degradative enzymes and cartilage biomarkers in equine joints with acute synovitis. *Equine Vet J.* 2009;41:693–699.
70. De Grauw JC, van Loon JPAM, van de Lest CHA, et al. In vivo effects of phenylbutazone on inflammation and cartilage-derived biomarkers in equine joints with acute synovitis. *Vet J.* 2014;201(1):51–56.
71. Smith RL, Kajiyama G, Schurman DJ. Staphylococcal septic arthritis: antibiotic and nonsteroidal anti-inflammatory drug treatment in a rabbit model. *J Orthop Res.* 1997;15(6):919–926.
72. Brusie RW, Sullins KE, White II NA, et al. Evaluation of sodium hyaluronate therapy in induced septic arthritis in the horse. *Equine Vet J.* 1992;24(Suppl 11):18–23.
73. Wysenbeek AJ, Volchek J, Amit M, et al. Treatment of staphylococcal septic arthritis in rabbits by systemic antibiotics and intra-articular corticosteroids. *Ann Rheum Dis.* 1998;57(11):687–690.
74. Honnas CM, Welch RD, Ford TS, et al. Septic arthritis of the distal interphalangeal joint in 12 horses. *Vet Surg.* 1992;21(4):261–268.
75. Groom LJ, Gaughan EM, Lillich JD, et al. Arthrodesis of the proximal interphalangeal joint affected with septic arthritis in 8 horses. *Can Vet J.* 2000;41(2):117–123.
76. Bramlage LR. Arthrodesis of the metacarpal/metatarsal phalangeal joint in the horse. *Proc Am Assoc Equine Pract.* 2009;55:144–149.
77. Kidd JA, Barr AR, Tarlton JF. Use of matrix metalloproteinases 2 and 9 and white blood cell counts in monitoring the treatment and predicting the survival of horses with septic arthritis. *Vet Rec.* 2007;161(10):329–334.
78. Cohen ND. Causes of and farm management factors associated with disease and death in foals. *J Am Vet Med Assoc.* 1994;204(10):1644–1651.
79. Neil KM, Axon JE, Begg AP, et al. Retrospective study of 108 foals with septic osteomyelitis. *Aust Vet J.* 2010;88(1-2):4–12.
80. Sanchez LC, Giguère S, Lester GD. Factors associated with survival of neonatal foals with bacteremia and racing performance of surviving Thoroughbreds: 423 cases (1982-2007). *J Am Vet Med Assoc.* 2008;233(9):1446–1452.
81. Firth EC, Dik KJ, Goedegebuure SA, et al. Polyarthritis and bone infection in foals. *Zentralbl Veterinarmed B.* 1980;27(2):102–124.
82. Firth EC, Goedegebuure SA. The site of focal osteomyelitis lesions in foals. *Vet Q.* 1988;10(2):99–108.
83. Firth EC. Current concepts of infectious polyarthritis in foals. *Equine Vet J.* 1983;15(1):5–9.

84. Gaschen L, LeRoux A, Trichel J, et al. Magnetic resonance imaging in foals with infectious arthritis. *Vet Radiol Ultrasound.* 2011;52(6):627–633.

85. Newquist JM, Baxter GM. Evaluation of plasma fibrinogen concentration as an indicator of physeal or epiphyseal osteomyelitis in foals: 17 cases (2002-2007). *J Am Vet Med Assoc.* 2009;235(4):415–419.

86. Collatos C, Clark ES, Reef VB, et al. Septicemia, atrial fibrillation, cardiomegaly, left atrial mass, and Rhodococcus equi septic osteoarthritis in a foal. *J Am Vet Med Assoc.* 1990;197(8):1039–1042.

87. Kawaguchi K, Church S. Clostridium septicum arthritis in three foals. *Aust Vet J.* 2004;82(10):612–615.

88. Theelen MJ, Wilson WD, Edman JM, et al. Temporal trends in in vitro antimicrobial susceptibility patterns of bacteria isolated from foals with sepsis: 1979-2010. *Equine Vet J.* 2014;46(2):161–168.

89. Hall MS, Pollock PJ, Russell T. Surgical treatment of septic physitis in 17 foals. *Aust Vet J.* 2012;90(12):479–484.

90. Kelmer G, Hayes ME. Regional limb perfusion with erythromycin for treatment of septic physitis and arthritis caused by Rhodococcus equi. *Vet Rec.* 2009;165(10):291–292.

91. Smith LJ, Marr CM, Payne RJ, et al. What is the likelihood that Thoroughbred foals treated for septic arthritis will race?. *Equine Vet J.* 2004;36(5). 452–426.

92. Steel CM, Hunt AR, Adams PL, et al. Factors associated with prognosis for survival and athletic use in foals with septic arthritis: 93 cases (1987-1994). *J Am Vet Med Assoc.* 1999;215(7):973–977.

8

Effects of Loading/Exercise on Articular Tissues and Developmental Aspects of Joints

P. René van Weeren and Pieter A. J. Brama

Joints are pivotal elements of the equine musculoskeletal system that enable locomotion, permitting physical exercise and hence allowing the horse to behave as the flight-and-fright animal it has evolved into and as the equine athlete we use for our equestrian activities (see Chapter 1 for an overview of general joint anatomy and physiology). However, this is not a one-way interaction. Physical exercise in the form of locomotion will generate forces that are exerted on the articular tissues. These forces are within the joint largely of compressive and shear nature, but tensile forces are important as well for the joint capsule and various intraarticular and extraarticular ligaments. This chapter deals largely with how the articular tissues cope with these forces and their role in joint homeostasis and in articular development.

In the living world there is, in general, equilibrium between the homeostasis of a given tissue and the functional challenges placed upon it. Gentle challenging will normally have a stimulating effect. In joints this is exemplified by the increase of synovial clearance after exercise, as was shown in case of technetium 99m medronate injection[1] and by increased radiopharmaceutical uptake in the carpus, metacarpophalangeal joint, proximal phalanx, and distal phalanx after treadmill exercise.[2] It is clear that excessive challenging is detrimental to tissues. At a certain moment the adaptive response will become insufficient and failure will occur in some form. As a general response, tissue loss, scar tissue formation, or even cancer may ensue. A good example is the development of liver cirrhosis after prolonged excessive alcohol intake. In articular tissues cancer formation is not a sequel to chronic overloading, but the same principle applies and excessive loading (or also less excessive but badly focussed loading, e.g., in case of joint malalignment) may lead to wear lines, cartilage erosions, and/or formation of osteophytes. However, it is not only overloading that may have detrimental effects; underuse of structures may equally lead to damage and pathologic situations. "Use it or lose it" is a slogan that has recently been used much in brain research, a tissue that was long thought to be immutable after childhood,[3] but that had already been known much longer to be true for most if not all parts of the body. Since the days of Julius Wolff, who formulated Wolff's Law at the end of the 19th century,[4] we know that bone needs a certain amount of stimulation to avoid osteoporosis. More recent research on tendons strongly suggests a similar effect

of stress-deprivation in this tissue.[5] The situation for articular tissues is not different.

In the interplay between biomechanical loading and tissue response, discrimination should be made between mature and juvenile tissues. Although in mature individuals the actual point on the scale of underuse/regular use/overuse may decide whether the effect on the tissues is beneficial or detrimental, in the juvenile situation there is an additional element. In the young and growing, individual tissues are still in development. This development is partially genetically determined, but also partially steered by environmental factors. The influence of conditions during prenatal and early postnatal life on the development of an organism and on its susceptibility for disorders later in life can be substantial. This is called the "Developmental Origins of Health and Disease" (DOHaD) principle.[6] The principle was first discovered when actual epidemiologic data on coronary heart disease in humans did not match with well-established risk factors, but appeared to be associated with infant mortality rates of the cohort under study, indicating that environmental conditions in early childhood or even prenatally influence the susceptibility for the development of disease later in life.[6] It is now a well-accepted concept that seems to have much wider applications than heart disease alone, many probably mediated by epigenetic mechanisms.[7] The musculoskeletal system is no exception, and research from the past decades has revealed some of the mechanisms through which the musculoskeletal tissues may be moulded in early life. Equine studies have been important in this respect.

This chapter describes the current state of knowledge of the effects of biomechanical loading on the principal components of the diarthrodial joint, articular cartilage, and subchondral bone (data on synovial tissues being virtually nonexistent). Starting with the mature joint, the chapter will conclude with a section on the more complex effects on the juvenile, still growing, and developing joint.

LOADING OF THE MATURE JOINT: BALANCING BETWEEN MAINTENANCE AND MORBIDITY

Data about the effects of exercise on articular tissues come from experimental, observational, and epidemiological studies. All types of investigations have their merits. Experimental studies are executed under well-controlled conditions, typically have an interventional character, and allow for a more reductionist approach in which causal relationships and mechanisms can be studied. However, they are always a simplification of reality and are extremely costly to carry out in a species like the horse. Not unimportantly, ethical aspects play a role here, too. Observational studies sample from existing cohorts with known exercise histories. They are much less expensive to carry out and ethics normally are not a point, but they are less strictly controlled, often suffer from small numbers, and are often retrospective in nature. Epidemiologic studies typically identify risk factors in a real-life environment. These studies yield highly valuable data, but need large numbers that are not always easy to generate when dealing with horses and are largely associative, rarely permitting the establishment of direct cause-consequence relationships or the discovery of mechanistic pathways.

Experimental Work

Most of the larger experimental studies have been conducted in the racing breeds, using either Standardbred Trotters or 2-year-old Thoroughbreds. Two-year-olds are beyond the phase of rapid growth and development they went through as foals, but cannot be considered as fully skeletally mature yet. They can be classified as "young-adult."

Little et al.[8] used musculoskeletal material from a study that was originally designed to investigate the phenomenon of overtraining. Twelve Standardbred horses were subjected to an 8-week moderate exercise program. After this, the horses were randomly assigned to two groups: one group continued moderate exercise and the other was subjected to strenuous exercise for 17 weeks. Horses were then rested for 16 weeks, after which full-depth cartilage explants were cultured. No histologic abnormalities were detected, but aggrecan synthesis was significantly less in the strenuously trained group and decorin production had gone up. It was concluded that strenuous exercise may have a (lasting) deleterious effect on metabolism, which then might affect the biomechanical resistance to injury of the tissue.

In a study designed to investigate the mechanical and histologic characteristics of middle carpal articular cartilage at specific locations in age- and sex-matched immature horses subjected to strenuous training or gentle exercise, which became known as the short-term Bristol study, 2-year-old Thoroughbreds were subjected to a 19-week exercise regimen. The experimental group had to gallop 3 times weekly on a treadmill, were trotted in a mechanical horse walker also 3 times per week, and were walked for 40 minutes 6 times per week. The control group only had to do the walking exercise.[9,10] Cartilage from the proximal articular surface of the radial, intermediate, and third carpal bone from the exercised animals had developed a thicker calcified layer than in non-exercised animals; however, the hyaline cartilage layer was similar in thickness.[9] The cartilage of the strenuously trained animals was biomechanically less stiff and showed more fibrillation and more chondrocyte clusters than the more

gently trained animals, suggesting exercise-induced deterioration of cartilage.[10] Exercise also influenced cartilage oligomeric matrix protein (COMP) distribution,[11] subchondral bone thickness and hardness,[12] and fibronectin.[13] However, an effect of treadmill training on modeling of the central and third tarsal bones could not be demonstrated.[14] Proteoglycan synthesis rates were measured after cartilage samples were brought into culture and appeared to be higher in the trained animals than in the controls.[15] This agreed with the fact that the strenuously exercised animals had higher glycosaminoglycan content than horses from the more gently trained group, which was most marked in the cartilage from the dorsal radial and dorsal intermediate carpal surfaces, sites known to be heavily loaded during exercise.[16] It further corroborated earlier work by Palmer et al.,[17] who had shown that exercise increases the amount of newly synthesized proteoglycans in cartilage, and it also influences the biomechanical behavior of the tissue.[18] In the horses from the Bristol study there were no overall effects on the collagen component of the extracellular matrix, but sites that are known to be predisposed to injury contained significantly less collagen in exercised horses.[16] It was hypothesized that there would be an upregulation of the proteinases cathepsin B and D in cartilage samples from these animals, as a prelude to the development of osteoarthritis, but this appeared to be not the case. It was found, however, that cathepsin D varied according to the topographic location within the joint, reflecting biomechanical differences experienced during a high-intensity compared with a low-intensity exercise regimen.[19] In conclusion, exercise has a direct and stimulating effect on proteoglycan metabolism of articular cartilage unless it is too heavy in which case the effect may be negative; the effect on the collagen component is less conclusive, but there are indications that (strenuous) exercise may activate catabolic enzymatic activity.

In the Massey University Grass Exercise Study (MUGES), conducted in New Zealand, seven 2-year-old Thoroughbreds were trained for 13 weeks on grass and sand tracks, after which the musculoskeletal tissues were thoroughly analyzed and compared with those of an untrained group of 7 animals.[20] Negligible clinical injury was detected and thus the study fulfilled the intention of investigating adaptive change rather than injury.[21] In contrast to the Bristol study, in this study a significant increase in thickness of (hyaline) cartilage was seen at certain sites of the third carpal bone (C3) after 13 weeks of training, in comparison to the pasture-raised controls.[22] A difference was only seen in the axial part of C3, an area that was used for mechanical testing in the Bristol study and not for histology, which may explain the difference. The response of the tissue was deemed adaptive rather than degenerative in nature, as at those sites no pathoanatomic damage could be detected. Biomechanically, stiffness of the metacarpal condylar subarticular calcified tissue, measured by nanoindentation, was not different between the groups.[23] However, in the metacarpophalangeal (MCP) joints of the MUGES animals wear lines and fibrillation were macroscopically visible and biochemical analyses indicated that water content had increased and hydroxylysylpyridinoline (HP) cross-links had decreased compared with the controls. These observations were interpreted as microdamage with ensuing loosening of the collagen network.[24]

Too much exercise is a more common phenomenon in the equine industry than too little, but articular tissues can be subject to stress deprivation, too. In a small study concerning 5 horses, cast immobilization for 7 weeks followed by a gradually increasing rehabilitation program for 8 weeks led to substantial loss of volumetric bone mineral density of subchondral bone that was not fully recovered during the rehab period.[25] Interestingly, in a functional sense, joint range of motion had not yet recovered after 8 weeks.[26]

In a study on the effects of superoxide dismutase (SOD) supplementation, repeated sprint exercise resulted in increased antioxidant defenses including endogenous erythrocyte SOD, total glutathione, glutathione peroxidase, gene transcripts for interferon-gamma, interleukin-10, and interleukin-1β in blood, and decreased plasma nitric oxide. Exercise increased the chondroitin sulfate content of synovial fluid (SF), as well as PGE_2. No effects of treatment with exogenous SOD were detected. It was concluded that the results reflected normal adaptive responses likely caused by exercise-induced tissue microdamage and oxidative stress.[27]

Some older studies have investigated the effect of exercise on the healing of artificially created lesions. In one of those studies, no effect was seen in ponies.[28] In an earlier study in 2- to 4-year-old horses, postoperative exercise led to thicker repair tissue; however, it was not of better (histologic) quality than that in nonexercised horses.[29] In the study by Todhunter et al.,[30] cartilaginous repair tissue from exercised ponies contained significantly more glycosaminoglycan and type-II collagen, and they concluded that postoperative exercise was beneficial. Of these studies, one was limited to walking exercise[28]; in both other studies exercise was more strenuous and included work at the faster gaits. It therefore seems likely that, like the overall effect of exercise on cartilage metabolism, the effect of exercise on healing is load-dependent.

Overall, the experimental studies indicate that articular tissues are responsive to exercise in mature animals. In the case of articular cartilage, the response is limited, but there is evidence of an adaptive increase in proteoglycan metabolism under the influence of exercise, which can result in an increase in proteoglycan content and even in a minimal increase in cartilage thickness. Too-heavy exercise can have an opposite effect. There are less data on the effects on the collagen network, but there are indications that (too) intense exercise may have a deleterious effect on this crucial structural component of articular cartilage as well. Moderate exercise therefore seems beneficial, but exercise may become too heavy. Many factors may determine the optimal level of exercise, including environmental factors and factors related to the individual horse, and no generalizations can be made to this respect at this moment.

Observational Studies

Exercise-induced loading has been shown to decrease COMP content at intermittently highly loaded areas; although,

regular lower level loading promotes COMP synthesis and/or retention.[31] In that same study a tendency towards thinner collagen fibrils in trained animals (Standardbred Trotters) was seen, suggesting some influence of exercise on the collagen component of articular cartilage too, either direct or indirect via the influence of COMP, which is known to play a role in the assembly of the collagen fibrils.[32]

In mature horses the articular cartilage has lost most of its plasticity and can hardly, if at all, be conditioned further, but (subchondral) bone remains responsive to exercise according to Wolff's law[4] and a certain degree of loading is necessary for maintenance. In an observational study of racing Thoroughbreds, radiographs were obtained from 17 horses 1 year after starting training (9 horses raced in a clockwise direction, and 8 in both clockwise and counterclockwise directions). There was no difference between the cortical bone in the right and left forelimbs at the start of the study, but after 1 year, the palmar cortex in the right forelimb was significantly thicker than that in the left forelimb, showing the effect of predominantly clockwise racing.[33] In a study comparing 106 Standardbred Trotters entering their first year of training (exercise group) and 7 age-matched Standardbreds at pasture (controls), which were clinically and radiographically examined at approximately 3-month intervals over 12 to 18 months, the horses in the exercise group showed a significant increase in sclerosis of the third carpal bone and middle carpal joint. Middle carpal joint lameness developed in 32/106 (30%) of the exercised horses and in none of the control horses. The incidence of lameness was lower in horses with mild (2/30, 6.7%) than moderate (10/32, 31.2%) and severe (20/44, 45.4%) sclerosis.[34] In a mixed population of racehorses and sport horses different types of high-intensity exercise appeared to be associated with different patterns of subchondral bone thickness in tarsal joints.[35] Exercise-induced microcracks are well-known to be the initial stages of condylar fractures of the metacarpus in racehorses.[36] In a detailed study on the metacarpophalangeal/metatarsophalangeal joints of racehorses,[37] defects on the condylar surface detected by macroscopic inspection ranged from cartilage fibrillation and erosion to focal cartilage indentations and cavitation in subchondral bone characteristic of traumatic osteochondrosis, which was thought to represent mechanically induced arthrosis provoked by (overload-induced) microdamage. Histologically, there was subchondral bone sclerosis. With advancing sclerosis an increased amount of osteocyte necrosis was present. Irregular trabecular microfractures developed at a depth of a few millimetres. The overlying articular cartilage was variably indented but remained largely viable with degeneration and erosion limited to the superficial layers. In the same line, a high-intensity treadmill exercise protocol resulted in functional adaptation of carpal bones with the increase in trabecular thickening and density localized to those regions underlying common sites of cartilage degradation,[38] fueling the age-old "chicken-or-egg" discussion[39] of what is the initial step in the development of osteoarthritis: changes in the articular cartilage or in the underlying subchondral bone? A similar mechanism may play a role in the development of navicular disease. Based on a histologic study comparing three groups of horses (young racing Thoroughbreds, young unshod ponies, and older horses with navicular syndrome), it was suggested that the navicular bone may experience habitual bending across the sagittal plane and that consequences of cumulative cyclic loading in horses with navicular syndrome include arthritic degeneration of adjacent joints and adaptive failure of the navicular bone, with accumulation of microdamage.[40]

In one of the few studies not conducted in racehorses, but in riding horses comparing pasture exercise to ridden exercise, Tranquille et al. found that exercise may, apart from its effect on subchondral bone, also affect thickness of both the calcified and hyaline cartilage layer and increase the risk of osteochondral lesions.[41,42]

In conclusion, most observational studies have focused on the effects of (strenuous) exercise on subchondral bone, corroborating the adaptive response of bone according to Wolff's law and demonstrating increased sclerosis and related pathology if exercise is very heavy. More recent work has also shown indications for an adaptive response of the articular cartilage, in line with the earlier mentioned experimental studies.

Biomarkers for Monitoring Loading

In the quest for early markers of joint disease, Cleary et al.[43] investigated the effects of exercise and osteochondral injury on concentrations of carboxy-terminal telopeptide fragments of type II collagen (CTX-II) in SF and serum of Thoroughbred racehorses and compared these with radiographic and arthroscopic scores of joint injury severity. The CTX-II concentrations in SF were significantly higher for horses with joint injuries, compared with preexercise and postexercise findings in noninjured horses, suggesting that SF CTX-II concentrations may be used to detect cartilage degradation in horses with joint injury. A similar effect of joint injury, but no effect of exercise, was found in a study investigating a type II collagen degradation product (collagenase cleavage neoepitope, commercially known as C2C) in SF from Thoroughbred racehorses that were trained for racing.[44] In general, the effects of exercise on levels of biomarkers in SF appear to depend on the amount of exercise given. In a study in which horses were experimentally subjected to strenuous treadmill exercise, Frisbie et al.[45] noted a significant increase in SF CS846 (an aggrecan marker), CPII (a marker of collagen synthesis), glycosaminoglycans (GAG), the C2C collagen degradation marker, osteocalcin, and collagen I concentrations. This is in line with other work on the effect of exercise on SF composition and concentrations of products of cartilage metabolism or inflammatory mediators. Moderate to strenuous exercise led to increases in plasma GAG levels and serum keratan sulfate and COMP.[46-48] Higher chondroitin sulfate peak chain lengths, but shorter hyaluronic acid chain lengths, were found in exercised versus rested horses.[49] Exercise increased PGE_2 content in SF and led to a TNF-α peak 2 hours after cessation of exercise,[50,51] but moderate exercise did not affect MMP-1 activity.[52] There is a mutual interaction between SF and articular cartilage. The former is not just a reflection of the status

of the latter, but may in itself influence cartilage metabolism. In fact, the effects of joint loading on cartilage are, at least in part, mediated by alterations in the SF. Cartilage explants cultured in postexercise SF showed enhanced GAG synthesis and diminished release when compared with cultures using preexercise SF.[53] A follow-up study concluded that insulin-like growth factor I (IGF-I) is an important contributor to the overall stimulating effect of SF on cartilage metabolism, but that it is unlikely that IGF-I is the only mediator causing this exercise-induced stimulating effect.[54]

It can be concluded that most of the currently used biomarkers in SF (see Chapter 10 for a review) will not react to minor or moderate exercise, but may increase significantly in case of strenuous exercise, reflecting the effect of heavy exercise on metabolism of the components of the articular cartilage extracellular matrix. The relationship is more complex than that, as change in SF composition may in itself affect cartilage metabolism.

Epidemiologic Studies

The metacarpophalangeal (MCP) joint is known to be the equine joint most susceptible to damage.[55] It is the MCP joint that, together with the carpal joint, has received most attention in terms of effect of exercise. This can be explained to a large extent by the high incidence of condylar fractures in the MCP joint and of third carpal bone slab fractures in the carpus in racehorses. Although most data come from Thoroughbred and Standardbred racing, in Quarter Horse racing the metacarpophalangeal/metatarsophalangeal (MCP/MTP) joints and the carpus are also the structures that are most often involved in (fatal) musculoskeletal injury.[56]

In a study by Reed et al. (2013),[57] a total of 647 racehorses spent 7785 months at risk of joint injury and 184 injuries were recorded. MCP/MTP injury risk decreased with increasing daily canter distance but increased with accumulation of canter or high-speed exercise since entering training. In contrast, accumulation of canter exercise was marginally associated with reduced carpal injury risk. Risk of all injury types varied significantly between trainers. Overall, the results of the study suggested that regular canter exercise is generally beneficial for joint health, although accumulation of high-speed exercise detrimentally affects MCP/MTP joints. A similar effect of high-speed training was seen in a study of carpal lameness in a population of 114 Standardbred Trotters, which were monitored clinically and radiographically for 12 to 18 months after entering their first year of training. Carpal lameness occurred in 28% of horses and was present in 56% with forelimb lameness. Apart from poor forelimb conformation, more intense speed training appeared to be a predisposing factor.[58]

In a modeling study based on exercise and injury data of 122 racing Thoroughbreds in California, it was again (high-intensity) sprint training that seemed to have a negative effect. Reduction by 20% of the number of sprints run at distances greater than 6 furlongs significantly reduced (by 9%) the modeled annual incidence of metacarpophalangeal condylar fracture (and of severe suspensory apparatus injury).[59]

Competing is of course equivalent to high-intensity exercise and has shown to increase the risk of injury. Lameness (either caused by joint or tendon problems) was increased during the 5 days after a race in a study performed in 256 Danish Standardbred Trotters. Interestingly, apart from the average intensity of exercise and the well-known trainer effect, the general set-up of training programs is also of importance. Horses were at higher risk 1.5 to 2.5 months after they had entered a given training regimen compared with the period where they had been trained by the same trainer for more than 3 months.[60]

Conclusion

From most if not all studies discussed previously the same overall picture emerges: in mature animals there is an effect of exercise (i.e., biomechanical loading) on the tissues of which diarthrodial joints are composed. As could be expected, the effect is most evident on (subchondral) bone, a tissue that is known to continue remodeling as a reaction to external stimuli throughout life. Further, it is important to realize that it is the intensity, rather than the duration or total exercise load, which determines whether the threshold between physiologic adaptation and pathologic deterioration is passed. Low-intensity to moderate-intensity exercise is beneficial, as it will stimulate proteoglycan synthesis and may lead to increase in cartilage thickness and glycosaminoglycan content. However, high-intensity exercise (including competition) may have a negative effect on chondrocyte metabolism (probably because of overstimulation or even direct cell damage), lead to proteoglycan depletion, and predispose to damage to the collagen network; this may become visible as erosion or wear lines and may eventually result in development of osteoarthritis. The microdamage will result in alterations in SF composition, which can have a negative effect on chondrocyte health, initiating a vicious cycle. Many equestrian activities are physically highly demanding and thus potentially harmful for joint health. It is a major challenge for trainers and riders to find the right balance between optimally stimulating joint metabolism through appropriate loading and avoiding excessive exercise that will cause tissue damage. This balance is one of the major determinants of longevity in the equine athlete.

LOADING OF THE JUVENILE JOINT: CRUCIAL CONDITIONING

The preceding paragraphs have given an overview of the effects of exercise on mature joints. In the adult animal, the two major components of the joint surface, subchondral bone and articular cartilage, are much different in character. Bone is known to remodel and adapt throughout life,[4] but articular cartilage (or at least the collagen component of it that provides the structural backbone of the tissue) is a much less reactive tissue because of the extremely long turnover times of mature collagen type II, which may extend to several hundreds of years.[61,62] (See also Chapter 1.) However, the situation is entirely different in juveniles that are still growing. In

these youngsters turnover times of all components of articular cartilage, including collagen, are by definition much lower and less at younger age when growth rate is highest. It can be anticipated that exercise will have major effects on juvenile joints, as it has on mature joints, but that in this case it will also influence the process of joint development. Given the relative immutability of mature articular cartilage alluded to above, it can therefore also be anticipated that effects of exercise at early age may have wide and long-lasting implications. In fact, there is now ample evidence that joints indeed are examples par excellence of the DOHaD principle.

The Process of Functional Adaptation

In the trajectory from newborn to adult an individual does not only grow (i.e., increase in size), but many anatomic and physiologic features also change in a functional sense. A good example is the changing role of the abomasum and the development of the forestomach in juvenile ruminants. Some of these changes are largely genetically determined (e.g., development of sexual maturity at a certain age), others are (also) driven by environmental factors (e.g., adaptation of the microbial flora in the equine intestinal system in foals through a gradual increase in intake of roughage and coprophagy). All these processes lead to an optimization of the growing youngster's adaptation to the living conditions in adult life. In joints a similar process takes place. Articular cartilage in mature individuals is not a homogeneous tissue; there are topographic differences, both over the joint area surface and with depth from the surface, in biochemical composition and consequently also in biomechanical characteristics. This topographic variation in characteristics makes the local tissue resistance match with the variations in biomechanical loading during locomotion[63] (see also Chapter 1). The question is whether this topographic heterogeneity, which represents an adaptation to meet the challenges posed by locomotion and athletic activity, is innate or is largely formed by environmental factors in the early juvenile period when cartilage metabolism is still high. The first indication for the latter option came from work by Little and Ghosh,[64] who showed that proteoglycan content was identical over the entire joint surface in neonatal lambs. Extensive work by Brama et al.[65] showed in foals that not only proteoglycan content, but also collagen including posttranslational modifications of collagen such as cross-links, were homogeneously distributed across the joint of the newborn animal as well. They called this neonatal situation the "blank joint." By sampling various age groups, they showed that most of the topographic heterogeneity that is characteristic of mature cartilage was already present at age 5 months. However, not all constituents of the extracellular matrix follow the same time path; HP cross-links (the most abundant pyridinoline cross-link in articular cartilage) did not reach a mature value until after 12 months[65,66] (Figure 8-1). Later, the underlying maturation process of articular cartilage in early life was indirectly confirmed with help of equine-specific cDNA microarrays. There was a distinct difference between neonatal and mature individuals in the expression of genes encoding for matrix proteins and matrix-modifying

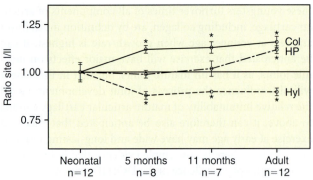

FIGURE 8-1 Age-related influence of different exercise levels on the development of topographical heterogeneity in collagen content (Col), hydroxylysine (Hyl) content and hydroxylysylpyridinoline (HP) crosslinks of the extracellular matrix of articular cartilage. The biochemical parameters are given as the ratio between two sites (mean ± s.e.). Site I is the dorsal margin of the proximal articular surface of the proximal phalanx; site II is the central fovea of that same joint. Site I is intermittently but heavily loaded; site II continuously but less intense. In the mature animal these sites have substantially different collagen contents (hence ratio different from one). In the newborn foal these differences do not exist yet but they develop under the influence of loading (hence ratio starting at 1, but digressing with increasing age).*P<0.05. (From: Brama P.A.J., TeKoppele J.M., Bank R.A., et al. (2002). Development of biochemical heterogeneity of articular cartilage: influences of age and exercise. Equine Vet J, 34(3), 265-269.)

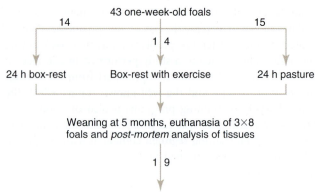

FIGURE 8-2 Experimental set-up of the EXOC study. A total of 43 Warmblood foals were divided into 3 different exercise groups at age 1 week. Exercise regimens consisted of either 24 hours/day box rest (N=14), a similar sedentary protocol but with additional high-intensity sprinting exercise for 30 minutes per day (N=14), or free-pasture exercise (N=15). After weaning at age 5 months, 8 foals from each group were euthanized and their tissues harvested. The remaining 19 foals were housed together and given a moderate exercise regimen. These animals were euthanized at age 11 months.

enzymes, with the former expressing more collagens, matrix-modifying enzymes, and provisional matrix noncollagenous proteins and the latter showing a transition from growth to homeostasis and tissue function related to coping with shear and compressive forces.[67]

The material properties of the extracellular matrix of cartilage are not only determined by the tissue components. The spatial arrangement and interconnections of these components, that is, the structure, plays an important role too. With respect to structure, similar developments take place during early life. The arcade structure of the collagen network, as originally described by Benninghoff,[68] is typical for mature cartilage, but not yet in its mature form present in the newborn. Investigations using polarized light microscopy have shown that collagen fibril orientation is predominantly parallel to the joint surface and subchondral bone at birth and gradually changes to the classic arcade structure after birth.[69]

This gradual transition from a blank, neonatal joint to a mature joint featuring topographic heterogeneity in biochemical and structural sense was termed the "process of functional adaptation" by Brama et al.[65]

The Driving Force behind the Process of Functional Adaptation

The first evidence that biomechanical loading is the main inciting factor in the process of functional adaptation came from a study that was originally designed to study the influence of exercise on the developmental orthopedic disease

osteochondrosis.[70] That study, commonly referred to as EXOC (for exercise and osteochondrosis), used a group of 43 Warmblood foals, which were divided into 3 subgroups with different exercise levels from the early age of 1 week. Foals and mares from 1 group (n=14) were kept in box stalls for 24 hours per day. The second group (n=14) was kept in identical box stalls, but additionally had to perform a number of short sprints during a restricted period, that is, in this group a basically sedentary lifestyle was supplemented with short bouts of heavy exercise. The third group (n=15) had free-pasture exercise for 24 hours/day and served as controls, as this was considered the most "natural" situation. These different exercise regimens were maintained until weaning at 5 months of age. After weaning, eight foals from each group were euthanized and their tissues harvested for detailed analyses. The remaining 19 foals were joined in a single group and subjected to a moderate-exercise regimen. These animals were euthanized at age 11 months. The aim was to see if any difference that might have resulted from the different exercise regimens during the first 5 months of their lives would be reversible or not. Figure 8-2 schematically depicts the experimental design of this study.

Bone is known to respond rapidly to changes in exercise and, as expected, the different training regimens were nicely reflected by differences in bone mineral density of both the proximal sesamoid bones[71] and the carpal bones,[72] measured with peripheral quantitative computed tomography (pQCT) and dual X-ray absorptiometry (DEXA), respectively. Microscopic measurement of relative bone volume in the small tarsal bones yielded similar results.[73] In all these cases the box-rested foals lagged behind in development with regard to both groups that had been trained. After 6 months of identical

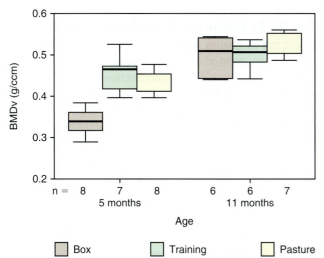

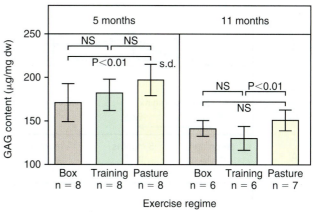

FIGURE 8-3 Box plot of bone mineral density (BMD), measured by DEXA scanning, of the medial dorsal area of the 3rd carpal bone in the groups of foals from the EXOC study. BMD was less in the box-rested group at age 5 months, but the difference with the other 2 groups had disappeared after 6 months of similar exercise. The overall increase is an age effect. (From: Firth E.C., van Weeren P.R., Pfeiffer D.U., et al. (1999). Effect of age, exercise and growth rate on bone mineral density (BMD) in third carpal bone and distal radius of Dutch Warmblood foals with osteochondrosis. Equine Vet J, 31 (Suppl 31), 74-78.)

FIGURE 8-4 Influence of the different exercise regimens on glycosaminoglycan (GAG) content (mean, error bars indicate SD) in cartilage from the metacarpophalangeal joint. There is a clear exercise effect at 5 months that has disappeared at 11 months with only a slightly, but significantly, lower GAG content in the foals subjected to a high-intensity exercise regimen imposed on a sedentary lifestyle. *NS*, Not significant. (From: Brama P.A., Tekoppele J.M., Bank R.A., et al. (1999). Influence of different exercise levels and age on the biochemical characteristics of immature equine articular cartilage. Equine Vet J, 31(Suppl 31), 55-61.)

exercise, these differences between animals of the original exercise groups had all disappeared (Figure 8-3). However, in some places bone density was a little less in the foals that had been subjected to the training protocol than in foals from the former box-rest and pasture groups, which was interpreted as a possible effect of overstimulation provoked by the combination of short bouts of heavy exercise with a basis of lack of exercise.[71,73]

There were also clear differences in articular cartilage composition. No effect of exercise on the water or DNA content was found, but GAG content increased with increasing exercise in the 5 months group (Figure 8-4). These differences had disappeared after 6 months of similar exercise.[74] In general, topographic heterogeneity, which was expressed as a significant difference from 1 in the ratio of two very differently loaded sites within the joint, appeared to develop in the pastured group and in the boxed/sprinted group alike. However, it did not do so in the boxed foals. This was direct proof of the steering effect of biomechanical loading on the process of functional adaptation.[65] As expected, not only the cartilage responded to exercise, but also the subchondral bone. In the 5-month-old foals from the EXOC study, exercise influenced calcium content and levels of lysylpyridinoline (LP) and HP cross-links at the more heavily loaded dorsal margin of the proximal phalanx, but not at the central fovea.[75] Calcium content and HP and LP cross-link levels increased significantly less over time in the subchondral bone of the proximal phalanx in box-rested foals.[76] The exercise level also had an effect on the amount and relative concentration of the bone

morphogenic enzymes alkaline phosphatase (ALP), tartrate resistant acid phosphatase (TRAP), and lysyl oxidase (LO).[77] However, there was a big and important difference between cartilage and the other tissues that were analyzed. Although proteoglycans and subchondral bone density became normal after the common training program from 5 to 11 months with foals from all former exercise groups showing similar levels, collagen and other collagen-related parameters such as hydroxylysine remained abnormal. These extracellular matrix components failed to "catch up" and to develop the characteristic topographic heterogeneity of mature individuals[65] (Figure 8-5). Apparently, for collagen there is a limited window in time during which the process of functional adaptation can take place. If this time window is not used, chances are over and no compensation is possible anymore. This phenomenon can be readily explained by the sharp rise in turnover time of collagen type II with increasing age and decreasing growth (see also Chapter 1). It is therefore very likely that, when the period of time when the collagen component of the extracellular matrix is still responsive to loading is not appropriately used, the joint will be left with inferior cartilage that may be less resistant to lifelong wear and tear and hence more susceptible to injury. This stresses the great importance of sufficient exercise in the early juvenile phase.

In the boxed/sprinted animals the degree of development of topographic heterogeneity was comparable to the pastured animals. However, when culturing chondrocytes harvested at age 11 months from animals from all former exercise groups, it appeared that chondrocytes from the former box/sprinted group could not be stimulated to increase metabolic activity, in contrast to samples from both other groups. Apparently, there was a deleterious long-term effect of the combination of

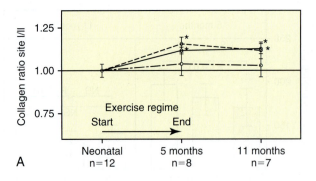

A

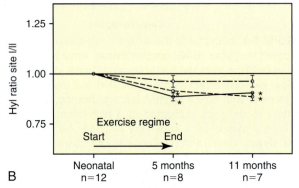

B

FIGURE 8-5 Influence of different exercise levels on the development of topographical heterogeneity in collagen (**A**) and hydroxylysine content (**B**). Site I is the dorsal margin of the proximal articular surface of the proximal phalanx; site II is the central fovea of that same joint. Site I is intermittently, but heavily loaded; site II continuously but less intense. In the mature animal these sites have substantially different collagen contents (hence ratio different from one). In the new-born foal these differences do not exist yet but they develop under the influence of loading (hence ratio starting at 1, but digressing with increasing age). Foals were trained for 5 months. (_ _ _ _ = pasture exercise 24 hours/day; ———— = box-rest with additional 30 minutes of intensive training; _._._._. = box-rest 24 hours/day). After 5 months exercise was equal for all groups. Note that the lack of exercise in the box group induced a delay in the development of topographic heterogeneity that was not compensated for when box confinement ceased in these collagen-related parameters, unlike the situation for proteoglycans (Figure 4) or bone mineral density (Figure 3). *, =Ratio significantly different from one, that is, existence of significant site differences ($P < 0.05$). (From: Brama P.A.J., TeKoppele J.M., Bank R.A., et al. (2002). Development of biochemical heterogeneity of articular cartilage: influences of age and exercise. Equine Vet J, 34(3), 265-269.)

sedentary lifestyle with bouts of high intensity exercise, possibly because of a kind of cellular exhaustion that might be caused by overstimulation during the first 5 months of life.[78] This would agree with data from analysis of serum markers (CPII and Ctx1) in live animals that showed indirectly a negative effect on collagen turnover in animals from this group, compared with pastured foals[79] and with the bone data mentioned above. Also in tendon tissue a similar phenomenon was observed.[80]

Can We Condition the Young Horse through Exercise at Young Age?

In the year 2000 the Global Equine Research Alliance (GERA) was formed. This is a consortium formed by equine orthopedic research groups from Massey University, Colorado State University, the Royal Veterinary College, and Utrecht University; its aim is to reduce musculoskeletal morbidity in performance horses through development of early detection systems for injury and preventive conditioning.[81] GERA conducted a large-scale study on the effect of early exercise on foals, which became known by its acronym, GEXA. It was clear from the EXOC study that the pasture group came out best in terms of conditioning of musculoskeletal tissues. This observation immediately raised the question of whether or not it would be possible to even better prepare the musculoskeletal system for future athletic performance through the combination of pasture exercise with, superimposed on this basis, additional exercise (Figure 8-6). In the GEXA study 33 Thoroughbred foals were allocated to one of 2 exercise groups directly after birth. One group (PASTEX, n=15) was raised on pasture and the other (CONDEX, n=18) was kept under identical circumstances, but was additionally subjected to an exercise protocol of gradually increasing intensity. The program implied cantering and sprinting; overall workload was increased by a moderate, but significant, 30%.[82] At age 18 months, 12 animals (6 from each group) were sacrificed for detailed tissue analyses, most of the others entered commercial racing and were not sacrificed (Figure 8-7).

The difference in exercise load in the GEXA study between groups was much less extreme than in the earlier EXOC study, as in this case there was no exercise level lower than "natural" pasture exercise. Therefore, less significant differences, if any, were to be expected. Biochemical and biomechanical analyses of full-thickness cartilage samples from the distal metacarpal bone showed site-related differences, but no exercise effect.[83] There was no difference in swelling behavior (as a measure of potential matrix damage) of articular cartilage from both exercise groups.[84] Also, the metabolic rate of chondrocytes (measured by ^{35}S-uptake) from third metacarpal cartilage was not different.[85] There also appeared to be no exercise effect on the thickness of calcified cartilage of the distal metacarpal condyle.[86] A detailed study on the calcified cartilage layer in particular and gross cartilage lesions in general in the midcarpal joint yielded similar results: several third or radial carpal bones had thickened calcified cartilage with microcracks, matrix and osteochondral junction changes, and increased vascularity, but there were no differences between exercise groups. Neither were there differences in prevalence of gross lesions. As most abnormalities of the calcified layer were not accompanied by histologic changes in the hyaline cartilage, this study concluded that calcified cartilage abnormalities beneath the undisrupted hyaline cartilage in the dorsoproximal aspect of the third carpal bone may represent the first changes in the pathogenesis of midcarpal osteochondral disease.[87]

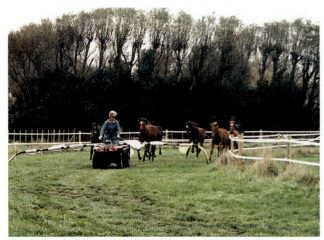

FIGURE 8-6 During the GEXA trial, foals were trained on a custom-made 500-m track constructed on the same grassland where the untrained group was housed. Foals were driven round with the help of modified farm bikes (there is another one at the rear of the group).

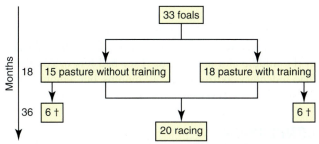

FIGURE 8-7 Experimental set-up of the GEXA study. A total of 33 Thoroughbred foals were divided into 2 different exercise groups from an average age of 3 weeks. Phase 1, the growth and conditioning phase, was the time from birth until age approximately 18 months, during which the conditioned group (CONDEX) was raised on pasture as well as subjected to a 16- to 18-month conditioning program of increasing exercise. The control group (PASTEX) exercised spontaneously at pasture only. At age 18 months, 6 foals from each group were subjected to euthanasia for postmortem analysis, to determine the effects of the conditioning program at tissue level. In phase 2, 20 animals were trained to race in a commercial setting as 2- and 3-year-olds (one animal from the PASTEX group suffered an unrelated accident and was euthanized).

However, notwithstanding the relatively marginal difference in exercise load, there was an effect on overall joint health. In a comprehensive study on the metacarpophalangeal joints it was shown that exercised horses had fewer gross lesions, less articular cartilage matrix staining in the dorsal aspect of the condyle, greater bone fraction in the dorsolateral aspect of the condyle, and higher bone formation rate. From this it was concluded that exercise at a young age may be safely imposed and may be protective to joints.[85] Also in other studies using the GEXA data effects of the exercise program were shown. Exercised horses had more viable chondrocytes in the more heavily loaded sites compared with

less loaded sites of the same metacarpal cartilage than their untrained counterparts.[88] Further, a detailed study of contiguous 100-μm thick slices taken from the proximal articular surface of the proximal phalanx down to the tidemark at differently loaded sites showed not only obvious site differences, but also exercise-related changes. In that study there was no exercise effect on proteoglycan content, which indicated that the exercise level had not been strenuous and confirmed the earlier work,[83,85] but the normal physiologic increase in collagen at the site located at the joint margin was shown to be significantly less in the CONDEX group.[89] The interpretation was that this represented early cessation of collagen remodeling at this site, because of the load-induced speeding up of the normal maturation process. Further, in the CONDEX animals, hydroxylysine content, HP cross-links, and pentosidine cross-links of similar slices from the same site in the metatarsophalangeal joint were all higher, which was again indicative of advancement of the normal process of functional adaptation of collagen.[90] In this context, the increased pentosidine levels in the CONDEX animals are of particular interest, because they indicate a lower metabolic activity in this group, giving further evidence of an advanced degree of maturation in the conditioned animals compared with the PASTEX animals (Figure 8-8).

Ultrastructural studies provided additional evidence for the exercise-induced difference in maturation rate. The parallelism index (PI, a measure of the degree to which the collagen fibrils are aligned to each other) and orientation index (OI, a measure of the average angle of collagen fibrils with respect to the articular surface), both measured using polarized light microscopy, appeared to be different between the two exercise groups. The PI was higher in the CONDEX animals, showing their temporal advancement in maturation of the collagen network.[91] An interesting observation was that the orientation of collagen fibrils in the deep zone of the cartilage was less perpendicular to the layer of calcified cartilage than expected according to the classic Benninghoff model. It was conjectured that this represented an adaptation of the direction of the collagen fibers to the high shear forces in the equine metacarpophalangeal joint. This equine joint is a heavily loaded joint with an exceptionally high range of motion. In these circumstances a more oblique insertion of the collagen fibers in the calcified cartilage layer may yield better resistance to shear than would a more perpendicular configuration. Based on this observation it is likely that the Benninghoff arcade model is more flexible than commonly thought and that a predominantly nonperpendicular direction of the collagen fibrils with respect to the tidemark can be expected in the deep zone of cartilage in certain joints, depending on the prevailing biomechanical circumstances.[91]

The extensive studies in the horse have provided compelling evidence for the large effect of exercise on the development of articular tissues with respect to biochemical composition and structural aspects and, consequently, on the biomechanical characteristics of tissue. This is of large clinical significance and fits very well with the DOHaD principle mentioned earlier in this chapter, especially with respect to the effect on the

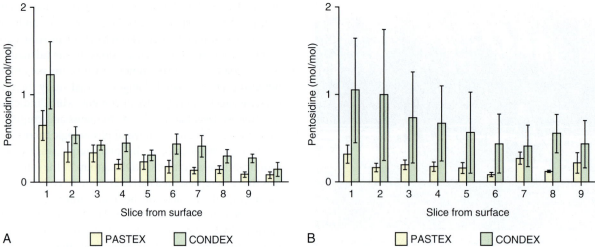

FIGURE 8-8 Mean values for pentosidine cross-link content (expressed as millimole per mole triple helix) for the slices produced at site 1 (**A**) and 2 (**B**) for both PASTEX and CONDEX animals. The most superficial layer (slice 1) is located at the joint surface; the deepest layer (slice 9 or 10) is adjacent to the calcified cartilage. Error bars indicate SD. (From: Van Weeren P.R., Firth E.C., Brommer H., et al. (2008). Early exercise advances the maturation of glycosaminoglycans and collagen in the extracellular matrix of articular cartilage in the horse. Equine Vet J, 40(2), 128-135.)

collagen component of cartilage that is known to be virtually immutable in mature individuals.

Other Species

Composition and basic reaction patterns of diarthrodial joints in large mammalian animals (including humans) seem to be surprisingly similar. Although most large-scale and long-term studies into the effect of exercise on the maturation process of juvenile joints (and other parts of the musculoskeletal system) have been carried out in horses, there is also evidence from other species that the exercise regimen at early age may profoundly affect cartilage properties and that this effect need not always be reversible. In a study in young Beagles in which one of the hind limbs was immobilized for 11 weeks, GAG content was shown to be reduced by almost 50% in the non-weight-bearing limb, and cartilage thickness and GAG content were increased in the contralateral limb.[92] When the study was repeated, but now followed by a 15-week rehabilitation program, the normal situation was not fully restored. The authors concluded that immobilization of skeletally immature joints may affect cartilage development, leading to a very slow recovery or even permanent alterations.[93] In humans the situation is comparable. Physical activity was shown to be a significant explanatory factor for cartilage thickness at all sites investigated by MRI in children in a cross-sectional study. The study concluded that "the current evidence supports a prescription of vigorous physical activity for optimum joint development in children."[94]

There is thus compelling evidence that early exercise affects the tissues of the musculoskeletal system and may do so in a permanent fashion. However, very little is known about the long-term effects on orthopedic health. Too little exercise may be detrimental, but too much exercise may have negative effects as well. Hamsters having free access to a running wheel during the first 3 months of life showed differences in the collagen network organization at age 5 months, especially in the middle and deep zones. They had less osteoarthritis than sedentary controls at age 12 months, but 3 months later the situation was reversed.[95]

CONCLUSION

Articular cartilage is responsive to biomechanical loading, and a well-balanced exercise program that avoids damage caused by both overloading and stress deprivation is crucial for joint health and longevity. This is obviously true in the young animal too, but in that case there is an extra dimension, as in the period of rapid growth there is an active process of functional adaptation of the equine musculoskeletal system.[96,97] There is now compelling evidence that the characteristic topographic heterogeneity in composition and ultrastructure of the extracellular matrix of mature cartilage is formed under the influence of loading, that is, through physical exercise, in the early phase of life. Compared with the situation in bone, it has been suggested[98] that the collagen network of rapidly growing juvenile animals responds to loading in a fashion similar to how trabecular bone responds to exercise.[4] However, there is a big and important difference with bone. Although bone will continue to respond to exercise throughout life under physiologic conditions, the collagen network can most probably do so only in the young, growing animal. After cessation of growth, the collagen remodelling rate falls to the extremely low level that is typical for mature individuals and is characterized by the very long collagen turnover times mentioned earlier. This concept is supported by scientific evidence. Although some studies have shown a response of the proteoglycan component of the extracellular matrix of cartilage to exercise in (young) adult horses, as mentioned in the first part of this chapter, no adaptive response of collagen has ever been demonstrated in this age group. This particular situation makes the early juvenile period into the only window of opportunity to manipulate the collagen network of articular cartilage through modification of loading, that is, differences in exercise. The recent studies cited above show that such manipulation is possible indeed and may either irreversibly delay the normal maturation process, as a result of lack of sufficient exercise level, or accelerate maturation. In both cases, this will result in a different topographic pattern in animals subjected to additional exercise on top of the "gold standard" of free-pasture exercise, or in animals deprived of exercise. It is likely, therefore, that the hypothesis—that variations in exercise regimens of juvenile persons or animals may influence the risk for the development of degenerative joint diseases later in life[99]—is true. In practical terms, this may mean support for the suggestion that athletic training of horses might better start earlier rather than later.[100] The first indications that this indeed may be the case come from the earlier mentioned GEXA study. Of the original 33 horses, 20 went into commercial racing. Follow-up of these animals showed that the incidence of orthopedic injuries was low in both former exercise groups and that there were no differences in the occurrence of orthopedic ailments, but animals that had received pasture exercise only tended to show signs of musculoskeletal disorders earlier than exercise-conditioned animals.[101] However, no definitive answer can be given yet about the possible beneficial effect of additional exercise, and even less can be said of the optimal exercise level. For this, long-term epidemiologic studies are necessary; they may establish the clinical effects of permanent modifications in the make-up of articular cartilage that can be provoked by exercise at early age in terms of injury risk and/or performance over the entire career of the equine athlete. The first data from this type of study are encouraging. In a population of 4683 racehorses Tanner et al.[102] showed that horses registered with a trainer, trialled, or raced as 2-year-olds were more likely to have won or been placed in a race than those that achieved these milestones as 3-year-olds or older. Further, horses that raced as 2-year-olds had significantly more years racing and thus better longevity. Exercise in general and early exercise in particular are likely the most important single factor for both maintenance and development of healthy joints.

REFERENCES

1. Dulin JA, Drost WT, Phelps MA, et al. Influence of exercise on the distribution of technetium Tc 99m medronate following intra-articular injection in horses. *Am J Vet Res.* 2012;73(3):418–425.
2. Foreman JH, Kneller SK, Twardock AR, et al. Forelimb skeletal scintigraphy responses in previously untrained Thoroughbreds undergoing initial treadmill training. *Equine Vet J.* 2002;34(Suppl 34):230–235.
3. Shors TJ, Anderson ML, Curlik II DM, et al. Use it or lose it: how neurogenesis keeps the brain fit for learning. *Behav Brain Res.* 2012;227(2):450–458.
4. Wolff J. *Das Gesetz der Transformation der Knochen.* Berlin: Hirschwald; 1892.
5. Arnoczky SP, Lavagnino M, Egerbacher M, et al. Loss of homeostatic strain alters mechanostat "set point" of tendon cells in vitro. *Clin Orthop Relat Res.* 2008;466(7):1583–1591.
6. Barker DJP. The origins of the developmental origins theory. *J Intern Med.* 2007;261(5):412–417.
7. Wadhwa PD, Buss C, Entringer S, et al. Developmental origins of health and disease: brief history of the approach and current focus on epigenetic mechanisms. *Semin Reprod Med.* 2009;27(5):358–368.
8. Little CB, Ghosh P, Rose R. The effect of strenuous versus moderate exercise on the metabolism of proteoglycans in articular cartilage from different weight-bearing regions of the equine third carpal bone. *Osteoarthritis Cartilage.* 1997;5(3):161–172.
9. Murray RC, Whitton RC, Vedi S, et al. The effect of training on the calcified zone of equine middle carpal articular cartilage. *Equine Vet J.* 1999;31(Suppl 30):274–278.
10. Murray RC, Zhu CF, Goodship AE, et al. Exercise affects the mechanical properties and histological appearance of equine articular cartilage. *J Orthop Res.* 1999;17(5):725–731.
11. Murray RC, Smith RK, Henson FM, et al. The distribution of cartilage oligomeric matrix protein (COMP) in equine carpal articular cartilage and its variation with exercise and cartilage deterioration. *Vet J.* 2001;162(6):121–128.
12. Murray RC, Vedi S, Birch HL, et al. Subchondral bone thickness, hardness and remodelling are influenced by short-term exercise in a site-specific manner. *J Orthop Res.* 2001;19(6):1035–1042.
13. Murray RC, Janicke HC, Henson FM, et al. Equine carpal articular cartilage fibronectin distribution associated with training, joint location and cartilage deterioration. *Equine Vet J.* 2000;32(1):47–51.
14. Whitton RC, Murray RC, Buckley C, et al. An MRI study of the effect of treadmill training on bone morphology of the central and third tarsal bones of young thoroughbred horses. *Equine Vet J.* 1999;31(Suppl 30):258–261.
15. Bird JL, Platt D, Wells T, et al. Exercise-induced changes in proteoglycan metabolism of equine articular cartilage. *Equine Vet J.* 2000;32(2):161–163.
16. Murray RC, Birch HL, Lakhani K, et al. Biochemical composition of equine carpal articular cartilage is influenced by short-term exercise in a site-specific manner. *Osteoarthritis Cartilage.* 2001;9(7):625–632.
17. Palmer JL, Bertone AL, Malemud CJ, et al. Site-specific proteoglycan characteristics of third carpal articular cartilage in exercised and non-exercised horses. *Am J Vet Res.* 1995;56(12):1570–1576.
18. Palmer JL, Bertone AL, Mansour J, et al. Biomechanical properties of third carpal articular cartilage in exercised and nonexercised horses. *J Orthop Res.* 1995;13(6):854–860.
19. Bowe EA, Murray RC, Jeffcott LB, et al. Do the matrix degrading enzymes cathepsins B and D increase following a high intensity exercise regime? *Osteoarthritis Cartilage.* 2007;15(3):343–349.
20. Firth EC, Rogers CW, Perkins NR, et al. Musculoskeletal responses of 2-year-old Thoroughbred horses to early training. 1. Study design and clinical, nutritional, radiological and histological observations. *N Z Vet J.* 2004;52(5):261–271.
21. Firth EC, Rogers CW. Musculoskeletal responses of 2-year-old Thoroughbred horses to early training. Conclusions. *N Z Vet J.* 2005;53(2):377–383.

22. Firth EC, Rogers CW. Musculoskeletal responses of 2-year-old Thoroughbred horses to early training. 7. Bone and cartilage response in the carpus. *N Z Vet J*. 2005;53(2):113–122.

23. Ferguson VL, Bushby AJ, Firth EC, et al. Exercise does not affect stiffness and mineralisation of third metacarpal condylar subarticular calcified tissues in 2 year old thoroughbred racehorses. *Eur Cell Mater*. 2008;16:40–46.

24. Brama PAJ, TeKoppele JM, Bank RA, et al. The influence of strenuous exercise on collagen characteristics of articular cartilage in Thoroughbreds age 2 years. *Equine Vet J*. 2000;32(6):551–554.

25. Van Harreveld PD, Lillich JD, Kawcak CE, et al. Effects of immobilization followed by remobilization on mineral density, histomorphometric features, and formation of the bones of the metacarpophalangeal joint in horses. *Am J Vet Res*. 2002;63(2):276–281.

26. Van Harreveld PD, Lillich JD, Kawcak CE, et al. Clinical evaluation of the effects of immobilization followed by remobilization and exercise on the metacarpophalangeal joint in horses. *Am J Vet Res*. 2002;63(2):282–288.

27. Lamprecht ED, Williams CA. Biomarkers of antioxidant status, inflammation, and cartilage metabolism are affected by acute intense exercise but not superoxide dismutase supplementation in horses. *Oxid Med Cell Longev*, Epub 2012 Aug 8; 2012.

28. Barr AR, Wotton SF, Dow SM, et al. Effect of central or marginal location and post-operative exercise on the healing of osteochondral defects in the equine carpus. *Equine Vet J*. 1994;26(1):33–39.

29. French DA, Barber SM, Leach DH, et al. The effect of exercise on the healing of articular cartilage defects in the equine carpus. *Vet Surg*. 1989;18(4):312–321.

30. Todhunter RJ, Minor RR, Wootton JA, et al. Effects of exercise and polysulfated glycosaminoglycan on repair of articular cartilage defects in the equine carpus. *J Orthop Res*. 1993;11(6):782–795.

31. Skiöldebrand E, Ekman S, Heinegård D, et al. Ultrastructural immunolocalization of cartilage oligomeric matrix protein (COMP) in the articular cartilage on the equine third carpal bone in trained and untrained horses. *Res Vet Sci*. 2010;88(2):251–257.

32. Halász K, Kassner A, Mörgelin M, et al. COMP acts as a catalyst in collagen fibrillogenesis. *J Biol Chem*. 2007;282(43):31166–31173.

33. Beccati F, Pepe M, Di Meo A, et al. Radiographic evaluation of changes in the proximal phalanx of Thoroughbreds in race training. *Am J Vet Res*. 2011;72(11):1482–1488.

34. Hopper BJ, Steel C, Richardson JL, et al. Radiographic evaluation of sclerosis of the third carpal bone associated with exercise and the development of lameness in Standardbred racehorses. *Equine Vet J*. 2004;36(5):441–446.

35. Murray RC, Branch MV, Dyson SJ, et al. How does exercise intensity and type affect equine distal tarsal subchondral bone thickness? *J Appl Physiol*. 2007;102(6):2194–2200.

36. Muir P, Peterson AL, Sample SJ, et al. Exercise-induced metacarpophalangeal joint adaptation in the Thoroughbred racehorse. *J Anat*. 2008;213(6):706–717.

37. Norrdin RW, Kawcak CE, Capwell BA, et al. Subchondral bone failure in an equine model of overload arthrosis. *Bone*. 1998;22(2):133–139.

38. Firth EC, Delahunt J, Wichtel JW, et al. Galloping exercise induces regional changes in bone density within the third and radial carpal bones of Thoroughbred horses. *Equine Vet J*. 1999;31(2):111–115.

39. Radin EL. Subchondral bone changes and cartilage damage. *Equine Vet J*. 1999;31(2):94–95.

40. Bentley VA, Sample SJ, Livesey MA, et al. Morphologic changes associated with functional adaptation of the navicular bone of horses. *J Anat*. 2007;211(5):662–672.

41. Tranquille CA, Blunden AS, Dyson SJ, et al. Effect of exercise on thicknesses of mature hyaline cartilage, calcified cartilage, and subchondral bone of equine tarsi. *Am J Vet Res*. 2009;70(12):1477–1483.

42. Tranquille CA, Dyson SJ, Blunden AS, et al. Histopathological features of distal tarsal joint cartilage and subchondral bone in ridden and pasture-exercised horses. *Am J Vet Res*. 2011;72(1):33–41.

43. Cleary OB, Trumble TN, Merritt KA, et al. Effect of exercise and osteochondral injury on synovial fluid and serum concentrations of carboxy-terminal telopeptide fragments of type II collagen in racehorses. *Am J Vet Res*. 2010;71(1):33–40.

44. Trumble TN, Scarbrough AB, Brown MP. Osteochondral injury increases type II collagen degradation products (C2C) in synovial fluid of Thoroughbred racehorses. *Osteoarthritis Cartilage*. 2009;17(3):371–374.

45. Frisbie DD, Al-Sobayil F, Billinghurst RC, et al. Changes in synovial fluid and serum biomarkers with exercise and early osteoarthritis in horses. *Osteoarthritis Cartilage*. 2008;16(10):1196–1204.

46. Okumura M, Kim GH, Tagami M, et al. Serum keratan sulphate as a cartilage metabolic marker in horses: the effect of exercise. *J Vet Med A Physiol Pathol Clin Med*. 2002;49(4):195–197.

47. Helal IE, Misumi K, Tateno O, et al. Effect of exercise on serum concentration of cartilage oligomeric matrix protein in Thoroughbreds. *Am J Vet Res*. 2007;68(2):134–140.

48. Calatroni A, Avenoso A, Feriazzo AM, et al. Transient increase with strenuous exercise of plasma levels of glycosaminoglycans in humans and horses. *Connect Tissue Res*. 2008;49(6):416–425.

49. Brown MP, Trumble TN, Plaas AH, et al. Exercise and injury increase chondroitin sulfate chain length and decrease hyaluronan chain length in synovial fluid. *Osteoarthritis Cartilage*. 2007;15(11):1318–1325.

50. Van den Boom R, Brama PA, Kiers GH, et al. The influence of repeated arthrocentesis and exercise on matrix metalloproteinase and tumour necrosis factor alpha activities in normal equine joints. *Equine Vet J*. 2004;36(2):155–159.

51. Van den Boom R, van de Lest CHA, Bull S, et al. Influence of repeated arthrocentesis and exercise on synovial fluid concentration of nitric oxide, prostaglandin E2 and glycosaminoglycans in healthy equine joints. *Equine Vet J*. 2005;37(3):250–256.

52. Brama PAJ, van den Boom R, DeGroot J, et al. Collagenase-1 (MMP-1) activity in equine synovial fluid: influence of age, joint pathology, exercise and repeated arthrocentesis. *Equine Vet J*. 2004;36(1):34–40.

53. Van den Hoogen BM, Van de Lest CHA, van Weeren PR, et al. Loading-induced changes in synovial fluid affect cartilage metabolism. *Br J Rheumatol*. 1998;37(1-2):671–676.

54. Van de Lest CH, van den Hoogen BM, van Weeren PR. Loading-induced changes in synovial fluid affect cartilage metabolism. *Biorheology*. 2000;37(1-2):45–55.

55. Kawcak CE, McIlwraith CW, Norrdin RW, et al. Clinical effects of exercise on subchondral bone of carpal and metacarpophalangeal joints in horses. *Am J Vet Res*. 2000;61(10):1252–1258.

56. Sarrafian TL, Case JT, Kinde H, et al. Fatal musculoskeletal injuries of Quarter Horse racehorses: 314 cases (1990-2007). J Am Vet Med Assoc. 2012;241:935–942.

57. Reed SR, Jackson BF, Wood JL, et al. Exercise affects joint injury risk in young Thoroughbreds in training. Vet J. 2013;196(3):339–344.

58. Steel CM, Hopper BJ, Richardson JL, et al. Clinical findings, diagnosis, prevalence and predisposing factors for lameness localised to the middle carpal joint in young Standardbred racehorses. Equine Vet J. 2006;38(2):152–157.

59. Hill AE, Carpenter TE, Gardner IA, et al. Evaluation of a stochastic Markov-chain model for the development of forelimb injuries in Thoroughbred racehorses. Am J Vet, Res. 2003;64(3): 328–37.

60. Vigre H, Chriél M, Hesselholt M, et al. Risk factors for the hazard of lameness in Danish Standardbred trotters. Prev Vet Med. 2002;56(2):105–117.

61. Maroudas A. Metabolism of cartilaginous tissues: a quantitative approach. In: Holborow EJ, Maroudas A, eds. Studies in joint disease. Vol. 1. Tunbridge Wells: Pitman Medical; 1980:59–86.

62. Maroudas A, Palla G, Gilav E. Racemization of aspartic acid in human articular cartilage. Connect Tissue Res. 1992;28(3): 161–169.

63. Brama PAJ, Karssenberg D, Barneveld A, et al. Contact areas and pressure distribution on the proximal articular surface of the proximal phalanx under sagittal plane loading. Equine Vet J. 2001;33(1):26–32.

64. Little CB, Ghosh P. Variation in proteoglycan metabolism by articular chondrocytes in different joint regions is determined by post-natal mechanical loading. Osteoarthritis Cartilage. 1997;5(1):49–62.

65. Brama PAJ, TeKoppele JM, Bank RA, et al. Development of biochemical heterogeneity of articular cartilage: influences of age and exercise. Equine Vet J. 2002;34(3):265–269.

66. Brama PAJ, TeKoppele JM, Bank RA, et al. Functional adaptation of articular cartilage: the formation of regional biochemical characteristics up to age one year. Equine Vet J. 2000;32(3):217–221.

67. Mienaltowski MJ, Huang L, Stromberg AJ, et al. Differential gene expression associated with postnatal equine articular cartilage maturation. BMC Musculoskelet Disord. 2008;9:149.

68. Benninghoff A. Form und Bau der Gelenkknorpel in ihren Beziehungen zur Funktion. Zweiter teil: Der Aufbau des Gelenkknorpels in seinen Beziehungen zur Funktion. Zsch Zelforsch Mikroskop Anat. 1925;2:783–862.

69. Van Turnhout MC, Haazelager MB, Gijsen MA, et al. Quantitative description of collagen structure in the articular cartilage of the young and adult equine distal metacarpus. Anim Biol. 2008;58:353–370.

70. Van Weeren PR, Barneveld A. Study design to evaluate the influence of exercise on the development of the equine musculoskeletal system of foals up to age 11 months. Equine Vet J. 1999;31(Suppl 31):4–8.

71. Cornelissen BPM, van Weeren PR, Ederveen AGH, et al. Influence of exercise on bone mineral density of immature cortical and trabecular bone of the equine metacarpus and proximal sesamoid bone. Equine Vet J. 1999;31(Suppl 31):79–85.

72. Firth EC, van Weeren PR, Pfeiffer DU, et al. Effect of age, exercise and growth rate on bone mineral density (BMD) in third carpal bone and distal radius of Dutch Warmblood foals with osteochondrosis. Equine Vet J. 1999;31(Suppl 31):74–78.

73. Barneveld A, van Weeren PR. Early changes in the distal intertarsal joint of Dutch Warmblood foals and the influence of exercise on bone density in the third tarsal bone. Equine Vet J. 1999;31(Suppl 31):67–73.

74. Brama PAJ, TeKoppele JM, Bank RA, et al. Influence of different exercise levels and age on the biochemical characteristics of immature equine articular cartilage. Equine Vet J. 1999;31(Suppl 31):55–61.

75. Brama PAJ, TeKoppele JM, Bank RA, et al. Training affects the collagen framework of subchondral bone in foals. Vet J. 2001;162(1):24–32.

76. Brama PAJ, TeKoppele JM, Bank RA, et al. Biochemical development of subchondral bone from birth until age eleven months and the influence of physical activity. Equine Vet J. 2002;34(2):143–149.

77. Van de Lest CH, Brama PA, van Weeren PR. The influence of exercise on bone morphogenic enzyme activity of immature equine subchondral bone. Biorheology. 2003;40(1-3):377–382.

78. Van den Hoogen BM, van de Lest CHA, van Weeren PR, et al. Effect of exercise on the proteoglycan metabolism of articular cartilage in growing foals. Equine Vet J. 1999;31(Suppl 31):62–66.

79. Billinghurst RC, Brama PAJ, van Weeren PR, et al. Significant exercise-related changes in the serum levels of two biomarkers of collagen metabolism in young horses. Osteoarthr Cartilage. 2003;11(10):760–769.

80. Cherdchutham W, Becker CK, Smith RKW, et al. Age-related changes and effect of exercise on the molecular composition of immature equine superficial digital flexor tendons. Equine Vet J. 1999;31(Suppl 31):86–94.

81. McIlwraith CW. Global Equine Research Alliance to reduce musculoskeletal injury in the equine athlete. Equine Vet Educ. 2000;12(5):260–262.

82. Rogers CW, Firth EC, McIlwraith CW, et al. Evaluation of a new strategy to modulate skeletal development in Thoroughbred performance horses by imposing track-based exercise during growth. Equine Vet J. 2008;40(2):111–118.

83. Nugent GE, Law AW, Wong EG, et al. Site- and exercise-related variation in structure and function of cartilage from equine distal metacarpal condyle. Osteoarthritis Cartilage. 2004;12(10):826–833.

84. Kim W, Kawcak CE, McIlwraith CW, et al. Influence of early conditioning exercise on the development of gross cartilage defects and swelling behavior of cartilage extracellular matrix in the equine midcarpal joint. Am J Vet Res. 2009;70(5):589–598.

85. Kawcak CE, McIlwraith CW, Firth EC. Effects of early exercise on metacarpophalangeal joints in horses. Am J Vet Res. 2010;71(4):405–411.

86. Doube M, Firth EC, Boyde A. Variations in articular calcified cartilage by site and exercise in the 18-month-old equine distal metacarpal condyle. Osteoarthritis Cartilage. 2007;15(11):1283–1292.

87. Kim W, Kawcak CE, McIlwraith CW, et al. Histologic and histomorphometric evaluation of midcarpal joint defects in Thoroughbreds raised with and without early conditioning exercise. Am J Vet Res. 2012;73(4):498–507.

88. Dykgraaf S, Firth EC, Rogers CW, et al. Effects of exercise on chondrocyte viability and subchondral bone sclerosis in the distal third metacarpal and metatarsal bones of young horses. Vet J. 2008;178(1):53–61.

89. Brama PAJ, Holopainen J, van Weeren PR, et al. Effect of loading on the organization of the collagen fibril network in juvenile equine articular cartilage. J Orthop Res. 2009;27(9):1226–1234.

90. Van Weeren PR, Firth EC, Brommer H, et al. Early exercise advances the maturation of glycosaminoglycans and collagen in the extracellular matrix of articular cartilage in the horse. *Equine Vet J.* 2008;40(2):128–135.

91. Brama PA, Holopainen J, van Weeren PR, et al. Influence of exercise and joint topography on depth-related spatial distribution of proteoglycan and collagen content in immature equine articular cartilage. *Equine Vet J.* 2009;41(6):557–563.

92. Kiviranta I, Jurvelin J, Tammi M, et al. Weight bearing controls glycosaminoglycan concentration and articular cartilage thickness in the knee joints of young beagle dogs. *Arthr Rheum.* 1987;30(7):801–809.

93. Kiviranta I, Tammi M, Jurvelin J, et al. Articular cartilage thickness and glycosaminoglycan distribution in the young canine knee joint after remobilization of the immobilized limb. *J Orthop Res.* 1994;12(2):161–167.

94. Jones G, Bennell K, Cicuttini FM. Effect of physical activity on cartilage development in healthy kids. *Br J Sports Med.* 2003;37:382–383.

95. Julkunen P, Halmesmäki EP, Livarinen J, et al. Effects of growth and exercise on composition, structural maturation and appearance of osteoarthritis in articular cartilage of hamsters. *J Anat.* 2010;217(3):262–274.

96. Firth EC. The response of bone, articular cartilage and tendon to exercise in the horse. *J Anat.* 2006;208(4):513–526.

97. Smith RK, Goodship AE. The effect of early training and the adaptation and conditioning of skeletal tissues. *Vet Clin North Am Equine Pract.* 2008;24(1):37–51.

98. Van Weeren PR, Brama PAJ. Equine joint disease in the light of new developments in articular cartilage research. *Pferde-heilk.* 2003;19:336–344.

99. Helminen HJ, Hyttinen MM, Lammi MJ, et al. Regular joint loading in youth assists in the establishment and strengthening of the collagen network of articular cartilage and contributes to the prevention of osteoarthrosis later in life: a hypothesis. *J Bone Miner Metab.* 2000;18(5):245–257.

100. Smith RK, Birch H, Patterson-Kane J, et al. Should equine athletes commence training during skeletal development? Changes in tendon matrix with development, ageing, function, and exercise. *Equine Vet J.* 1999;31(Suppl 30):201–209.

101. Rogers CW, Firth EC, McIlwraith CW, et al. Evaluation of a new strategy to modulate skeletal development in racehorses by imposing track-based exercise during growth: the effects on 2- and 3-year-old racing careers. *Equine Vet J.* 2008;40(2):119–127.

102. Tanner JC, Rogers CW, Firth EC. The association of 2-year-old training milestones with career length and racing success in a sample of Thoroughbred horses in New Zealand. *Equine Vet J.* 2013;45(1):20–24.

Principles of Diagnosis

Christopher E. Kawcak, Myra F. Barrett, Natasha M. Werpy, and Kurt Selberg

Clinical lameness examination and diagnostic imaging of the limbs are commonly performed in practice with the goal of providing an objective characterization of the cause of lameness. However, with the development of volumetric imaging techniques (those techniques that can be used to image in 3 dimensions, that is, computed tomography [CT] and magnetic resonance imaging [MRI]) came better understanding of tissue lesions that lead to pain and lameness. As our understanding improved, there has been incentive to identify lame horses earlier and to better understand the interpretation of diagnostic techniques that provide insight into therapeutic and rehabilitation recommendations. However, recent studies indicate that in cases of mild lameness, defined as horses being ≤1.5 grade on the American Association of Equine Practitioners (AAEP) lameness scale,[1] there was poor agreement among clinicians on the painful limb, necessitating the need for more objective means of characterizing lameness in horses.[2] It appears that the identification of the lame limb(s) and site of pain within a limb are now the weak links in characterizing disease in horse limbs. Some of this is likely because each clinician has his own personal means of examining a horse and interpreting findings. As more objective measures of lameness are developed and volumetric imaging is used on a more consistent basis, these findings can help clinicians focus their attention on those subjective parameters that are most consistent. However, the ultimate goal is to identify the site/sites that is/are painful and to best characterize the location and severity of tissue damage so as to render an accurate prognosis and institute the best treatment for horse and client. This chapter will provide an overview of clinical and imaging examinations that lead to diagnosis and offer recommendations for treatment.

CLINICAL EXAMINATION

Documentation of the history of the lameness is important, as are the expectations by the owner and trainer for the horse's

level of use. It is important to document the rider's experience and any previous lamenesses and treatments that have been used. The clinical lameness examination is the cornerstone for appropriate diagnosis of equine musculoskeletal disease. Veterinarians need to be able to recognize abnormal findings on visual and physical examination and to understand the influences of various conformational abnormalities on the horse's capacity to fulfill its function. Veterinarians must also be able to recognize if a horse is lame and in which leg or legs the horse is lame. Further, they must be able to grade the degree of lameness consistently for comparison with examination findings after diagnostic analgesia is used and for assessment at follow-up examinations. In addition, clinicians must be able to recognize pain in the upper body (neck, back, and pelvis), which may not lead to overt lameness but rather to poor performance. The goal of this section is to discuss subjective and objective changes in a horse's gait during lameness and clinical tools that can be used to characterize lameness subjectively.

Static Examinations
Conformation
The first phase of the lameness examination is evaluation of the conformation, in which both experience and science play a role. The horse should be evaluated from all sides and the conformation of the horse should be characterized in light of the intended use. Conformation of the horse has been well characterized subjectively by both veterinarians and horsemen over the last couple of centuries. In the last several years, more objective assessments of conformation and its impact on soundness have been evaluated. Most recently, a direct association has been made between good conformation at a young age and longevity in competition.[3] In addition, certain conformational characteristics have been associated with injury in racing Thoroughbreds.[4] Distal limb conformation can be influenced during growth; however, there are certain conformational types that are breed-specific and that must be understood when evaluating foals.

In addition, conformation in foals changes during development, and an understanding of this change is absolutely necessary to make correct recommendations for optimization of conformation.[5,6] Although there are undoubtedly horses with poor conformation that have been exceptional athletes, in general abnormal conformation can lead to chronic lameness that can limit the athletic career. Conformation analysis is a subjective interpretation; still, there are some studies in which objective characterization has been correlated to athletic longevity. Anderson and McIlwraith characterized the longitudinal development of equine limbs in proportion to size and concluded that growth rate plateaued in Thoroughbred racehorses at 2 years of age.[5] They also correlated conformational abnormalities to problems within the forelimbs and concluded that offset knees contributed to fetlock problems and that the odds of a forelimb fracture increased with pastern length. Another interesting finding is that carpal valgus, which is commonly considered an abnormal finding in young horses, was shown to be a protective mechanism as demonstrated through a decrease in the odds of carpal fracture and effusion with increased carpal angle. Thus, some conformational traits that were once thought to be abnormal may be protective.[5]

The second phase of the lameness examination is the static examination. During this examination, hoof testers should be applied to the feet, especially around the nail holes, sole, frog, and hoof wall. It must be noted, however, that hoof testers have been shown to be about 50% accurate when correlated with caudal heel pain.[7] In addition, findings may vary between operators, as there is considerable variation in the force a person will apply to various parts of the hoof.[8] The hoof capsule should also be statically examined for conformation and coronary band characteristics. On occasion changes in hoof wall characteristics can be a sign of joint problems. Wear pattern of the shoe should also be characterized and digital pulse should be appreciated both before and after walking and trotting. In some instances, subtle hoof pain can cause a significant increase in digital pulse after walking or trotting, when it was fairly normal before.

Joints and tendon sheaths should also be palpated and synovial effusion should be differentiated from joint capsule or tendon sheath thickening. In joints with synovial effusion, the synovial fluid can be balloted between different parts of the joint in most instances. However, significant synovial effusion can be present yet not have a clinical impact on the presenting lameness; conversely, in some cases, especially those with subchondral bone disease, synovial effusion may not be present. Significant synovial effusion may also be difficult to palpate in a joint or tendon sheath that has chronic capsular or sheath thickening (Figure 9-1). Synovial effusion must also be distinguished from synovial hernia or hygroma. For instance, in the dorsal aspect of the carpus a synovial hernia may palpate no differently from synovial effusion, except for the fact that it is usually isolated to either the dorsomedial or dorsolateral aspects of the joint and on occasion the defect in the joint capsule can be palpated. A hygroma, on the other hand, is more diffuse in nature than effusion and the fluid cannot be palpated across various aspects of the joint. In some instances, contrast arthrography may be needed to further characterize and differentiate these problems. Joints should also be palpated for pain response, which is usually only significant in cases of septic synovitis. Joints should also be assessed for pain during flexion and crepitus should be appreciated and noted. Some synovial structures are often complicated in their anatomy and this causes confusion when interpreting clinical results. For instance, carpal effusion must be differentiated from tendon sheath swelling and carpal canal swelling. An in-depth understanding of anatomy will help to differentiate swelling of these structures. In addition, palpation of the three joints in the stifle can be confusing to some clinicians. The three joints must be distinguished based on normal landmarks and care must be taken to differentiate synovial effusion from joint capsule swelling.

Muscle symmetry should be appreciated and soft tissues and bones should be palpated to determine geometry and pain during palpation. Isolated pain on palpation is of value for further investigation. However, for proximal suspensory ligaments, for example, there can be significant damage at the origin, especially in the bone component, without much

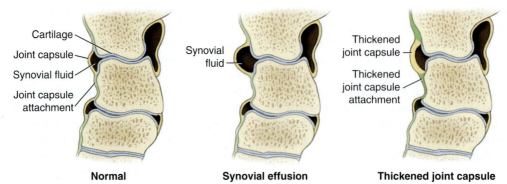

| Normal | Synovial effusion | Thickened joint capsule |

Cartilage
Joint capsule
Synovial fluid
Joint capsule attachment

Synovial fluid

Thickened joint capsule
Thickened joint capsule attachment

FIGURE 9-1 Palpation of synovial joints can present in one of three ways. *Left,* normal in which synovial effusion is not apparent; *middle,* synovial effusion in which synovial fluid can easily be palpated and balloted between different areas of the joint; and *right,* joint capsule thickening, which can be palpated as soft tissue thickening with or without the perception of significant fluid feeling. Synovial effusion can often be difficult to palpate through a thickened joint capsule.

response to palpation. Conversely, significant pain can sometimes be elicited in the proximal suspensory area without significant damage. In the latter case some have speculated that the pain response is caused by manual stimulation of the adjacent nerves. Range of motion of the joints and limbs should be appreciated, although reduction in range of motion is not always a source of pain. It must be remembered that some young horses in active work can respond dramatically to passive flexion such as the fetlock joints of Thoroughbreds and the hind limbs of Western Performances horses. The degree of pain on palpation and with flexion can be subjectively graded. We categorize these responses as normal, mild, moderate, or severe. Crepitus of the joint can also be appreciated on flexion and extension and should again be characterized.

There are certain areas within the limb that can be confusing to inexperienced practitioners during palpation. Distal interphalangeal effusion is best appreciated in the 1- to 2-cm area proximal to the coronary band. The fetlock joint and the tendon sheath are closely associated with each other and synovial effusion in one site can be confused with synovial effusion in another. Basic anatomy understanding is necessary to characterize the difference between the two. For the carpus, not only are the two high motion joints (antebrachiocarpal and middle carpal) prone to effusion but they are surrounded by multiple tendon sheaths and the carpal canal. Swelling in any of these structures can be confused with carpal joint swelling. However, the tendon sheaths around the cranial and lateral aspects of the joint are often covered by a retinaculum over the dorsal aspect of the carpus, limiting their synovial effusion and swelling to areas proximal and distal to the carpal joints. Synovial effusion or swelling of the carpal canal is most visible on the lateral aspect of the distal radius proximal to the accessory carpal bone. Tarsocrural joint effusion is readily appreciated in the dorsal medial aspect of the joint as well as in the lateral and medial plantar pouches located caudal to the tibia. However, in some horses, especially Western Performance horses, significant swelling can occur in the lateral plantar pouch of the tarsocrural joint. Often this is more soft tissue thickening than fluid and is not always directly related to lameness. The stifle is another area that is confusing to palpate for the novice practitioner. Landmarks that must be appreciated to palpate the joints appropriately are the medial aspect of the tibial plateau, the medial collateral ligament, and the patellar ligaments. An understanding of their location and easy identification of their presence will help the clinician in identifying the synovial structures. Effusion of the medial femoral tibial joint can be appreciated cranial to the medial collateral ligament starting approximately 1 cm proximal to the medial aspect of the tibial plateau. There is a large synovial pocket in this area in which fluid can accumulate. The femoropatellar joint is the easiest in which to identify synovial effusion as the swelling will be often between the medial and middle patellar ligaments and oftentimes quite significant. Effusion of the lateral femorotibial joint can be readily appreciated on ultrasound over the lateral aspect of the joint, surrounding the peroneus tertius. There are some joints in which synovial effusion is not readily appreciated. It is difficult to appreciate synovial effusion in such joints as the proximal interphalangeal joint and elbow, shoulder, and distal tarsal joints.

The third phase of the lameness examination is the dynamic examination. The clinician should observe the horse from the front, back, and sides, and the horse should be initially walked to evaluate hoof landing and limb movement. Stride length and the cranial and caudal phase of the stride should also be characterized. A neurologic assessment should also be made at that time. In addition, it is a good idea to walk the horse on both hard and soft footing to see if any change in limb use can be appreciated.

Limb movement and lameness in the horse are best characterized at the trot. This 2-beat gait allows for appreciation of consistent abnormalities in limb and body movement that can indicate that a horse is lame in a specific limb(s). Horses should be trotted under control but without restrictive control of the head to allow for free head, neck, and axial skeletal movement. Often, axial skeletal motion, including head and neck motion, best allows characterization of the lameness because their movement is often compensatory in nature. It is best to trot the horses on both hard and soft footing, in straight lines, and in circles in both directions. Good footing is necessary as it appears that horses are often tentative to the integrity of the footing and may compensate for subtle lamenesses.

Objective Assessment of Lameness

Limb movement and use can be assessed either by analysis of ground reaction force (kinetics) or limb movement (kinematics), or a combination of both.[9] Pain in a limb typically causes reduced weight bearing in the affected limb or limbs, thereby causing reduced ground reaction force by the ground with the limb at hoof contact. Ground reaction force is typically measured with a force plate, the gold standard, but the environment in which this is done is confining and not practical for routine lameness use. However, ground reaction force is now being measured with force shoes,[10] pressure-sensitive mats,[11] and force-measuring treadmills.[12] Each has its own issues that sometime limits use. Shoes require a cable to be attached to the limbs, pressure-sensitive mats can fail over time and have poor correlation with force plate measurement, and horses move differently on treadmills than they do over ground.[13,14] In addition, inertial sensors attached to the limb have shown acceleration data that correlate to vertical force in lame horses.[15] Although measurement of ground reaction force may be a sensitive means of assessing limb use in the horse, its practical application is still limited at this time.

Kinematic measurement of lameness involves two- or three-dimensional (2D and 3D, respectively) evaluation of limb and body motion. Stationary kinematic volumes are created in a laboratory where several acquisition media, usually video cameras, can be used to observe limb and body motion. To enhance the accuracy of the measurements, reflective spheres can be attached to the horse at fixed points so as to objectively measure movement of that area. For 2D measurement, a single camera can be used to measure sagittal plane parameters: joint flexion, hoof height and flight, head movement, etc. For 3D analysis, at least two cameras must be able to track a reflective sphere at any one time. Consequently this requires dedicated facilities and personnel, which is not clinically practical, and the analysis technique needed depends on whether a forelimb or hindlimb is being evaluated.[16] However, inertial sensor technology can be used to measure specific kinematic parameters to aid in characterization of lameness. Kinematics can be assessed using a single sensor on a limb,[17-20] the head, withers, and/or body,[21] or in combination with gyroscopes to assess head motion with limb loading.[22] Limb-mounted inertial sensors have shown good agreement with kinematic analyses in the cranio-caudal and vertical planes, but they are relatively poor in the lateral-medial plane.[23] Body-mounted inertial sensors on the head, withers, and/ or pelvis have been shown to be helpful in characterizing body motion during normal lunging and circling,[24,25] during lunging or circling with lameness,[26,27] during movement both in hand and under saddle,[28] in response to hindlimb flexion tests,[29,30] for segmenting limb contact timing,[31] in response to hindlimb analgesia,[32] and when assessing the influence of speed on subtle lameness.[33] However, a combination of sensors across the pelvis are needed to best characterize hindlimb lameness.[21] Keegan et al. found that results from subjective lameness examinations and inertial sensors placed on the body and limbs had good correlations, but agreement was fair in most cases.[34] However, in an experimental model of lameness, results from the inertial sensor identified subtle lameness sooner than subjective evaluation by experienced clinicians.[35] Therefore, it appears that inertial sensor technology may aid in early detection of lameness.

Subjective Measures of Lameness

It is essential to understand that a lameness examination is an artistic experience acquired by years of clinical practice along with integration of objective information about horse movement. Although recommendations can be made to help an individual better characterize lameness, a clinician needs to develop his or her own set of skills to optimize the ability to see and characterize lameness in horses. It is also important to know that obvious lameness oftentimes may not need to be present to be performance limiting. Some lamenesses are not amenable to diagnostic analgesia for full characterization of site of injury, and alleviation of some subtle lamenesses, although treatable, may not solve the performance-limiting problem. With experience comes the ability to characterize the lameness as it relates to pain and specific body parts. Although some insist that they can characterize the site of lameness subjectively, our approach usually has been to use this as an indicator to drive diagnostic analgesia to confirm the diagnosis, not in place of diagnostic analgesia. Similar gait deficits can exist for various conditions but it is important to document those specific movements that may indicate pain in a particular area.

Most of the assessment of lame horses is done at a trot; in North America a 0 to 5 grading scale is used and in Europe a 0 to 10 grading scale is used. The same scales can also be used during an examination in circles and in response to flexion. The AAEP lameness grading scale is most typically used in the United States; grade 0 is sound; grade 1 is difficult to observe and not consistently apparent regardless of circumstances (such as weight carrying, circling, inclines, and hard surfaces); grade 2 is difficult to observe at a walk or trotting a straight line but is consistently apparent under certain circumstances (such as weight carrying, circling, inclines, and hard surfaces); grade 3 is consistently observable at a trot under all circumstances; grade 4 is an obvious lameness with marked head nodding, hitching, or shortened stride; and a horse with a grade 5 lameness typically shows minimal weight bearing.[1] At a trot, stride characteristics should be characterized, although overall stride length cannot differ between limbs or else the horse would be moving in a circle. Therefore, if a horse has a decreased cranial phase, then the caudal phase usually makes up for the difference in both limbs. In some instances the stride may differ in its lateral to medial motion; for example, horses with carpal pain typically abduct the forelimbs to reduce flexion in the carpi. Hoof placement should be characterized as well. The hardness of the surface can stimulate a pain response variable with the site of pain within the limb. Hard ground is thought to make horses with foot, bone, and joint pain worse; whereas, soft ground is felt to make the lameness worse in a horse with soft tissue pain, including those with soft tissue problems in the foot.

Flexion tests are commonly used to subjectively characterize the site of pain and the severity. The use of flexion tests has at times been contentious; however, they are still used commonly in practice. Response to flexion tests can be variable depending on the level of lameness, the use of the horse, and uncontrollable factors within a horse. Although Pfau et al. have shown that the asymmetry induced by subtle lameness can be worsened with flexion, they also demonstrated considerable variability in flexion response between horses.[29]

It is impossible to isolate just one area, joint, or tissue with flexion tests. For instance, digital flexion can aggravate pain in the proximal suspensory ligament region, and "stifle flexion" will include the tarsus and digit to some extent. That is not to say that these flexion tests are not of value, but rather that they should not be solely relied upon for identifying the site of lameness. Some level of worsening lameness in response to flexion is normal usually for 3 to 5 steps and it must be remembered that in some young athletes flexion response may be worse without that site being the primary site of pain. One method of assessing response is to grade lameness as normal, mild, moderate, or severe. The lameness can also be rescored after the flexion test.

Moving a horse in a circle is often beneficial. Good control and consistent circles are needed on both hard and soft ground. Some generalizations include foot pain in a limb making the lameness in that limb worse on the inside of the circle and on hard ground; soft tissue pain in a limb making the lameness worse with the limb on the outside of the circle; and lameness caused by lesions on the medial side of the limb making the lameness worse with the limb on the outside of the circle. In some cases the lameness seen on the circle can be worse than baseline, or visa versa.

With hindlimb lameness the entire pelvis rises before the lame limb contacts the ground. Differences in hip motion commonly occur with increased push off from the sound limb at the end of the stride. In horses with more severe lameness, grade 3 and above, the head will often go forward, and sometimes this is confused with forelimb lameness.

Multiple limb lesions can sometimes be difficult to see at a trot. In general, horses with bilateral forelimb lameness will show a shuffling gate with short strides. Horses with bilateral hind-limb lameness will appear "short strided" with almost a smooth rocking horse appearance. Horses with contralateral limb lameness will typically demonstrate a rough rocking horse lameness, and horses with ipsilateral limb lameness look very similar with the head nod consistent with lameness in both limbs. However, it should be noted that horses with hind end lameness may drift away from the lame leg. Lameness in one limb can also cause worsening lameness in another. For instance, a horse with right hind lameness may not become totally sound until the lameness in the left front is completely blocked.

Diagnostic Analgesia

In most cases it is best to use diagnostic analgesia to further characterize the site(s) of pain. Diagnostic analgesia is performed and then the lameness is recharacterized sometime later. After diagnostic analgesia, horses should be reexamined within a few minutes and in some cases reexamined again outwards of 30 minutes after. Significant migration of the local anesthetic can be observed as the postblock duration increases.

The two main types of local anesthetic used are lidocaine hydrochloride and mepivacaine hydrochloride. Bupivacaine hydrochloride may also be used when a longer duration of analgesia is needed (4 to 6 hours). Mepivacaine is typically used more often because it is longer lasting and less irritating than lidocaine. The tolerance for and duration of effect of mepivacaine can vary significantly. Although mepivacaine typically wears off between 1 and 2 hours, there can be a significant prolonged effect on the lameness. Besides the variability in chemical effect, the regional anatomy being injected can also play a large role in the variability of the response. The biggest concern is that injection of a blocking agent into one structure may affect another significant structure. There are three ways that this can happen. The first is that a synovial structure may share a physical or physiologic communication with an associated joint or structure. For instance, in some horses, injection into the distal interphalangeal joint can affect the navicular bursa and/or the palmar digital nerves, which traverse closely to the joint.[36,37] The second means of diffusion is physical extravasation of blocking agent from a joint to desensitize local nerves. As mentioned, there is some concern that this can happen in the distal interphalangeal joint. In other cases, it has been speculated that mepivacaine can extravasate from the injection site in a fetlock to the local nerves in the area of the fetlock joint. This was demonstrated by case in which an MRI showed a foot lesion in a horse that had blocked sound to a metacarpophalangeal joint injection (M.F. Barrett, personal communication, 2010). It was speculated that mepivacaine had extravasated from the joint to block the palmar nerves

at the level of the proximal sesamoid bones. The third way in which blocks can be confusing is caused by proximal migration of anesthetic agent through a neurovascular bundle. There has long been a concern based on volumetric imaging techniques that lesions existed well proximal to the site of blocking. As an example, proximal P1 lesions have been seen in horses that block sound to a palmar digital nerve block.[38] Horses that improve significantly to low 4-point nerve blocks yet have proximal suspensory lesions with nothing distally are another example. Seabaugh et al. have shown that the administration of contrast agent at the site of a low 4-point nerve block can demonstrate direct deposit of contrast agent into a synovial structure, spread of the contrast agent through the soft tissues over time into associated synovial structures, and/or movement of contrast and dye either through the neurovascular bundle or the lymphatics to a more proximal site.[39] Therefore, care must be taken in interpretation of nerve and joint blocks. In some cases, when a lesion is found more proximal than the diagnostic analgesic procedures have demonstrated, conformation of that lesion as a site of pain is needed. For instance, when a proximal P1 lesion is seen in a horse that goes sound with a palmar digital nerve block, intraarticular analgesia can be administered to further confirm the significance of that lesion.

In some cases, because of trainers' schedules and the mild level of lameness, trainers may ask that the basic lameness examination be performed with flexion tests and possibly some basic perineural blocks; however, a thorough examination may not be possible. In this case, the goal is to treat the horse and monitor its response to treatment. A further goal with this method is to reduce the risk of further injury as much is as possible. With this technique, however, there is some inherent danger that an undiagnosed injury would not be appropriately treated or characterized, and the risk of worsening of the injury should be considered.

Overall, it is best to stay consistent, determined, and disciplined when evaluating the lame horse. There is often some bias in saying that a horse is better after diagnostic analgesia especially in very prolonged lameness examinations when a horse does not block out consistently. Discipline must be used to continue aggressively working up these cases to eliminate that bias. Although the literature can be useful for helping to characterize lameness, not all horses respond the same as those in the literature. Individual clinicians should develop their own guidelines for management of these cases as lameness characteristics and response to treatment can change quickly.

PRINCIPLES OF IMAGING

Radiographs

Digital radiography has exploded in the veterinary market. The advantages of digital radiography are the ability to centrally store and easily search patient images and to allow images to be sent instantly through the internet. This has positively affected radiology workflow, eliminating much of the manual steps such as retrieving prior studies and improving both efficiency and point of care for the patient on the farm. Digital radiography has made veterinary medicine radiographic examinations more transmissible and accessible for consultation and allows easier distribution of images for purchase examinations. Because of these advantages, digital radiography has been widely accepted in the veterinary profession and is deployed throughout academia and private practice alike.

The basics of radiographic exposure and technique selection do not change just because a different form of image receptor is used. When producing images using digital technologies, the veterinarians/technicians must still determine the radiation exposure needed to produce quality images for diagnostic interpretation. However, digital radiography as opposed to screen film has a larger acceptable range of radiation to create a diagnostically acceptable image. A quality image has sufficient brightness to visualize anatomic structures, subject contrast that allows differentiation among anatomic structures, and maximum spatial resolution.

There are two main types of digital radiography commonly used in veterinary medicine: direct digital radiography and computed radiography. Direct digital radiography is more widely used in the equine environment and will be discussed. It typically uses an indirect conversion of the photons (x-rays) to visible light with scintillation material such a gadolinium-based or cesium iodide in the detector. Cesium iodide is becoming more widely used in veterinary medicine, offering 30% to 40% more speed than other mediums. This ultimately allows for less radiation to make a diagnostic exposure. The visible light from the scintillation is then converted to an electrical charge using a photodiode. The electrical charge is sent to a thin film transistor array or a charged-coupled device that digitizes the charges before sending it to the computer for display. If the detector is using a charged-coupled device, a lens focuses the light before the charge-coupled device converts the light into digital signal. In charged-coupled devices, some photons are lost during optical reduction. This results in lost light and may produce increased noise in the image compared with those systems that use thin film transistors.[40]

Image panel sizes vary. The most common configurations in veterinary medicine are 10×12, 11×14, and 14×17 inches (width × length). Depending on the frequency of larger body parts imaged, the larger panel sizes may be more versatile. Similar to digital cameras, the megapixel values are also included in the sensor's specification, which is a measure of resolution or how many pixels are in an area. The space between these pixels is also included, known as pixel pitch. The smaller this number, the better, and most x-ray panels range from 100 to 140 microns. The number of bits used to define each pixel determines bit depth; the greater the bit depth, the greater the number of tones (grayscale or color) that can be represented. Currently, most flat panel displays use 10 to 16 bits. When comparing bit depth, higher numbers may allow for greater accuracy.[41]

The configurations of the flat panel detectors include wired and wireless. Wireless configurations are becoming more widespread and offer more freedom while obtaining radiographs. There are currently generation 1 and generation 2 configurations in wireless x-ray detectors. The distinct advantage of the generation 2 devices is that they sense a radiation source without syncing to the x-ray source. This is similar in principle to a digital camera detecting a visible light to make an exposure. This allows for any radiation source to be used without additional setup. Both of these systems transmit their images from the detector to the computer through (ad hoc wifi) wireless channels in the range of 5 mHz.

Once the image has been made, it is transformed from the raw data to the image displayed. This subject has been reviewed in depth.[42,43] Preprocessing takes place out of the user's hands and is often vendor-specific.[42] Ultimately the digital x-ray images are processed to enhance diagnostic information and reduce irrelevant detail. It is important to realize that images may be processed in such a way that image quality is degraded and diagnostic information is lost. Radiograph detectors should be tested using the most common anatomic areas as well as difficult areas such as the cervical spine for thorough evaluation before purchase. Consultation with an experienced radiologist may also be helpful to avoid systems that are not durable, are difficult to use, or have subpar digital image processing. Image processing may also be adjusted to the user's liking. It is important to fine-tune the images once the x-ray system is purchased if there are anatomic areas not to the equine practitioner's liking.

Digital x-ray panel technologies and the software that runs them continue to advance at a rapid rate. The machines are becoming more portable, producing superior images, and allowing for easier consultation.

Ultrasonography

Machines and Technical Principles

Ultrasonography is a mainstay of musculoskeletal imaging. There has been much advancement in ultrasound technology that has allowed for great improvement in image quality. Additionally, with great experience and multimodality comparison studies, the diagnostic capability of ultrasound has expanded considerably.

Ultrasound uses pulse-echo technology to produce images by sending a high-frequency sound wave through the tissue and then listening for the returning echo. Different tissue types affect the sound waves differently depending on their stiffness and density, and this allows the computer to map the returning sound waves to make an image.[44] Advances that have helped improve image quality include harmonic imaging and spatial compounding. Harmonic imaging filters unwanted frequencies to help reduce image noise and improve resolution.[45] Harmonic imaging can improve image quality, but it can also decrease tissue penetration. Therefore, its usefulness in equine imaging can be limited to more superficial structures, although this is somewhat machine-dependent as some have greater beam attenuation than others. Most modern ultrasound machines allow for harmonic imaging, which can be easily turned on and off. If the operator finds insufficient penetration and an overly dark image while scanning with harmonics turned on, it is usually just a simple press of a button to turn harmonics off to allow for greater beam penetration.

Spatial compounding sends sound waves in multiple beams that are being steered in different directions. The information is collected and averaged together. Compound imaging improves the ultrasound image by reducing artifacts, creates a smoother image with better margin definition, and allows for visualization of structures deep to highly attenuating structures.[45] Spatial compounding, beam steering, other manipulations of the sound beam, and postprocessing can significantly alter image appearance. Different brands often have proprietary names for the forms of spatial compounding and image manipulation that is used, such as M-View (Esaote, Genova, Italy), ApliPure (Toshiba, Tokyo, Japan), and CrossXBeam (GE Healthcare, Wauwatosa, WI), among others. The degree to which these applications change the image will depend on the number of manipulations included in the function. Overall, these functions work to reduce artifact and speckle and to make an image look smoother. To the unaccustomed eye, these changes can sometimes seem blurry or overly smooth. However, these functions actually help to represent the tissue characteristics more accurately and to reduce artifact. With time, most operators will find that they prefer the images produced using these applications.

Other advances in ultrasound include 3D imaging, fusion imaging, and elasticity imaging. Although not commonly used in equine practice, these technologies are increasing in availability. Fusion imaging in particular is an exciting frontier for the evaluation of joints. Fusion imaging allows for combination of cross-sectional imaging (CT or MRI) with ultrasound imaging. The CT or MR image is displayed on one portion of the screen and the live ultrasound on the other. As the transducer moves, the corresponding cross-sectional image is displayed. This technology has great potential for helping detect lesions with ultrasound that were originally found with advanced imaging and for guiding treatment.[46] Elastic imaging includes elastography and acoustic radiation force.[47] Elastography and acoustic radiation force are methods of evaluating tissue stiffness in humans to help distinguish benign from malignant breast tumors, monitor atherosclerosis, and evaluate tendon and ligament injury.[48,49] Elastography is just starting to gain traction in equine imaging, and the elastographic characteristics of normal equine tendons have been described.[50] Changes in stiffness can help detect injury and track healing. Traditional ultrasound machines are used in conjunction with special software for elastography, alleviating the need to buy a special unit purely for this evaluation. It is likely that, as continued research makes the results of elastic imaging more clinically applicable, elastic imaging will grow in popularity.

The types of ultrasound machines that are available to equine practitioners vary greatly from very small portable units with minimal options for image manipulation to larger, high-quality in-house units. The selection of the appropriate machine will depend on the caseload and needs of the individual practitioner (Table 9-1). The image quality of different units varies significantly, with some small portable units allowing for very good image quality and others producing poor-to-limited-quality images. In general, the larger in-house units produce better images than the portable units, although a poor-quality in-house unit will not rival some of the better portable units. Although the price of the unit is often correlated with image quality, this does not always apply; therefore, testing multiple systems is important before purchase. If possible, try multiple machines over several examination types before deciding on which to buy. Test the machine on difficult structures and thicker-skinned horses. Another important factor to consider before purchase is whether or not the clientele generally allows for clipping hair. Show horse practices often cannot clip their patients and some machines are much

TABLE 9-1	Selection Factors to Consider When Purchasing an Ultrasound Unit
Ultrasound location	In-hospital, if all the ultrasounds will be performed in-house, a console unit is recommended as they generally have superior image quality Field work, if a portable unit is required, consider portability and ergonomics. Is it lightweight, easy to carry and set up?
Image quality	Does the machine provide easily reproducible good quality images? Is there adequate resolution so that small lesions can be identified? Consultation with a radiologist or dedicated equine imager is recommended.
Cost	What is the best possible unit in the price range? Not all units priced similarly have the same quality. Do not base purchase on price alone. Shop around; many vendors offer discounts at the end of the year or on demo equipment. Some offer package deals with radiography equipment.
Type of imaging	Musculoskeletal vs reproduction vs abdominal vs cardiac. Certain machines produce better musculoskeletal images than others. The ultrasound of choice may differ for primarily abdominal vs primarily musculoskeletal imaging. The choice of probes will differ as well.
Settings and ergonomics	Are the function keys easy to find and manipulate? Can they be easily reached when sitting low to perform an exam on the distal limb? Can the depth be manipulated at intervals less than 1 cm? (This is important for musculoskeletal imaging.)
User-friendliness	How much manipulation is needed to produce a good quality image? For practitioners who do not want to engage in a lot of image manipulation, the more automated machines may be better suited.

better at others in producing a quality image through hair. In fact, some of the highest quality digital machines are actually quite sensitive to hair and do not produce good images with clipping, even on thin-coated horses. Ultrasound machines should be tested in the most realistic daily scanning environment (not just what looks good on the trade show floor) for thorough evaluation before purchase. Consultation with an experienced equine imager can also be helpful.

Proficiency in machine manipulation is essential to image quality. There are machines on the market that automatically adjust the settings and do not allow the practitioner to change them. Although these machines have the advantage of being straightforward and user-friendly, there is some limit to image quality because images cannot be fine-tuned. Standard ultrasound machines have numerous settings and knobs that operators have to learn how to use. Presets simplify imaging by allowing for the user's preferred settings to be stored and automatically selected during a scan; however, even when using presets there is a constant dynamic flow of image manipulation to maximize quality. Even the best machines on the market will not produce good quality images without an educated operator.

For musculoskeletal imaging, the linear probe is the most frequently used. Linear probes provide excellent resolution and can range in frequency, usually from 6 to 14 MHz, allowing for greater leeway in the depth of structure images. Linear probes are used for the majority of joints, such as the stifle and fetlock, as well as the metacarpus, metatarsus, and pastern. Microconvex probes do not have as good resolution but have the advantage of a small surface or footprint, which means they can have greater contact with irregular surfaces and fit in smaller spaces than the linear probe. A microconvex probe is essential for examining the navicular apparatus between the heel bulbs and can also sometimes be helpful for examining the lateral meniscus and lateral cranial meniscal ligament of the stifle. Macroconvex probes have the lowest frequency and are used for examining deep structures, such as the caudal aspect of the stifle and the pelvis. The higher the probe frequency, the better the resolution, but the trade-off is decreased tissue penetration. In general, all examinations should be performed with the highest frequency that allows sufficient penetration and the best resolution. Therefore, for the practitioner who will routinely be scanning musculoskeletal structures, having all three of the above-mentioned probes is important.

Standoff pads are used in musculoskeletal imaging to improve probe contact to the limb and improve resolution of the near-field structures. The typical standoff pad is made of thick rubbery material and conforms to the transducer. The disadvantages of standoff pads are that they require increased probe pressure, create artifacts, and sometimes require decreasing the frequency because of beam attenuation. An alternative to the traditional standoff is a product called Superflab (Mick Radio-Nuclear Instruments, Inc., Mount Vernon, NY). This product is used for radiation therapy but also works very well as standoff material. It is thin and conforms to the limb, improving probe contact and near-field imaging, without the artifact and increased probe pressure of traditional pads.

A high-quality ultrasound study requires adequate time and an appropriate setting. Ultrasound should be performed in dim light whenever possible to maximize image quality, as too much light will result in overly bright images (similar to the autobrightness function of a smart phone in bright sunlight). Overly bright images risk masking more subtle injuries. Ultrasound exams should be standardized and all structures in the area of interest should be examined. For example, the lateral aspect of the stifle joint is often overlooked but should be included as part of the standard examination, as injuries can occur there. Additionally, non-weight-bearing imaging is important in many studies. The cranial meniscal ligaments of the stifle, weight-bearing surface of the medial femoral tibial joint, and dorsal metacarpal condyles are all structures that must be examined in a non-weight-bearing position. Non-weight-bearing studies also allow for manipulation of the ergot to better evaluate the palmar/plantar aspect of the fetlock. The use of blocks and farrier stands can help provide limb stabilization while these studies are performed. Taking joints through a range of motion while scanning can also provide information about joint instability or other dynamic pathologic changes.[51] Many high-quality continuing education courses and wet labs are available and recommended for practitioners wishing to improve their ultrasound skills.

In summary, ultrasound technology is continuing to improve at a rapid rate. Machines are becoming more portable, streamlined, and faster and have better image quality. Even with increasing availability and use of advanced imaging, ultrasound will continue to play a crucial role in equine musculoskeletal imaging.

Nuclear Medicine

Nuclear scintigraphy uses radionuclides attached to various molecules that are specific for various body systems and tissue types. Bone scans are the most common type of nuclear scintigraphic examination performed in the horse. For bone scans, methylene diphosphonate (MDP) and hydroxymethylene diphosphonate (HDP) are the most common radionuclides; HDP may have better bone distribution.[52] Nuclear scintigraphy camera design incorporates a thallium-doped sodium iodine crystal that scintillates in response to gamma photons emitted during decay after intravenous injection of the radioisotope. Light, in the form of small bursts, is produced at the crystal when a photon strikes it (scintillation). The photomultipliers detect the light and convert it to electrical signals. Finally, the attached computer creates an image from the electrical signals.

Nuclear scintigraphy of the skeletal system has 3 phases once the radionuclide has been injected intravenously. Immediate to 30 seconds postinjection is the vascular phase. Three to 5 minutes postinjection is the soft tissue phase. The bone phase occurs when the patient is imaged approximately 2 hours postinjection.[53]

Scintigraphic examination of the extremities should include a minimum of cranial/dorsal and lateral images. Most if not all images are acquired with standing sedation.

The image matrix is generally set to 256 × 256 with image counts between 150,000 and 300,000. Timed scans may also be used for static images; however, as the scan progresses the number of counts may reduce because of decay. Thus, imaging with specific counts per region of interest is recommended.

Indications for skeletal nuclear scintigraphy as a diagnostic aid are numerous. Soft tissue phase images should be considered for acute lameness and cases of trauma. Abnormal radiopharmaceutical uptake in soft tissues during this phase is often caused by hyperemia. Delayed uptake (that which persists in the bone phase) in the soft tissues is present only if there is necrosis or calcification or if the area of concern is in close proximity to adjacent bony structures.[54] Sometimes there is no uptake if the tissue is necrotic. Rarely does the presence of soft tissue uptake during the soft tissue phase not persist to some degree in the bone phase. It is our opinion that most if not all of the soft tissue phase is early bone uptake and that soft tissue phase contributes little to the outcome of a case, except in rare cases of trauma or infection. Bone phase imaging is often employed for acute or chronic lameness, multilimb lamenesses, avoidance behaviors in athletics, poor performance, suspected axial skeletal pathologic change, lamenesses that are localized to a specific region not seen with other diagnostic imaging techniques, and/or areas that are difficult to image with other techniques.[53,55,56] Radiopharmaceutical uptake in an area of pathologic change is typically characterized by focal to diffuse uptake and noted as mild to severe in the affected anatomy. Additionally, lack of radiopharmaceutical uptake (photopenia) may also be indicative of pathologic change.[57]

Increased radiopharmaceutical uptake reflects an area of bone turnover and may not reflect pathologic change or clinical significance.[58] For instance, the physes of young animals have markedly increased uptake, in particular the distal radial physis, and may continue to have uptake well beyond radiographic closure.[59,60] Additionally, significant radiopharmaceutical uptake may be associated with normal bone adaptation that occurs with athletic work, again without clinical relevance.[61,62] This concept is exemplified in the distal metacarpal/tarsal subchondral bone when a horse returns to or just starts to work.[63]

As with all imaging and diagnostic tests, using a systematic approach during interpretation is recommended. Symmetry between limbs, expected pattern, and amount of uptake are assessed and correlated with anatomy and type of work the horse does and related to the clinical signs. From this information a list of differential diagnoses is made. Displaying the images in the same order will help to avoid missing views and ensure all views are present for the desired study and are of diagnostic quality. Abnormal radiopharmaceutical uptake in bone scans is typically described as focal or diffuse and qualified as mild, moderate, or intense. In general, there is good correlation between severity of clinical signs and radiopharmaceutical uptake. For instance, fractures are generally focal, intense areas of radiopharmaceutical uptake and often cause a pronounced lameness.

Quality control checks and gamma camera function tests are often used to ensure quality diagnostic images. The operating procedure for these tests may be different for the variety of systems available and should be obtained from the system's representative. In general, to ensure the proper sensitivity of the gamma camera, the peak and uniformity of the camera should be checked monthly and weekly, respectively. This can be done with technetium or gallium without the collimator on the camera. The dose should be centered. The peak should be within 4 numbers of 140 KeV, as the gamma emission of technetium is 140 KeV.

A variety of artifacts can occur with nuclear scintigraphy and have been reviewed.[64] Some common artifacts are reviewed here. The most commonly encountered is a "dead" photomultiplier tube, which manifests as a circular or hexagonal area or is void of signal. The urinary bladder often impedes full evaluation of the sacroiliac region as technetium 99 is primarily excreted by the renal system. Administering furosemide 1 hour before the scan often alleviates superimposition of the urinary bladder. Urine contamination is most often encountered in the feet and along the inside of the hind legs in mares. This is characterized by linear radiopharmaceutical uptake along the sole of the foot and multifocal linear radiopharmaceutical uptake along the medial hind legs/tarsus. Urine may be washed off in both instances. Feet contamination may be avoided by wrapping them in duct tape. Image nonuniformity may be encountered even with a normal functioning gamma camera. One common cause of image nonuniformity is edge packing. This is seen as increased counts at the edge of the field camera. Edge packing is caused by internal reflection of light at the edge of the crystal and absence of photomultiplier tubes beyond the crystal edge. Diffuse decreased or poor bone uptake is often encountered in older horses, cold climates, and large-body horses. Poor bone uptake may be offset by working horses for 30 to 45 minutes before imaging, working daily for 2 weeks before imaging (especially if they have not been working), and keeping them in a heated area.

Nuclear scintigraphy is a sensitive diagnostic tool for athletic injury. However, it can produce false-negative as well as false-positive results. As with all imaging, nuclear scintigraphy is used to confirm clinical suspicion of disease. The keys to getting the most information from nuclear scintigraphic scans are a thorough physical examination, lameness evaluation, and diagnostic anesthesia.

Advanced Diagnostics: Magnetic Resonance Imaging and Computed Tomography

Advanced imaging is becoming more readily available in veterinary medicine for the diagnosis of joint injury. Increased numbers of MRI and CT units designated for equine patients have become available in private and university practices. The use of advanced imaging allows the diagnosis of injuries that may not be identified using standard imaging modalities, because of the nature, subtlety, or location of the injury. When earlier diagnosis of these injuries can be achieved with advanced imaging, it may provide a greater chance of impacting the outcome and return to athletic function. Both MRI and CT provide advantages over standard imaging modalities because of their volumetric nature. Both are forms of cross-sectional imaging that allow the acquisition of slices from an anatomic region that can subsequently be viewed in multiple planes without superimposition of structures.[65-69] However, there are important fundamental differences between MRI and CT. Understanding these differences is important relative to case selection because MRI and CT will provide different information about a case, especially in regard to specific types of pathologic change in a joint and the periarticular structures. Therefore, an imaging modality should be selected with knowledge of the information that can be gained from it and used in combination with a list of most likely differential diagnoses, based on clinical assessment of the horse.

Although CT can be considered as either a series of individual, thinly sliced radiographs or a volume of radiographic data, MRI is proton-based, which provides a different level of soft tissue detail and fluid sensitivity. CT will excel at osseous detail, except in regard to the presence of fluid, while MRI will produce superior soft tissue imaging and allows detection of osseous fluid. The development of newer CT technology may allow for fluid detection. Extrapolating from the basic strengths of these two modalities, predominantly soft tissue versus bone, makes the potential information gained from each modality quite apparent. Although CT will be less sensitive in demonstrating certain types of soft tissue injury and less accurate in characterizing fluid-based soft tissue lesions, it provides information about the stage of the repair process based on the assessment of contrast enhancement and vascular ingrowth (S. Puchalski, personal communication). Furthermore, it is important to understand the differences between various MRI systems as well as how the use of contrast can affect CT and MR images. The addition of contrast to these modalities can further impact case selection and the information that can be obtained.

Terminology

Having a basic knowledge of terminology specific to each modality can be helpful when reading imaging reports and trying to understand the findings as well as their clinical significance. This basic knowledge would include the terms that are used to describe the appearance of tissues on MR and CT images as well as the names and general characteristics of the MRI sequences used to create the images.

Magnetic Resonance Imaging Terminology. "Signal intensity" is used to describe the shade of gray of a specific tissue on an MR image.[70] Tissues that are bright or white are described as hyperintense or as having high signal intensity. Hypointense, or low signal intensity, describes tissues that appear dark or black. Isointense is used as a comparative term for two tissues that have the same signal intensity. For example, cortical bone and tendons, when normal, have similar signal intensities on MR images using certain sequences and can therefore be considered isointense when compared with each other. Additionally, hyperintense and hypointense

can be used as relative terms to describe the signal intensity of a structure compared with a different structure. On certain images, muscle will have a brighter signal intensity than tendons and would be considered hyperintense in comparison to a tendon. Intermediate signal intensity can be used to describe tissue that is gray. The multiple different uses of terminology can be confusing. However, the tremendous number of shades of gray on MR images requires a basis for comparison of various structures.

Magnetic Resonance Imaging Sequences

An MRI sequence produces a series of images that were obtained using certain machine settings.[71-73] These settings create images with a specific characteristic appearance relative to the signal intensity of the tissues. There are three major categories of sequences: spin echo (fast or turbo), gradient echo, and inversion recovery. The category of sequence has a direct impact on the image appearance and quality. Within the three categories, numerous MR sequences are available, and when comparing the images made using different sequences, it is important to recognize that the same exact tissue can have a different shade of gray because of the manner in which the images were acquired. Therefore, the same area of fluid in the distal interphalangeal joint can appear from bright white to dark gray depending on the sequence selected to acquire the images.[74,75]

Knowing the characteristic appearance of the different MR sequences is imperative for proper image interpretation. The most frequently used MR sequences in the equine patient are T1-weighted, T2-weighted, proton density, and short tau inversion recovery (STIR), each of which has a characteristic appearance (Table 9-2). Although the appearance of the images obtained when using a given sequence can be characterized, it is important to recognize that there is a range of different signal intensities within this characteristic appearance. Furthermore, the image appearance can be easily changed by the person performing the examination, by simply altering the sequence settings on the computer.

Computed Tomography Terminology. Density (sometimes referred to as hyperintensity or hypointensity) is used to describe different shades of gray on CT images, and the term can often be applied relative to a reference structure. Areas of white are referred to as hyperdense, although dark areas are hypodense. Similar to MRI, isodense refers to tissues of similar density. Although the density can be evaluated subjectively based on a tissue's shade of gray on the images, the density is often measured using image software that produces a number providing specific information about the tissue density. In CT the density of the tissue is measured using Hounsfield units (HUs). Reference ranges of the HUs for different tissues (see Table 9-2), which are measured relative to water, have been established, and measuring the density of different tissues on CT images can provide clinically relevant information.

Factors that Determine Magnetic Resonance Image Quality

Image quality is largely determined by three factors: the signal-to-noise ratio (SNR), the contrast-to-noise ratio (CNR),

TABLE 9-2

MRI Sequences	Dense Bone	Trabecular Bone/Fat	Fluid	Tendon	Ligament
T1	Black	Light gray	Medium gray	Dark gray to black	Medium to dark gray
T2	Black	Light to medium gray	White to light gray	Black	Medium to dark gray
PD	Black	Light gray	Light gray	Black	Medium to dark gray
STIR	Black	Dark gray to black	White to light gray	Black	Medium to dark gray
CT HU Values (kV dependent)	+1000*	100 to 300 (trabecular bone) -60 to -100† (fat)	0 (water)*	75 to 115*,† (tendon) 250* (collagen)	76 to 109‡

CT, Computed tomography; *HU*, Hounsfield units.

*Whitehouse R.W. (2003). Computed tomography (CT) and CT arthrography. Imaging of the knee (pp. 23-40). Medical Radiology. Springer Berlin Heidelberg, Berlin, Germany.

†Weissman B.N.W. (2009). Imaging of arthritis and metabolic bone disease: expert consult online (p. 203). Elsevier Health Sciences. Accessed May 9, 2003. http://nuclmed.web.auth.gr/magazine/eng/jan13/6.pdf

‡Kaser-Hotz B., Sartoretti-Schefer S., Weiss R. (1994). Computed tomography and magnetic resonance imaging of the normal equine carpus. Vet Radiol Ultrasound 35(6), 458.

and artifacts. Of these three factors, the SNR has the largest impact on image quality. In this context, signal is defined as information generated from the tissues that is representative of the anatomy and is used to produce an image. Noise is false information produced from the tissues or the MR system that is also incorporated into the image. The SNR demonstrates the amount of true information in an image relative to the amount of noise. It is readily apparent when evaluating images acquired using different field strengths that the SNR increases with field strength.[76,77]

As the field strength increases, the MR system is able to acquire more information from the imaged tissues. The additional information is integrated into each pixel, producing a higher resolution image with better detail. This is especially apparent when comparing the appearance of small structures imaged with high- and low-field MRI systems. Images with a comparatively lower SNR will appear grainy, and smaller structures will be difficult to delineate clearly.[78,79]

Within each type of MR system, steps can be taken to increase the SNR, resulting in improved image resolution. Generally, these modifications will increase the image acquisition time. Increased acquisition time increases motion artifact in both standing and anesthetized cases, and it can be prohibitive in anesthetized cases because of increased risk of anesthetic complications from prolonged anesthesia. Although many factors can affect the SNR, the most significant factor is the field strength of the MRI system.

The CNR is largely determined by sequence selection. However, field strength does impact the CNR. The CNR is the difference in the signal intensity of two different regions in the image, scaled to image noise. Increasing the CNR ratio between different structures or tissue types creates a greater difference in their relative signal intensities. The CNR is important relative to differentiating different structures or tissue types, which is quite pertinent to lesion detection.

Artifacts are signal intensities or signal voids that were not produced from and do not represent the imaged anatomy. They are inherent in MR images as a result of MR physics and the process of image acquisition, as well as a consequence of translating 3D tissue into a 2D image. Artifacts occur even when the images are properly acquired and the MR system is functioning correctly. Furthermore, artifacts are produced from the tissue and the MR system, both contributing to false information in the image. When MR sequences are properly designed and the images are correctly obtained, artifacts are minimized as much as possible. In general, the longer scan times required for low-field systems will result in increased motion artifacts compared with high-field systems. The difference in the SNR, in combination with motion artifacts, has the biggest impact on image quality when comparing MR images from high- and low-field systems.

Factors that Determine Image Quality in Computed Tomography

The hardware, software, and x-ray tube settings selected affect the image quality produced by a CT system.[80] Most systems in use today have a CT table that moves the patient through the gantry with great precision, collecting information about the tissue density from a volume of tissue that is then recorded by an x-ray detector. That information is translated into numerical values specific for that tissue (HUs). Multirow or multislice CT scanners were an important advancement in CT. The transition from one row of detectors to multiple rows allows very thin and overlapping slices, increasing image resolution with a reduced number of rotations, and more effective use of the x-ray beam. This, in combination with helical scanning, allows higher quality images with extremely rapid scan times, a substantial advantage of CT versus MRI. Reconstructions are a pivotal part of CT imaging. The quality of reconstructions is influenced by the hardware (the quality of the data obtained) and by the software (the computer's ability to manipulate the data). Surface and volume rendering, which produces a 3D image, provides an additional component of information that is the direct benefit of all the hardware and software advancements resulting in the acquisition of more and better quality data from tissue.

Similar to MRI, noise and artifacts affect the quality of CT images. Image acquisition and the specific setting used to acquire the study affect both the noise and artifacts in images.[81-85] Common CT artifacts are the result of the modality's x-ray basis. Underexposure can increase noise, similar to conventional radiography. Very high-density tissues can cause beam hardening artifacts in the surrounding tissue that can be most pronounced in the adjacent soft tissues.

Clinical Applications of Advanced Imaging in Regard to Joint Disease

In regard to the specific application of these modalities in the diagnosis of joint disease, the strengths and weaknesses of the individual modalities must be considered. CT has superior bone detail and will far exceed MRI in the detection of fine bone proliferation or lysis of the periarticular margins and at the joint capsule or other soft tissue attachments. Fine bone detail can be very challenging to identify using MRI, as the appearance of bone and soft tissue can overlap. Joint-associated osseous proliferation can have adjacent soft tissue thickening, such as enthesophyte formation at a joint capsule attachment with associated joint capsule scarring. When these tissues are confluent and have the same signal intensity, differentiating between them can be difficult to impossible. This specific overlap of tissue types at osseous interfaces does not occur with CT. However, certain MR sequences will have less overlap than others. Knowing what sequences will highlight different types of pathologic change is important when selecting a musculoskeletal protocol for joint imaging as well as pivotal for accurate image interpretation.

MRI is the only modality that can definitely identify fluid in bone, which is frequently present with certain types of joint injury. There are multiple different types of fat-suppressed images that are designed to highlight the presence of fluid in bone and soft tissue. The STIR sequence and the fat-suppression technique, which can be used in conjunction with fast or turbo spin echo and gradient echo sequences, are most frequently incorporated into musculoskeletal protocols to aid in the detection of pathologic change that has associated abnormal fluid. In addition, the resolution or persistence of osseous fluid can be an important factor in determining the treatment and prognosis of joint disease, thus making its identification pertinent. However, a recheck MRI examination is required to make this delineation. In many cases determining the nature of osseous fluid, relative to the type of pathologic change, is not possible on an initial MR study. Recheck MRI examination is used to determine the efficacy of treatment and/or a rehabilitation program and to more clearly define if the bone or soft tissue structure can "heal" or resolve the injury. If there is not a clear indication on the initial examination, then the MRI results are used in conjunction to distinguish degenerative bone injury from something that can be repaired or can resolve.

CT will be inferior to MRI in characterizing soft tissue lesions such as abnormalities affecting the joint capsule or injury to the supporting soft tissue structures. However, the conspicuity of soft tissue lesions can be improved with the use of intravascular CT contrast, and a technique for this has been described.[86]

Intravascular contrast can also provide information about vascular ingrowth and tissue permeability that may not be obvious with MRI and requires special software that is not necessarily part of a standard MRI software package. Contrast use is also a consideration in MRI as it can enhance the visibility of subtle lesions, similar to CT. However, it is less cost effective than contrast use with CT.

Quite a bit of interest has been generated regarding the development of an equine-specific CT that would allow imaging of regions not currently able to be imaged, such as the back and pelvis. In addition, CT imaging of the cervical spine could be performed in the standing sedate horse. This would obviously be a great advantage in the diagnosis of joint-related injury in regions that are difficult or impossible to diagnose with standard imaging modalities.

MRI is superior at articular cartilage imaging as it can demonstrate surface abnormalities and defects or fissures as well as abnormalities within the articular cartilage despite an intact surface. There are limits to what can be identified within the articular cartilage using standard MRI sequences, and this can be improved with both contrast and cartilage-specific sequences. Articular cartilage imaging is severely limited with low-field MRI systems. With the currently available techniques, high-field MRI is required for the definitive diagnosis of articular injury. Even at 1.0 T and 1.5 T, clearly differentiating the cartilage articular–synovial fluid interface is challenging in joints where the articular cartilage is quite thin relative to the subchondral bone thickness and in joints with marked curvature of the articular surfaces. In these joints, such as the carpus, tarsus, and fetlock, partial volume averaging can obscure the articular cartilage margins.

Contrast CT arthrography can be used to identify articular cartilage defects that communicate with the joint and will demonstrate cartilage thinning. However, even with standard intraarticular CT contrast, intrasubstance articular cartilage abnormalities will not be identified. The development of new contrast agents may alter the detection of intrasubstance articular cartilage abnormalities with CT.[87]

In cases with articular cartilage defects or thinning, the contrast distribution in the joint will be abnormal. Following intraarticular administration, the contrast fills articular cartilage defects, causing focal pooling of hyperdense material that can be easily identified. Diffuse articular cartilage thinning can be more difficult to identify, depending on the severity. However, the contrast will line the articular surface of the cartilage and provide a clear measure of cartilage thickness. Contrast agents are being investigated that allow correlation between glycosaminoglycan content and articular cartilage contrast enhancement following intraarticular administration.[88] Certainly this would be of great clinical benefit given the current limitations of articular cartilage imaging.

Conclusions

CT and MRI offer multiplanar imaging without superimposition of structures, allowing the diagnosis of certain types of joint injury that would not be visible with standard imaging modalities. CT offers rapid imaging with superior bone detail. The fast scan times are extremely beneficial when combining imaging with another general anesthesia procedure, such as surgery. However, the benefits of rapid scanning are offset by the lack of soft tissue detail and tissue contrast that is achieved with MRI. A limited series of images can be done to allow the combination of an MR study with another general anesthesia procedure. However, even with a limited study the MR scan time will exceed the CT scan time. Using CT and MRI in conjunction can maximize the advantages and minimize the weaknesses of the two modalities. MRI allows the identification of osseous fluid, which is a significant benefit in conjunction with soft tissue detail and superior articular cartilage imaging. Having a specific idea about what tissues are affected and what types of pathologic change are of greatest concern can aid in the selection process when considering these two modalities. A nonbiased person with knowledge of the available advanced imaging systems and all the pertinent case information should be consulted if there are questions regarding the most appropriate advanced modality to use.

REFERENCES

1. Guide for veterinary service and judging of equestrian events. 4 ed Lexington, KY: American Association of Equine Practitioners; 1991.
2. Keegan KG, Dent EV, Wilson DA, et al. Repeatability of subjective evaluation of lameness in horses. *Equine Vet J.* 2010;42(2):92–97.
3. Jônsson L, Engenvall A, Roepstorf L, et al. Associations of health status and conformation with longevity and lifetime competition performance in young Swedish Warmblood riding horses: 8,238 cases (1983-2005). *J Am Vet Med Assoc.* 2014;244(12):1449–1461.
4. Anderson TM, McIlwraith CW. The role of conformation and musculoskeletal problems in the Racing Thoroughbred. *Equine Vet J.* 2004;36(7):571–575.
5. Anderson TM, McIlwraith CW. Longitudinal development of equine conformation from weanling to age 3 years in the Thoroughbred. *Equine Vet J.* 2004;36(7):563–570.
6. Robert C, Valette J-P, Denoix J-M. Longitudinal development of equine forelimb conformation from birth to weaning in three different horse breeds. *Vet J.* 2013;198(Suppl 1):e75–e80.
7. Turner TA. Predictive value of diagnostic tests for navicular pain. *Proc AAEP.* 1996;42:201–204.
8. Arndt JL, Pfau T, Day P, et al. Forces applied with a hoof tester to cadaver feet vary widely between users. *Vet Rec.* 2013;172(7):182.
9. Keegan KG. Objective assessment of lameness. In: Baxter GM, ed. *Adams and Stachak's lameness in horses.* Wiley-Blackwell; 2011:154–164.
10. Roland ES, Hull ML, Stover SM. Design and demonstration of a dynamometric horseshoe for measuring ground reaction loads of horses during racing conditions. *J Biomech.* 2004;38(10):2102–2112.
11. Perino VV, Kawcak CE, Frisbie DD, et al. The accuracy and precision of an equine in-shoe pressure measurement system as a tool for gait analysis. *J Equine Vet Sci.* 2007;27(4): 161–166.
12. Weishaupt MA, Hogg HP, Wiestner T, et al. Instrumented treadmill for measuring vertical ground reaction forces in horses. *Am J Vet Res.* 2002;63(4):520–527.
13. Gómez Alvarez CB, Rhodin M, Byström A, et al. Back kinematics of healthy trotting horses during treadmill versus over ground locomotion. *Equine Vet J.* 2009;41(3):297–300.
14. Buchner HH, Savelberg HH, Schamhardt HC, et al. Kinematics of treadmill versus overground locomotion in horses. *Vet Q.* 1994;16(Suppl 2):S87–90.
15. Keegan KG, MacAllister CG, Wilson DA, et al. Comparison of an inertial sensor system with a stationary force plate for evaluation of horses with bilateral forelimb lameness. *Am J Vet Res.* 2012;73(3):368–374.
16. Boye JK, Thomsen MH, Pfau T, et al. Accuracy and precision of gait events derived from motion capture in horses during walk and trot. *J Biomech.* 2014;47(5):1220–1224.
17. Moorman VJ, Reiser RF, Peterson ML, et al. Effect of forelimb lameness on hoof kinematics of horses at a walk. *Am J Vet Res.* 2013;74(9):1192–1197.
18. Moorman VJ, Reiser RF, Peterson ML, et al. Effect of forelimb lameness on hoof kinematics of horses at a trot. *Am J Vet Res.* 2013;74(9):1183–1191.
19. Moorman VJ, Reiser RF, McIlwraith CW, et al. Validation of an equine inertial measurement unit system in clinically normal horses during walking and trotting. *Am J Vet Res.* 2012;73(8):1160–1170.
20. Olsen E, Andersen PH, Pfau T. Accuracy and precision of equine gait event detection during walking with limb and trunk mounted inertial sensors. *Sensors (Basel).* 2012;12(6):8145–8156.
21. Pfau T, Starke SD, Tröster S, et al. Estimation of vertical tuber coxae movement in the horse from a single inertial measurement unit. *Vet J.* 2013;198(2):498–503.
22. Keegan KG, Kramer J, Yonezawa Y, et al. Assessment of repeatability of a wireless, inertial sensor-based lameness evaluation system for horses. *Am J Vet Res.* 2011;72(9):1156–1163.
23. Olsen E, Pfau T, Ritz C. Functional limits of agreement applied as a novel method comparison tool for accuracy and precision of inertial measurement unit derived displacement of the distal limb in horses. *J Biomech.* 2013;46(13):2320–2325.
24. Pfau T, Stubbs NC, Kaiser LJ, et al. Effect of trotting speed and circle radius on movement symmetry in horses during lunging on a soft surface. *Am J Vet Res.* 2012;73(12):1890–1899.
25. Brocklehurst C, Weller R, Pfau T. Effect of turn direction on body lean angle in the horse in trot and canter. *Vet J.* 2014;199(2):258–262.
26. Rhodin M, Pfau T, Roepstorff L, et al. Effect of lunging on head and pelvic movement asymmetry in horses with induced lameness. *Vet J.* 2013;198(Suppl 1):e39–e45.
27. Starke SD, Willems E, May SA, et al. Vertical head and trunk movement adaptations of sound horses trotting in a circle on a hard surface. *Vet J.* 2012;193(1):73–80.
28. Robartes H, Fairhurst H, Pfau T. Head and pelvic movement symmetry in horses during circular motion and in rising trot. *Vet J.* 2013;198(Suppl 1):e52–e58.
29. Starke SD, Willems E, Head M, et al. Proximal hindlimb flexion in the horse: effect on movement symmetry and implications for defining soundness. *Equine Vet J.* 2012;44(6):657–663.
30. Marshall JF, Lund DG, Voute LC. Use of a wireless, inertial sensor-based system to objectively evaluate flexion tests in the horse. *Equine Vet J Suppl.* 2012;43:8–11.

31. Starke SD, Witte TH, May SA, et al. Accuracy and precision of hind limb foot contact timings of horses determined using a pelvis-mounted inertial measurement unit. *J Biomech.* 2012;45(8):1522–1528.

32. Pfau T, Spicer-Jenkins C, Smith RK, et al. Identifying optimal parameters for quantification of changes in pelvic movement symmetry as a response to diagnostic analgesia in the hindlimbs of horses. *Equine Vet J.* 2014;46(6):759–763.

33. Starke SD, Raistrick KJ, May SA, et al. The effect of trotting speed on the evaluation of subtle lameness in horses. *Vet J.* 2013;197(2):245–252.

34. Keegan KG, Wilson DA, Kramer J, et al. Comparison of a body-mounted inertial sensor system-based method with subjective evaluation for detection of lameness in horses. *Am J Vet Res.* 2013;74(1):17–24.

35. McCracken MJ, Kramer J, Keegan KG, et al. Comparison of an inertial sensor system of lameness quantification with subjective lameness evaluation. *Equine Vet J.* 2012;44(6):652–656.

36. Keegan KG, Wilson DA, Kreeger JM, et al. Local distribution of mepivacaine after distal interphalangeal joint injection in horses. *Am J Vet Res.* 1996;57(4):422–426.

37. Pleasant RS, Mall HD, Legg WB, et al. Intraarticular anesthesia of the distal interphalangeal joint alleviates lameness associated with the navicular bursa in horses. *Vet Surg.* 1997;26(2):137–140.

38. Contino EK, Werpy NM, Morton A, et al. Metacarpophalangeal joint lesions identified on magnetic resonance imaging with lameness that resolves using palmar digital nerve and intra-articular analgesia. *Proc AAEP.* 2012;58:534.

39. Seabaugh KA, Selberg KT, Valdes-Martinez A, et al. Assessment of the tissue diffusion of anesthetic agent following administration of a low palmar nerve block in horses. *J Am Vet Med Assoc.* 2011;239(10):1334–1340.

40. Widmer W. Acquisition hardware for digital imaging. *Vet Radiol Ultrasound.* 2008;49(1 Suppl 1):S2–S8.

41. Heo M-S, Han D-H, An B-M, et al. Effect of ambient light and bit depth of digital radiograph on observer performance in determination of endodontic file positioning. *Oral Surg Oral Med Oral Pathol Oral Radiol Endodontol.* 2008;105(2):239–244.

42. Lo WY, Puchalski SM. Digital image processing. *Vet Radiol Ultrasound.* 2008;49(1 Suppl 1):S42–47.

43. Barnes GT, Lauro K. Image processing in digital radiography: basic concepts and applications. *J Digit Imag.* 1989;2(3):132–146.

44. Abu-Zidan FM, Hefny AF, Corr P. Clinical ultrasound physics. *J Emerg Trauma Shock.* 2011;4(4):501–503.

45. Powers J, Kremkau F. Medical ultrasound systems. *Interface Focus.* 2011;1:477–489.

46. Klauser AS, Peetrons P. Developments in musculoskeletal ultrasound and clinical applications. *Skeletal Radiol.* 2009;39(11):1061–1071.

47. Palmeri ML, Nightingale KR. Acoustic radiation force-based elasticity imaging methods. *Interface Focus.* 2011;1:553–564.

48. Treece G, Lindop J, Chen L, et al. Real-time quasi-static ultrasound elastography. *Interface Focus.* 2011;1:540–552.

49. Duenwald S, Kobayashi H, Frisch K, et al. Ultrasound echo is related to stress and strain in tendon. *J Biomech.* 2011;44(3):424–429.

50. Lustgarten M, Redding WR, Labens R, et al. Elastographic characteristics of the metacarpal tendons in horses without clinical evidence of tendon injury. *Vet Radiol Ultrasound.* 2013;55(1):92–101.

51. Brenner S, Whitcomb MB. Ultrasonographic diagnosis of coxofemoral subluxation in horses. *Vet Radiol Ultrasound.* 2009;50(4):423–428.

52. Arndt J, Pauwels E, Camps J, et al. Clinical differences between bone-seeking agents. *Eur J Nucl Med.* 1985;11(8):330.

53. Lamb C, Koblik P. Scintigraphic evaluation of skeletal disease and its application to the horse. *Vet Radiol.* 1988;29(1):16–27.

54. Van der Wall H, Fogelman I. Scintigraphy of benign bone disease. *Semin Musculoskelet Radiol.* 2007;11(4):281–300.

55. Archer DC, Boswell JC, Voute LC, et al. Skeletal scintigraphy in the horse: current indications and validity as a diagnostic test. *Vet J.* 2007;173(1):31–44.

56. Hoskinson J. Equine nuclear scintigraphy: indications, uses, and techniques. *Vet Clin North Am Equine Pract.* 2001;17(1):63–74.

57. Levine DG, Ross BM, Ross MW, et al. Decreased radiopharmaceutical uptake (photopenia) in delayed phase scintigraphic images in three horses. *Vet Radiol Ultrasound.* 2007;48(5):467–470.

58. Dyson SJ. Subjective and quantitative scintigraphic assessment of the equine foot and its relationship with foot pain. *Equine Vet J.* 2002;34(2):164–170.

59. Uhlhorn H, Eksell P, Carlsten J. Scintigraphic characterization of distal radial physeal closure in young Standardbred racehorses. *Vet Radiol Ultrasound.* 2000;41(2):181–186.

60. Twardock AR. Equine bone scintigraphic uptake patterns related to age, breed, and occupation. *Vet Clin North Am Equine Pract.* 2001;17(1):75–94.

61. Ehrlich PJ, Seeherman HJ, O'Callaghan MW, et al. Results of bone scintigraphy in horses used for show jumping, hunting, or eventing: 141 cases (1988-1994). *J Am Vet Med Assoc.* 1998;213(10):1460–1467.

62. Bailey RE, Dyson SJ, Parkin TD. Focal increased radiopharmaceutical uptake in the dorsoproximal diaphyseal region of the equine proximal phalanx. *Vet Radiol Ultrasound.* 2007;48(5):460–466.

63. Kawcak C, McIlwraith C, Norrdin R, et al. Clinical effects of exercise on subchondral bone of carpal and metacarpophalangeal joints in horses. *Am J Vet Res.* 2000;61(10):1252–1258.

64. Gentili A, Miron SD, Adler LP. Review of some common artifacts in nuclear medicine. *Clin Nucl Med.* 1994;19(2):138–143.

65. Abragam A. *The principles of nuclear magnetism.* London, UK: Oxford University Press; 1961.

66. Farrar TC, Becker ED. *Pulse and Fourier transform nuclear magnetic resonance.* New York, NY: Academic Press; 1971.

67. Bottomley PA, Foster TH, Argersinger RE, et al. A review of normal tissue hydrogen NMR relaxation times and relaxation mechanisms from 1-100 MHz: dependence on tissue type, NMR frequency, temperature, excision and age. *Med Physics.* 1984;11(4):425–448.

68. Bottomley PA, Hardy CJ, Argersinger RE, et al. A review of H nuclear magnetic resonance relaxation in pathology: are T1 and T2 diagnostic? *Med Physics.* 1987;14(1):1–37.

69. Baxter GM. *Manual of equine lameness.* Chichester, West Sussex, UK: Wiley-Blackwell; 2011:216–219.

70. Stark DD, Bradley WG. *Magnetic resonance imaging.* St. Louis, MO: Mosby-Year Book; 1992:44–45.

71. Beutel J, Kundel HL, Van Metter RL. *Handbook of medical imaging: physics and psychophysics;* volume 1. Bellingham, WA: SPIE; 2000:398–414.

72. Elmaoglu M, Celik A. *MRI handbook: MR physics, patient positioning, and protocols.* New York, NY: Springer; 2012:69–89.

73. Brown MA, Semelka RC. *"16.1-16.3.4 Clinical Applications." MRI basic principles and applications.* New York, NY: Wiley-Liss; 1999:224–232.

74. Mitchell DG, Cohen M. *MRI principles.* Philadelphia, PA: Saunders; 2004:375–378.

75. Stark DD, Bradley WG. *Magnetic resonance imaging.* St. Louis, MO: Mosby-Year Book; 1992:43–44.

76. Rutt BK, Lee DH. The impact of field strength on image quality in MRI. *J Mag Res Imag.* 1996;6(1):57–62.

77. Mitchell DG, Cohen M. *MRI principles.* Philadelphia, PA: Saunders; 2004:133–137.

78. Beutel J, Kundel HL, Van Metter RL. Handbook of medical imaging. *physics and psychophysics.* Bellingham, WA: SPIE; 2000;1:415–419.

79. Mitchell DG, Cohen M. *MRI principles.* Philadelphia, PA: Saunders; 2004:117–120.

80. Marshall CH, Goodenough DJ, Bergeron RT. *The physical basis of computed tomography.* St. Louis, MO: W.H. Green; 1982:93.

81. Buzug TM. *Computed tomography: from photon statistics to modern cone-beam CT.* Berlin, Germany: Springer Science & Business Media; 2008:445–462.

82. Edelstein WA, Bottomley PA, Hart HR, et al. Signal, noise, and contrast in nuclear magnetic resonance (NMR) imaging. *J Comput Assist Tomogr.* 1983;7(3):391–401.

83. Hendrick RE, Nelson TR, Hendee WR. Optimizing tissue contrast in magnetic resonance imaging. *Magn Reson Imaging.* 1984;2(3):193–204.

84. Robb RA, Morin RL. Principles and instrumentation for dynamic x-ray computed tomography. In: Marcus JL, et al., ed. *Cardiac imaging: a companion to Braunwald's heart disease.* Philadelphia, PA: WB Saunders; 1991.

85. Mayo JR. High-resolution computed tomography: technical aspects. *Radiol Clin North Am.* 1991;29(5):1043–1048.

86. Puchalski SM, Galuppo LD, Hornof WJ, et al. Intraarterial contrast-enhanced computed tomography of the equine distal extremity. *Vet Radiol Ultrasound.* 2007;48(1):21–29.

87. Nelson B, Kawcak CE, Goodrich LR, et al. Use of CT and CT arthrography as a multimodal diagnostic approach to stifle disease in quarter horses (abstract). *Vet Surg.* 2013;42:E102–E103.

88. Stewart RC, Nelson BB, Kawcak CE, et al. Development of a clinical contrast-enhanced computed tomography scoring system for distinguishing osteoarthritis disease state. *Sci. Trans. Med.* 2015. Submitted.

The radiographs listed below appear on the following pages. Each radiograph is shown twice; both with labels and without. A master list of labels is presented before each region.

REGION 1: FOOT AND PASTERN

1a. Lateromedial
1b. Palmaroproximal-palmarodistal oblique
1c. Horizontal dorsopalmar
1d. Skyline
1e. Dorso 45° lateral-palmaromedial oblique

REGION 2: FETLOCK

2a. Lateromedial
2b. Flexed lateromedial
2c. Dorso 20° proximo-palmarodistal
2d. Dorso 45° lateral-palmaromedial oblique
2e. Latero 30° dorsal 70° proximal-mediopalmarodistal oblique
2f. Latero 45° proximal-distomedial oblique
2g. Dorsoproximal-dorsodistal oblique (skyline)

REGION 3: CARPUS

3a. Lateromedial
3b. Flexed lateromedial
3c. Dorsoproximal
3d. Dorsolateral-palmaromedial oblique
3e. Dorsomedial-palmarolateral oblique
3f. Skyline view of the distal radius
3g. Proximal row skyline
3h. Distal row skyline

REGION 4: ELBOW

4a. Lateromedial
4b. Craniocaudal

REGION 5: SHOULDER

5a. Lateromedial
5b. Caudo 45° lateral-craniomedial oblique

REGION 6: TARSUS

6a. Lateromedial
6b. Dorsoplantar
6c. Dorsolateral-plantaromedial oblique
6d. Dorsomedial-plantarolateral oblique
6e. Calcaneal skyline

REGION 7: STIFLE

7a. Lateromedial
7b. Caudocranial
7c. Caudo 45° lateral-craniomedial oblique
7d. Flexed latero 10° cranio 10° distal-mediocaudo proximal oblique
7e. Cranioproximal-craniodistal oblique (skyline of the patella)

REGION 8: HIP

8a. Ventro 15°-30° medial-dorsolateral
8b. Dorso 30° lateral-lateroventral oblique

PROXIMAL PHALANX-a

1. Palmar aspect of the medial (a) and lateral (b) condyles on the distal aspect of the proximal phalanx
2. Distal dorsal articular surface of the proximal phalanx
3. Distal articular surface of the proximal phalanx
4. Eminences for attachment of the medial (a) and lateral (b) collateral ligaments of the proximal interphalangeal joint on the distal aspect of the proximal phalanx
5. Articular cartilage in the proximal interphalangeal joint space, approximately half the thickness of the articular cartilage in the distal interphalangeal joint

MIDDLE PHALANX-b

6. Proximal articular surface of the middle phalanx
7. Extensor process of the middle phalanx
8. Dorsal aspect of the distal articular surface of the middle phalanx
9. Medial (a) and lateral (b) eminences on the dorsal aspect of the middle phalanx for collateral ligament attachments of the distal interphalangeal joint
10. Medial (a) and lateral (b) eminences for the ligamentous and tendinous attachments on the proximal palmar aspect of the middle phalanx
11. Palmar border of the middle phalanx
12. Proximal Palmar border of the middle phalanx
13. Articulation between the navicular bone and middle phalanx
14. Distal medial condyle of the middle phalanx
15. Distal articular margin of the middle phalanx
16. Articular cartilage of the DIPJ, approximately twice the thickness of the articular cartilage in the proximal interphalangeal joint

DISTAL PHALANX-c

17. Dorsal surface of the distal phalanx
18. Extensor process of the distal phalanx
19. Dorsal articular border of the distal phalanx
20. Palmar articular margin of the distal phalanx
21. Flexor surface of the distal phalanx; attachment site of the deep digital flexor tendon and impar ligaments
22. Semilunar line on the solar surface of the distal phalanx (axial surface of the palmar process)
23. Medial (a) and lateral (b) aspects of the solar border of the distal phalanx
24. Palmar articular border of the distal phalanx
25. Medial (a) and lateral (b) fossae of the distal phalanx, attachment sites of insertions of collateral ligaments of the distal interphalangeal joint
26. Vascular channels of the distal phalanx
27. Solar canal of the distal phalanx
28. Distal solar margin of the distal phalanx
29. Medial (a) and lateral (b) palmar processes of the distal phalanx

NAVICULAR BONE-d

30. Dorsal articular surface of the navicular bone
31. Sagittal ridge on the flexor surface of the navicular bone
32. Proximal border of the navicular bone
33. Flexor surface of the navicular bone
34. Trabecular bone of the navicular bone
35. Articular surface of the navicular bone
36. Medial extremity of the navicular bone, slightly more rounded in appearance than the lateral extremity
37. Lateral extremity of the navicular bone, less rounded than the medial extremity
38. Distal palmar border of the navicular bone
39. Synovial invaginations

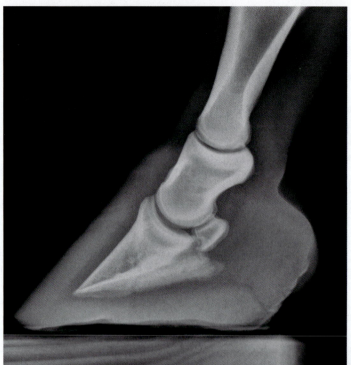

1a. Lateromedial

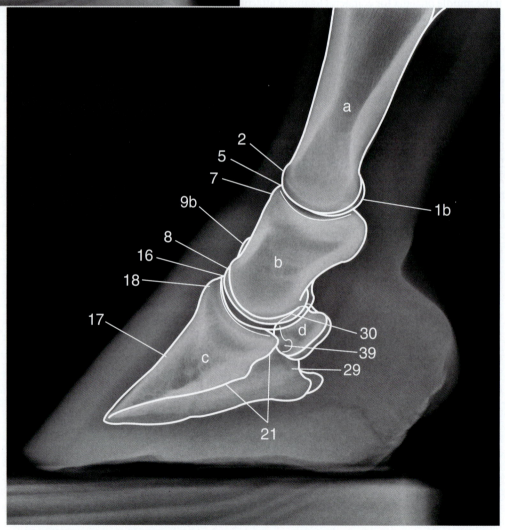

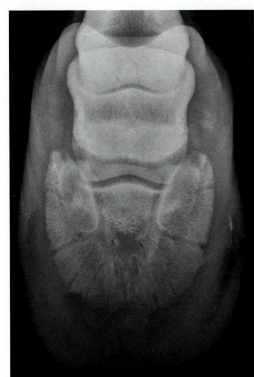

1b. Palmaroproximal-palmarodistal oblique

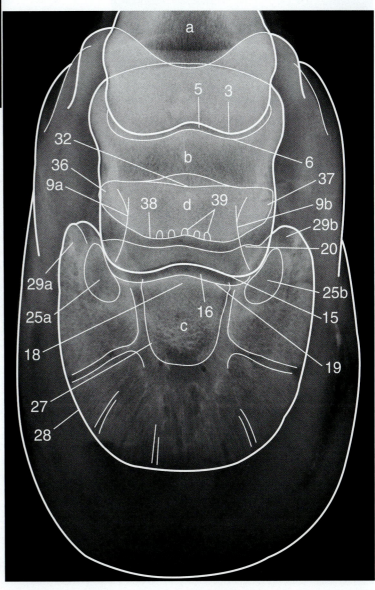

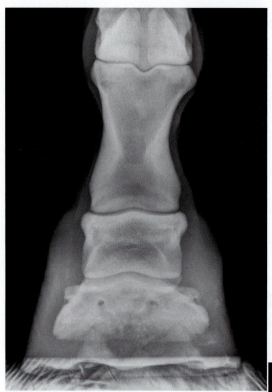

1c. Horizontal dorsopalmar

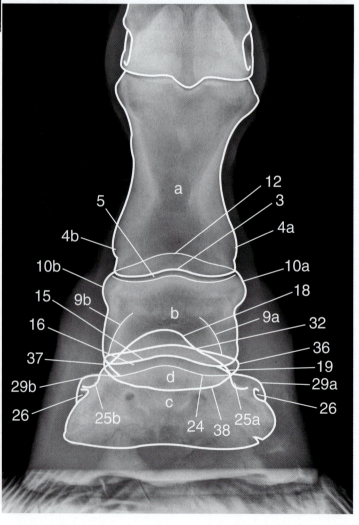

1d. Skyline palmaro 55 proximal-palmarodistal

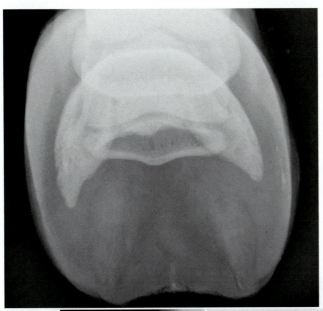

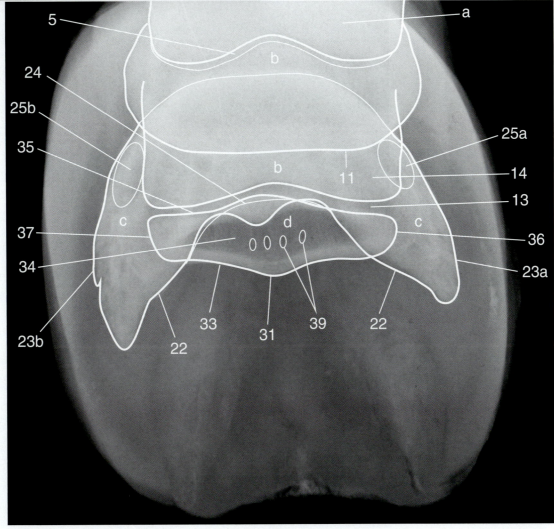

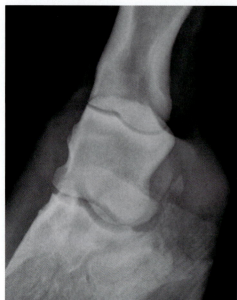

1e. Dorso 45° lateral-palmaromedial oblique

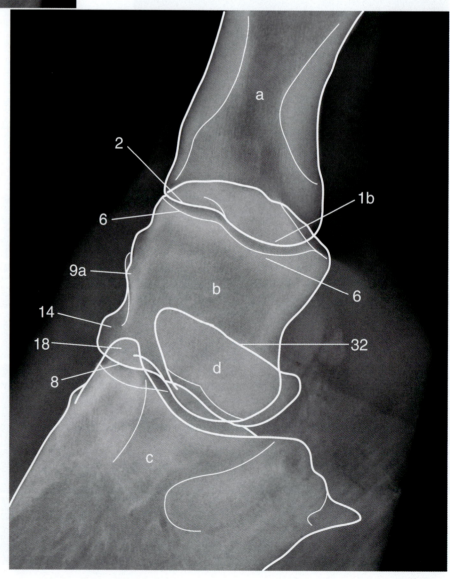

FETLOCK

Third metacarpal bone (a)

Proximal phalanx (b)

Proximal sesamoid bones (c)

1. Sagittal ridge of the third metacarpal bone (dorsal [a] and palmar [b] margins)
2. Medial condyle of the third metacarpal bone (dorsal a, palmar b)
3. Lateral condyle of the third metacarpal bone (dorsal a, palmar b)
4. Dorsal proximal joint attachment of the third metacarpal bone
5. Palmar proximal joint capsule attachment of the third metacarpal bone
6. Parasagittal groove of the third metacarpal bone (medial a, lateral b)
7. Attachment site of long collateral lig of the third metacarpal bone (medial a, lateral b)
8. Fossa and attachment of short collateral lig of the third metacarpal bone (medial a, lateral b)
9. Proximal articular margin of proximal phalanx (dorsal a, palmar b, medial c, lateral d)
10. Sagittal groove of proximal phalanx
11. Medial palmar eminence of proximal phalanx
12. Lateral palmar eminence of proximal phalanx
13. Mid palmar surface of proximal phalanx
14. Attachment site of superficial (long) collateral ligaments on proximal phalanx (medial a, lateral b)
15. Attachment site of the deep (short) collateral ligaments on proximal phalanx (medial a, lateral b)
16. Medial sesamoid bone
17. Lateral sesamoid bone
18. Dorsal articular surface of the sesamoid bones—medial (a) and lateral (b)
19. Distal margin (base) of the sesamoid bones (attachment of distal sesamoidean ligaments) (medial a, lateral b)
20. Proximal margin (apex) of the sesamoid bones—attachment of suspensory ligament branches (medial a, lateral b)
21. Axial surface of the sesamoid bones (attachment of intersesamoidean ligament) branches
22. Palmar proximal abaxial margin of the sesamoid bones (medial a, lateral b)
23. Dorsal proximal abaxial margin sesamoid (attachment site of suspensory ligament branches—medial [a] lateral [b])

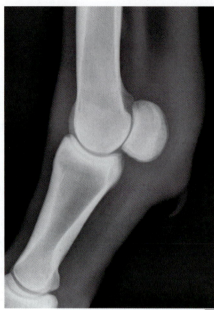

2a. Lateromedial

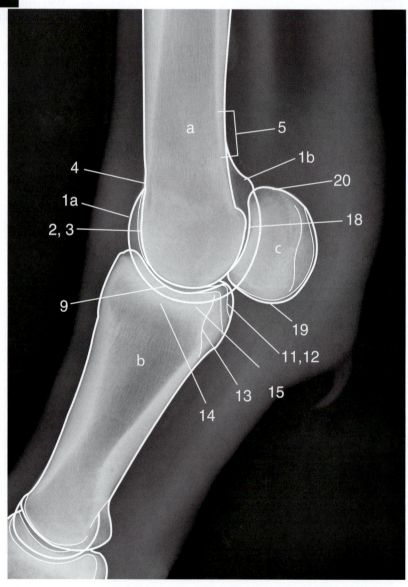

2b. Flexed lateromedial

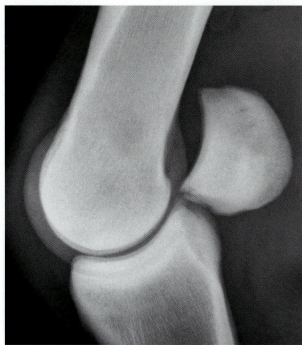

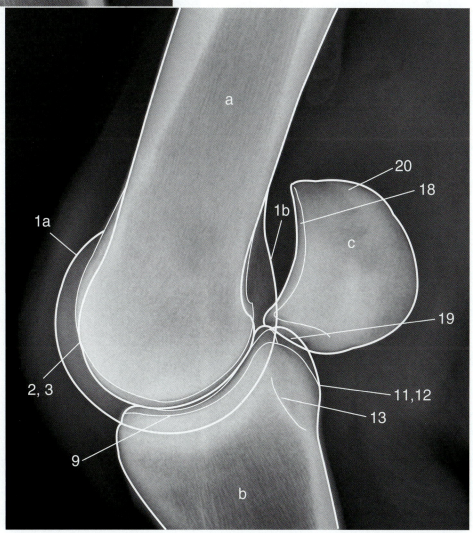

2c. Dorso 20° proximo-palmarodistal

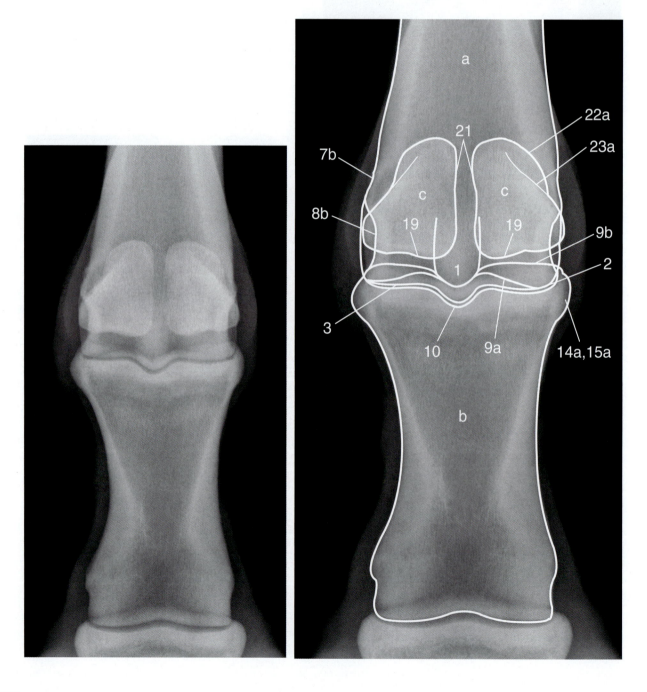

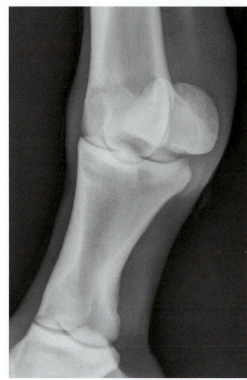

2d. Dorso 45° lateral-palmaromedial oblique

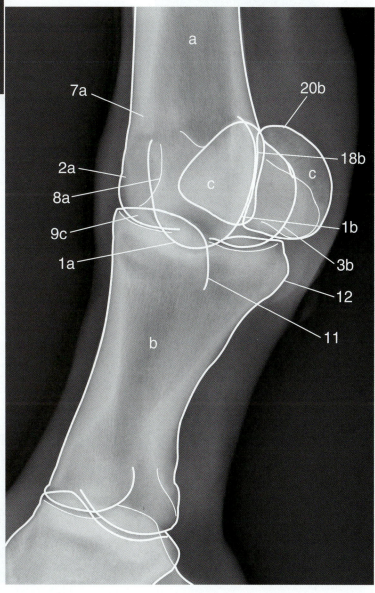

2e. Latero 30° dorsal 70° proximal-mediopalmarodistal oblique

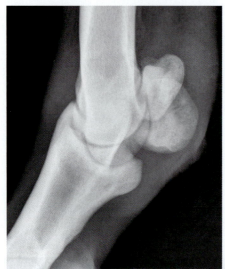

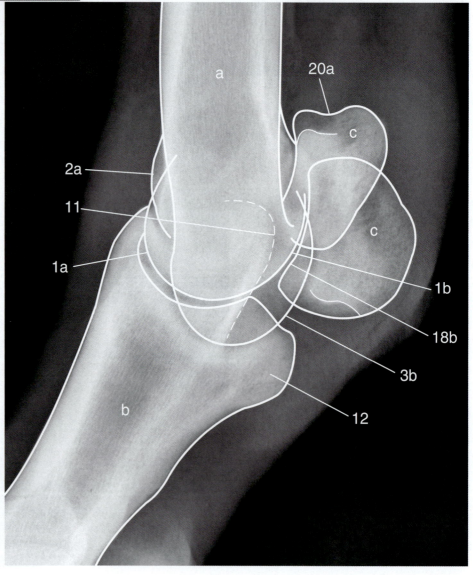

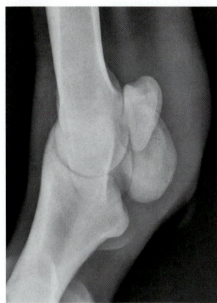

2f. Latero 45° proximal-distomedial oblique

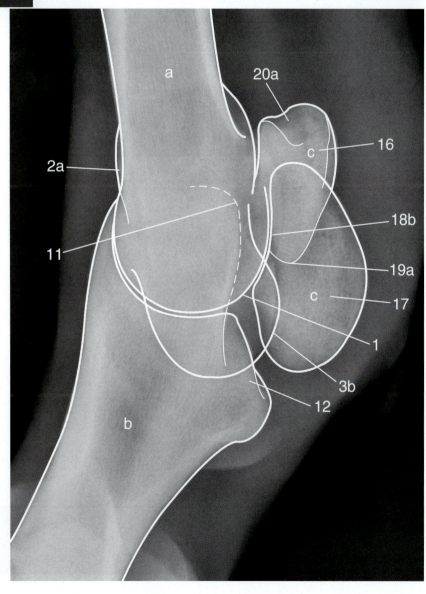

2g. Dorsoproximal-dorsodistal oblique (skyline)

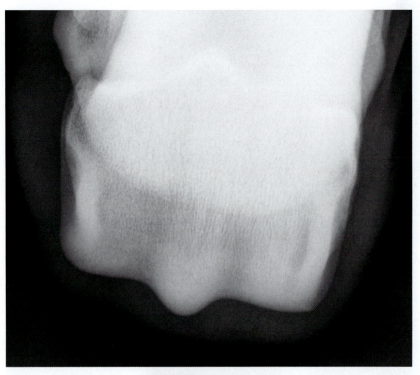

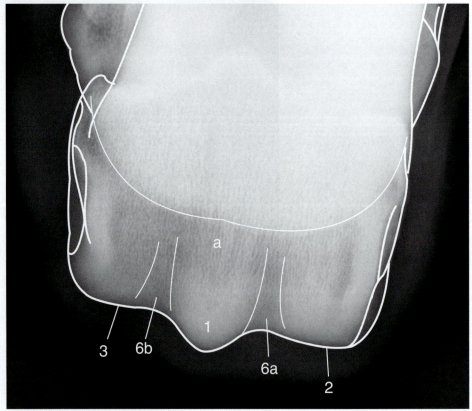

RADIUS

1. Radius
   a. Dorsal articular margin radial trochlea
2. Radiocarpal joint
   a. Dorsomedial aspect of radiocarpal joint
3. Depressions in the medial and lateral styloid processes for attachment of medial (a) and lateral (b) collateral ligaments. Appearance can change with obliquity
4. Lateral tuberosity of distal radius, for attachment of collateral ligaments

PROXIMAL CARPAL ROW

5. Closely superimposed palmar borders of intermediate, radial and ulnar carpal bones
6. Accessory carpal bone
7. Middle carpal joint
   a. Dorsomedial aspect of middle carpal joint
   b. Dorsolateral aspect of middle carpal joint
   c. Articulation of radial carpal and third carpal bones
8. Radial carpal bone
   a. Dorsal border of radial carpal bone,
   b. Palmar border of radial carpal bone
   c. Medial and lateral borders of radial carpal bone
   d. Palmaromedial borders of radial carpal bone
   e. Joint capsule attachment on radial carpal bone
9. Intermediate carpal bone
   a. Dorsal border of intermediate bone
   b. Palmar border of intermediate carpal bone
   c. Medial and lateral borders of intermediate carpal bone
   d. Dorsolateral border of the intermediate carpal bone
10. Ulnar carpal bone
    a. Dorsal border of ulnar carpal bone
    b. Medial and lateral borders of ulnar carpal bone

DISTAL CARPAL ROW

11. Location of 1st carpal bone when present
    a. Location of the first carpal bone superimposed over second and third carpal bones
12. Second carpal bone
    a. Medial and lateral borders of the second carpal bone
    b. Dorsomedial border of second carpal bone
    c. Palmaromedial border of second metacarpal bone
13. Third carpal bone
    a. Dorsomedial and lateral borders of the third carpal bones
    b. Palmarolateral border of 3rd carpal bone
    c. Radial facet
    d. Intermediate facet
14. Fourth carpal bone
    a. Medial and lateral borders of fourth carpal bone
    b. Dorsomedial border of fourth carpal bone
    c. Palmaromedial border of fourth metacarpal bone
15. Carpometacarpal joint
    a. Articulation between third carpal bone and third metacarpal bone

METACARPALS

16. Second metacarpal bone
    a. Medial border of the second metacarpal bone
17. Third metacarpal bone
    a. Medial and lateral borders of the third metacarpal bone
    b. Palmaromedial border of third metacarpal bone
18. Fourth metacarpal bone
    a. Palmarolateral border of fourth metacarpal bone

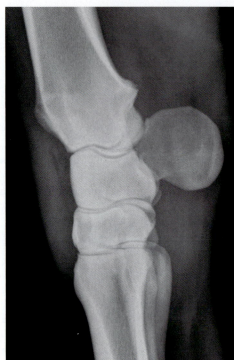

3a. Lateromedial

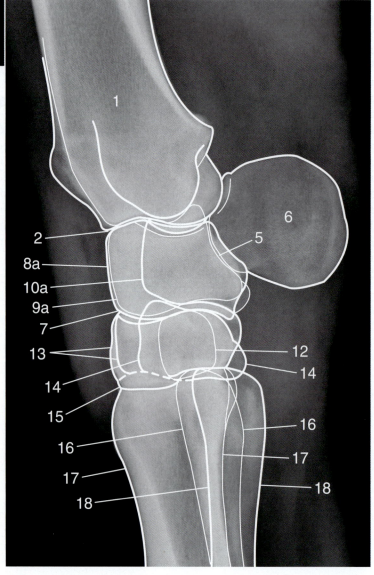

3b. Flexed lateromedial

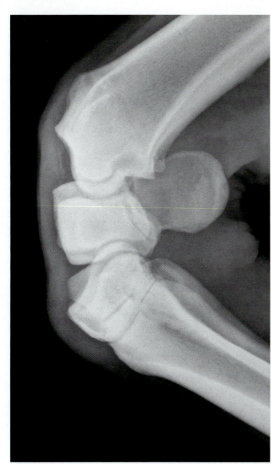

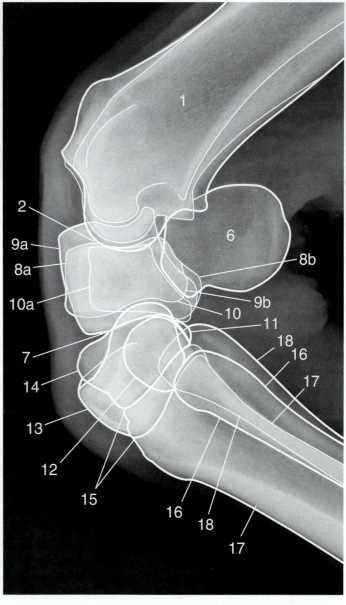

3c. Dorsopalmar

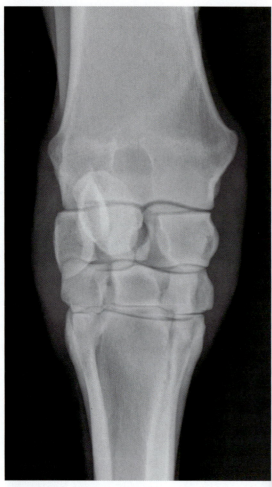

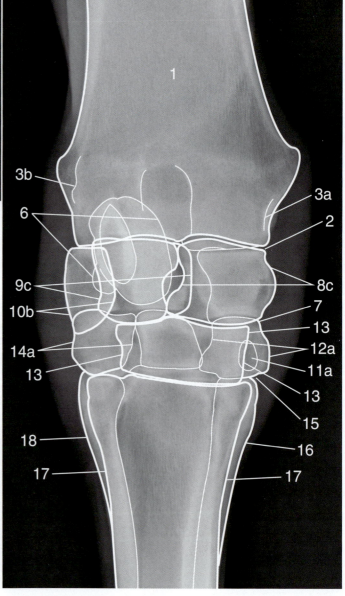

3d. Dorsolateral-palmaromedial oblique

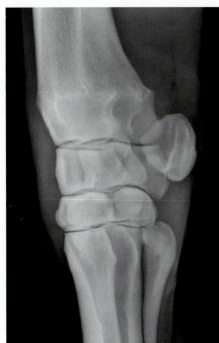

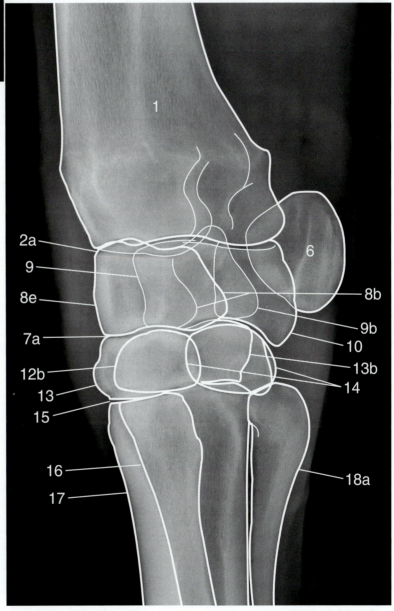

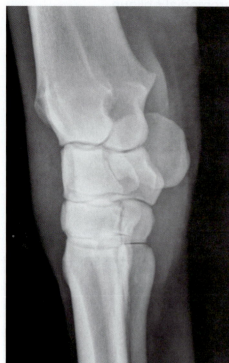

3e. Dorsomedial-palmarolateral oblique

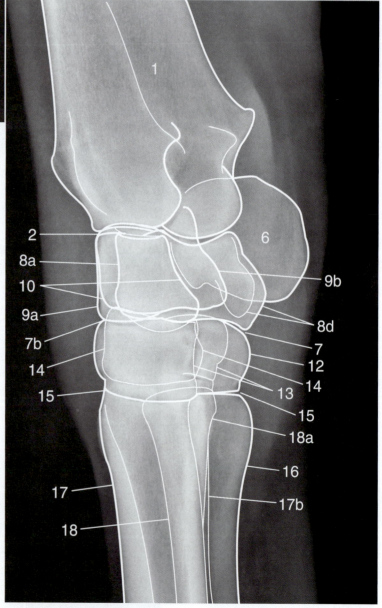

3f. Skyline view of the distal radius

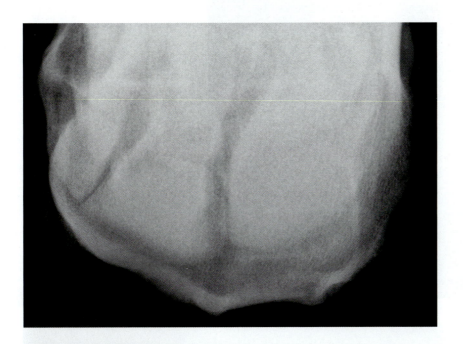

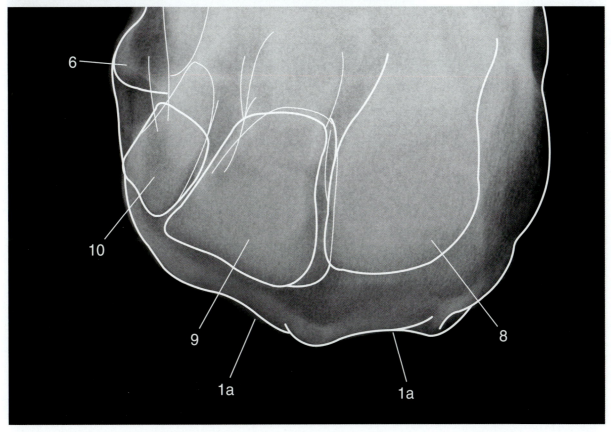

3g. Proximal row skyline

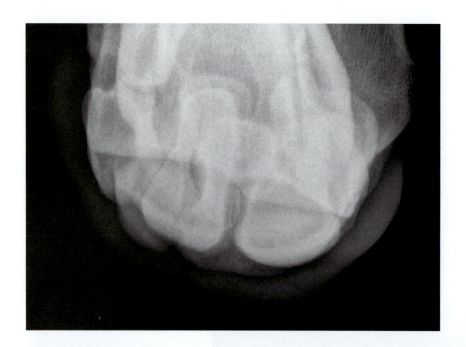

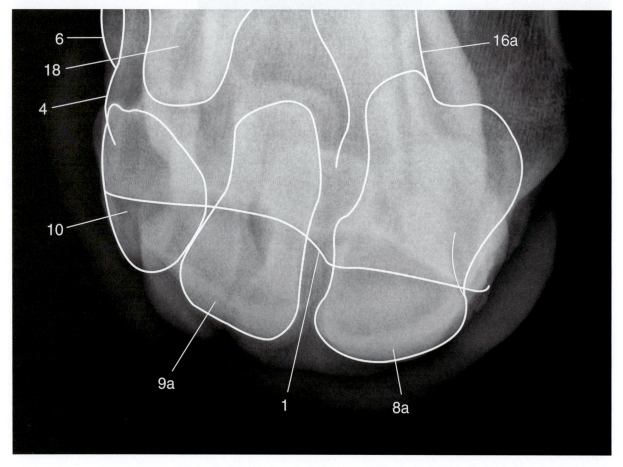

3h. Distal row skyline

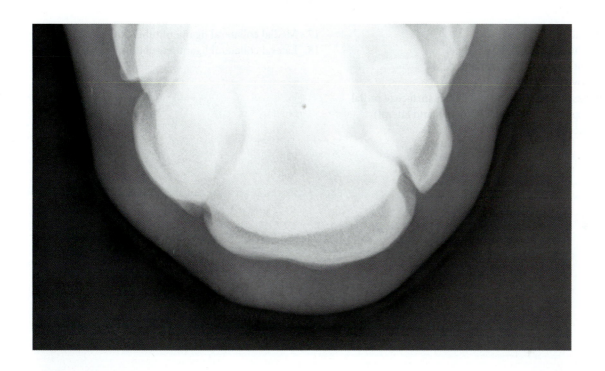

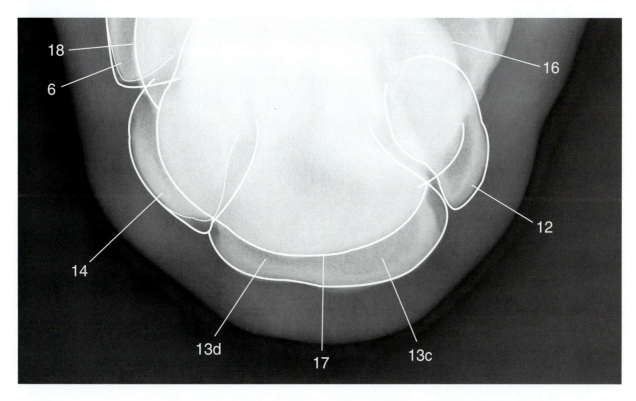

HUMERUS (a)

1. Lateral epicondyle
2. Medial epicondyle
3. Olecranon fossa
4. Coronoid fossa
5. Radial fossa
6. Lateral supracondylar crest
7. Trochlea of humerus (medial condyle)
8. Capitulum of humerus (lateral condyle)
9. Sagittal groove of humerus
10. Fovea capitis: Medial and lateral articular surface of radial head (corresponding to humerus medial and lateral)
11. Trochlear incisure of ulna

RADIUS (b)/ULNA (c)

12. Olecranon
13. Anconeal process
14. Medial coronoid process of ulna
15. Lateral coronoid process of ulna
16. Radial tuberosity
17. Medial collateral ligament tuberosity (radius)
18. Lateral collateral ligament tuberosity (radius)

4a. Lateromedial

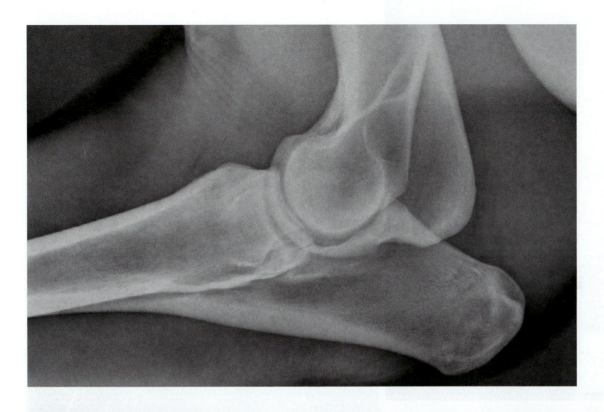

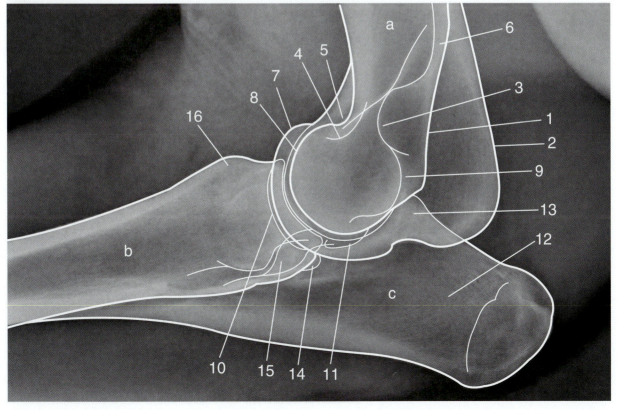

4b. Craniocaudal

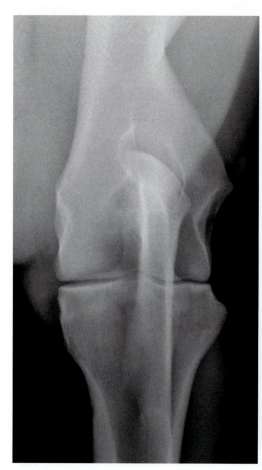

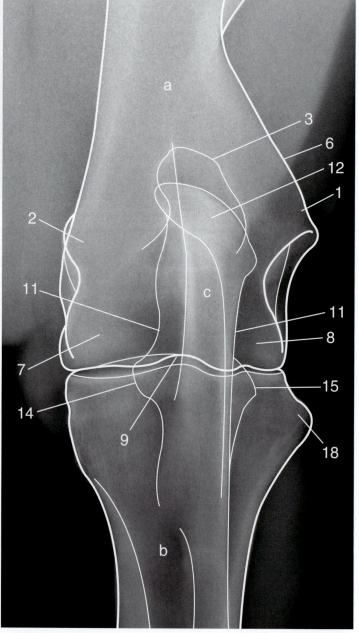

HUMERUS (a)

1. Humeral head
2. Greater tubercle
   a. Caudal part
   b. Cranial part
3. Lesser tubercle
4. Intermediate tubercle
5. Intertubercular groove
6. Deltoid tuberosity
7. Humeral neck
8. Fossa between tubercles and humeral head

SCAPULA (b)

9. Supraglenoid tubercle
10. Infraglenoid tubercle
11. Coracoid process
12. Glenoid notch
13. Glenoid

5a. Lateromedial

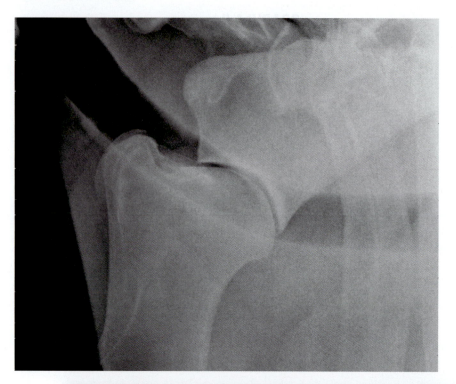

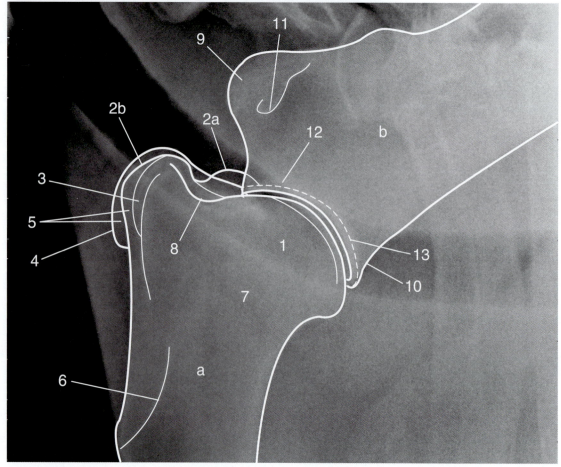

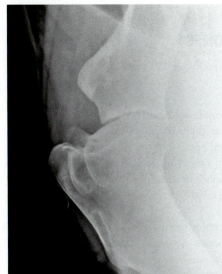

5b. Caudo 45° lateral-craniomedial oblique

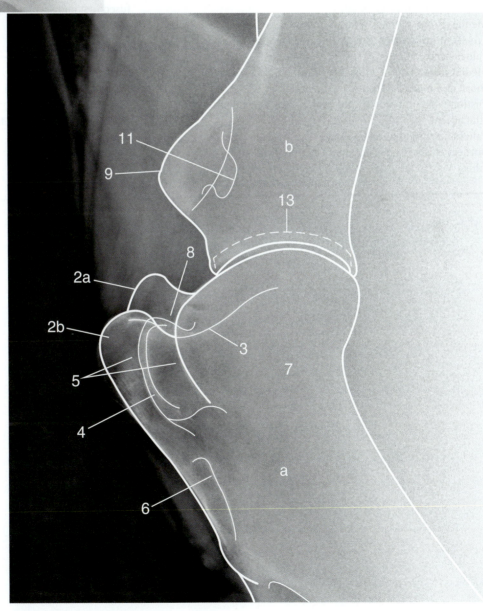

TIBIA-a

1. Distal intermediate ridge of tibia
2. Caudal aspect of distal intermediate ridge of tibia
3. Medial malleolus of the tibia
4. Medial malleolus of tibia superimposed on talus and calcaneus
5. Lateral malleolus of the tibia
6. Tibiotarsal joint
7. Articulation of the medial trochlear ridge of talus and medial tibia.

TALUS-c/CALCANEUS-b

8. Sustentaculum tali
9. Lateral trochlear ridge of talus
10. Medial trochlear ridge of talus
11. Trochlear groove between trochlear ridges on talus
12. Talocalcaneal joint
13. Medial tuberosity of talus, the insertion of superficial, short, and medial collateral ligaments
14. Distomedial tuberosity of talus for ligamentous attachment
15. Talus superimposed on calcaneus
16. Borders of sinus tarsi: the space between calcaneus and talus

TARSAL BONES

17. Central tarsal bone
18. PIT joint
19. DIT joint
    a. Articulation of third and central tarsal bones
20. First and second tarsal bones
21. Third tarsal bone
22. Prominent ridge for ligamentous attachments on dorso-medial surface of third tarsal bone
23. Fourth tarsal bone
24. TMT joint
    a. Articulation between fourth tarsal and fourth metatarsal bones
    b. Articulation between second metatarsal bone and fused first and second tarsal bone

METATARSAL

25. Second metatarsal bone
    a. Plantar border of second metatarsal bone
26. Third metatarsal bone
    a. Dorsoproximal ridge of third metatarsal bone, insertion of tibialis cranialis
27. Fourth metatarsal bone

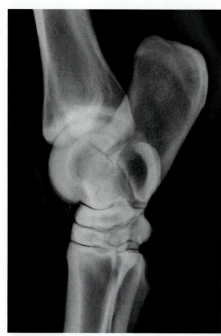

6a. Lateromedial

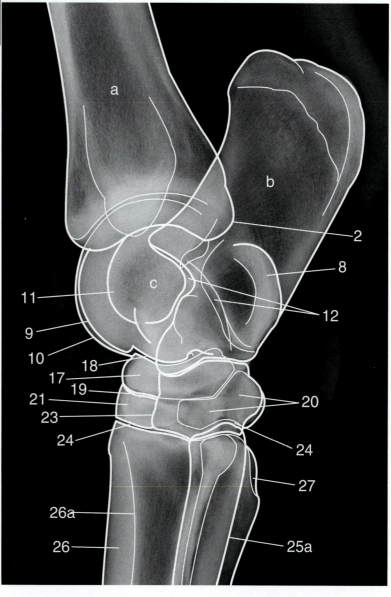

6b. Dorsoplantar

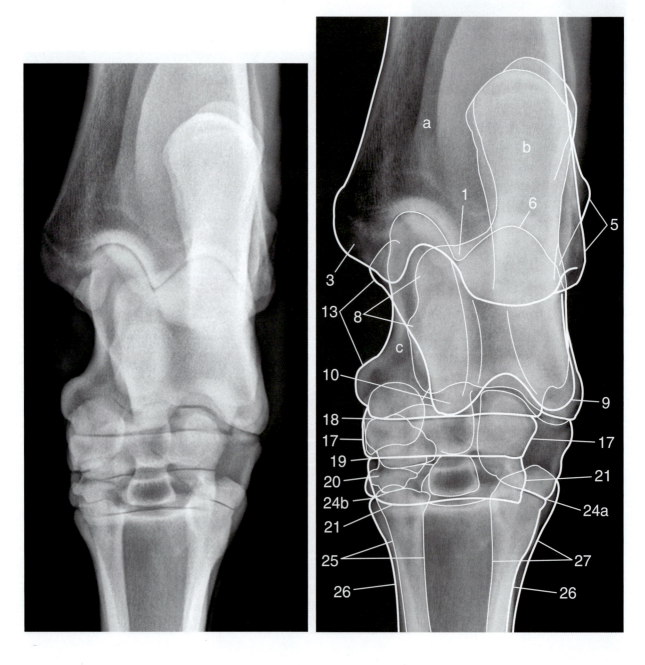

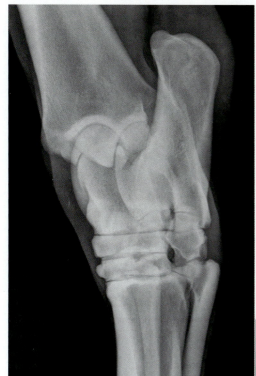

6c. Dorsolateral-plantaromedial oblique

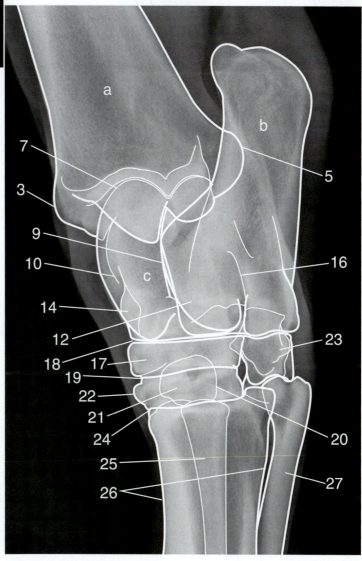

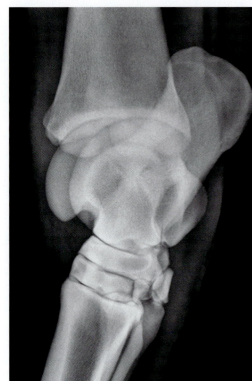

6d. Dorsomedial-plantarolateral oblique

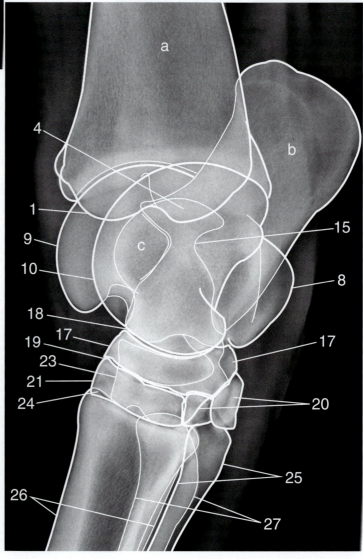

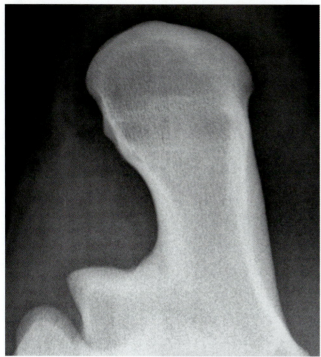

6e. Calcaneal skyline

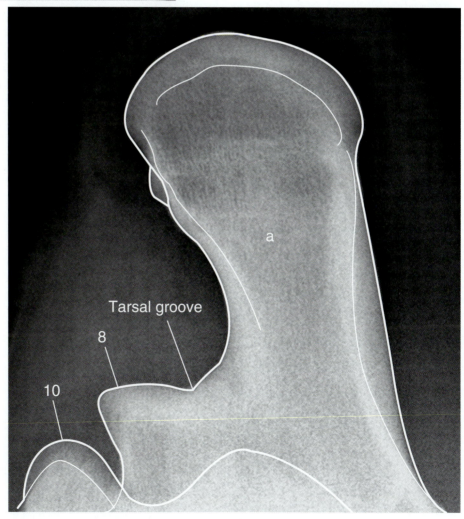

a) Femur
b) Tibia
c) Patella

1. Medial trochlear ridge of the femur
2. Lateral trochlear ridge of the femur
3. Intertrochlear groove of the femur
4. Medial femoral condyle (weight-bearing articular surface 4a) of the femur
5. Lateral femoral condyle of the femur
6. Medial epicondyle of the femur and collateral ligament attachment
7. Lateral epicondyle of the femur and collateral ligament attachment
8. Intercondylar groove of the femur
9. Attachment of cranial cruciate ligament (femoral a, tibial b)
10. Extensor fossa femur
11. Intercondylar eminence of the tibia (medial a, and lateral b)
12. Tibial tuberosity (medial a, lateral b)
13. Medial tibial condyle
14. Lateral tibial condyle
15. Fibular head
16. Site of insertion of medial (a) and lateral (b) cranial meniscal ligament on the proximal tibia
17. Lateral articular surface of patella
18. Medial articular surface of patella
19. Apex of patella
20. Base of patella

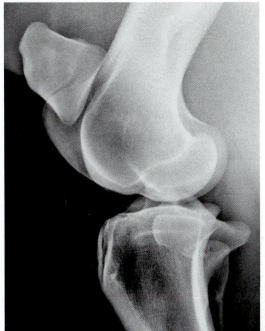

7a. Lateromedial

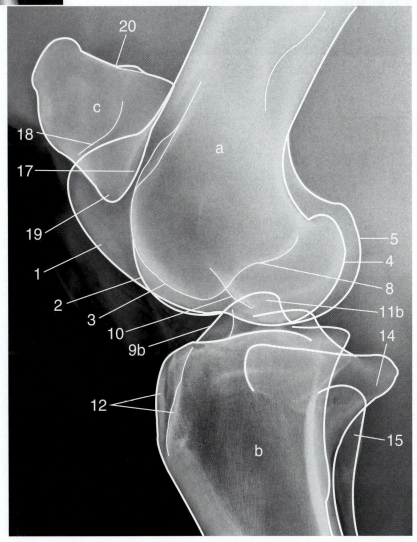

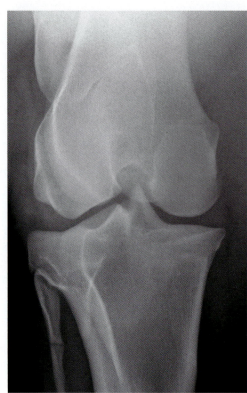

7b. Caudocranial

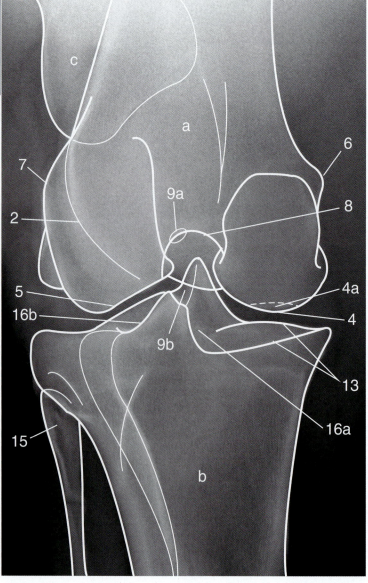

7c. Caudo 45° lateral-craniomedial oblique

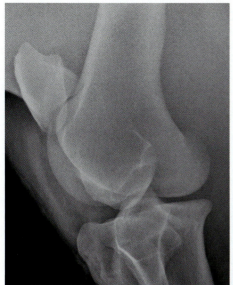

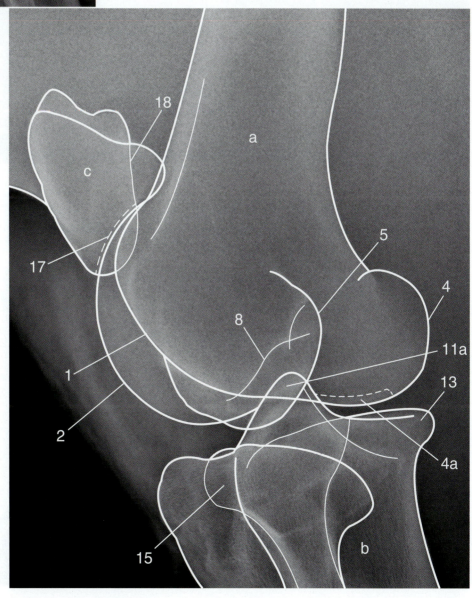

7d. Flexed latero 10° cranio 10° distal-mediocaudo proximal oblique

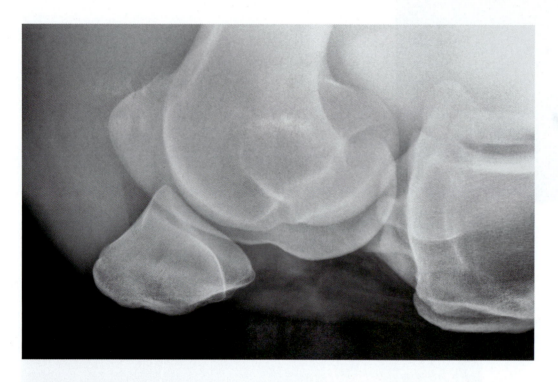

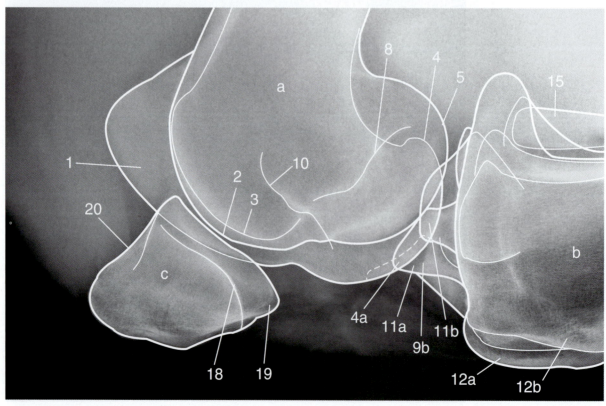

7e. Cranioproximal-craniodistal oblique (skyline of the patella)

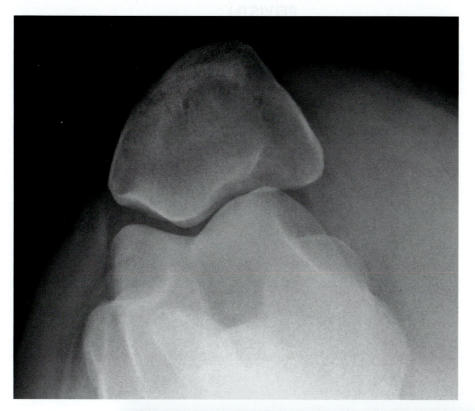

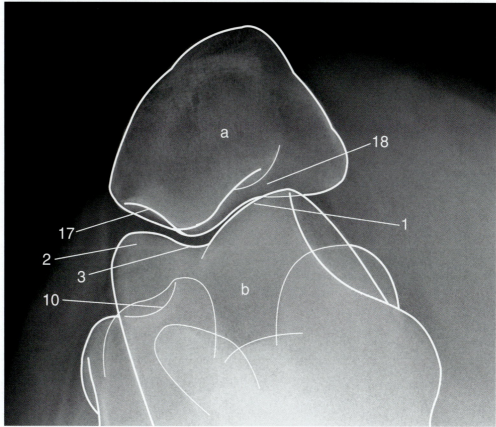

FEMUR (a)

1. Femoral head (shaded)
2. Fovea capitis
3. Neck
4. Greater trochanter
   a. Cranial part
   b. Caudal part
   c. Trochanteric incisure
5. Trochanteric fossa

PELVIS (b)

6. Acetabulum
   a. Acetabular rim
7. Fossa of acetabulum
8. Ischium
9. Ilium
10. Obturator foramen

8a. Ventro 15°-30° medial-dorsolateral

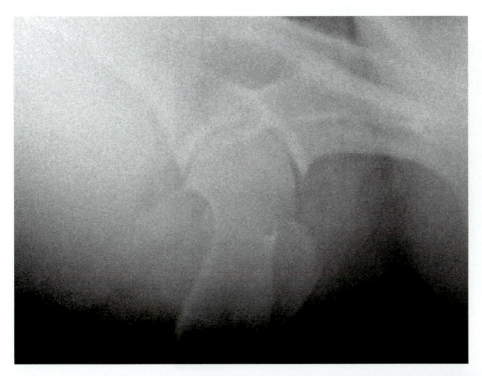

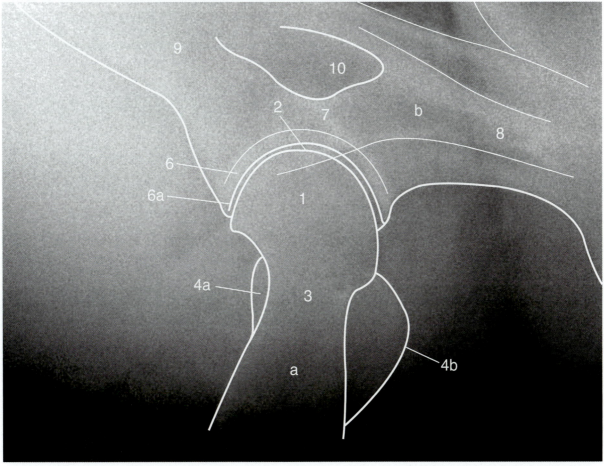

8b. Dorso 30° lateral-lateroventral oblique

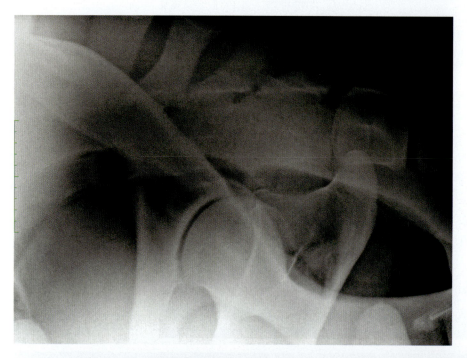

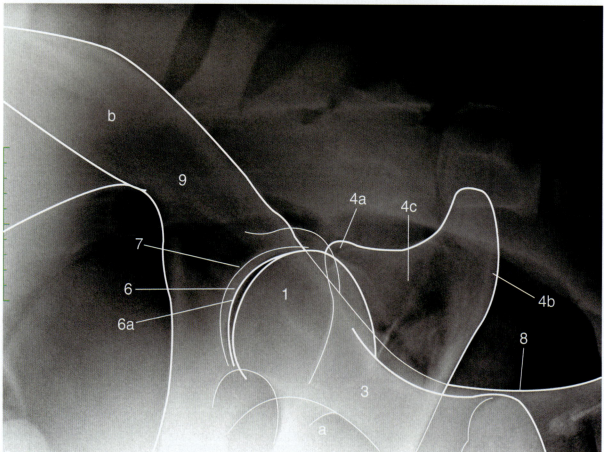

Synovial Fluid and Serum Biomarkers

David D. Frisbie, C. Wayne McIlwraith, and Janny C. de Grauw

Joint disease in horses is currently diagnosed using routine clinical methods such as musculoskeletal examination and diagnostic imaging; however, more accurate and earlier diagnoses may lead to identification of osteoarthritis (OA) before irreversible changes occur within joint tissues. The potential for such earlier diagnoses is available in a research setting through measuring levels of molecular signals and (by) products of tissue turnover, which may act as disease biomarkers. It has been recognized that early structural changes may remain asymptomatic for many years and that such putative biomarkers offer a potential to more easily monitor disease, especially in response to novel therapeutic agents. Extensive work with biomarkers of articular cartilage and bone as well as markers of joint inflammation and pain in both human and equine OA patients has yielded promising results. This chapter discusses some of the markers that have been and are being evaluated in synovial fluid and serum samples, with particular focus on those of potential relevance to equine practitioners and/or benefit to the equine industry.

WHAT IS A BIOMARKER?

The definition of a biomarker is ever changing, but the Biomarker Definitions Working Group[1] defines a biomarker as a "characteristic that is objectively measured and evaluated as an indicator of normal biologic processes, pathogenic processes, or pharmacologic responses to a therapeutic intervention."[2] The group further states that "Biomarkers can be anatomic, physiologic, biochemical or molecular parameters associated with the presence and severity of specific diseases and are detectable by a variety of methods including physical examination, laboratory assays, and imaging." Kraus et al. further differentiate the use of "dry" and "wet" biomarkers in OA.[3] Dry biomarkers include imaging parameters (i.e., from radiographs, magnetic resonance imaging, and ultrasound), questionnaires, and data from visual analog scales, for example, pain scores or quality of life indicators. Wet biomarkers include genetic (RNA, DNA) markers as well as biochemical molecules (carbohydrates, proteins, protein fragments, peptides, metabolites) that can be measured in a variety of sample matrices including blood, serum, urine and synovial fluid (SF) as well as tissue sources. Further distinction within the category of wet biomarkers can be made by using the terms "direct" and "indirect" molecular markers.

Direct molecular markers can be used as measures of tissue synthesis or breakdown, as they specifically reflect known anabolic or catabolic processes. For example, fibrillar collagens, such as collagen types I and II, are synthesized as immature procollagens that undergo proteolytic changes before conversion to mature collagen fibrils. Peptides at either end of the procollagen molecule are cleaved before the procollagen is incorporated into a mature collagen fibril. Estimations of type II collagen synthesis have been obtained from synovial fluid and serum samples by using a specific antibody that recognizes the propeptides cleaved from the carboxy termini (Figure 10-1).[4]

Conversely, indirect biochemical markers include molecules such as cytokines, inflammatory mediators, growth factors, and enzymes that are released with trauma and disease processes, affect tissue turnover, but are not themselves generated in the process of tissue synthesis or breakdown. Depending also on the sample type in which they are measured (SF, serum, or urine), such indirect markers can be seen as indicative of the degree of homeostatic imbalance within the joint at the moment of sampling and may represent contributions from several events and tissue sources (cartilage, bone, and synovium).

In the past 3 decades, the field of OA marker research has evolved rapidly and has yielded many candidate markers that have so far proven more or less useful in fulfilling each of five potential roles biomarkers may play. These roles have been conveniently classified in the human Osteoarthritis Biomarkers Network "BIPED" classification scheme[5] as follows: **B**urden of disease markers (markers that can be used to assess disease severity and thus stage disease), **I**nvestigative (markers for which a role in the disease process is likely but which are as yet insufficiently proven to be included in the other classes), **P**rognostic (markers that bear a relation to prognosis in individuals with OA or that can determine disease risk), **E**fficacy of intervention (markers that may be used to monitor response to pharmacologic treatment), and finally **D**iagnostic markers (those that can reliably distinguish between OA-affected and healthy individuals).

At the current time, no single marker can be classified as diagnostic for early-stage OA, whether in humans or animals.[6] Although human OA research has yielded several promising burden of disease and prognostic markers, most candidate markers are still at an experimental "investigative" stage. This is also true in equine OA biomarker research,

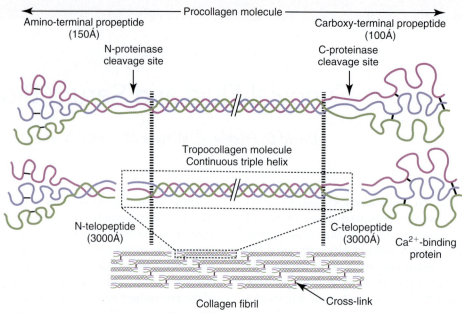

FIGURE 10-1 Type II procollagen synthesis and fibril formation, showing removal of propeptides as the triple helix is formed. The released propeptides form the basis of the carboxypropeptide of type II collagen (CPII) marker. (Reproduced with permission from Ray C.S., et al. (1996). Use of synovial fluid and serum markers in articular disease. In: McIlwraith C.W., Trotter G.W. (Eds.) Joint disease in the horse (pp. 203-216). Philadelphia, PA: Saunders.)

where long-term intervention and outcome studies in individuals with spontaneous disease are lacking. The importance of biomarkers in equine joint disease at present lies in their potential use for early diagnosis of disease including "prefracture" disease, clarification of pathobiologic processes as well as surrogate outcome measures for monitoring response to treatment in clinical and experimental trials. This chapter will cover selected direct and indirect "wet" biomarkers that are being investigated for use in diagnosis and monitoring of equine joint disease.

UNDERSTANDING JOINT STRUCTURE AND METABOLISM IN HEALTH AND DISEASE

Synovial joints may be considered complex organs in which all constituent tissues (articular cartilage, subchondral bone, and synovial membrane) interact with each other, both directly and via the SF, in health and disease. Details of these aspects have been previously presented in Chapter 1.

Osteoarthritis is generally characterized by degradation of articular cartilage and associated changes in the subchondral bone and fibrous joint capsule. These changes are not always concurrent in all joint tissues, and the extent of involvement in the disease process may vary from individual to individual. Some horses may present with minimal subchondral bone involvement but gross synovitis; in others extensive cartilage fibrillation is the main feature. Although joint inflammation alone does not suffice for a diagnosis of OA, it does feature prominently in clinical presentation (pain, joint effusion) and as a target for symptomatic treatment with antiinflammatories and analgesics.[7] More importantly, ongoing inflammation may drive tissue degradation and thus contribute to

disease progression.[8] To monitor disease status in individuals with OA, multiple biomarkers are therefore likely to be needed, with the panel reflecting tissue anabolic and catabolic changes as well as joint inflammatory status.

In a recent review entitled "Value of biomarkers in osteoarthritis: current status and perspectives" a group of experts in the human field identified 66 "relevant" published works between 1994 and 2012 to include in their discussions.[9] Although most biomarkers have been shown to cross species lines, the following review will be tailored to biomarkers the authors feel are pertinent to the horse, and thus should be noted not to be fully inclusive of the field of study.

INDIVIDUAL DIRECT BIOMARKERS OF ARTICULAR CARTILAGE METABOLISM IN OSTEOARTHRITIS

Anabolic Processes

The carboxy propeptide of type II collagen is a useful measure of the anabolic process of type II collagen synthesis. Previous studies have shown that levels of carboxy propeptide of type II collagen were significantly higher in SF from people with OA versus those without OA. Levels peaked early in the radiographic progression of the disease and declined in patients with severe radiographic changes.[10,11] This biomarker has also been shown to change significantly in serum samples from people with OA and rheumatoid arthritis.[4,12] In horses, the serum level of carboxy propeptide of type II collagen was significantly elevated in both experimental and clinical cases of joint disease.[13,14] Similar to the SF levels in people, equine serum levels were higher early in the disease

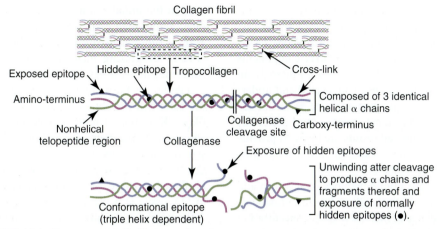

Collagen fibril

FIGURE 10-2 Structures of fibrillar type II collagen to show the composition of a collagen fibril with cross-links between the nonhelical telopeptide regions of individual tropocollagen molecules and the helical regions of adjacent molecules. Each tropocollagen molecule is composed of a triple helix of triple identical α chains. The cleavage site of collagenase is indicated. The cleaved triple helix unwinds to expose "hidden" epitopes on α chains that are not detectable by antibodies in the native triple helix. Nonhelical (telopeptide) and conformational (triple helical-dependent) epitopes are also indicated. (Reprinted with permission from Poole A.R. (1992). Immunology of cartilage. In: Moskowitz R.W., Howell D.S., Goldberg V.M., et al. (Eds.). Osteoarthritis diagnosis and management (2nd ed.) (pp. 155-189). Orlando, FL: Saunders.)

process and declined with advanced disease.[13] As mature cartilage has a very low basal collagen II turnover rate, it is hard to study the impact of therapeutic interventions (medical or surgical) on the cartilage collagen network, unless animals are sacrificed and cartilage is harvested and analyzed after treatment. Measurement of SF CPII concentration at baseline and with treatment over time can help identify in vivo local effects on cartilage collagen turnover that would otherwise go unnoticed. In this way, SF CPII has proven its use as an efficacy of intervention marker in multiple human studies.[15-18] Although intuitively both sustained reductions and possibly increases in SF CPII concentration following treatment may be interpreted as detrimental because they signal altered cartilage metabolic balance,[16,18] the long-term clinical significance of such changes still remains to be established.

Chondroitin sulfate (CS) is a major glycosaminoglycan (GAG) of aggrecan, and measuring specific CS epitopes on newly synthesized proteoglycan (PG) molecules provides a useful biomarker for aggrecan synthesis. An epitope called CS-846 that normally is found only in fetal tissues but is almost absent in healthy adult articular cartilage, has been measured in many species. Levels of CS-846 epitope are increased in SF in people after injury or primary OA compared with levels in SF from normal joints. Serum levels are also elevated in joint disease but to a lesser extent than SF levels.[19,20] CS-846 levels were significantly elevated in SF from horses with experimental and clinical joint disease.[13,14] CS-846 was also significantly elevated in serum and had a significant relationship to grade of disease following a quadratic curve like carboxy propeptide of type II collagen described above.[13] SF CS-846 levels peaked in parallel with GAG release after experimental induction of synovitis, and they were not affected by oral NSAID treatment.[17,21] Correct interpretation of CS-846 or other putative

anabolic aggrecan epitope levels as markers of aggrecan anabolic response requires one to realize that, for the epitope to be measured in SF or serum, it must (after synthesis) also undergo cleavage from the cartilage matrix. In other words, they might not be anabolic markers per se, but rather may indicate an activated metabolic state in which cleavage and repair mechanisms are both occurring at a higher rate. Other CS epitopes such as 3B3 and 7D4 were shown to be useful in assessing cartilage injury in animal models and in people with clinical disease[22] but have not been used in the horse.

Catabolic Processes

Measuring the degradation of type II collagen is of potential benefit in monitoring OA. Antibodies have been developed to identify exposed but previously inaccessible cleaved or denatured type II collagen fragments (Figure 10-2). Several different antibody-based marker assays are available, each detecting a distinct conformational (and sometimes proprietary) epitope on cleaved collagen II fragments that may have different in vivo fates; this complicates biologic interpretation of data obtained with one collagen cleavage marker versus another and interpretation of levels in SF versus serum or urine.

Collagen II cleavage markers that have been studied more or less extensively in equine SF and serum samples include C2C,[16,17,21,23-27] CTX-II,[28-30] and Col2-1 and Col2-1NO2.[31,32] Significant elevations in levels of degraded type II collagen were demonstrated in SF and serum samples from horses, dogs, and rabbits with experimental OA.[33] Significant increases were also detected in the serum of people with OA, with a correlation to disease activity.[33] Further, in foals with osteochondrosis, type II collagen fragments were significantly different compared to normal foals, suggesting potential use of this biomarker in early identification of osteochondrosis.[34]

Since an imbalance between cartilage catabolism and compensatory matrix synthesis is at the core of progressive cartilage destruction in OA, measuring ratios of anabolic versus catabolic markers for specific cartilage matrix components (e.g., for type II collagen: CPII/C2C ratio, or for proteoglycan balance: CS-846/GAG ratio) has been advocated and undertaken.[26,35] The rationale is that when anabolic and catabolic markers are measured in the same samples (and preferably repeatedly over time), combined results are likely to provide a more comprehensive picture of cartilage health status than single biomarker measurements.

Glycosaminoglycans are a building block of aggrecan and can be easily measured in both the SF and serum of patients with joint disease. Evidence of increased GAG concentration in the SF of horses with clinical joint issues has been documented for some time and has also been confirmed in experimental studies.[36] Although a seemingly nonspecific marker when measured in serum, as GAGs are present from numerous tissue sources (i.e., tendon, bone, eye), it is a sensitive marker of change; elevated levels are detected in the serum of horses with experimental joint disease as early as 14 days postinduction.[14] Glycosaminoglycan levels in SF samples may vary depending on inflammatory activity and degree of joint effusion[21] as well as cartilage OA status[37]; hence, for this marker as for many others, cross-sectional comparisons based on single sample measurements are likely much less informative than are serial samples used to monitor response to treatment.[17,18,38]

Analysis of specific subpopulations of aggrecan components including keratan and chondroitin sulfate (KS and CS) has been undertaken, as changes in relative SF composition of these may occur with disease[39] and/or may exist naturally between joints.[40] KS, one of the GAGs found on proteoglycan molecules of aggrecan, has been evaluated extensively. In people, elevations in serum levels of KS were associated with OA in some, but not all, studies.[20,41,42] Lack of correlation of serum[43] and SF[22] KS levels with cartilage damage compromises the value of serum KS as a biomarker of joint disease in people. In dogs, a specific KS epitope (5D4) was of limited value in experimentally induced and naturally occurring cruciate injury.[44,45] The usefulness of KS in serum and synovial fluid of horses with osteochondral fragmentation is also questionable.[13] Other aggrecan epitopes, most notably ARGS(V), that are generated by specific enzymatic cleavage, have recently become popular as a means to study aggrecanase-mediated aggrecan cleavage in OA.[46,47]

Cartilage oligomeric protein (COMP) is an abundant noncollagenous protein constituent of cartilage. COMP was once thought to be cartilage-specific, but it has also been localized in tendons and synovium. Serum and synovial fluid concentrations of COMP are increased in people with OA.[48,49] A positive correlation exists between COMP levels and radiographic grading of OA, progression of radiographic changes,[50] and results of nuclear scintigraphy.[51] Unlike COMP levels in people, initial work in the horse demonstrated that serum and SF levels of COMP were significantly lower in diseased joints.[52] It appears that this discrepancy was caused by the antibody used in the initial equine studies, which recognized mainly intact rather than intact and breakdown products of COMP. Thus, a subsequent study[53] in the horse using an antibody (14G4) recognizing intact and breakdown fragments also confirmed increase in COMP immunoreactivity with disease.

Fibulin peptides are a group of proteins associated with the basement membrane of the extracellular matrix of cartilage. This class of proteins has shown promise in people where proteomic methods identified Fib3-1 and Fib3-2 to be significantly elevated in cartilage and serum of humans with OA.[54] Further, these proteins were localized to the surface of fibrillated cartilage, providing specific evidence of their role in OA tissue at a site where early damage is concentrated. Although these biomarkers have not yet been tested in equine patients their promise is exciting.

INDIVIDUAL DIRECT BIOMARKERS OF BONE METABOLISM IN JOINT DISEASE

Anabolic and catabolic cascades exist in bone, but specific biomarkers in normal and disease states are not clearly defined. In part this is because bone is largely composed of type I collagen, which is highly abundant in all connective tissues in the body. This section deals only with bone markers thought to be significant in joint disease in horses.

Anabolic Processes

Osteocalcin (OC) is a small noncollagenous protein associated with bone assembly and turnover and has been measured in serum and synovial fluid samples from people with OA. Levels of OC correlated with bone scan findings and markers of cartilage metabolism.[51,55] However, because OC levels are higher in serum than in SF, OC in synovial fluid may be derived from peripheral blood and may not reflect local joint disease.[55] Osteocalcin levels were measured in horses, and, as in people, they appear to vary with age and with the administration of corticosteroids,[55,56] but the effect of gender remains unclear.[56] General anesthesia affects serum OC levels for 4 days.[57] As an efficacy of intervention marker, OC was included in a panel of markers measured in SF of horses receiving 10 days oral treatment with phenylbutazone; treatment increased SF but not serum OC levels over 4 weeks,[27] with as yet unknown clinical significance.

Bone-specific alkaline phosphatase is an isoform of alkaline phosphatase that is expressed at high levels on the cell surface of the bone-forming osteoblasts and plays an important role in bone formation. In a recent equine study a correlation was found between SF levels of bone-specific alkaline phosphatase, KS-5D4 epitope, and total GAG, as well as among all three biomarkers and the amount of joint damage defined arthroscopically.[58] This supports a putative role for altered subchondral bone metabolism in equine OA.

Catabolic Processes

Type I collagen C-telopeptides (CTX-I) may be useful markers of bone resorption. CTX-I levels in people with rheumatoid arthritis were positively correlated with indices of disease activity and joint destruction.[59,60] CTX is present in equine serum, though in studies performed in the authors' laboratory (DDF and CWM), it has not provided additive information in predicting OA or OA from changes associated with exercise, at least when analyzed with other articular cartilage biomarkers. Its potential usefulness as a marker of pathologic processes involving altered bone turnover remains unknown.[61,62]

Human bone sialoprotein (BSP) is found only in adult bone, and levels are seven times higher at the interface of cartilage and bone compared with other locations in bone. Serum levels are elevated significantly in people with clinical OA and those with bone scans consistent with OA.[63,64] Detection of equine BSP has been reported in bone tissue samples,[65] but the potential use of equine BSP measurement in SF or serum for identifying subchondral bone damage in horses with OA remains unknown.

INDIRECT BIOMARKERS OF JOINT HOMEOSTASIS

Given the anatomic and functional interdependence of subchondral bone, articular cartilage, and synovial membrane, it would be an oversimplification of synovial joint biology to try and measure joint health status based only on markers of cartilage or bone turnover. An important factor in the maintenance of joint homeostasis is the presence or absence of acute or chronic synovial inflammation. Debate is ongoing as to whether OA should be considered a primary degenerative disease of individual joints or a low-grade inflammatory (driven/accompanied) disease.[5] Regardless, cartilage damage will elicit an inflammatory response through release of detritus and altered biomechanics, and vice versa inflammatory mediators and enzymes released by irritated synovium can affect cartilage matrix integrity. Measuring indirect markers of joint tissue turnover, that is, those molecular signals that are involved in maintaining homeostatic balance or in the disruption thereof, can provide clues to the intraarticular environment that would not be obtained if only direct markers of bone or cartilage turnover were measured. For this purpose, SF is arguably the sample type of choice, as SF reflects real-time local concentrations of such molecular signals, whereas serum or urine does not.

Although tissue degradation is central to OA pathogenesis, it is known that structural changes in joint tissues (cartilage loss, subchondral bone changes) are poorly correlated to clinical symptoms of disease.[66] In part, this disparity may be caused by the important contribution of active inflammation to clinical presentation of disease. It has in fact been found that indirect inflammatory markers are among the best performing as burden of disease, prognostic, and treatment efficacy markers.[6] Their use in evaluating efficacy of treatment also owes to the fact that many indirect markers (enzymes, cytokines, mediators) themselves constitute potential target molecules for therapeutic intervention. Hence longitudinal measurement of such markers during experimental treatment allows for identification of relevant pharmacologic actions.[17,27,67,68] In this way, indirect molecular markers

measured in SF can help identify local antiinflammatory or possible disease-modifying effects of treatment.

Inflammatory and Pain-related Mediators

The synovial membrane is well-vascularized and innervated, and activated synoviocytes release a range of inflammatory mediators, including kinins, leukotrienes, prostaglandins, and acute-phase proteins like serum amyloid A. Many of these can act on polymodal nociceptors (free C-fiber and A-δ nerve endings) in the joint capsule and marginal periosteum to sensitize and directly stimulate them, causing action potential propagation. Upon stimulation, peripheral sensory neurons can in turn respond with retrograde release of neuropeptides like substance P into SF, thus contributing to the intraarticular "inflammatory soup" and to disease progression.[69] Multiple inflammatory mediators have been investigated for their potential role as indirect markers of disease activity, pain and joint function in OA.

Bradykinin (BK) is one of the most potent endogenous pain-producing mediators known to date, and enhanced BK levels in SF have been found in humans with painful TMJ disease[70]; BK concentrations in SF also correlate with direct markers of cartilage degradation and inflammation in human knee OA.[71] Although SF BK concentration was not increased in horses with pain referable to the MTP or MCP joint[23] and could not be detected in SF samples of horses with clinical OA (de Grauw et al. 2008, unpublished data), in an equine LPS-induced model of noninfectious synovitis, local BK release surged within 24 hours after LPS injection and responded to treatment with meloxicam or intraarticular morphine.[17,21,67] At this stage, SF BK seems more useful as an indicator of joint inflammatory status in experimental rather than clinical joint disease in horses.

Serum amyloid A (SAA) is the major acute-phase protein in horses. Serum SAA concentrations increase caused by liver synthesis of SAA during systemic or severe local inflammatory states, and SAA in SF may largely derive from extraarticular sources.[72,73] However, SAA is also moderately expressed by equine synovial membrane.[74] Dramatic increases in SF (and serum) SAA are seen during severe acute joint inflammation as in LPS-induced synovitis[72,75] and infectious arthritis.[76] Although SAA may be useful to help discriminate between infectious and noninfectious joint conditions, it appears to be of little value as a biomarker in noninfectious arthropathies including OA.[75]

A report in horses that substance P and prostaglandin E_2 (PGE_2) concentrations were elevated in OA versus control joints,[77] and early work in human knee OA where preoperative SF substance P levels predicted postoperative pain relief [78] prompted investigations in horses with pain referable to the fetlock region by perineural nerve blocks and with a positive or negative response to intraarticular (MCP or MTP joint) anesthesia. Higher SF substance P concentrations were indeed found in joints that responded to intraarticular anesthesia versus those that did not,[23] suggesting a relation between SF SP levels and intraarticular pain. Also, in an LPS-induced synovitis model, substance P levels consistently rose and fell with onset and resolution of inflammation and lameness,[17,21,67] and substance P was elevated in inflamed but not denervated equine joints.[79] Importantly, measurement of this mediator in SF by ELISA carries some inherent difficulties, and different commercial assay kits may give widely varying results.[80] Thus, absolute values obtained in different studies using different assay kits cannot be directly compared.[21,23,80] However, within a study, serial samples analyzed using the same assay method may be very valuable in monitoring effects of analgesic and antiinflammatory therapy.[17,67]

PGE$_2$ is one of the many arachidonic acid derivatives that are locally released into SF by inflamed synovial membrane and in lesser part by the articular cartilage.[81] It forms the principal target of NSAID therapy and may act as a sensitive indicator of joint alteration and active synovitis in various joint conditions.[14,15,77,82,83] As such, SF PGE$_2$ concentration is commonly included as a surrogate outcome measure in clinical trials that seek to establish antiinflammatory and/or potential analgesic activity of novel or existing joint therapies.[17,38,84] In an early clinical study, PGE$_2$ concentrations were elevated in MCP or MTP SF of lame horses versus sound controls, but were not related to the response to intraarticular anesthesia.[23] This highlights two problems when trying to correlate SF mediator levels to estimates of joint pain and function. First, we lack a gold standard assessment of presence or absence of articular pain in veterinary patients with spontaneous disease (here, intraarticular anesthesia may have had its limitations in detecting articular pain). Second, because of the simultaneous contribution of various anatomic and pathologic sources to pain in naturally occurring OA, SF levels of individual mediators simply are unlikely to bear a direct linear relation to the amount of pain and lameness displayed. The importance of PGE$_2$ as a pain-related mediator in OA is however well established, and a reduction in SF PGE$_2$ in response to therapy has consistently been associated with clinical improvements in lameness.[17,67,85] Hence, SF PGE$_2$ is one of the most useful treatment efficacy markers when investigating antiinflammatory and potential analgesic effects of joint therapy.

Growth Factors and Cytokines

Given the very limited capacity of adult articular cartilage for functional repair, cartilage preservation based on the maintenance of a balance between tissue anabolism and degradation is paramount to joint function. Growth factors like insulin-like growth factor 1 (IGF-1) and transforming growth factor β1 (TGF-β1) as well as cytokines like interleukin-1β (IL-1β), interleukin-6 (IL-6), tumor necrosis factor α (TNF-α), and high mobility group box protein 1 (HMGB-1) are major orchestrators of the molecular events involved in both physiologic cartilage remodeling and pathologic tissue degradation. Several studies have targeted the potential role of dysregulation of these factors in equine joint disease including developmental orthopedic disease (mainly osteochondrosis) and OA.

Studies of IGF-1 in joint function have found that it is an important anabolic factor in promoting cartilage repair[86]; hence, dysregulation may contribute to cartilage pathology.

Although plasma concentrations of IGF-1 were found to be lower in a group of foals with osteochondrosis[87] and horses with juvenile proximal interdigital OA[88], serum or plasma IGF-1 levels are influenced by many systemic factors (including age, sex, and diet) and so interindividual variation may obscure relations with disease. It could be argued that even SF concentrations of growth factors that act in nanomolar to picomolar quantities, may not reflect their actions at various tissue depths within the cartilage.[81] For these reasons, growth factors are unlikely to be useful as indirect biomarkers in OA. However, SF growth factor concentrations can conveniently be used to evaluate the efficacy of intraarticular therapies that aim to replenish intraarticular anabolic factors (like platelet rich plasma [PRP] or autologous conditioned serum [ACS]).[89,90]

Although IL-1β is known as a central culprit in cartilage degradation in human and equine OA, SF levels of IL-1 in OA-affected joints are in fact quite variable and often not significantly higher than in control joints.[91,92] Again, this may be illustrative of a common problem with the measurement in body fluids of labile protein molecules that act in a paracrine fashion at nanometer distances within tissues; body fluid (even SF) levels simply may not reflect local tissue concentrations or actions. One early equine study found SF IL-1β to be a good predictor of joint disease,[82] but this has not been corroborated since. Despite the lack of a consistent association of SF IL-1β levels with disease presence or severity, given the overwhelming evidence of the catabolic role of IL-1 in the OA disease process it is still sometimes included as a surrogate efficacy marker in clinical trials (SF IL-1 levels all below detection limits in canine experimental OA).[93] Experimental induction of cartilage degradation by exposure to LPS or IL-1 is particularly common in in vitro studies, where attenuation of IL-1-induced changes in response to exogenous therapy is generally perceived as a positive treatment effect.[94,95] However, beneficial effects seen in vitro may or may not translate to the in vivo situation.

In human OA research, serum IL-6 has shown some promise as an indirect marker of inflammatory activity that importantly correlates with pain and physical function scores in OA.[96,97] In horses, some work has been done on SF but not on serum IL-6 as a marker of joint disease. Experimentally, IL-1β was shown to induce IL-6 release in equine joints[79] and in an equine LPS-induced synovitis model SF IL-6 levels showed a sustained increase upon onset of inflammation and lameness.[98] In horses with spontaneous (i.e., naturally occurring) disease, one study found dramatic increases in SF IL-6 in carpal joints with osteochondral lesions.[99] Early work by Bertone et al.[82] in OA versus control horses categorized SF IL-6 as an excellent predictor of joint disease in general. Others also identified higher SF IL-6 levels in OA joints of racehorses compared with controls.[100] Although this indicates there may be potential for SF IL-6 to act as an indirect marker of inflammation and pain in OA horses, more (longitudinal) studies in larger, well-defined patient populations are needed to corroborate this. Cross-sectional serum IL-6 measurement in small groups of (equine) patients versus controls is unlikely to be useful, as interindividual variation because of differences in age and sex would likely obscure any correlation of serum IL-6 with OA disease activity.[101]

Tumor necrosis factor-α (TNF-α) is a key mediator of mechanical joint hyperalgesia.[102,103] An early experimental study in equine LPS-induced synovitis demonstrated local TNF-α release,[104] although a more recent study failed to consistently identify SF TNF-α in LPS-induced synovitis samples.[105] As for naturally occurring OA, an early study reported SF TNF-α concentration to be a good predictor of spontaneous joint disease in horses.[82] However, Ley et al. found SF TNF-α levels to be low and not associated with any specific joint lesion.[99] Yet another report found SF TNF-α to be elevated only in equine carpal joints with advanced OA.[106] It remains to be seen whether these conflicting data are mainly because of differences in analytical methods or because of differences in clinical patient populations and disease severity. Until these matters are resolved, the potential added value of SF TNF-α as a marker of equine OA remains questionable.

HMGB-1 is a nuclear chaperone protein that is rapidly released into SF but not serum with the onset of local joint inflammation.[105] Increased HMGB-1 immunostaining has been demonstrated in equine OA joints with naturally occurring osteochondral fragments[107] and significantly higher SF HMGB-1 concentrations were found in 45 thoroughbred racehorses with osteochondral injury compared with 40 sound controls.[108] Although these preliminary findings show some promise for SF HMGB-1 as a marker of inflammation associated with osteochondral injury, it remains to be established whether measurement of SF HMGB-1 levels has added value as a diagnostic or prognostic marker for OA.

Enzyme Activity

When synoviocytes and/or chondrocytes are activated by noxious stimuli, they increase expression and release of several enzymes that can affect cartilage matrix degradation, including numerous members of the matrix metalloproteinase (MMP) family, as well as A disintegrin and thrombospondin-like motifs (ADAMTS) and serine proteases. Leukocyte influx and activation also contribute highly to the net overall proteolytic activity in inflammatory SF.[109] Many of these enzymes are present in a latent inactive form, and/or are bound to endogenous enzyme inhibitors in normal SF, and are only activated in inflammatory conditions. Hence, simply measuring protein levels of the enzymes may not reflect the actual potential for matrix degradation.[109] Activity assays, which measure the conversion rate of an exogenously added substrate that is cleaved by the enzyme in question, provide a better reflection of true SF degrading enzyme activity. As cartilage maintenance depends largely on a balance between matrix synthesis and catabolism, sustained excessive catabolic enzyme activity may be devastating to synovial joints.

Many members of the MMP family have been implicated in the OA disease process. Since sustained rises in collagenase (MMP-1, -8, -13) and/or gelatinase (among others, MMP-2 and -9) activities are likely to cause cartilage collagen II damage, they have received much attention as indirect

markers of cartilage turnover and as potential efficacy markers (therapeutic targets) for enzyme-inhibitory treatments. In a study of amphotericin-induced joint inflammation, MMP-2 and MMP-9 activity rose sharply, with SF MMP-2 activity remaining elevated for the duration of the study (5 weeks) to an extent that could well contribute to cartilage damage.[110] Models of LPS-induced synovitis likewise show dramatic increases in SF MMP activity,[21] which may largely be leukocyte-derived. In spontaneous disease, Fietz et al. found SF MMP-2 and MMP-9 activities to be elevated in equine joints with infectious versus noninfectious joint disease, although MMP-2 was also higher in joints with noninfectious joint disease versus healthy controls.[111] A study in equine cadaveric MCP joints found general MMP activity to increase in line with increasing severity of cartilage degeneration,[112] indicating a link between elevated MMP activity and structural joint damage. Used as a surrogate "efficacy of intervention" marker in an experimental trial, SF collagenase activity was found to be reduced by oral treatment with meloxicam[17] but not phenylbutazone.[18] Although MMP inhibition may be a very useful attribute of antiarthritic medications, studies using SF markers alone cannot establish chondroprotectivity, as markers only provide a reflection of cartilage status as opposed to direct cartilage macroscopic or microscopic evaluation. However, the use of these markers as surrogate outcome measures may help to identify previously unknown drug actions that may be relevant to joint health.

FUTURE OF BIOMARKERS IN OSTEOARTHRITIS

So far, limited but promising data are available regarding the use of wet biomarkers to diagnose and monitor equine joint disease. An important obstacle to progress in biomarker research has been the less than simple relation between the production of a candidate marker at the target site (i.e., inside the joint) and the concentration measured in body fluids at a distance from this site. An important distinction to be made is between measurement of putative markers in serum or urine versus SF; the former sample types cannot, by their nature, discriminate between contributions from individual joints or in fact from other tissue sources (tendon sheaths, bone, skin, vitreous of the eye, etc.), and thus will reflect systemic "whole body" marker production, metabolism, and clearance. SF arguably provides the closest reflection of individual joint status; however, SF aspiration carries greater risk than urine or serum collection, and concentrations of markers in SF may be highly influenced by the level of active joint inflammation (marker dilution or "washout"). In addition, many commercial assay kits are intended for use in culture supernatant, serum, or plasma and are consequently not validated for use in SF. Assurance of reliable assay performance is imperative if meaningful results are to be obtained, and in the past this has sometimes been questionable. Assay validation is likewise paramount whenever markers are measured using antibody-based assays intended for other (e.g., human or rodent) species. Unless the antibody was raised against the equine marker epitope (e.g., specific antiequine IL-6 and TNF-α antibodies are available) or in case of 100% sequence homology (as with human or equine substance P), antibody-cross reactivity must be ascertained.

The factors influencing concentrations of biomarkers in various body fluids differ for individual markers but include liver and kidney clearance, circadian rhythms, intestinal peristalsis, exercise level, age, breed, diet, sex, drug administration, surgery, and general anesthesia. Methods of sample collection and storage also may be influential, particularly when labile peptides or proteins are concerned. In addition, the in vivo metabolic fate of many candidate biomarkers is still not fully known, which means that a low concentration of a marker measured by an (immuno)assay that only detects the intact molecule may be caused by the assay not picking up metabolites of the marker molecule (see also COMP above).

Although biomarkers may have a future role in diagnosing and monitoring equine joint disease, a combination of markers, as noted, will likely be required, especially because so many factors influence disease activity. Proof of principle work has shown that biomarkers significantly change in the face of experimentally induced OA, and this change is significantly greater than that seen with exercise alone.[14,113] Specifically, SF concentrations for 8/8 biomarkers were significantly increased in OA-affected joints of horses undergoing exercise versus sham-operated joints of similarly exercised horses. Likewise, serum from OA-affected horses showed a significant increase in 6/8 biomarkers versus serum from similarly exercised control horses. Using biomarker levels from either SF or serum, horses could be correctly categorized into the appropriate group (OA-affected or sham) 100% of the time within 14 days of OA induction using discriminant analysis, suggesting great promise for the use of such biomarker panels for detecting and monitoring disease.

Initially, clinical studies on SF and serum OA biomarkers tended to focus on the ability of individual markers or panels of markers to diagnose or stage disease, that is, to distinguish between patients and controls or among patients with various stages of disease. These studies are often cross-sectional in design, in that they attempt to correlate joint status as measured by routine diagnostic methods to marker concentrations measured at a single time point in patients and controls. However, even when strict inclusion criteria are used, clinical cases are likely to vary with regard to age, weight, inciting cause and duration of disease, severity of symptoms, and synovial inflammatory activity at the time of sampling.[58] Each of these factors can act as a confounder and hence obscure any relation that might otherwise have been found between marker levels and disease status. To overcome these limitations, large numbers of patients tend to be needed, for instance, to allow for stratification. Importantly, as we still lack gold standard means of diagnosing "early OA," correct classification of arguably the most interesting clinical cases is often also debatable.

To date, in a clinical setting, several cross-sectional studies have looked at a variety of candidate biomarkers in both SF and serum for potential use in non-invasive prediction of disease severity. Specifically, COMP has been shown to have

significantly altered serum levels in horses with clinical OA versus control horses.[114] Differences in COMP levels in SF have also been identified when making similar comparisons in clinical cases with joint disease.[53,115,116] Another cross-sectional study[58] using the contralateral limb as a control demonstrated that concentrations of BAP (bone-specific alkaline phosphatase), KS, KS:GAG ratio, and HA were significantly different between early OA joints and control joints. Importantly, they also observed that KS and the KS:GAG ratio had good correlation with articular cartilage pathology. These cross-sectional studies provide promising examples for the potential use of biomarkers in equine orthopedics; prospective longitudinal studies are the next step to provide further proof of principle. The advantages of longitudinal versus cross-sectional study designs are multiple, but perhaps most importantly longitudinal analysis provides a baseline and thus some frame of reference within which changes in serum or SF marker levels in an individual over time can be interpreted.[117] Because no normal values or ranges for experimental SF and serum biomarkers have been established, low- or high-marker levels in a single sample are often hard to interpret biologically in terms of the extent of joint damage. For example, low glycosaminoglycan (GAG) levels in an individual SF sample may indicate any number of things, ranging from little release of GAG from the cartilage or dilution of GAG levels caused by joint effusion to such extensive depletion of GAG from the cartilage (in late-stage disease) that, despite high catabolic activity, levels of GAG in SF will not be elevated.[118] In a longitudinal study, SF GAG levels measured at a certain time point could be related to previous or subsequent events (e.g., induction of synovitis/creation of a cartilage lesion in an experimental setting or initiation of treatment or injury occurrence in a clinical setting), allowing for much more meaningful interpretation.

One such study using serum markers has been completed through collaboration of the Equine Research Center at Colorado State University and equine veterinarians practicing at Southern California Thoroughbred race tracks. Race horses that were 2 and 3 years old were entered in the study (N=238).[28] Horses had monthly musculoskeletal examinations and blood drawn and stored for later biomarker examination. They were followed for a maximum of 10 months and were considered to have sustained an injury if they were out of training for more than 30 days. Horses with solitary musculoskeletal injuries and completion of more than 2 months in the study were analyzed for biomarker levels along with a randomly selected uninjured control population. The following were considered musculoskeletal injury: intraarticular fragmentation, tendon or ligamentous injury, stress fractures, and dorsal metacarpal disease. Fifty-nine horses sustained a single musculoskeletal injury; 71 acted as uninjured controls. Interestingly, the greatest change in biomarker levels appeared to occur 4 to 6 months before injury. Using sophisticated statistical modeling, it was possible, based on biomarker levels in this group of horses, to accurately predict horses that would sustain an injury 73.9% of the time. Given these promising results, another study in Western performance horses has also shown promise in predicting soft tissue injury. Unfortunately, the high cost of this kind of study and thus the commercialization of this technology remain the most challenging aspect of bringing biomarkers into routine clinical use in horses.

Biomarker research to date has largely been hypothesis-driven, meaning that specific candidate molecules have been investigated as potential biomarkers of disease based on existing knowledge of their role in joint biology and pathology. Another exciting approach uses techniques developed within the various "-omics" disciplines. It is based on analytical platforms that can measure up to thousands of analytes (genes, gene products, metabolites, etc.) simultaneously in a single biologic sample, thus generating molecular "fingerprints" that can be compared between healthy and diseased states.[90,119] These so-called "shot-gun" approaches enable true biomarker "discovery" (i.e., identification of novel biomarkers without *a priori* hypotheses about likely candidates), but they pose major statistical and bioinformatics challenges inherent to dealing with huge datasets. Also, the validity of conclusions depends heavily on sensitivity and specificity of the analytical method, stability of individual analytes, and very importantly, on correct definition of diseased versus healthy states (sample selection and clinical diagnosis). In this respect, progress in biomarker research is likely to go hand in hand with improvements in the field of advanced diagnostic imaging modalities. In this field too we will benefit from well-designed in vivo experimental studies in which longitudinal responses to well-defined experimental stimuli can be monitored over time.[120]

In conclusion, the field of biomarkers for joint research has so far produced some exciting and promising data, but the implementation of these data into a commercially viable platform that is available to the equine practitioner and the patient is yet to be realized. Until this occurs, it is important for practitioners to understand and appreciate the possibilities, but also the limitations of SF and serum biomarker measurement, whenever they are used in scientific publications for the investigation of disease or response to treatment.

REFERENCES

1. Downing GJ, ed. *Office of Science Policy National Institutes of Health.* Bethesda, Maryland, USA. Amsterdam: Elsevier; 2000.
2. Downing GJ. *National Institutes of Health United States Food and Drug Administration. Biomarkers and surrogate endpoints: clinical research and applications.* Bethesda, Maryland: Proceedings of the NIH-FDA Conference; 1999. April 15-16, 1999.
3. Kraus VB, Burnett B, Coindreau J, et al. Application of biomarkers in the development of drugs intended for the treatment of osteoarthritis. *Osteoarthritis Cartilage.* 2011;19(5):515–542.
4. Nelson F, Dahlberg L, Lavery S, et al. Evidence for altered synthesis of type II collagen in patients with osteoarthritis. *J Clin Invest.* 1998;102(12):2115–2125.
5. Bauer DC, Hunter DJ, Abramson SB, et al. Classification of osteoarthritis biomarkers: a proposed approach. *Osteoarthritis Cartilage.* 2006;14(8):723–727.
6. Lafeber FP, van Spil WE. Osteoarthritis year 2013 in review: biomarkers: reflecting before moving forward, one step at a time. *Osteoarthritis Cartilage.* 2013;21(10):1452–1464.
7. Kidd JA, Fuller CJ, Barr AR. Osteoarthritis in the horse. *Equine Vet Educ.* 2001;13(3):160–168.
8. Sutton S, Clutterbuck A, Harris P, et al. The contribution of the synovium, synovial derived inflammatory cytokines and neuropeptides to the pathogenesis of osteoarthritis. *Vet J.* 2007;179(1):10–24.
9. Lotz M, Martel-Pelletier J, Christiansen C, et al. Value of biomarkers in osteoarthritis: current status and perspectives. *Ann Rheum Dis.* 2013;72(11):1756–1763.
10. Ishiguro N, Ito T, Ito H, et al. Relationship of matrix metalloproteinases and their inhibitors to cartilage proteoglycan and collagen turnover: analyses of synovial fluid from patients with osteoarthritis. *Arthritis Rheum.* 1999;42(1):129–136.
11. Shinmei M, Ito K, Matsuyama S, et al. Joint fluid carboxy-terminal type II procollagen peptide as a marker of cartilage collagen biosynthesis. *Osteoarthritis Cartilage.* 1993;1(2):121–128.
12. Månsson B, Carey D, Alini M, et al. Cartilage and bone metabolism in rheumatoid arthritis. Differences between rapid and slow progression of disease identified by serum markers of cartilage metabolism. *J Clin Invest.* 1995;95(3):1071–1077.
13. Frisbie DD, Ray CS, Ionescu M, et al. Measurement of synovial fluid and serum concentrations of the 846 epitope of chondroitin sulfate and of carboxy propeptides of type II procollagen for diagnosis of osteochondral fragmentation in horses. *Am J Vet Res.* 1999;60(3):306–309.
14. Frisbie DD, Al-Sobayil F, Billinghurst RC, et al. Changes in synovial fluid and serum biomarkers with exercise and early osteoarthritis in horses. *Osteoarthritis Cartilage.* 2008;16(10):1196–1204.
15. Robion FC, Doizé B, Bouré L, et al. Use of synovial fluid markers of cartilage synthesis and turnover to study effects of repeated intraarticular administration of methylprednisolone acetate on articular cartilage in vivo. *J Orthop Res.* 2001;19(2):250–258.
16. Céleste C, Ionescu M, Poole AR, et al. Repeated intraarticular injections of triamcinolone acetonide alter cartilage matrix metabolism measured by biomarkers in synovial fluid. *J Orthop Res.* 2005;23(3):602–610.
17. de Grauw JC, van de Lest CH, Brama PA, et al. In vivo effects of meloxicam on inflammatory mediators, MMP activity and cartilage biomarkers in equine joints with acute synovitis. *Equine Vet J.* 2009;41(7):693–699.
18. de Grauw JC, van Loon JP, van de Lest CH, et al. In vivo effects of phenylbutazone on inflammation and cartilage-derived biomarkers in equine joints with acute synovitis. *Vet J.* 2014;201(1):51–56.
19. Lohmander LS, Ionescu M, Jugessur H, et al. Changes in joint cartilage aggrecan after knee injury and in osteoarthritis. *Arthritis Rheum.* 1999;42(3):534–544.
20. Poole AR, Dieppe P. Biological markers in rheumatoid arthritis. *Semin Arthritis Rheum.* 1994;23(6 Suppl 2):17–31.
21. de Grauw JC, van de Lest CH, van Weeren PR. Inflammatory mediators and cartilage biomarkers in synovial fluid after a single inflammatory insult: a longitudinal experimental study. *Arthritis Res Ther.* 2009;11(2):R35.
22. Bello AE, Garrett Jr WE, Wang H, et al. Comparison of synovial fluid cartilage marker concentrations and chondral damage assessed arthroscopically in acute knee injury. *Osteoarthritis Cartilage.* 1997;5(6):419–426.
23. de Grauw JC, van de Lest CH, van Weeren PR, et al. Arthrogenic lameness of the fetlock: synovial fluid markers of inflammation and cartilage turnover in relation to clinical joint pain. *Equine Vet J.* 2006;38(4):305–311.

24. Lettry V, Sumie Y, Mitsuda K, et al. Divergent diagnosis from arthroscopic findings and identification of CPII and C2C for detection of cartilage degradation in horses. *Jpn J Vet Res.* 2010;57(4):197–206.

25. Trumble TN, Scarbrough AB, Brown MP. Osteochondral injury increases type II collagen degradation products (C2C) in synovial fluid of Thoroughbred racehorses. *Osteoarthritis Cartilage.* 2009;17(3):371–374.

26. Donabédian M, van Weeren PR, Perona G, et al. Early changes in biomarkers of skeletal metabolism and their association to the occurrence of osteochondrosis (OC) in the horse. *Equine Vet J.* 2008;40(3):253–259.

27. Fradette ME, Céleste C, Richard H, et al. Effects of continuous oral administration of phenylbutazone on biomarkers of cartilage and bone metabolism in horses. *Am J Vet Res.* 2007;68(2):128–133.

28. Frisbie DD, McIlwraith CW, Arthur RM, et al. Serum biomarker levels for musculoskeletal disease in two- and three-year-old racing Thoroughbred horses: a prospective study of 130 horses. *Equine Vet J.* 2010;42(7):643–651.

29. Nicholson AM, Trumble TN, Merritt KA, et al. Associations of horse age, joint type, and osteochondral injury with serum and synovial fluid concentrations of type II collagen biomarkers in Thoroughbreds. *Am J Vet Res.* 2010;71(7):741–749.

30. Cleary OB, Trumble TN, Merritt KA, et al. Effect of exercise and osteochondral injury on synovial fluid and serum concentrations of carboxy-terminal telopeptide fragments of type II collagen in racehorses. *Am J Vet Res.* 2010;71(1):33–40.

31. Verwilghen DR, Enzerink E, Martens A, et al. Relationship between arthroscopic joint evaluation and the levels of Coll2-1, Coll2-1NO(2), and myeloperoxidase in the blood and synovial fluid of horses affected with osteochondrosis of the tarsocrural joint. *Osteoarthritis Cartilage.* 2011;19(11):1323–1329.

32. Verwilghen DR, Martens A, Busschers E, et al. Coll2-1, Coll2-1NO2 and myeloperoxidase concentrations in the synovial fluid of equine tarsocrural joints affected with osteochondrosis. *Vet Res Commun.* 2011;35(7):401–408.

33. Poole AR. *NIH white paper: biomarkers, the osteoarthritis initiative a basis for discussion.* Bethesda, Maryland: Proceedings NIH conference; 2000.

34. Billinghurst RC, Brama PA, van Weeren PR, et al. Evaluation of serum concentrations of biomarkers of skeletal metabolism and results of radiography as indicators of severity of osteochondrosis in foals. *Am J Vet Res.* 2004;65(2):143–150.

35. de Grauw JC, Donabédian M, van de Lest CH, et al. Assessment of synovial fluid biomarkers in healthy foals and in foals with tarsocrural osteochondrosis. *Vet J.* 2011;190(3):390–395.

36. McIlwraith CW. Use of synovial fluid and serum biomarkers in equine bone and joint disease: a review. *Equine Vet J.* 2005;37(5):473–482.

37. Alwan WH, Carter SD, Dixon JB, et al. Interleukin-1-like activity in synovial fluids and sera of horses with arthritis. *Res Vet Sci.* 1991;51(1):72–77.

38. Pearson W, Orth MW, Lindinger MI. Evaluation of inflammatory responses induced via intraarticular injection of interleukin-1 in horses receiving a dietary nutraceutical and assessment of the clinical effects of long-term nutraceutical administration. *Am J Vet Res.* 2009;70(7):848–861.

39. Machado TS, Correia da Silva LC, Baccarin RY, et al. Synovial fluid chondroitin sulphate indicates abnormal joint metabolism in asymptomatic osteochondritic horses. *Equine Vet J.* 2012;44(4):404–411.

40. Fuller CJ, Barr AR, Dieppe PA, et al. Variation of an epitope of keratan sulphate and total glycosaminoglycans in normal equine joints. *Equine Vet J.* 1996;28(6):490–493.

41. Caterson B, Christner JE, Baker JR. Identification of a monoclonal antibody that specifically recognizes corneal and skeletal keratan sulfate. Monoclonal antibodies to cartilage proteoglycan. *J Biol Chem.* 1983;258(14):8848–8854.

42. Sweet MB, Coelho A, Schnitzler CM, et al. Serum keratan sulfate levels in osteoarthritis patients. *Arthritis Rheum.* 1988;31(5):648–652.

43. Brandt KD, Thonar EJ. Lack of association between serum keratan sulfate concentrations and cartilage changes of osteoarthritis after transection of the anterior cruciate ligament in the dog. *Arthritis Rheum.* 1989;32(5):647–651.

44. Innes JF, Sharif M, Barr AR. Changes in concentrations of biochemical markers of osteoarthritis following surgical repair of ruptured cranial cruciate ligaments in dogs. *Am J Vet Res.* 1999;60(9):1164–1168.

45. Innes JF, Sharif M, Barr AR. Relations between biochemical markers of osteoarthritis and other disease parameters in a population of dogs with naturally acquired osteoarthritis of the genual joint. *Am J Vet Res.* 1998;59(12):1530–1536.

46. Larsson S, Lohmander LS, Struglics A. An ARGS-aggrecan assay for analysis in blood and synovial fluid. *Osteoarthritis Cartilage.* 2014;22(2):242–249.

47. Struglics A, Hansson M, Lohmander LS. Human aggrecanase generated synovial fluid fragment levels are elevated directly after knee injuries due to proteolysis both in the inter globular and chondroitin sulfate domains. *Osteoarthritis Cartilage.* 2011;19(8):1047–1057.

48. Clark AG, Jordan JM, Vilim V, et al. Serum cartilage oligomeric matrix protein reflects osteoarthritis presence and severity: the Johnston County Osteoarthritis Project. *Arthritis Rheum.* 1999;42(11):2356–2364.

49. Lohmander LS, Saxne T, Heinegard DK. Release of cartilage oligomeric matrix protein (COMP) into joint fluid after knee injury and in osteoarthritis. *Ann Rheum Dis.* 1994;53(1):8–13.

50. Conrozier T, Saxne T, Fan CS, et al. Serum concentrations of cartilage oligomeric matrix protein and bone sialoprotein in hip osteoarthritis: a one year prospective study. *Ann Rheum Dis.* 1988;57(9):527–532.

51. Sharif M, George E, Dieppe PA. Correlation between synovial fluid markers of cartilage and bone turnover and scintigraphic scan abnormalities in osteoarthritis of the knee. *Arthritis Rheum.* 1995;38(1):78–81.

52. Misumi K, Vilim V, Clegg PD, et al. COMP in equine synovial fluids and sera. In: Price J, ed. *Symposium on markers in the horse.* Northampton, UK: Highgate; 2000.

53. Arai K, Misumi K, Carter SD, et al. Analysis of cartilage oligomeric matrix protein (COMP) degradation and synthesis in equine joint disease. *Equine Vet J.* 2005;37(1):31–36.

54. Henrotin Y, Gharbi M, Mazzucchelli G, et al. Fibulin 3 peptides Fib3-1 and Fib3-2 are potential biomarkers of osteoarthritis. *Arthritis Rheum.* 2012;64(7):2260–2267.

55. Salisbury C, Sharif M. Relations between synovial fluid and serum concentrations of osteocalcin and other markers of joint tissue turnover in the knee joint compared with peripheral blood. *Ann Rheum Dis.* 1997;56(9):558–561.

56. Lepage OM. Physiological variation in bone markers in horses: Molecular markers of cartilage and bone metabolism in the horse (p. 9). In: Price J, ed. *Symposium on markers in the horse.* Northampton, UK: Highgate; 2000.

57. Grafenau P, Eicher R, Uebelhart B, et al. General anesthesia decreases osteocalcin plasma concentrations in horses. *Equine Vet J.* 1999;31(6):533–536.

58. Fuller CJ, Barr AR, Sharif M, et al. Cross-sectional comparison of synovial fluid biochemical markers in equine osteoarthritis and the correlation of these markers with articular cartilage damage. *Osteoarthritis Cartilage.* 2001;9(1):49–55.

59. Bonde M, Garnero P, Fledelius C, et al. Measurement of bone degradation products in serum using antibodies reactive with an isomerized form of an 8 amino acid sequence of the C-telopeptide of type I collagen. *J Bone Miner Res.* 1997;12(7):1028–1034.

60. Garnero P, Jouvenne P, Buchs N, et al. Uncoupling of bone metabolism in rheumatoid arthritis patients with or without joint destruction: assessment with serum type I collagen breakdown products. *Bone.* 1999;24(4):381–385.

61. Billinghurst RC, Brama PAJ, van Weeren PR, et al. Significant exercise-related changes in the serum levels of two biomarkers of collagen metabolism in young horses. *Osteoarthritis Cartilage.* 2003;11(10):760–769.

62. Frisbie DD, Al-Sobayil F, Billinghurst RC, et al. Serum markers differentiate exercise from pathology and correlate to clinical parameters of pain in an osteoarthritic model. *Osteoarthritis Cartilage.* 2002;10(Suppl A):553.

63. Petersson IF, Boegård T, Svensson B, et al. Changes in cartilage and bone metabolism identified by serum markers in early osteoarthritis of the knee joint. *Br J Rheumatol.* 1998;37(1):46–50.

64. Petersson IF, Boegård T, Dahlström J, et al. Bone scan and serum markers of bone and cartilage in patients with knee pain and osteoarthritis. *Osteoarthritis Cartilage.* 1998;6(1):33–39.

65. Ekman S, Skiöldebrand E, Heinegård D, et al. Ultrastructural immunolocalisation of bone sialoprotein in the osteocartilaginous interface of the equine third carpal bone. *Equine Vet J.* 2005;37(1):26–30.

66. Zhang W, Doherty M, Peat G, et al. EULAR evidence-based recommendations for the diagnosis of knee osteoarthritis. *Ann Rheum Dis.* 2010;69(3):483–489.

67. van Loon JP, de Grauw JC, van Dierendonck M, et al. Intra-articular opioid analgesia is effective in reducing pain and inflammation in an equine LPS induced synovitis model. *Equine Vet J.* 2010;42(5):412–419.

68. Frisbie DD, Stewart MC. Cell-based therapies for equine joint disease. *Vet Clin North Am Equine Pract.* 2011;27(2):335–349.

69. Coutaux A, Adam F, Willer JC, et al. Hyperalgesia and allodynia: peripheral mechanisms. *Joint Bone Spine.* 2005;72(5):359–371.

70. Suzuki T, Segami N, Nishimura M, et al. Bradykinin expression in synovial tissues and synovial fluids obtained from patients with internal derangement of the temporomandibular joint. *Cranio.* 2003;21(4):265–270.

71. Bellucci F, Meini S, Cucchi P, et al. Synovial fluid levels of bradykinin correlate with biochemical markers for cartilage degradation and inflammation in knee osteoarthritis. *Osteoarthritis Cartilage.* 2013;21(11):1774–1780.

72. Lindegaard C, Gleerup KB, Thomsen MH, et al. Anti-inflammatory effects of intra-articular administration of morphine in horses with experimentally induced synovitis. *Am J Vet Res.* 2010;71(1):69–75.

73. de Seny D, Cobraiville G, Charlier E, et al. Acute-phase serum amyloid A in osteoarthritis: regulatory mechanism and proinflammatory properties. *PLoS One.* 2013;8(6):e66769.

74. Berg LC, Thomsen PD, Andersen PH, et al. Serum amyloid A is expressed in histologically normal tissues from horses and cattle. *Vet Immunol Immunopathol.* 2011;144(1-2):155–159.

75. Jacobsen S, Niewold TA, Halling-Thomsen M, et al. Serum amyloid A isoforms in serum and synovial fluid in horses with lipopolysaccharide-induced arthritis. *Vet Immunol Immunopathol.* 2006;110(3-4):325–330.

76. Jacobsen S, Thomsen MH, Nanni S. Concentrations of serum amyloid A in serum and synovial fluid from healthy horses and horses with joint disease. *Am J Vet Res.* 2006;67(10):1738–1742.

77. Kirker-Head CA, Chandna VK, Agarwal RK, et al. Concentrations of substance P and prostaglandin E2 in synovial fluid of normal and abnormal joints of horses. *Am J Vet Res.* 2000;61(6):714–718.

78. Pritchett JW. Substance P level in synovial fluid may predict pain relief after knee replacement. *J Bone Joint Surg Br.* 1997;79(1):114–116.

79. Hardy J, Bertone AL, Weisbrode SE, et al. Cell trafficking, mediator release, and articular metabolism in acute inflammation of innervated or denervated isolated equine joints. *Am J Vet Res.* 1998;59(1):88–100.

80. Campbell DE, Raftery N, Tustin R, et al. Measurement of plasma-derived substance P: biological, methodological, and statistical considerations. *Clin Vaccine Immunol.* 2006;13(11):1197–1203.

81. de Grauw JC, van de Lest CH, van Weeren PR. A targeted lipidomics approach to the study of eicosanoid release in synovial joints. *Arthritis Res Ther.* 2011;13(4):R123.

82. Bertone AL, Palmer JL, Jones J. Synovial fluid cytokines and eicosanoids as markers of joint disease in horses. *Vet Surg.* 2001;30(6):528–538.

83. van den Boom R, van de Lest CH, Bull.S, et al. Influence of repeated arthrocentesis and exercise on synovial fluid concentrations of nitric oxide, prostaglandin E2 and glycosaminoglycans in healthy equine joints. *Equine Vet J.* 2005;37(3):250–256.

84. Frisbie DD, Kawcak CE, McIlwraith CW. Evaluation of the effect of extracorporeal shock wave treatment on experimentally induced osteoarthritis in middle carpal joints of horses. *Am J Vet Res.* 2009;70(4):449–454.

85. Kawcak CE, Frisbie DD, Trotter GW, et al. Effects of intravenous administration of sodium hyaluronate on carpal joints in exercising horses after arthroscopic surgery and osteochondral fragmentation. *Am J Vet Res.* 1997;58(10):1132–1140.

86. Goodrich LR, Hidaka C, Robbins PD, et al. Genetic modification of chondrocytes with insulin-like growth factor-1 enhances cartilage healing in an equine model. *J Bone Joint Surg Br.* 2007;89(5):672–685.

87. Sloet van Oldruitenborgh-Oosterbaan MM, Mol JA, Barneveld A. Hormones, growth factors and other plasma variables in relation to osteochondrosis. *Equine Vet J.* 1999;31(Suppl 31):45–54.

88. Lejeune JP, Franck T, Gangl M, et al. Plasma concentration of insulin-like growth factor I (IGF-I) in growing Ardenner horses suffering from juvenile digital degenerative osteoarthropathy. *Vet Res Commun.* 2007;31(2):185–195.

89. Chiaradia E, Pepe M, Tartaglia M, et al. Gambling on putative biomarkers of osteoarthritis and osteochondrosis by equine synovial fluid proteomics. *J Proteomics.* 2012;75(14):4478–4493.

90. Textor JA, Willits NH, Tablin F. Synovial fluid growth factor and cytokine concentrations after intraarticular injection of a platelet-rich product in horses. *Vet J.* 2013;198(1):217–223.

91. Kokebie R, Aggarwal R, Lidder S, et al. The role of synovial fluid markers of catabolism and anabolism in osteoarthritis, rheumatoid arthritis and asymptomatic organ donors. *Arthritis Res Ther.* 2011;13(2):R50.

92. McNulty AL, Rothfusz NE, Leddy HA, et al. Synovial fluid concentrations and relative potency of interleukin-1 alpha and beta in cartilage and meniscus degradation. *J Orthop Res.* 2013;31(7):1039–1045.

93. Rhouma M, de Oliveira El, Warrak A, Troncy E, et al. Anti-inflammatory response of dietary vitamin E and its effects on pain and joint structures during early stages of surgically induced osteoarthritis in dogs. *Can J Vet Res.* 2013;77(3):191–198.

94. Fenton JI, Chlebek-Brown KA, Caron JP, et al. Effect of glucosamine on interleukin-1-conditioned articular cartilage. *Equine Vet J.* 2002;34(Suppl 34):219–223.

95. Bertone AL, Ishihara A, Zekas LJ, et al. Evaluation of a single intraarticular injection of autologous protein solution for treatment of osteoarthritis in horses. *Am J Vet Res.* 2014;75(2):141–151.

96. Stannus OP, Jones G, Blizzard L, et al. Associations between serum levels of inflammatory markers and change in knee pain over 5 years in older adults: a prospective cohort study. *Ann Rheum Dis.* 2013;72(4):535–540.

97. Shimura Y, Kurosawa H, Sugawara Y, et al. The factors associated with pain severity in patients with knee osteoarthritis vary according to the radiographic disease severity: a cross-sectional study. *Osteoarthritis Cartilage.* 2013;21(9):1179–1184.

98. Hawkins DL, Cargile JL, MacKay RJ, et al. Effect of tumor necrosis factor antibody on synovial fluid cytokine activities in equine antebrachiocarpal joints injected with endotoxin. *Am J Vet Res.* 1995;56(10):1292–1299.

99. Ley C, Ekman S, Elmén A, et al. Interleukin-6 and tumour necrosis factor in synovial fluid from horses with carpal joint pathology. *J Vet Med A Physiol Pathol Clin Med.* 2007;54(7):346–351.

100. Billinghurst RC, Fretz PB, Gordon JR. Induction of intraarticular tumour necrosis factor during acute inflammatory responses in equine arthritis. *Equine Vet J.* 1995;27(3):208–216.

101. Suagee JK, Corl BA, Crisman MV, et al. Relationships between body condition score and plasma inflammatory cytokines, insulin, and lipids in a mixed population of light-breed horses. *J Vet Intern Med.* 2013;27(1):157–163.

102. Inglis JJ, Notley CA, Essex D, et al. Collagen-induced arthritis as a model of hyperalgesia: functional and cellular analysis of the analgesic actions of tumor necrosis factor blockade. *Arthritis Rheum.* 2007;56(12):4015–4023.

103. Richter F, Natura G, Löser S, et al. Tumor necrosis factor causes persistent sensitization of joint nociceptors to mechanical stimuli in rats. *Arthritis Rheum.* 2010;62(12):3806–3814.

104. Hawkins DL, MacKay RJ, Gum GG, et al. Effects of intraarticularly administered endotoxin on clinical signs of disease and synovial fluid tumor necrosis factor, interleukin 6, and prostaglandin E2 values in horses. *Am J Vet Res.* 1993;54(3):379–386.

105. de Grauw JC, Heinola T, van Weeren R, et al. Rapid release of high mobility group box protein-1 (HMGB-1) in transient arthritis. *Clin Exp Rheumatol.* 2010;28(2):292–293.

106. Kamm JL, Nixon AJ, Witte TH. Cytokine and catabolic enzyme expression in synovium, synovial fluid and articular cartilage of naturally osteoarthritic equine carpi. *Equine Vet J.* 2010;42(8):693–699.

107. Ley C, Ekman S, Ronéus B, et al. Interleukin-6 and high mobility group box protein-1 in synovial membranes and osteochondral fragments in equine osteoarthritis. *Res Vet Sci.* 2009;86(3):490–497.

108. Brown MP, Trumble TN, Merritt KA. High-mobility group box chromosomal protein 1 as a potential inflammatory biomarker of joint injury in Thoroughbreds. *Am J Vet Res.* 2009;70(10):1230–1235.

109. Simard N, Boire G, de Brum-Fernandes AJ, et al. A novel approach to measure the contribution of matrix metalloproteinase in the overall net proteolytic activity present in synovial fluids of patients with arthritis. *Arthritis Res Ther.* 2006;8(4):R125.

110. Marttinen PH, Raulo SM, Suominen MM, et al. Changes in MMP-2 and -9 activity and MMP-8 reactivity after amphotericin B induced synovitis and treatment with bufexamac. *J Vet Med A Physiol Pathol Clin Med.* 2006;53:311–318.

111. Fietz S, Einspanier R, Hoppner S, et al. Determination of MMP-2 and -9 activities in synovial fluid of horses with osteoarthritic and arthritic joint diseases using gelatin zymography and immunocapture activity assays. *Equine Vet J.* 2008;40:266–271.

112. van den Boom R, van der Harst MR, Brommer H, et al. Relationship between synovial fluid levels of glycosaminoglycans, hydroxyproline and general MMP activity and the presence and severity of articular cartilage change on the proximal articular surface of P1. *Equine Vet J.* 2005;37(1):19–25.

113. Kawcak CE, Frisbie DD, Werpy NM, et al. Effects of exercise vs experimental osteoarthritis on imaging outcomes. *Osteoarthritis Cartilage.* 2008;16(12):1519–1525.

114. Misumi K, Vilim V, Hatazoe T, et al. Serum level of cartilage oligomeric matrix protein (COMP) in equine osteoarthritis. *Equine Vet J.* 2002;34(6):602–608.

115. Skiöldebrand E, Heinegård D, Eloranta ML, et al. Enhanced concentration of COMP (cartilage oligomeric matrix protein) in osteochondral fractures from racing Thoroughbreds. *J Orthop Res.* 2005;23(1):156–163.

116. Taylor SE, Weaver MP, Pitsillides AA, et al. Cartilage oligomeric matrix protein and hyaluronan levels in synovial fluid from horses with osteoarthritis of the tarsometatarsal joint compared to a control population. *Equine Vet J.* 2006;38(6):502–507.

117. Lohmander LS, Dahlberg L, Eyre D, et al. Longitudinal and cross-sectional variability in markers of joint metabolism in patients with knee pain and articular cartilage abnormalities. *Osteoarthritis Cartilage.* 1998;6(5):351–361.

118. Ratcliffe A, Doherty M, Maini RN, et al. Increased concentrations of proteoglycan components in the synovial fluids of patients with acute but not chronic joint disease. *Ann Rheum Dis.* 1988;47(10):826–832.

119. Ritter SY, Subbaiah R, Bebek G, et al. Proteomic analysis of synovial fluid from the osteoarthritic knee: comparison with transcriptome analyses of joint tissues. *Arthritis Rheum.* 2013;65(4):981–992.

120. Kraus VB, Nevitt M, Sandell LJ. Summary of the OA biomarkers workshop 2009 – biochemical markers: biology, validation, and clinical studies. *Osteoarthritis Cartilage.* 2010;18(6):742–745.

11

Nonsteroidal Antiinflammatory Drugs

C. Wayne McIlwraith and David D. Frisbie

Although nonsteroidal antiinflammatory drugs (NSAIDs) are sometimes defined as those substances other than steroids that suppress one or more components of the inflammatory response,[1] the term NSAID tends to be used more restrictively to describe antiinflammatory agents that inhibit some component of the enzyme system that converts arachidonic acid into prostaglandins and thromboxane, especially the prostaglandin E (PGE) series. The latter are thought to be intimately involved in pain, altered cartilage metabolism, and ongoing inflammation in damaged joints. Elevation of prostaglandin E2 (PGE2) levels are always associated with synovial inflammation of horses with osteoarthritis (OA) and cartilage matrix depletion.[2] The use of NSAIDs to inhibit the arachidonic acid cascade has been a mainstay for the treatment of joint disease for decades.[3,4] NSAIDs are typically used in cases of acute injury and are often accompanied by other treatments. The renal and gastrointestinal side effects associated with NSAIDs, however, limit their long-term use for the treatment of joint disease.

Traditionally, inhibition of PGE2 and the resulting symptomatic pain relief has been viewed as a beneficial goal in treating OA (Figure 11-1). Although some recent research has suggested that this inhibition may have long-term unfavorable effects on cartilage metabolism, this is controversial, and based on current knowledge it is not expected to alter the continued use of NSAIDs in clinical practice.[5] Research has also suggested that NSAIDs may have a role in mediating joint pain at the level of the spinal cord as well as locally, although specific research in this area has not yet been conducted in the horse.[6] It is generally expected that medication blocking cyclooxygenase (COX) would affect prostaglandins alone and this could therefore be considered focused antiinflammatory therapy.

Phenylbutazone is the most commonly used NSAID in the horse; it is often given at a dose of 4.4 mg/kg once or twice daily (Figure 11-2). Phenylbutazone is considered one of the more potent NSAIDs for symptom-modifying effects in equine musculoskeletal disease. In experimental trials using an equine OA model developed at Colorado State University (CSU), phenylbutazone had significant symptom-modifying effects and decreased the synovial fluid PGE2 levels; however, significant detrimental effects, including bone changes documented using magnetic resonance imaging (MRI), were seen.[7] In horses with naturally occurring OA, variable results have been noted.[8] Lameness scores were lowest after administration of the combination of phenylbutazone with flunixin meglumine (Figure 11-3) versus phenylbutazone alone, but concerns about secondary side effects (including acute necrotizing colitis) have been raised.[7]

All NSAIDs inhibit COX activity to some degree,[2,4] but in the early 1990s the identification of isoenzymes for the COX pathway (COX-1 and COX-2) had implications for more specific therapy. COX-1 has been associated with the housekeeping functions of the COX pathway. It is known to be constitutively produced and important in the balance of normal physiologic function of the gastrointestinal and renal systems, although it has a lesser role in the inflammatory cascade. COX-2 has mainly been associated with inflammatory events, especially those driven by macrophages and synovial cells and has only minor roles in normal physiology, thus its "bad" or inducible role.

The protective role of COX-1 for the gastroduodenal mucosa has been shown both experimentally in laboratory animals and in human clinical trials. Furthermore, studies have shown that the greatest degree of damage to the gastroduodenal mucosa is generally caused by NSAIDs that preferentially inhibit COX-1.[9] In fact, the preferential COX-2 inhibitor rofecoxib (Vioxx) was shown in human patients to induce ulceration at a lower incidence than that seen in a randomized placebo group.[10]

As with most biologic systems, complete inhibition of COX-2 may not be optimal for the joint or the horse; some value, albeit minimal, has been shown from expression of COX-2 as well as some demonstrable negative effects of COX-1 expression.[5,11,12] More specifically, a low level of COX-1 expression is inducible during stress or inflammatory periods. Likewise, some constitutive expression of COX-2

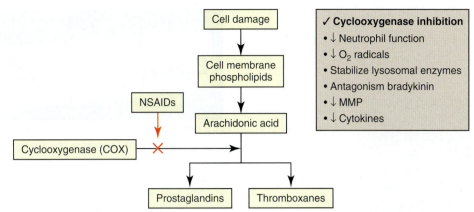

FIGURE 11-1 The location on the prostaglandin cascade where NSAIDs inhibit cyclooxygenase, demonstrating the principal effects of cyclooxygenase inhibition.

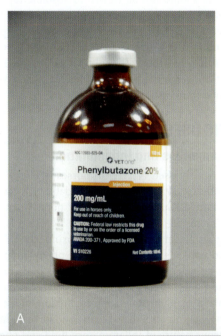

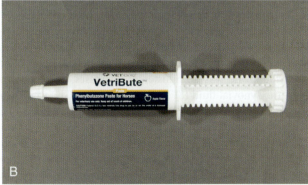

FIGURE 11-2 Phenylbutazone, the most commonly used NSAID, is available for intravenous (**A**) and oral use (**B**).

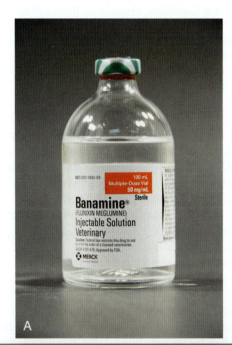

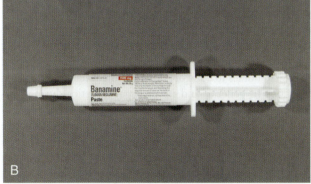

FIGURE 11-3 Flunixin meglumine is available for intravenous (**A**) and oral use (**B**).

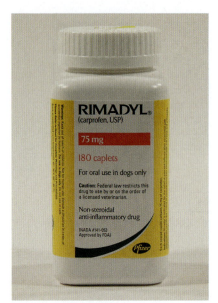

FIGURE 11-4 Carprofen, available as Rimadyl® in the United States, is licensed for small animals, but it has been used in horses where phenylbutazone is causing side effects. Carprofen is also available and licensed as Zenecarp® tablets and injection for use in dogs and horses in New Zealand, and an oral formulation is licensed in Europe.

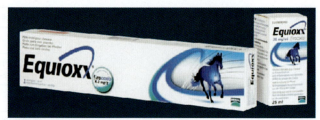

FIGURE 11-5 Equioxx® (firocoxib) is the first-COX-2-specific NSAID licensed for horses in the United States. (Courtesy: Equioxx, Merial.)

has been demonstrated by the brain, kidney, and pancreatic islet cells, and it has a function in bone resorption. Furthermore, COX-2 suppression has been shown to delay gastric ulcer healing in rats. Thus, as Oscar Wilde said, "The pure and simple truth is rarely pure and never simple." Whereas COX-1 is mainly responsible for the protective functioning of prostaglandins, COX-2 may play an accessory constitutive role in the COX pathway.

The mainstream view is still that the beneficial effects of selective COX-2 inhibition in OA are ideal. Anecdotally, carprofen (Rimadyl) (Figure 11-4) was used at CSU in horses that developed high serum creatinine levels and diarrhea in association with phenylbutazone use. These side effects disappeared when horses were given carprofen; a protective effect was seen, implying there may be more preferential COX-2 inhibition than with phenylbutazone therapy. Firocoxib (Equioxx) (Figure 11-5), a member of the class of drugs that selectively inhibits the COX-2 isoenzyme, is now approved for use in horses to control pain and inflammation associated with OA in general, and its pharmacokinetics during prolonged use have been determined.[13]

Although prostaglandin inhibition provides effective symptomatic relief, there may be long-term deleterious effects of some NSAIDs on cartilage metabolism.[5] In vitro work in the horse had initially shown no evidence of deleterious effects on cartilage metabolism.[14] However, in a more recent study phenylbutazone was given to horses for 14 days, and serum was tested on articular cartilage explants in vitro. There was decreased proteoglycan synthesis to a degree similar to that with recombinant human interleukin-1β.[15] However, in the absence of any clinical associations between phenylbutazone

use and articular cartilage degeneration, continued appropriate use of NSAIDs is justified.

In summary NSAIDs remain the standard of care for first-line treatment of traumatically induced inflammation; they are routinely given preorthopedic and postorthopedic surgery; phenylbutazone and flunixin meglumine are the most commonly used; newer COX-2 preferential inhibitors are available but should not be viewed as absolute replacements to phenylbutazone and flunixin meglumine; NSAIDs are not corticosteroids; COX-1 is mainly responsible for protective prostaglandins; COX-2 plays some accessory role but is more important than previously thought. However, these facts still might not outweigh the beneficial effects of selective COX-2 inhibition in joint disease.

SPECIFIC USES OF NSAIDs

Use in Lameness and Inflammation

The most widely used NSAID in horses is phenylbutazone, based on efficacy, availability, and affordability. It can be given orally or intravenously. It is relatively nontoxic at repeated doses of 2.2 mg/kg twice daily or less.[16] With a single dose of 4.4 mg/kg plasma half-life is approximately 5.5 hours in horses and ponies.[17] However, a single phenylbutazone dose of 4.4 mg/kg markedly reduced PGE2 and PGI2 production in exudate for up to 24 hours.[18,19] This is explained by the accumulation of phenylbutazone in inflammatory exudate, leading to an elimination half-life in exudate of 24 hours (the proteinaceous nature of inflammatory fluid and phenylbutazone's high degree of protein binding probably explain this).[20] This has led to a general recommendation of once-daily dosing. There was a significant reduction of lameness in horses with experimentally induced synovitis for 8 to 10 hours after phenylbutazone was administered; decreases in joint temperature, synovial fluid (SF) volume, and SF PGE2 were also noted. In a comparison with ketoprofen, phenylbutazone effects were significantly greater.[21]

The mechanism of pain reduction is interesting, and it has been proposed that hyperalgesia is induced by lowering the nociceptive threshold level and allowing a pain response to a typically nonpainful stimuli. It has also been shown that NSAIDs inhibit prostaglandin production thereby returning nociceptive threshold towards normal.[22] Differentiation of nociceptive pain versus inflammatory pain was done in horses by looking at thermal invoked hoof withdrawal reflexes. Phenylbutazone (7.3 mg/kg) did not alter normal cutaneous pain perception (nociception), and it was concluded that the antiinflammatory effects provide the benefit.[23] The majority of studies in other species have shown that phenylbutazone is a weaker and effective analgesic at antiinflammatory doses in response to noxious thermal stimuli. Studies with a single dose of phenylbutazone (4.4 mg/kg) versus saline after 1 hour of experimentally induced lameness (adjustable Heart Bar shoe model creating a 4/5 grade lameness) showed that lameness scores were lower 2 to 8 hours posttreatment and heart rate was lower from 2 to 6 hours posttreatment ($P < 0.05$).[24] An evaluation of the effects of phenylbutazone in chronic forelimb (clinical) lameness, using a controlled crossover design in 9 horses, compared saline versus 4.4 mg/kg versus 8.8 mg/kg phenylbutazone once daily for 4 days with a minimum of 14 days between treatments. The mean peak vertical force (mPVF) increased at all posttreatment evaluation times with phenylbutazone (reflection of analgesia) and there was no advantage with higher doses (this agrees with the findings of Toutain et al.[25]). The clinical lameness scores significantly decreased at 6 and 8 hours but only at 24 hours with the high dose. There was no significant difference with mPVF at high or low doses.[26] As mentioned before when phenylbutazone and ketoprofen were compared in experimentally induced synovitis, the effects of phenylbutazone were significantly greater (Figure 11-6).[27] The authors propose that NSAIDs usually do not completely block pain; instead, they primarily reduce the hyperalgesia associated with the painful conditions, and these effects include reducing peripheral afferent discharge from hyperalgesic areas as well as having central antihyperalgesic effects.

Flunixin meglumine is also commonly used clinically at a dose of 1.1 mg/kg given once daily by intravenous (IV) or oral routes. Its half-life is relatively short. The onset of analgesia occurs within 2 hours and can persist up to 30 hours (it has been theorized that rapid accumulation at inflammatory foci is responsible for a longer duration of action versus short half-life).[28] Phenylbutazone and flunixin meglumine have been compared in navicular syndrome.[29] Twelve horses with navicular syndrome received phenylbutazone (4.4 mg/kg), flunixin meglumine (1.1 mg/kg), or saline IV once daily for 4 days with a 14-day washout. At 6, 12, and 24 hours after the fourth treatment, both lameness (American Association of Equine Practitioners grade) and peak vertical force (force plate) significantly improved versus saline. There was no significant difference between phenylbutazone and flunixin meglumine.

Another comparison was done between phenylbutazone alone or concurrent administration of phenylbutazone and flunixin meglumine in 29 horses with naturally occurring lameness (lameness measured by kinematic evaluation while trotting on treadmill 0 and 12 hours after NSAID administration). The combination (oral administration of phenylbutazone and IV administration of flunixin) for 5 days resulted in better clinical improvement of the lameness condition 12 hours after the last dose than phenylbutazone alone. After, horses that did not improve were excluded (5 horses), both regimens significantly alleviated

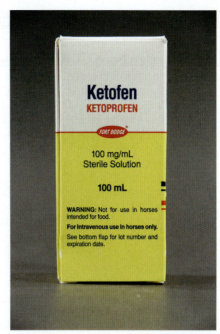

FIGURE 11-6 Ketoprofen (Ketofen®) is available for intravenous use in horses.

lameness. However, one horse in the combination group died of necrotizing colitis.[8] It was also noted that all posttreatment plasma concentrations of NSAIDs were less than those allowed by the USEF for a single NSAID at that time, and this led to concern over "stacking" of NSAIDs. A partial listing of available NSAIDs is illustrated in Table 11-1.

In an in vitro study looking at COX-1 and COX-2 inhibition in equine blood by phenylbutazone, flunixin, carprofen, and meloxicam (Figure 11-7), levels of COX were measured by in vitro enzyme-linked analyses. As expected comparisons of IC50 indicated that meloxicam and carprofen are more selective inhibitors of COX-2 than phenylbutazone and flunixin; of the four NSAIDs examined, meloxicam was the most advantageous for horses.[30] However, at IC80 phenylbutazone (+134.4%) and flunixin (+29.7%) had greater COX-2 selectivity than at IC50, and meloxicam (−41.2%) and carprofen (−12.9%) had lower COX-2 selectivity than at IC50. The authors propose that selectivity of NSAIDs should be assessed at the 80% as well as the 50% inhibition level. Further, that the therapeutic margins were not particularly high signifies that further work is needed to clarify the effect of COX-2 inhibitors in horses. The pharmacokinetics and safety of single and multiple oral doses of meloxicam in adult horses have been described.[31] In a comparative study of meloxicam versus phenylbutazone, it was shown that there was a decreased deleterious effect on gastric mucosal integrity with meloxicam.[32] Meloxicam was administered at the recommended daily dose of 0.6 mg/kg orally.

The one selective COX-2 inhibitor that has been licensed in the U.S. (firocoxib) was compared with oral phenylbutazone in a randomized controlled trial with 253 horses.[33] Horses were treated with firocoxib (0.1 mg/kg) or phenylbutazone (4.4 mg/kg) every 24 hours for 14 days. There was

TABLE 11-1	Partial Listing of Currently Available NSAIDs*				
Generic Name	Product Name	Formulations	Recommended Dose (mg/kg)	Standard Availability	Cost
Phenylbutazone	EQUI-PHAR Phenyl-butazone (Vedco, Inc.)	1 g tablet	4.4 bid for 1 day, 2.2 bid for 4 days, 2.2 sid	100 tabs	$12.35/100 tabs
	EQUI-PHAR (phenyl-butazone) injection 20% (Vedco, Inc.)	Injectable 20% 200 mg/mL	2.2-4.4 bid for 5 days	100 mL	$9.22/100 mL
	Phenylzone paste (Intervet/Merck Animal Health)	Paste	1-2.2 bid for 4 days	20 g syringe	$18.62/20 g syringe
Carprofen	Rimadyl (Zoetis)	Injectable 50 mg/mL	0.7 sid (IV)	20 mL	$96.80/20 mL
		Tablets 100 mg	4.4 sid (PO)	180 tabs	$185/180 tabs
Flunixin meglumine	Flu-Nix D (AgriLabs)	Injectable 50 mg/mL	1.1 sid for 5 days (IV, IM)	100 mL 250 mL	$12.64/100 mL $25.82/250 mL
	Banamine Paste (Intervet/Merck Animal Health)	Paste	1.1 sid for 5 days	30 g syringe	$23.98/30 g syringe
Ketoprofen	Ketofen (Zoetis)	Injectable 100 mg/mL	2.2 sid for 5 days (IV)	50 mL 100 mL	$90.52/50 mL $151.47/100 mL
Firocoxib	EQUIOXX Oral Paste (Merial)	Paste	0.1 mg/kg sid for up to 14 days	6.93 g syringe (box of 20 or 72)	$2.81/syringe

*Availability and costs are as of 2014.
bid, Twice daily; *IM*, intramuscular; *IV*, intravenous; *PO*, by mouth; *sid*, daily.

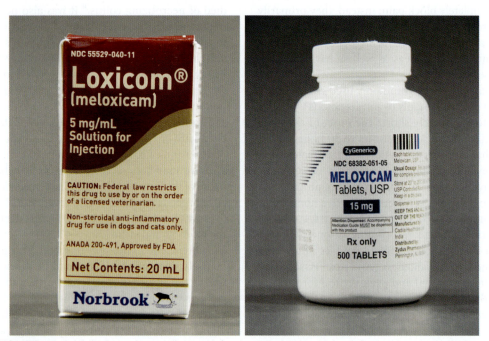

FIGURE 11-7 Meloxicam is not licensed for horses in the United States but is elsewhere. A recent comparison with phenylbutazone showed there was a lesser effect on gastric mucosal integrity with meloxicam.

no significant difference in overall clinical lameness score but the improvement was greater in firocoxib-treated horses for pain or manipulation on palpation ($P = 0.028$), joint circumference score ($P = 0.26$), and range of motion score ($P = 0.012$). Details on the pharmacokinetics and metabolism of orally administered firocoxib have also been presented.[34] In a study evaluating oral administration of firocoxib for the management of musculoskeletal pain and lameness associated with OA in horses, 390/429 horses from 80 sites and 20 states met the criteria for analysis. Signs of musculoskeletal pain or lameness attributed to OA were diagnosed in 197/360 (50.5%) horses and in multiple joints in 193/390 (49.5%). In those with involvement of a single joint, the tarsus was the most frequently affected joint 79/197 (40.1%) among the 390 horses with complete lameness data; improvement was reported in approximately 80% by day 14. Investigators rated 307 (78%) of horses improved, and owners or handlers rated 316 (81%) horses as improved at termination of the study. Horses treated with firocoxib paste had significant improvement in lameness scores from baseline values. Improvement was most rapid within the first 7 days after starting treatment and continued, albeit a slower rate, through treatment day 14. This study concluded that firocoxib significantly improved lameness scores throughout the 14-day period with few adverse reactions and is a safe COX-2-specific NSAID for the treatment of musculoskeletal pain and lameness associated with OA.[35] In another study of synovitis induced with lipopolysaccharide (LPS), upregulation of μ-opioid receptor (MOR) expression was demonstrated in equine synovial membrane.[36] Although upregulation of MOR-like protein was demonstrated in the inflamed synovial membrane of the placebo-treated horses, it was not apparent in the phenylbutazone-treated animals. Thus, the conclusion was that acute inflammation in the joint will upregulate MOR although phenylbutazone antiinflammatory treatment will attenuate this response.

The complexities of the effects of PGE2 were increased by a report that exogenous PGE2 significantly reduced equine IL-1β-induced expression of MMP-1, -3, -13, and TIMP-1. Abrogation of cytokine induction with PGE2 was comparable to that with dexamethasone.[37] The authors concluded that the potential for physiologically relevant regulation of expression of these genes by PGE2 is a consideration when considering drugs that inhibit prostanoid synthesis in the treatment of equine arthropathies. They also mentioned that, although certain studies suggest a catabolic effect of prostaglandin in joints, other data suggest that the E series prostaglandins are protective of cartilage matrix synthesis.[38] They also noted that these findings are similar to those of DiBattista et al., who showed that progressively higher doses of PGE2 essentially eliminated MMP-1 expression by synovial fibroblasts, but similar concentrations of prostanoids were only capable of reducing stromelysin expression to a certain level after which it was uninfluenced by further increases in dose.[39]

Postoperative Use of NSAIDs for Horses

In a study of postoperative analgesia using phenylbutazone, flunixin, or carprofen (another COX-2-selective drug), there was a significant difference in time after surgery during which further analgesia was needed. For flunixin (n=72) the mean time before further analgesia was needed was 12.8 ± 4.3 hours (mean ± SD), for carprofen 11.7 ± 6.9 hours, and for phenylbutazone 8.4 ± 4.6 hours.[40] Because there was no control group, it was possible that postoperative pain was minimal and all were ineffective. In another study comparing phenylbutazone or placebo postoperatively, 15 horses received phenylbutazone (4 mg/kg) IV before surgery and 2 mg/kg every 12 hours after up to 60 hours. Ten controls received saline at the same time. The total postoperative pain severity index was higher in the placebo group than the phenylbutazone group, suggesting some analgesic effect.[41] However, there was no difference in plasma β-endorphin, catecholamine concentrations, or

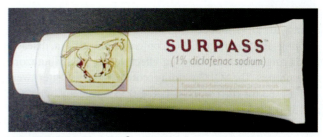

FIGURE 11-8 Surpass® (1% diclofenac sodium) is the only topical NSAID available and licensed for horses.

anesthetic recovery time and a low level of discomfort in the controls.

The usefulness of naproxen sodium (another COX-2-preferential NSAID) after arthroscopic meniscectomy in humans was evaluated in a randomized, double-blind prospective study. It was concluded that there was less pain, less synovitis, less effusion, more rapid return of movement in quadriceps function, and more rapid return to work and sport.[42] Whether or not these data can be extrapolated to assume long-term function improvement in horses is not clear. In another post-arthroscopy human study, there was no benefit from the intramuscular (IM) NSAID diclofenac sodium at surgery and with 100 mg daily for 7 days versus physiotherapy or no treatment (this was a prospective, randomized, controlled trial). At 42 days there was also no significant difference and complications were recorded in 9.6% of patients.[43] In a second study evaluating the clinical effects of naproxen sodium after human knee arthroscopy in a randomized controlled trial, 550 mg of naproxen once daily was compared with placebo. At 10 days in surgical arthroscopy cases, naproxen-treated patients had significant improvement in synovial effusion ($P < 0.01$), range of motion ($P < 0.001$), quadriceps strength ($P < 0.05$), pain ($P < 0.001$), walking activity ($P < 0.05$), and use of crutches ($P < 0.01$). In addition, at 20 days there were improvements in synovial effusion ($P < 0.05$), range of motion ($P < 0.01$), and pain ($P < 0.05$). In diagnostic arthroscopy there was a benefit in pain at 10 days ($P < 0.01$) and no benefit at 20 days.[44]

Evaluation of Topical Diclofenac

A licensed topical NSAID preparation, 1% diclofenac sodium cream (Surpass) (Figure 11-8) is now available in the U.S. but not in Europe. Previous human research indicated that topical NSAIDs could be clinically beneficial while reducing systemic side effects. Antiinflammatory effects were demonstrated experimentally in the horse using an induced subcutaneous inflammation model.[45] More recently, its value was demonstrated in equine OA using an osteochondral fragment-exercise model.[7] Using the carpal OA model, baseline lameness in OA joints was 2.52 ± 0.83 versus 0.40 ± 0.57 in the sham operated ($P < 0.001$). There was a significant treatment effect with change of lameness score: 20.27 ± 0.05 for phenylbutazone, 0.13 ± 0.05 for diclofenac cream (DLC), and 0.12 ± 0.05 for no treatment. The PGE2 concentration was significantly increased with OA: 217.06 ± 29.39 pg/mL versus 33 ± 3.80 pg/mL in the sham-operated joint, and treatment with phenylbutazone induced a significant decrease in SF PGE2 concentration versus both DLC and controls. However, treatment with DLC induced significant improvement in SOFG staining and cartilage GAG content, indicating a disease-modifying osteoarthritic drug effect versus phenylbutazone and controls. The SOFG staining scores (higher is better) were 0.71 ± 0.33 for the controls, 4.48 ± 0.33 for phenylbutazone, and 5.56 ± 0.33 for DLC.[7]

WHAT ARE THE NEGATIVE EFFECTS WITH USE OF NSAIDs?

The principal toxic effects with NSAIDs are gastrointestinal complications (particularly gastric ulceration) and negative effects on renal function. NSAIDs affect endogenous prostaglandin-associated cytoprotective mechanisms.[2] There is also evidence that all NSAIDs may have a direct toxic effect on the gastrointestinal mucosa.[46] Prostaglandins are involved in maintaining normal renal function and vascular hemostasis and coordinating actions of circulating hormones.[47] Provided that the drugs are used at clinical dose rates, however, such problems are uncommon in the horse.[1,48]

The question of whether or not phenylbutazone is harmful to articular cartilage has been addressed in the horse through in vitro studies, and the data are contradictory. Two in vitro studies found no evidence that phenylbutazone was harmful to cartilage.[14,49] In the latter study, induced proteoglycan loss was reduced by phenylbutazone at clinically relevant concentrations but not by Depo Medrol. Depo Medrol caused a dose-dependent suppression of proteoglycan synthesis in all concentrations.

In another combined in vivo/in vitro study, healthy 1- to 2-year-old horses were randomly assigned to the control (n=5) or treated group (4 mg of phenylbutazone/kg of body weight, orally, every 12 hours; n=6). Articular cartilage specimens were collected before treatment was initiated (day 0), after 14 days of treatment, and 2 weeks after cessation of treatment (day 30). Proteoglycan synthesis and stromelysin concentration in cartilage extracts were assessed after 72 hours of culture in medium alone or with recombinant human interleukin-1beta (IL-1β; 0.1 ng/mL). On day 0, proteoglycan synthesis was significantly less in cartilage explants cultured in IL-1β compared with medium alone. Mean proteoglycan synthesis in explants collected on days 14 and 30 was significantly less in treated horses versus controls. However, incubation of explants from treated horses with IL-1β did not result in a further decrease in proteoglycan synthesis. The authors concluded that oral administration of phenylbutazone for 14 days significantly decreased proteoglycan synthesis in articular cartilage explants from healthy horses to a degree similar to that induced by in vitro exposure to IL-1β. They therefore stated that phenylbutazone should be used judiciously in athletic horses with OA, because chronic administration may suppress proteoglycan synthesis and potentiate cartilage damage.[15] It is to be noted that 4.4 mg/kg twice daily for 30 days is a dose rate that far exceeds use in clinical practice.

In another study to determine the effects of phenylbutazone on bone activity and bone formation in horses, 6 healthy 1- to 2-year-old horses received phenylbutazone (4.4 mg/kg of body weight, orally, every 12 hours) and 6 healthy 1- to 2-year-old horses were used as controls. Biopsies were performed to obtain unicortical bone specimens from one tibia on day 0 and from the contralateral tibia on day 14. Fluorochromic markers were administered IV 2 days before and on days 0, 10, 15, and 25 after biopsy was performed, and all horses were euthanized at day 30 and tissues from biopsy sites with adjacent cortical bone were collected. The mineral apposition rate (MAR) and regional acceleratory phenomenon (RAP) were significantly reduced in phenylbutazone horses and filling of cortical defects significantly greater in control horses,[50] signifying that we need to pay attention to the science but no in vivo clinical associations have been made. In a review of the effects of NSAIDs on bone healing,[51] Barry noted that research using rodent and rabbit models provides strong evidences that NSAIDs negatively affect bone healing, but whether or not this effect is clinically important is controversial in both human and veterinary medicine. The study cited above[50] is the only equine study that insinuates anything and further work is needed to guide veterinarians as to appropriate dose and length of time for prescription of NSAIDs in general. In a study of the effect of oral administration of phenylbutazone on biomarkers of cartilage and bone metabolism in horses, there were no significant differences between control and treatment groups for the biomarkers chondroitin sulfate 846, procollagen type IIC propeptide, collagen II cleavage, and C-terminal telopeptide of type II collagen in serum or synovial fluid,[52] indicating minimal effects on articular cartilage. However, there was a significant increase in osteocalcin concentration in SF in the treatment group but no change for serum osteocalcin, which may suggest an anabolic effect of phenylbutazone on periarticular bone and which would not be considered a negative effect. In humans, MRIs of knee cartilage in older adults were compared with those of nonusers of NSAIDs (n=334), users of COX-2 inhibitors (n=40), and users of conventional NSAIDs (n=21). Compared with the first two groups, users of conventional NSAIDs had increased defects in both medial and lateral compartments of the knee.

POTENTIAL ANALGESIC EFFECTS OF NSAIDs WITH REGARD TO WITHDRAWAL FROM COMPETITION

A historical perspective of the genesis of regulated medication in the U.S. racing industry with phenylbutazone as the focus was recently provided.[53] In their introduction, the authors stated that "the impact of sustained effect on the health and welfare of the horse and its contribution to injuries during competition remains problematic." A thorough review is presented but the authors' interpretation of the literature, particularly the potential of causing musculoskeletal problems, is at some variance with what we feel the literature says. They cite a study by Sabaté et al.[54] where phenylbutazone and suxibuzone, a prodrug of phenylbutazone, were shown to be equally effective in the treatment of 155 lame horses in a multicenter, controlled, randomized, double-blind study. There were no significant differences in alleviating lameness in horses, but suxibuzone had better acceptability when administered orally with some food and the authors concluded that it was a good therapeutic alternative. Soma et al. noted that approximately 50% of the horses showed an improvement in 3 days of treatment with 30% showing an additional improvement at 6 days and stated that "this study illustrated the concern of many veterinarians as to the duration of administration of phenylbutazone."[53] We question the amount of concern from veterinarians regarding therapeutic doses of 4.4 mg/kg once daily. There is indeed a study that associated NSAID use and musculoskeletal injury in Thoroughbred racehorses in Kentucky.[55] It looked at the plasma levels of NSAIDs in injured horses at Kentucky racetracks from January 1, 1995, to December 1, 1996. During that period there were 84 catastrophic cases (euthanized horses) and 126 noncatastrophic musculoskeletal injuries. The plasma concentrations of phenylbutazone and flunixin were higher in injured horses than in control horses. Most injured and control horses did not have a detectable level of naproxen in their plasma samples. The authors recognize that further studies must be carried out to determine whether horses with higher plasma concentrations of NSAIDs have an altered risk of musculoskeletal injury compared with other horses. They also acknowledge that other possible risk factors (age, racetrack surface, length of race, gender, training program, preexisting pathologic conditions, etc.) contribute to musculoskeletal injuries of horses, and these must be eliminated and/or must be similar for each individual horse in future studies to determine the real role of NSAIDs as a possible risk factor for musculoskeletal injuries of racehorses.

Having acknowledged that, enforcement of a limit to administration of phenylbutazone in racehorses is certainly appropriate. The Racing Medication and Testing Consortium (RMTC) voted for a model rule change to reduce the threshold for phenylbutazone from 5 µg/mL to 2 µg/mL. This decision was based on a White Paper since published as a refereed article by Soma et al.[53] The article was based on studies that were conducted to determine PBS concentrations following various dosing schedules.[56-58] A dosing schedule of 4.4 mg/kg (2 g) for 3 to 4 days followed by a single IV dose of 4.4 mg/kg 24 hours before racing would result in a plasma phenylbutazone concentration that would not exceed 5 µg/mL.

There are marked differences between racehorses and sport horses in that fatal injuries in racehorses in 2009 were approximately 2/1000 starts (892 fatal injuries in 446,196 racing starts [Jockey Club Welfare Safety Summit 2009]). On the other hand, Shoemaker 2010 reported that USEF in 2009 recorded 1,717,352 starts and 18 deaths (6 were orthopedic) across all breeds and disciplines, which approximates to 1/100,000 starts. Despite this the British Equine Veterinary Association made a submission on the use of NSAIDs in competition horses in August 2010 protesting a recent announcement by FEI that it was going to adopt a "progressive list" of medications permissible for horses in competition to be an extremely retrograde step for equine welfare. The study used considerable extrapolation from racing. Ironically, the World AntiDoping Agency permits the unrestricted use of NSAIDs during competition in human athletes (www.wada). In contrast, FEI prohibits the use of NSAIDs at any level (FEI prohibited substance list, www.feicleansport.org).

REFERENCES

1. Lees P, Higgins AJ. Clinical pharmacology and therapeutic uses of non-steroidal antiinflammatory drugs in the horse. *Equine Vet J.* 1985;17(2):83–96.
2. May SA, Lees P. Non-steroidal anti-inflammatory drug. In: McIlwraith CW, Trotter GW, eds. *Joint disease in the horse.* Philadelphia, PA: Saunders; 1996:223–237.
3. Frisbie DD. Musculoskeletal system: medical treatment of joint disease. In: Auer JA, Stick JA, eds. *Equine surgery* (4th ed.). Philadelphia, PA: Elsevier Saunders; 2011:1114–1122.
4. Vane JR. Inhibition of prostaglandin synthesis as a mechanism of action for aspirin-like drugs. *Nature.* 1971;231(25):232–235.
5. Dingle DJ. Prostaglandins in human articular cartilage metabolism. *J Lipid Med.* 1993;6(2):303–312.
6. Malmberg AB, Yaksh TL. Hyperalgesia mediated by spinal glutamate or substance P receptor blocked by spinal cyclooxygenase inhibition. *Science.* 1992;257(5074):1276–1279.
7. Frisbie DD, McIlwraith CW, Kawcak CE, et al. Evaluation of topically administered diclofenac liposomal cream for treatment of horses with experimentally induced osteoarthritis. *Am J Vet Res.* 2009;70(2):210–215.
8. Keegan KG, Messer NT, Reed SK, et al. Effectiveness of administration of phenylbutazone alone or concurrent administration of phenylbutazone and flunixin meglumine to eliminate lameness in horses. *Am J Vet Res.* 2008;69(2):167–173.
9. Wallace JL, Reuter BK, McKnight W, et al. Selective inhibitors of cyclooxygenase-2: are they really effective, selective, and GI-safe? *J Clin Gastroenterol.* 1998;27(Suppl 1):S28.
10. Laine L, Harper S, Simon T, et al. A randomized trial comparing the effect of rofecoxib, a cyclooxygenase 2-specific inhibitor, with that of ibuprofen on the gastroduodenal mucosa of patients with osteoarthritis. Rofecoxib Osteoarthritis Endoscopy Study Group. *Gastroenterology.* 1999;117(4):776–783.
11. Frisbie DD. Current state of treatment of equine joint disease. In: *Proc Am Assoc Equine Pract FOCUS on Joints Meeting.* 2004:157–176.
12. Kunkel S, Chensue S. Arachidonic acid metabolites regulate interleukin-1 production. *Biochem Biophys Res Commun.* 1985;128(2):892–897.
13. Legendre LT, Tessmin RK, McClure SR, et al. Pharmacokinetics of firocoxib after administration of multiple consecutive daily doses to horses. *Am J Vet Res.* 2008;69(11):1399–1405.
14. Jolly WT, Whittem T, Jolly AC, et al. The dose-related effects of phenylbutazone and methylprednisolone acetate formulation (Depo-Medrol) on cultured explants of equine carpal articular cartilage. *J Vet Pharmacol Ther.* 1995;18(6):429–437.
15. Beluche LA, Bertone AL, Anderson DE, et al. Effects of oral administration of phenylbutazone to horses on in vitro articular cartilage metabolism. *Am J Vet Res.* 2001;62(12):1916–1921.
16. Collins LG, Tyler DE. Phenylbutazone toxicosis in the horse: a clinical study. *J Am Vet Med Assoc.* 1984;184(6):699–703.
17. Lees P, Taylor JB, Maitho TE, et al. Metabolism, excretion, pharmacokinetics and tissue residues of phenylbutazone in the horse. *Cornell Vet.* 1987;77(2):192–211.

18. Higgins AJ, Lees P. Phenylbutazone inhibition of prostaglandin E2 production in equine acute inflammatory exudate. *Vet Rec.* 1983;113:622–623.

19. Higgins AJ, Lees P, Taylor JB. Influence of phenylbutazone on eicosanoid levels in equine acute inflammatory exudate. *Cornell Vet.* 1984;74(3):198–207.

20. Lees P, Taylor JB, Higgins AJ, et al. Phenylbutazone and oxyphenbutazone distribution into tissue fluids in the horse. *J Vet Pharmacol Ther.* 1986;9(2):204–212.

21. Owens JG, Kamerling SG, Stanton SR, et al. Effects of pretreatment with ketoprofen and phenylbutazone on experimentally induced synovitis in horses. *Am J Vet Res.* 1996;57(6):866–874.

22. Johnston SA, Fox SM. Mechanisms of action of anti-inflammatory medications used for the treatment of osteoarthritis. *J Am Vet Med Assoc.* 1997;210(10):1486–1492.

23. Kamerling SG, Weckman TJ, DeQuick DJ, et al. A method for studying cutaneous pain perception and analgesia in horses. *J Pharmacol Methods.* 1985;13(3):267–274.

24. Foreman JH, Barange A, Lawrence LM, et al. Effects of single-dose intravenous phenylbutazone on experimentally induced, reversible lameness in the horse. *J Vet Pharmacol Ther.* 2007;31(1):39–44.

25. Toutain PL, Autefage A, Legrand C, et al. Plasma concentrations and therapeutic efficacy of phenylbutazone and flunixin meglumine in the horse: pharmacokinetic/pharmacodynamic modeling. *J Vet Pharm Ther.* 1994;17(6):459–469.

26. Hu HH, MacAllister CG, Payton ME, et al. Evaluation of the analgesic effects of phenylbutazone administered at a high or low dosage in horses with chronic lameness. *J Am Vet Med Assoc.* 2005;226(3):414–417.

27. Owens JG, Kammerling SG, Stanton SR, et al. Effects of ketoprofen and phenylbutazone on chronic hoof pain and lameness in the horse. *Equine Vet J.* 1995;27(4):296–300.

28. Houdeshell JW, Hennessey PW. A new non-steroidal anti-inflammatory analgesic for horses. *J Equine Med Surg.* 1977;1(2):57–63.

29. Erkert RS, MacAllister CG, Payton ME, et al. Use of force plate analysis to compare the analgesic effects of intravenous administration of phenylbutazone and flunixin meglumine in horses with navicular syndrome. *Am J Vet Res.* 2005;66(2):284–288.

30. Beretta C, Garavaglia G, Cavalli M. COX-1 and COX-2 inhibition in horse blood by phenylbutazone, flunixin, carprofen and meloxicam: an in vitro analysis. *Pharmacol Res.* 2005;52(4):302–306.

31. Noble G, Edwards S, Lievaart J, et al. Pharmacokinetics and safety of single and multiple oral doses of meloxicam in adult horses. *J Vet Intern Med.* 2012;26(5):1192–1201.

32. Arcy-Moskwa ED, Noble GK, Weston LA, et al. Effects of meloxicam and phenylbutazone on equine gastric mucosal permeability. *J Vet Intern Med.* 2012;26(6):1494–1499.

33. Doucet MY, Bertone AL, Hendrickson D, et al. Comparison of efficacy and safety of paste formulations of firocoxib and phenylbutazone in horses with naturally occurring osteoarthritis. *J Am Vet Med Assoc.* 2008;232(1):91–97.

34. Kvaternick V, Pollmeier M, Fischer J, et al. Pharmacokinetics and metabolism of orally administered firocoxib, a novel second generation coxib, in horses. *J Vet Pharmacol Ther.* 2007;30(3):208–217.

35. Orsini JA, Ryan WG, Carithers DS, et al. Evaluation of oral administration of firocoxib for the management of musculoskeletal pain and lameness associated with osteoarthritis in horses. *Am J Vet Res.* 2012;73(5):664–671.

36. Van Loon JP, de Grauw JC, Brunott A, et al. Upregulation of articular synovial membrane μ-opioid-like receptors in an acute equine synovitis model. *Vet J.* 2013;196(1):40–46.

37. Tung JT, Arnold CE, Alexander LH, et al. Evaluation of the influence of prostaglandin E2 on recombinant equine interleukin-1beta-stimulated matrix metalloproteinases 1, 3 and 13 and tissue inhibitor of matrix metalloproteinase 1 expression in equine chondrocyte cultures. *Am J Vet Res.* 2002;63(7):987–993.

38. Goldring MB, Suen L-F, Yamin R, et al. Regulation of collagen gene expression by prostaglandins and interleukin-1 beta in culture chondrocytes and fibroblasts. *M J Ther.* 1996;3(1):9–16.

39. DiBattista JA, Martel-Pelletier J, Fujimoto N, et al. Prostaglandins E2 and E1 inhibit cytokine induced metalloproteinase expression in human synovial fibroblasts. *Lab Invest.* 1994;71(2):270–278.

40. Johnson CB, Taylor PM, Young SS, et al. Postoperative analgesia using phenylbutazone, flunixin or carprofen in horses. *Vet Rec.* 1993;133(14):336–338.

41. Raekallio M, Taylor PM, Bennett RC. Preliminary investigations of pain and analgesia assessment in horses administered phenylbutazone or placebo after arthroscopic surgery. *Vet Surg.* 1997;26(2):150–155.

42. Ogilvie-Harris DJ, Bauer M, Corey P. Prostaglandin inhibition and the rate of recovery after arthroscopic meniscectomy. A randomised double-blind prospective study. *J Bone Joint Surg Br.* 1985;67(4):567–571.

43. Birch NC, Sly C, Brooks S, Powles DP. Anti-inflammatory drug therapy after arthroscopy of the knee. A prospective, randomised, controlled trial of diclofenac or physiotherapy. *J Bone Joint Surg Br.* 1993;75(4):650–652.

44. Rasmussen S, Thomsen S, Madsen SN, et al. The clinical effect of naproxen sodium after arthroscopy of the knee: a randomized, double-blind, prospective study. *Arthroscopy.* 1993;9(4):375–380.

45. Caldwell FJ, Mueller PO, Lynn RC, et al. Effect of topical application of diclopenac liposomal suspension on experimental induced subcutaneous inflammation in horses. *Am J Vet Res.* 2004;65(3):271–276.

46. Lichtenberger LM, Wang ZM, Romero JJ, et al. Non-steroidal anti-inflammatory drugs (NSAIDs) associated with Zwitterionic phospholipids: insight into the mechanism and reversal of NSAID-induced gastrointestinal injury. *Nat Med.* 1995;1(2):154–158.

47. Meade EA, Smith WL, DeWitt DL. Differential inhibition of prostaglandin endoperoxide synthase (cyclooxygenase) isozymes by aspirin and other non-steroidal anti-inflammatory drugs. *J Biol Chem.* 1993;268(9):6610–6614.

48. Fennell LC, Franklin RP. Do nonsteroidal anti-inflammatory drugs administered at therapeutic dosages induce gastric ulceration in horses? *Equine Vet Edu.* 2009;21(12):660–662.

49. Frean SP, Cambridge H, Lees P. Effects of anti-arthritic drugs on proteoglycan synthesis by equine cartilage. *J Vet Pharmacol Ther.* 2002;25(4):289–298.

50. Rohde C, Anderson DE, Bertone AL, et al. Effects of phenylbutazone on bone activity and formation in horses. *Am J Vet Res.* 2000;61(5):537–543.

51. Barry S. Non-steroidal anti-inflammatory drugs inhibit bone healing: a review. *Vet Comp Orthop Traumatol.* 2010;23(6):385–392.

52. Fradette ME, Céleste C, Richard H, et al. Effects of continuous oral administration of phenylbutazone on biomarkers of cartilage and bone metabolism in horses. *Am J Vet Res.* 2007;68(2):128–133.

53. Soma LR, Uboh CE, Maylin GM. The use of phenylbutazone in the horse. *J Vet Pharmacol Ther*. 2012;35(1):1–12.

54. Sabaté D, Homedes J, Salichs M, et al. Multicentre, controlled, randomized and blinded field study comparing efficacy of suxibuzone and phenylbutazone in lame horses. *Equine Vet J*. 2009;41(7):700–705.

55. Dirikolu L, Woods WE, Boyles J, et al. Nonsteroidal antiinflammatory agents and musculoskeletal injuries in Thoroughbred racehorses in Kentucky. *J Vet Pharmacol Ther*. 2009;32(3):271–279.

56. Soma LR, Gallis DE, Davis WL, et al. Phenylbutazone kinetics and metabolite concentrations in the horse after five days of administration. *Am J Vet Res*. 1983;44(11):2104–2109.

57. Houston T, Chay S, Woods WE, et al. Phenylbutazone and its metabolites in plasma and urine of Thoroughbred horses: population distributions and effects of urinary pH. *J Vet Pharmacol Ther*. 1985;8(2):136–149.

58. Soma LR, Sams R, Duer W, et al. Plasma and serum concentrations of phenylbutazone and oxyphenbutazone in racing Thoroughbreds 24 hours after treatment with various dosage regimens. *Am J Vet Res*. 1985;46(4):932–938.

12

Intraarticular Corticosteroids*

C. Wayne McIlwraith

The use of corticosteroids for musculoskeletal conditions in horses was first reported in 1955.[1] The use of intraarticular (IA) corticosteroids is commonplace and an important part of the armamentarium of practitioners caring for equine sport horses (racing and otherwise), but it also continues to incite controversy. The Thoroughbred horse racing industry has come under renewed scrutiny in recent years in the United States because of horses suffering catastrophic injury during high-profile events. Consequently, the public outcry over these events has led to Congressional oversight and investigation, which in turn has led to significant scrutiny of medications that are used in the sport. Anabolic steroids were banned in 2008[2] and now other medications are also being critically reviewed. Intraarticular use of corticosteroids has become a recent focus (or refocus) of attention. Proponents of IA corticosteroid treatment argue that such therapy is needed to decrease inflammation and musculoskeletal pain, which is common in the Thoroughbred race horse, and more importantly, to avoid overloading the other limbs, possibly leading to catastrophic injury. However, opponents of corticosteroid use feel that it is merely masking pain and leads to joint deterioration. Much of this perception of harm is based on opinion and has been passed on down through the literature.[3]

EARLY HISTORY OF CORTICOSTEROID USE IN EQUINE JOINT DISEASE

The use of hydrocortisone in the treatment of a variety of musculoskeletal conditions in 94 horses and cattle was first reported in 1955.[1] The author cited profound improvements in clinical signs in most cases, but also cautioned that treated animals should be rested after injection to allow healing of affected tissues. This report was followed by a series of investigations by Van Pelt and co-workers in the 1960s and early 1970s evaluating certain effects of various corticosteroid preparations in a wide variety of clinical conditions.[4-8] A small number of clinical trials were also reported in the mid-1970s.[9-13] Mostly favorable results were reported, but

these studies were poorly controlled, which compromised the interpretation of the results.

To the author's knowledge, the first paper indicting corticosteroids as harmful in the horse was written by O'Conner.[14] This review addressed some important points but was based solely on human literature. The statement "An endless destructive cycle is set into motion which, if continued, will produce a steroid arthropathy which can render the horse useless." was referenced to an abstract written by an anonymous author.[15] Six other human-based references (four textbook chapters and two journal articles) were quoted, and one of them alluded to corticosteroids producing Charcot-like arthropathy. Charcot arthropathy is a human neurogenic disease that results in the loss of sensation, loss of proprioceptive control, instability, and arthritis and is most often a sequel to syphilis. There has never been any scientific demonstration of a comparable response associated with corticosteroid usage in horses but some authors continue to perpetuate the concept of analogy to Charcot arthropathy.[16-18] Salter et al., however, commented that "as yet, no absolute proof exists that the reported deterioration of human joints following repeated IA injections of hydrocortisone is caused by the hydrocortisone."[18] In the chapter on steroidal antiinflammatory agents in his textbook, Tobin's quotes included "A patient on corticosteroids can walk all the way to the autopsy room" and "A horse can wear a joint surface right down to the bone running on a glucocorticoid-injected joint."[19] Instances of degenerative joint disease caused by corticosteroids were presented without proof of such a pathogenesis.[19]

EARLY EVALUATIONS OF DIRECT EFFECTS

A number of studies have evaluated the effect of methylprednisolone acetate (MPA) injected into normal equine joints. In the first study, Marcoux injected 80 mg of 6-alpha-methylprednisolone acetate into equine carpal joints and compared the response to repeated injections of blood (simulating hemarthrosis).[20] He concluded that repeated injections into normal equine articulations did not have any direct toxic effects on the articular tissue, and that the injection of the vehicle of MPA did not alter the articular structures. He also noted that the volume of synovial fluid was diminished in joints receiving corticosteroids and questioned whether or not lesions might have occurred if the animals had been under forced exercise.

*The author wishes to acknowledge a previous publication, from which much of the information in this chapter has been drawn: McIlwraith C.W. (2010). The use of intra-articular corticosteroids in the horse: what is known on a scientific basis? *Equine Vet J* 42(6), 563-571.

In another study, eight mature horses with no prior signs of joint disease or history of IA therapy were treated with eight weekly IA injections of MPA.[21] Treatments were given at a dose of 120 mg/joint into the right antebrachiocarpal and middle carpal joints with the left joints used as untreated controls. Decreased staining for glycosaminoglycan (GAG) was seen in the articular cartilage, as was increased chondrocyte necrosis, hypocellularity, and articular cartilage fibrillation. The proteoglycan content of the articular cartilage was reduced to 56.52% of the control values, and the proteoglycan content decreased further at the 4- and 8-week recovery periods to 40.77% and 35.17% of the control values, respectively. The rate of proteoglycan synthesis as measured by $^{35}SO_4$ uptake was reduced to 17.04% of the control values after the last injection, and 4 weeks later increased to 55.31% and 71.28% of the control values, respectively, but these synthetic rates are still less than the controls. The doses used in this study were high by clinical standards, and with both joints injected could be considered particularly high.

In a third study, Trotter et al. evaluated the effect of MPA on normal equine articular cartilage by injecting 100 mg 3 times at 14-day intervals into middle carpal joints.[22] Horses remained clinically normal during the study and significant radiographic changes were not observed. Articular cartilage fibrillation was not evident in any joint, but Safranin O matrix staining intensity and uronic acid content (a measure of GAG content) were significantly lower in the treated joints.

Meagher looked at the effects of MPA and continued exercise in horses with carpal fractures that measured 1 cm wide and 2.5 cm in length (more like a slab fracture).[23] There was one control horse and five horses with bilateral fractures created with arthrotomy, making this a particularly severe model. One middle carpal joint received MPA 120 mg; the other one was an untreated control. The horses were galloped for 4.5 to 5 miles daily from the 22nd day until the 78th day. Cartilage erosion and periarticular proliferation occurred in the nontreated joints (probably related to instability and arthrotomy), with changes more severe in the joints injected with MPA. This study was considered to confirm previous statements that adequate rest is required after injection of IA corticosteroids. Degenerative changes were also reported following IA corticosteroid administration in a horse with a clinical slab fracture.[24] In this particular study, both the joint with the slab fracture and the opposite middle carpal joint were treated with 120 mg MPA, and the horse exercised on the track. The degenerative changes were considered to be typical of "steroid-induced arthropathy."[24]

There has been long-standing controversy surrounding the use of IA corticosteroids because of the concern that overuse of a pain-free joint could result in accelerated cartilage degeneration and this impression has been compounded by reports of negative effects of corticosteroids on chondrocyte metabolism.[25] It is to be noted that all studies discussed in this section were conducted with one specific corticosteroid, MPA.

MORE RECENT RESEARCH ON BENEFICIAL AND DELETERIOUS EFFECTS IN IN VIVO AND IN VITRO EQUINE MODELS

The use of IA corticosteroids for equine joint disease was extensively reviewed in 1996,[26] and the specific benefits and deleterious side effects of IA corticosteroids in the horse have been further clarified since then. Corticosteroids are potent antiinflammatory agents, and they inhibit the inflammatory process at all levels. Although traditional thinking has ascribed corticosteroid antiinflammatory effects to stabilization of lysosomal membranes with a concomitant release of lysosomal enzymes, the antiinflammatory effect is now known to be much more complex and far reaching.[27] Glucocorticoids exert their effects through cytoplasmic receptors. In addition to the well-known general effects of reducing capillary dilation, margination, migration, and accumulation of inflammatory cells, glucocorticoids inhibit the synthesis and release of several soluble mediators, including acting on the prostaglandin cascade. They have been shown to inhibit interleukin-1 (IL-1), considered the most important mediator of cartilage degradation and tumor necrosis factor (TNFα) at low concentrations.[28] Pain relief is attributed to inhibition of prostaglandin synthesis in large measure, specifically by inhibiting the enzyme phospholipase A2 and cyclooxygenase (COX)-2 expression in the arachidonic cascade.[25] Some more recent work with equine cartilage explants explored corticosteroid activities. The plasma serum protease activator protein C (APC) has been shown to be synthesized by human chondrocytes in sites of pathologic cartilage fibrillation and in vitro work had shown that APC synergizes with interleukin-1 beta (IL-1β) to promote degradation from articular cartilage.[29] In this study examining possible disease modification with corticosteroids, APC synergized with IL-1 or TNFα, promoting significant collagen degradation from equine cartilage explants within 4 days, but it did not augment GAG release. APC activated promatrix metalloproteinases (MMP-2) but not pro-MMP-9 as assessed by gelatin cymography. APC did not directly activate pro-MMP-13. Dexamethasone, triamcinolone, and MPA were evaluated at concentrations between 10^{-5} M and 10^{-10} M, and high concentrations significantly increased GAG release from IL-1 plus APC-treated explants. With the exception of MPA 10^{-10} M, all concentrations of corticosteroids caused significant decreases in IL-1 plus APC-driven hydroxyproline loss. Treatment with corticosteroids also decreased expression of MMP-1, -3, and -13 mRNA.[29] This attenuation of degradative response in the cartilage by corticosteroids commonly used in clinical practice supported in vivo studies that showed disease-modifying activity with triamcinolone acetonide (TA). The results with MPA differed somewhat from those seen in in vivo studies showing degradative effects on articular cartilage.

Controlled studies have been done in the horse in vivo to clarify therapeutic response, as well as deleterious effects of three commonly used corticosteroids (Figure 12-1). Based on the author's observation of an apparent lack of correlation

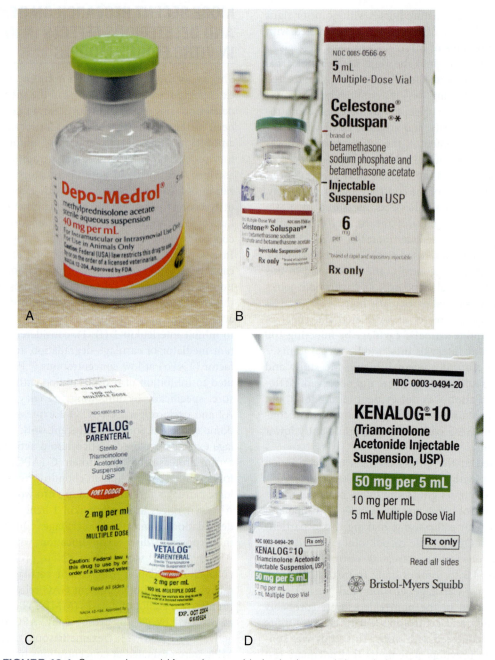

FIGURE 12-1 Commonly used IA corticosteroids in the horse: (**A**) methylprednisolone acetate (Depo-Medrol), (**B**) betamethasone sodium phosphate and betamethasone acetate (Celestone Soluspan), (**C**) triamcinolone acetonide (Vetalog), (**D**) triamcinolone acetonide (Kenalog-10; this is a higher concentration of 10 mg/mL licensed for human use but commonly used in horses).

between prior use of betamethasone esters (Betavet Soluspan®) and articular cartilage degradation during arthroscopic surgery for osteochondral chip removal in the early 1980s, experimental studies of betamethasone esters (Betavet Soluspan) followed by the other two commonly used IA corticosteroids MPA [Depo-Medrol®] and TA [Vetalog®] were initiated using an osteochondral fragment model developed at Colorado State University (CSU).[30-32]

Osteochondral fragments were created arthroscopically on the distal aspect of both middle carpal joints in 12 horses and one joint was treated with 2.5 mL of Betavet Soluspan®

(now available as Celestone Soluspan®) at 14 days after surgery and repeated in 35 days.[30] The opposite joint was injected with saline as a control. No deleterious side effects to the articular cartilage (based on histology, histochemistry, and uronic acid content) were demonstrated. In addition, comparison of exercise versus nonexercise on injected joints showed that exercise also did not have any harmful effects in the presence of corticosteroid administration.

In subsequent studies with IA corticosteroids (as well as other treatments) the model was modified so that the opposite joint was a sham-operated control instead of a chip

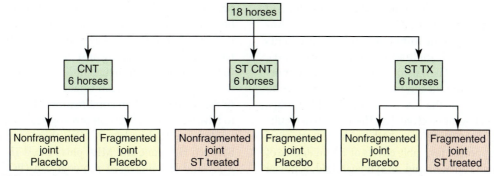

FIGURE 12-2 Design of experiments to assess the value of direct IA injection of a corticosteroid into an osteoarthritic joint (ST TX) and injection of IA corticosteroid in a remote joint (ST CNT) versus a saline-injected control (CNT). *ST,* Steroid; *TX,* therapy.

fragment. The model was also modified to more effectively produce early osteoarthritic change by leaving bone and cartilage debris within the joint. Depo-Medrol and Vetalog were tested using three groups and the test system is depicted in Figure 12-2.[31,32] Eighteen horses were randomly assigned to each of 3 groups (6 horses/group). Both middle carpal joints in the placebo control group (CNT) horses were injected intraarticularly with polyionic fluid. The corticosteroid control group horses (ST CNT) were injected with corticosteroid in the middle carpal joint without an osteochondral fragment and the opposite middle carpal joint was injected with a similar volume of polyionic fluid. The corticosteroid-treated group horses (ST TX) were treated with corticosteroid in the joint that contained the osteochondral fragment and the opposite middle carpal joint was injected with a single volume of polyionic fluid. All horses were treated intraarticularly on days 14 and 28 after surgery and exercised on a high-speed treadmill for 6 weeks, starting on day 15.

In joints containing an osteochondral fragment and treated with MPA there was reduction, although not significant, in the degree of lameness; however, there was a significant effect on PGE2 levels in the synovial fluid and lower scores for intimal hyperplasia and vascularity (no effect on cellular infiltration) in the synovial membrane compared to placebo-treated joints.[32] Of more importance, modified Mankin scores (a score of negative histopathologic change in the articular cartilage) were significantly increased in association with MPA, confirming deleterious effects of IA administration of MPA on articular cartilage.[32] All of these changes were observed at 70 days, which is 42 days after the second and last injection of MPA. Synovial aspiration was difficult (low volume, high viscosity) after treatment with MPA, which was not seen with other corticosteroids tested. In other work, repetitive IA administration of MPA to exercising horses altered the mechanical integrity of articular cartilage, but there was no effect on subchondral or cancellous bone.[33] In an earlier publication investigating joint function and healing after IA administration of 120-mg MPA, it inhibited the development and maturation of repair tissue of surgically-created full-thickness articular cartilage defects in exercised horses at 42 days and incited potential long-term (180 days) detrimental synovial membrane

inflammation.[34] However a single dose of MPA did not cause long-term detrimental effects (180 days) in the quality of the repair tissue (percentage of fibrocartilage).

In vitro studies have also demonstrated negative effects with IA MPA. Byron et al.[35] showed a significant decrease in proteoglycans in chondrocytes after MPA administration in vitro. Fubini et al.[36] showed a similar response in that MPA led to a decrease in matrix protein markers and chondrocyte differentiation. Murphy et al.,[37] however, showed that in the face of an inflammatory environment, MPA was beneficial to the articular cartilage. Galon et al.[38] examined gene expression of peripheral blood monocytes and hypothesized that the beneficial effects of MPA on inflammation may be more positive than the direct negative effects to the articular cartilage. However, as previously presented, the one controlled in vivo study in the horse confirmed that MPA caused deleterious effects that exceeded the benefits from inhibiting inflammation.[32]

A more recent study examined both MPA and lidocaine for their potential toxicity to bovine articular chondrocytes cultured in alginate beads and exposed to either 0.9% saline solution (negative control) MPA (4, 8, and 16 mg/mL), MPA (8 mg/mL) with 1% lidocaine, or MPA (8 mg/mL) and saline solution in a simulated inflammatory environment (IL-1β exposure).[39] Flow cytometry was used to assess chondrocyte viability. The results showed a dose- and time-dependent decrease in chondrocyte viability after exposure to clinically relevant doses of MPA. The combination of MPA and lidocaine was the most toxic with virtually no cells surviving after treatment. In addition, MPA did not mitigate the inflammatory effects of IL-1β; rather, it further potentiated the chondrotoxicity. As with humans, IA corticosteroids and local anesthetics are used together in equine practice and these findings are quite relevant. The combined use of IA administered local anesthetic solutions and nonsteroidal antiinflammatory drugs (NSAIDs) has been reported in horses,[40,41] but potential side effects of IA local analgesia and IA corticosteroids have not been tested.

Examination of TA (Vetalog) in the CSU model showed entirely different results from those seen with MPA. Horses that were treated intraarticularly with 12 mg TA (at days 14 and 28) in a joint containing a fragment were less lame than horses in the CNT and ST CNT groups (see Figure 12-1).

Horses treated with TA in either joint had lower protein and higher hyaluronan (HA) and GAG concentrations in synovial fluid. Synovial membrane from CNT and ST CNT joints had less inflammatory cell infiltration, intimal hyperplasia, and subintimal fibrosis. Analysis of articular cartilage morphologic parameters showed the modified Mankin score to be significantly better in the TA CNT and TA TX groups irrespective of which joint received TA. These positive results were observed 48 days after the second and last injection of TA. The results supported favorable effects of TA on degree of clinically detectable lameness and on synovial fluid, synovial membrane, and articular cartilage morphologic parameters, both with direct IA administration and remote site administration versus placebo injections.[31] Additionally, evaluation of the effects of IA TA on subchondral bone showed no deleterious effects.[42]

These studies, coupled with some recent in vitro work demonstrating protective effects of TA,[43] have fueled the recommendation that the use of TA is ideal, especially in high motion joints. There have been some opinions that low-dose administration alleviates the negative effects of MPA; however, based on in vitro titration studies in our laboratory, it appears that the lower doses commonly used are unlikely to have the same effects and a greater concentration of MPA (equivalent to 100 mg in middle carpal joint) is needed to inhibit the catabolic compared to the anabolic effects in articular cartilage.[44] Some clinicians feel that the "low" dose is clinically effective, but it has not been supported by in vitro work. A study of the commonly used dose of 40 mg in the osteochondral model will be an interesting comparison.

Recently, IA administration of TA and mepivacaine was combined both to confirm the site of lameness and treat synovitis at the same time.[45] Lameness and joint inflammation were produced in a short-term model of inflammation with IA injection of lipopolysaccharide (LPS). Mepivacaine alone effectively eliminated lameness for 45 minutes after injection, regardless of whether TA was also administered, and 9 mg of TA reduced lameness and concentration of synovial fluid protein after the second LPS injection regardless of whether or not mepivacaine was also injected. TA could be detected in synovial fluid samples for at least 10 days following drug administration (detected in serum at low concentrations 12 hours after administration regardless of whether mepivacaine was coadministered). These findings are in accordance with another pharmacodynamic study, in which 6 mg of TA could be detected at low concentrations in those joints for up to 14 days and in plasma for at least 24 hours.[46]

CAN ADJUNCTIVE USE OF HYALURONAN IN CONJUNCTION WITH METHYLPREDNISOLONE ACETONIDE MITIGATE THE DELETERIOUS EFFECTS?

IA corticosteroids have commonly been combined with HA, and there is a perception that HA might be protective against any deleterious effects of MPA. This perception has been based on tradition rather than scientific proof, but has become quite common among equine practitioners.[47] Two in vitro equine studies have addressed whether HA might have a mitigating effect against the deleterious effects of MPA. In the first, HA addition had little effect on MPA-induced cartilage matrix proteoglycan catabolism in cartilage explants.[48] In the second, MPA in combination with HA was considered to have beneficial effects on proteoglycan metabolism in IL-1-treated equine chondrocytes (but there were no comparisons between HA alone and MPA plus HA).[49] The combination of MPA and HA increased proteoglycan (PG) synthesis compared with untreated IL-1-insulted explants. It needs to be recognized that increase in proteoglycan synthesis can be an early part of OA and that in vitro studies do not necessarily mimic the in vivo situation.

COMBINED USE OF HYALURONAN AND TRIAMCINOLONE ACETONIDE

There is some support that the combination of TA and HA is beneficial based on a study of 16 human patients with knee osteoarthritis (OA). This was a 1-year, single-blind, randomized study in which 24 patients were treated with IA HA once weekly for 3 weeks and then again at 6 months (total of 6 injections).[50] Sixteen of these patients also had 1 mL of TA before the first and fourth HA injections and evaluation using the WOMAC index (used to assess patients with OA of the hip or knee using 24 parameters including 5 indices of pain, 2 of stiffness, 7 of social function, and 10 of emotional function). Results were better with the combination of these two products. There was no progression of OA on MRI in either group.

There is indirect evidence that the use of HA with TA could provide clinical benefit in the horse. In a recent study the use of IA HA as well as IA Adequan® was assessed in the CSU chip fragment model. IA injection of 20 mg of HA was done at 14, 21, and 28 days.[51] There was significantly less cartilage fibrillation with HA at day 70 despite less impressive reduction of synovial effusion and synovial membrane vascularity and subintimal fibrosis versus Adequan.[52] The combination of the potent antiinflammatory effects of TA and the chondroprotective effects of HA is, therefore, logical. However, a very recent paper assessed intraarticular treatment with triamcinolone combined with hyaluronate compared to triamcinolone alone.[52] This was a randomized open-label multicenter clinical trial in 80 lame horses from 13 clinics with the primary outcome parameter being clinical success rate defined as greater or equal to 2 grades lameness reduction (on a 0-5 scale) at three weeks. The success rate of IA TA three weeks after treatment was 87.8% while that of TA plus HA was 64.1% ($P = 0.01$). At three months half the horses in each group were back in full work regardless of treatment assignment. This study did not provide any evidence that a combination of TA with high MW HA is more effective than TA alone for treatment of joint related lameness but recognized limitations in that only a single clinical sign was assessed.[52] Another recent study combining TA with Adequan had inferior results to each product alone[53] and, therefore, broad generalizations on combination therapy should not be made.

LAMINITIS: A SUGGESTED POTENTIAL COMPLICATION OF INTRAARTICULAR CORTICOSTEROID USE

Fear of laminitis has also caused less use of TA by some equine practitioners, despite scientific studies demonstrating its effectiveness as well as its chondroprotective properties. There have been anecdotal associations made and maximum doses established based on a report of no cases of laminitis in 1200 horses treated when a dose did not exceed 18 mg.[54] A more recent follow-up study with data on the potential for TA to produce laminitis concludes that there was no association between the occurrence of laminitis and the IA use of TA.[55]

A legal case in the United Kingdom, where a horse developed laminitis after receiving 80 mg of TA in each tarsus and 20 mg of dexamethasone in its back,[56] led to a review of the literature[57] and a retrospective study of one clinician's cases.[58] The literature review revealed that good evidence linking laminitis to corticosteroid injection was lacking and that a large-scale multicenter trial was needed.[57] In a third publication,[58] the clinician reported that laminitis associated with IA injection of corticosteroids had occurred in 3/2000 (0.15%) cases. TA was most often used and the upper total dose ranged from 20 to 45 mg.[58] In general, the literature supports the use of total body doses of 45 mg as safe. Having said that, there have been individual reports of laminitis associated with lower doses, but in cases that the author is aware of there have been additional factors, including stress through transportation, preparation for sales, or adjunctive administration of other corticosteroids systemically or into nonarticular areas.

Use of Corticosteroids in Low-motion versus High-motion Joints

Another traditional concept has been that, although it is better not to use MPA (Depo-Medrol) in high-motion joints, its use in low-motion joints (such as the distal tarsal joints) is appropriate. The implication is that the state of the articular cartilage in these joints is not as important and may be able to promote ankylosis. There is no evidence yet that we can promote ankylosis in this fashion, and the other side of this argument is that we should preserve articular cartilage whenever we can. A retrospective study of the effect of IA treatment of OA in the distal tarsal joints with MPA or TA (with or without HA) led to a positive outcome in only 38% of horses.[59] The entry requirement for the study was a 50% or better improvement after IA analgesia. The authors recognized that because of diffuse analgesia, including in the proximal suspensory area, some of the cases that did not respond may have had clinical problems other than OA of the distal tarsal joints. Also, horses with OA of the distal intertarsal or tarsal metatarsal joint responded better than horses with disease in the proximal intertarsal joint. Horses treated once with IA MPA or TA either with or without HA improved after a median of 56 days ($P < 0.001$) and there was no significant difference between MPA and TA. These findings

of clinical effectiveness at 56 days are supported by our studies with the CSU chip fragment model when effectiveness was still observed at day 70 when treatments with TA and MPA had been given at days 14 and 28. Our experimental studies have indicated that there is a systemic or remote effect with corticosteroids, and even with MPA in a low-motion joint there could still be negative effects on other high-motion joints.

WHAT ARE EQUINE VETERINARIANS USING IN PRACTICE?

To determine the most common uses of these medications, members of the American Association of Equine Practitioners (AAEP) were surveyed.[60] A total of 831 survey responses were submitted and tabulated. The majority of respondents (77%) use TA to treat high-motion joints and 73% use MPA to treat low-motion joints. Veterinarians treating the Western performance and sport horse were significantly more likely to use TA than MPA in high-motion joints ($P = 0.0201$ and $P < 0.0001$, respectively). TA use versus MPA use in high-motion joints by racehorse veterinarians was significantly lower compared with other veterinarians ($P < 0.0001$).

Since the data were accumulated in 2009, it is the author's perception that the use of MPA has continued to decrease. The use in this AAEP survey certainly had variance with what is done overseas and new regulations in the US (see above-mentioned stricter drug restrictions in the racehorse) that can decrease and potentially curtail the use of MPA. As noted in 2013,[61] in the author's native country of New Zealand, there is currently a 48-day withholding period for MPA; there is no use of MPA in racehorses and it is not missed (A. Ritmeester, personal communication, 2013).

THE ASSOCIATION OF INTRAARTICULAR CORTICOSTEROIDS AND CATASTROPHIC INJURY

An interesting pathway of rationalization led to a concept that corticosteroids cause racetrack breakdown more correctly considered as catastrophic injury.[62] Several premises are involved in the development of this association. A study of New York Racing Association's fracture incidence concluded that there was no effect of track or weather condition on the incidence of fractures in Thoroughbred racehorses during races,[63] and therefore the fractures were not traumatic. In addition, changes of osteopetrosis, osteonecrosis, and osteochondrosis in the developing femoral epiphysis in pony foals receiving daily intramuscular injections of dexamethasone (either 0.5 or 5.0 mg/100 kg body weight) for either 3, 8, or 11 months have been shown.[64] Lastly, lesions of bone remodeling similar to those identified above[64] have been found postmortem (including macroscopic, microradiographic, and microscopic assessments) in racehorses that fractured.[62] In their microscopic examination of fracture cases, Krook and Maylin also concluded that the lesions of osteochondrosis, chondroosteonecrosis, and degenerative lesions of tendons and ligaments were closely similar to those resulting from IA and intratendinous injections of corticosteroids and proposed a cause and effect relationship.[62] It should be pointed out that the bone can only react in so many ways, and some similar histologic changes seen in experimental research can hardly be extrapolated to the pathologic appearance of clinical lesions.

This argument is not to diminish the importance of catastrophic injury. It is a serious problem and all possible pathogenetic pathways must be investigated. However, a role for osteochondrosis or corticosteroids in the pathogenesis of catastrophic injury has never been proven. Work by Kawcak,[42] Murray,[33] and their co-workers refutes any harmful effects of TA or MPA on subchondral bone. It is now well recognized that microdamage in the subchondral bone occurs early in the exercising athlete and this microdamage can lead to pathologic fractures.[65,66]

A recent study on musculoskeletal injury (MSI) rates in Thoroughbred racehorses following local corticosteroid injection merits attention.[67] This was a retrospective cohort study comparing the rates of MSI in horses receiving local corticosteroid injection with those in untreated horses and those in horses before such treatment. Of 1911 study horses over a long time period, 392 had been treated. An MSI was defined as any limb injury identified by a veterinarian following which the horse did not race for at least 6 months or was retired. There were 219 MSIs; carpal injuries (47%), fore fetlock (22%), and forelimb tendon injuries (16%) were the most common. There was a positive association between local corticosteroid injection and subsequent MSI rates, which was considered most likely caused by progression of the musculoskeletal condition that prompted treatment. The International Federation of Horse Racing Authorities has acknowledged this study through its welfare committee and is recommending a 14-day stand-down period. It also stated that the risk was gone by 49 days, which, in this author's opinion, supports the need for threshold levels to be defined.

PHARMACOLOGY OF CORTICOSTEROIDS AND DURATION OF PHARMACOLOGIC EFFECTS

Cortisol (hydrocortisone) and cortisone are among the natural antiinflammatory corticosteroids, but they also have substantial effects on sodium and water retention. Because of early clinical observations suggesting antiinflammatory actions of this group of agents, cortisone was tested in rheumatoid arthritis and proved dramatically effective. Consequent to this, Kendall, Reichstein, and Hench, the scientists who synthesized cortisone and directed its therapeutic application, were awarded the Nobel Prize.[17] Since these initial findings, companies selectively modified the basic glucocorticoid molecule to develop glucocorticoid analogs with more antiinflammatory activity and less mineralocorticoid activity. The basic steroid molecule is a 4-ring structure. Chemical alterations, such as adding a double bond between C_1 and C_2 (as with prednisolone), improved glucocorticoid activity and reduced mineralocorticoid activity. Methylation at C_6 (as with MPA) further augments these effects. As a result, research has produced synthetic corticosteroids with 700 times the antiinflammatory action of cortisol.

The antiinflammatory actions of the glucocorticoids are mediated through cytoplasmic receptors.[26] This in turn leads to signaling pathways and gene regulation changes to cause changes in protein expression. Equine veterinarians use corticosteroids for their antiinflammatory properties, but this does not mean they are "antianabolic."[17] That author's contention was generated by the results of treating children during the growth period. Extrapolation to adult horses, however, where increased synthesis of critical components of the articular cartilage has been demonstrated in association with TA and betamethasone injections[30,31] is inappropriate.

It has been traditionally assumed that the duration of response after corticosteroid injection correlates inversely with the solubility of the corticosteroid preparation in water.[68] Triamcinolone hexacetonide is the most insoluble corticosteroid ester and has been generally considered to have the longest duration of action in people.[68,69] However, triamcinolone hexacetonide is quite different from the TA that veterinarians use. Other suggested determinants of the duration of action have included the drug's rate of hydrolysis by synovial tissue enzymes and the binding affinity of the corticosteroid to the steroid receptors in the cytoplasm of target cells.[70] The relative contribution of these suggested determinants to the duration of action remains unclear; however, the duration of action caused by lower solubility and slower absorption should not be confused with either the onset of action or the potency of the drug. Steroid esters are considered prodrugs, as the active moiety is the free alcohol or steroid base resulting from hydrolysis.[70-73] Therefore the local effect of a corticosteroid used intraarticularly is also dependent on the rate of hydrolysis within the joint.

In a pharmacokinetic study using MPA given intraarticularly in horses, the drug was found to hydrolyze rapidly to the active moiety methylprednisolone (MP), with higher synovial fluid MP concentration found within 2 hours of MPA injection.[71,74] Measurable concentrations of MP were present in synovial fluid between 5 and 39 days, but MPA was measurable for only 2 to 6 days postinjection.[71] Systemically MPA was never detected in plasma, and MP in plasma was detected at very low concentrations from only 24 hours after joint injection. Depression of systemic hydrocortisone concentration was noted for 3 to 4 days and considered an indicator of pharmacodynamic effects. The study concluded that MPA needs to be considered rapidly acting when given intraarticularly. However, the potential variability in the duration of action with a wide range of times in which MP could be measured in the joint is relevant.[75]

In a more recent study, 200 mg of MPA was injected intraarticularly into an equine carpal joint, and plasma MP levels, as well as the endogenous glucocorticoids hydrocortisone (Hyd) and cortisone (Cor) concentrations, were determined via liquid chromatography mass spectrometry. The median transfer half-life of MP from the joint to plasma and elimination half-life from plasma were 1.7 and 19.2 hours, respectively. Plasma concentrations of MP peaked at 8 hours (mean ± SD 7.26 ± 3.3 ng/mL) and decreased to 0.11 ± 0.8 ng/mL at 144 hours after injection.[74] Cor and Hyd concentrations were significantly decreased from baseline values and remain suppressed for as long as 240 hours after injection. Plasma MPA concentrations were still quantifiable in horses between 144 and 192 hours (6 and 8 days). This was in contrast to previous reports[71] using high-performance liquid chromatography (HPLC) where only trace concentrations of MP were detected in plasma following IA injection of MPA, but in samples taken from the joint, MP was detected for as long as 39 days and MPA was detected for 3 to 6 days after administration.

Although available pharmacokinetic data indicate corticosteroid suspensions have relatively short IA half-lives,[73] there is considerable variation in their clearance. One study showed that intraarticularly administered MPA can liberate its active moiety for up to 1 month.[71] The specific reasons for divergent pharmacokinetic profiles, as well as the well-known phenomenon of the duration of symptomatic relief far exceeding that predicted by IA half-lives of these preparations, are unclear. Based on the work of Frisbie et al.,[32] however, positive clinical effects could still be seen 42 days after the second and last injection of MPA in vivo.

Further variability from conventionally held beliefs was shown in another study with TA in horses.[46] In a study using radioimmunoassay, TA was shown to be absorbed from equine joints very rapidly with peak serum levels occurring within 4 hours of IA administration of 6 mg of TA into three joints. Synovial fluid concentrations were highest 1 day after injection (7.5 ng/mL), decreased to a steady state concentration by day 4 (10 ng/mL), and became undetectable by day 15. Serum levels of TA increased to 3 ng/mL within 1 hour and further increased to a peak of 4.3 ng/mL at 4 hours. The level then decreased to 2 ng/mL at 24 hours and was nearly undetectable in 48 hours. Because esterification of a corticosteroid prolongs the antiinflammatory effect,[76] it is somewhat surprising that TA clears the joint so quickly. However, as has been pointed[68] out before, persistence and effectiveness are also related to other factors in addition to hydrolysis. Adrenal suppression for 5 days following IA administration of TA was reported by Chen et al. after serum cortisol levels were measured.[46]

It is difficult to directly transpose pharmacokinetic data into biologic potency or activity. The latter depends on total dose administered, duration of action, duration of treatment, rate of conversion to biologically active metabolites, the crystal size of the suspension, and other difficult to define variables.[27,70,77] Corticosteroid crystals have been identified in the cytoplasm of chondrocytes, as well as in synovial fluid leukocyte.[68,78] The active form of the drug presumably binds to a cytoplasmic glucocorticoid receptor after release from the crystal.[78] The erratically active steroid metabolites could be released from these chondrocytic crystals long after measurable concentrations of the parent drug are absent in synovial fluid. Corticosteroid crystals also seem to concentrate preferentially in chondrocytes from osteoarthritic cartilage rather than those from normal cartilage.[78]

To evaluate whether methylprednisolone (MP) diffuses into the centrodistal (CD) joint after MPA is administered into the tarsometatarsal (TMT) joint, the concentration of MP in the CD joint after MPA was administered into the TMT joint was evaluated.[79] Eighty milligrams of MPA was administered into the left TMT joint of 7 horses, and the concentration of MP in the ipsilateral CD joint measured in tissue at 0.5, 1, 3, 6, 9, 12, or 24 hours later in one of the test horses. Using HPLC, a therapeutic concentration of MP was demonstrated in all CD joints sampled 6 hours after administration of MPA into the TMT joint.[79] Another study documented plasma, urine, and synovial fluid disposition of MPA and isoflupredone acetate (IPA). Horses were injected with 100 mg of MPA or 4 mg of IPA. Both corticosteroids appeared to be rapidly hydrolyzed to their respective esters forms as detected by HPLC. Synovial fluid from the contralateral joint contained no detectible MPA or IPA in any sample collection time (collection times were 8, 24, 48, 72, 240, and 672 hours). The median half-life for MPA in plasma as detected by HPLC was 10.3 hours in the synovial space.[80]

CLINICAL EFFECTIVENESS (PHARMACODYNAMICS) RELATIVE TO PHARMACOLOGIC PRESENCE (PHARMACOKINETICS) AND POTENTIAL TO QUANTITATE THIS ACTIVITY

Results of in vivo studies have led to in vitro studies of the effects of corticosteroids on articular cartilage to identify specific cellular events. Measuring gene expression using pharmacogenomic methods, however, provides the potential of more global assessment of all pharmacodynamic responses after IA corticosteroid injection. An example of this technique has been published using MPA administration in rats.[81,82] MPA was administered using two routes and the effect on mRNA gene expression from muscle cells was monitored over time using microarrays. This work demonstrated the ability of measuring gene expression (either upregulated or downregulated) as a pharmacodynamic (pharmacogenomic) method. As expected a host of genes were differentially expressed (upregulated or downregulated) as a consequence to corticosteroid administration. Also differential gene expression occurred even after the pharmacokinetic effects were gone. This may explain why exogenous corticosteroids have both acute and chronic effects.

Galon et al. evaluated gene expression in blood mononuclear cells caused by systemic corticosteroid administration using microarray followed by real-time polymerase chain reaction.[38] Antiinflammatory genes such as IL-10, TGF-β, and IL-lRa were all upregulated as were those genes that are responsible for stimulating cell trafficking, stimulating scavenger systems, and upregulating matrix metalloproteinase. However, at the same time there was a significant decrease in genes that are responsible for cellular immune response because of decreased antigen presentation and T-cell activation. This led the group to conclude that the disease state of the tissues may dictate the corticosteroid sensitivity. It is proposed that using such methods in the horse would be a novel means of objectively evaluating pharmacodynamic effects relative to pharmacokinetics after IA injection of corticosteroids in the horse. This would allow for the development of methods not only to better identify the significance of corticosteroids during routine drug testing, but also to identify those cases that may be most responsive to treatment, those factors that may lead to laminitis, and possibly development of drugs that may influence more specific targets in joint injury and disease.

THE INFLUENCE OF REST FROM EXERCISE AFTER INTRAARTICULAR CORTICOSTEROID INJECTION

As mentioned previously, rest from exercise after IA corticosteroid injection is commonly recommended. This recommendation could be an adaptation of a similar practice among human rheumatologists.[25] A substantially protracted duration of symptomatic efficacy (increase of nearly 70%) was reported to accompany a strict regimen of rest and gradual return to use of the injected limb in human patients with rheumatoid synovitis of the knee.[83] In a more recent report, a prolonged clinical response in patients resting for 24 hours after corticosteroid injection was seen.[84] The potential explanations for postinjection rest leading to length and response to corticosteroid injections have not been investigated, but Caron suggested that a period of restricted joint motion would likely reduce clearance of the medication and enable better penetration of IA tissues.[25] Relevant to the equine situation, it does give another reason for a longer time period between IA injection and racing. However, the author feels that threshold periods designed to minimize IA injection within 7 days of racing are appropriate and can be defended scientifically.

AN EVOLUTION OF STRICTER DRUG RESTRICTIONS

Although a role for corticosteroids in the pathogenesis of catastrophic injury has never been proven (see the section on association of IA corticosteroids in catastrophic injury), the potential for masking of pain by the presence of pharmacologic concentrations of corticosteroids sufficient to hide early anatomic disruption is of major concern.[85] The Racing Medication and Testing Consortium (RMTC) stated that "the use of corticosteroids in performance horses is, in some circumstances, dictated by trainers and based upon the entry of a horse in a race. This scenario emphasizes the masking of clinical signs rather than the mitigation of disease. However, it is undesirable to have treatment too close to the performance event in which the response to treatment and the resolution of clinical signs are important for clarification that there is no serious anatomic disruption being masked. Our primary concern must be for the safety of the horse and rider."

In October 2010 the AAEP issued a White Paper on clinical guidelines for veterinarians practicing in a pari-mutuel environment, in which it was stated that "the AAEP recognizes that the practice of veterinary medicine, particularly in a pari-mutuel, does not take place in a vacuum devoid of

TABLE 12-1   The Products, Doses Investigated, and their Corresponding Plasma or Serum Thresholds

Product	Dose	Threshold
Methylprednisolone acetate (e.g., Depo-Medrol)	100 mg	100 pg of methylprednisolone/mL of serum or plasma
Triamcinolone acetonide (e.g., Vetalog)	9 mg	100 pg of triamcinolone-acetonide/mL of serum or plasma
Betamethasone sodium phosphate and betamethasone acetate	9 mg	10 pg of betamethasone/mL of serum or plasma

These are not clinical dosing recommendations; rather, the doses represent those administered when making threshold recommendations.
(Reprinted with permission from RMTC.)

economic consideration.[86] However, from a medical standpoint, the AAEP believes that entry-driven procedures are generally not in the best interest of the horse. It is with this goal in mind, that clinicians in a pari-mutuel environment are encouraged to make sound treatment decisions particularly with reference to the use of IA corticosteroids that allow for adequate time to properly diagnose, treat, and evaluate the horse's response to IA therapy before racing. Additionally, until such time as security and testing technology can insure proper adherence to scientifically validated withdrawal times, practitioners in a pari-mutuel environment should make these treatment decisions with the health and welfare of the horse as the uppermost concern."

In November 2013 the RMTC hosted a corticosteroid experts conference in Anaheim, California, and this meeting brought together qualified individuals with professional expertise in key areas with the goal of providing a comprehensive plan for regulating corticosteroid use in horseracing to protect equine health and welfare. Participants included analytical chemists, veterinary pharmacologists, veterinary surgeons, racing regulatory veterinarians, and racetrack veterinarians. Among the recommendations was a prohibition on IA use of corticosteroids within 7 days of a race, taking into considerations the concerns expressed by many participants about the proximity of IA injections to race day. The experts also recommended a 72-hour withdrawal time for dexamethasone, a commonly used short-acting corticosteroid that can be administered intravenously, intramuscularly, and orally. Recommendations were discussed based on recent pharmacokinetic data on elimination of synthetic corticosteroids following IA administration including MPA,[87,88] TA,[89,90] and unpublished data on betamethasone. These studies were based on a single joint injection to get consistency between horses in achieving threshold recommendations. As a result there was a table with threshold levels for MPA, TA, and betamethasone esters in the RMTC position statement on corticosteroids (Table 12-1). The RMTC also

TABLE 12-2 Threshold of Four Different Corticosteroids Recommended by the RCI. This Allows Assessment of Flexibility at a Given Dose

Corticosteroid	Maximum Cumulative Dose (range)	Time Until Below RCI Recommended Threshold				
		Day 7	Day 10	Day 14	Day 17	Day 21
Triamcinolone acetonide (n=17)	18 mg (9-18)	17/17				
Methylprednisolone acetate (n=24)	600 mg (40-600)	7/24	16/24	19/24	20/24	24/24
Betamethasone (n=10)	60 mg (12-60)	7/10	10/10			
Isoflupredone (n=7)	18 mg (4-18)	7/7				

(Pilot study performed by Blea et al. and reported by McIlwraith C.W. (2013). Managing joint disease in the racehorse in the face stricter drug restrictions. In: *Proc Am Assoc Equine Pract* 59, 436-442.)

recommended that the Association of Racing Commissioners International (RCI) remove its initial restricted administration times. The existing thresholds would prevent IA administrations close to the race while allowing appropriate treatment with smaller doses of corticosteroids. The RCI determined that an implementation period with feedback of laboratory results to practitioners was also recommended to allow veterinarians to adjust their protocols and adapt to changes in the regulations with regard to administration times and varying administration doses.

As an example of this, a practitioners study on Thoroughbred racehorses in California tested dosages not previously studied, as well as multiple IA injections and combinations of IA corticosteroids, with follow-up venous blood samples 0, 7, 10, 14, 17, 21, 28, and 35 days after administration. The author presented results at the 2013 AAEP Annual Convention (Table 12-2).[61] As it can be seen with a maximum dose averaging 18 mg (range 9 to 18 mg) 17/17 samples were below RCI recommended threshold at day 7. On the other hand with MPA (24 samples with a dose range of 40 to 600 mg), all 24 samples fell below RCI recommended threshold at day 21 (16/24 at day 10, 19/24 at day 14, and 20/24 at day 17, respectively). With betamethasone at a dose of 60 mg, 7/10 fell below the RCI recommended threshold at day 7 and 10/10 at day 10. Similarly with 18 mg of isoflupredone 7/7 samples fell below RCI recommended threshold at day 7 (see Table 12-2).

Investigative work is continuing and in 2014 a study commenced in racing Quarter horses in Southern California. In the meantime, a number of opportunities exist. Decrease in dose of MPA to 40 mg and 20 mg has happened in the US; whereas, as mentioned previously, use in racehorses has essentially stopped in Australia and New Zealand. One prominent equine veterinarian practicing in the UK and France limits all doses to 0.1 to 0.5 mL in a low-motion joint or bursa combined with other corticosteroids and only once every 6 months. With TA many people are using 3 mg/joint and some people 1 to 2 mg.

The preliminary data reveal this will enable multiple joint usage. With betamethasone esters, better information on dosage is necessary but doses of 6 to 15 mg usually fall within threshold restrictions.

SUMMARY

IA corticosteroids are potent antiinflammatory agents. Different products vary in their benefits versus deleterious effects. Betamethasone esters (Celestone Soluspan) have no deleterious side effects, and TA (Vetalog) is in fact chondroprotective and can promote cartilage health. In contrast, MPA (Depo-Medrol) has been consistently shown to have deleterious effects. Generalization about harmful effects of IA corticosteroids is inappropriate and research has defined beneficial and deleterious effects. IA corticosteroids have prolonged effectiveness; there was significant clinical benefit seen at 56 days in one clinical study, and controlled clinical studies in the chip fragment model documented persistent clinical effects at 70 days after IA therapy at 14 and 28 days. Prolonged effectiveness is hypothesized to be caused by IA corticosteroids interacting with cytoplasmic receptors and initiating upregulation of prolonged effects. There is some evidence that a period of rest facilitates improved absorption of IA corticosteroids and therapeutic efficacy, but exercise per se does not promote negative effects. There is no evidence that IA corticosteroids cause harm to subchondral bone or promote catastrophic injury. Good evidence linking laminitis to corticosteroid injection is lacking, and current clinical evidence argues against generalizations of potential risk. In vitro work has helped to define the minimum doses necessary, and with MPA effective therapeutic doses have deleterious effects on articular cartilage. There is no evidence at this stage that combination therapy with HA can mitigate against negative effects with MPA, but recent work shows that HA does have chondroprotective effects and combination therapy with TA or betamethasone esters is appropriate.

REFERENCES

1. Wheat JD. The use of hydrocortisone in the treatment of joint and tendon disorders in large animals. *J Am Vet Med Assoc.* 1955;127(940):64–67.

2. Racing Medication and Testing Consortium. RMTC Board recommends policy on the implementation of anabolic/androgenic steroid regulations March 26, 2008. www.rmtcnet.com/content_pressreleases.asp?id=&s=&article=336.

3. McIlwraith CW. The usefulness and side effects of intra-articular corticosteroid: what do we know? In: *Proc Am Assoc Equine Pract.* 1992;38:21–30.

4. Van Pelt RW. Clinical and synovial fluid response to intra-articular synovial injection of 6α-methylprednisolone acetate into horses and cattle. *J Am Vet Med Assoc.* 1963;143:738–748.

5. Van Pelt RW. Clinical and synovial fluid response to intra-articular synovial injection of 6 alpha-methyl, 17-alpha-hydroxyprogesterone acetate in tarsal hydrarthrosis (bog spavin) in the horse. *J Am Vet Med Assoc.* 1967;151:1159–1171.

6. Van Pelt RW, Riley WF. Therapeutic management of tarsal hydrarthrosis (bog spavin) in the horse by intra-articular injection of prednisolone. *J Am Vet Med Assoc.* 1967;151(3):2328–2337.

7. Van Pelt RW, Riley WF. Tarsal hydrarthrosis in the horse: response to intra-articular injection of synthetic steroids. *Can Vet J.* 1969;10(5):130–135.

8. Van Pelt RW, Tillotson PJ, Gertsen KE. Intra-articular injection of betamethasone in arthritis in horses. *J Am Vet Med Assoc.* 1970;156(11):1589–1599.

9. Houdeshell JW. Field trials of a new long-acting corticosteroid in the treatment of equine arthropathies. *Vet Med Small Anim Clin.* 1969;64(9):782–784.

10. Houdeshell JW. The effect of a corticosteroid combination on blood and synovial fluid in horses. *Vet Med Small Anim Clin.* 1970;65(10):963–966.

11. McKay AG, Milne JF. Observations of the intra-articular use of corticosteroids in the racing Thoroughbred. *J Am Vet Med Assoc.* 1976;168(11):1039–1041.

12. Swanstrom OG, Dawson HA. Intra-articular betasone and Depo-Medrol: a comparative study. In: *Proc Am Assoc Equine Pract.* 1974;20:249–254.

13. Vernimb GD, Van Hoose LM, Hennessey PW. Effects of intra-articular Flumethasone suspension on synovial effusion enzyme activity of arthritic horses. *J Am Vet Med Assoc.* 1977;160(2):186–190.

14. O'Conner JT. The untoward effects of the corticosteroids in equine practice. *J Am Vet Med Assoc.* 1968;153(12):1614–1617.

15. Anonymous. Abstracts of medical literature. *JAMA.* 1958;173:2302.

16. Chandler GN, Wright V. Deleterious effects of intra-articular hydrocortisone. *Lancet.* 1958;272:661–663.

17. Harkins JD, Carney JM, Tobin T. Clinical use and characteristics of the corticosteroids. *Vet Clin North Am Equine Pract.* 1993;9(3):543–562.

18. Salter RB, Gross A, Hall JH. Hydrocortisone arthropathy — an experimental investigation. *Can Med Assoc J.* 1967;97(8):374–377.

19. Tobin T. Steroidal-anti-inflammatory agents: the corticosteroids and ACTH. In: *Drugs and the performance horse.* Springfield, IL;1981:(pp. 132–148).

20. Marcoux M. The effect of methylprednisolone in blood on equine articular structures. In: *Proc Am Assoc Equine Pract.* 1977;23:333–341.

21. Chunekamrai S, Krook LP, Lust G, et al. Changes in articular cartilage after intra-articular injection of methylprednisolone acetate in horses. *Am J Vet Res.* 1989;50(10):1733–1741.

22. Trotter GW, McIlwraith CW, Yovich N, et al. Effects of intra-articular administration of methylprednisolone acetate on normal equine articular cartilage. *Am J Vet Res.* 1991;52(1):83–87.

23. Meagher DM. The effect of intra-articular corticosteroids and continued training on carpal chip fractures of horses. In: *Proc 25th Ann Conv Am Assoc Equine Pract.* 1979;25:405–412.

24. Owen RA, Marsh JA, Hallett FR, et al. Intra-articular corticosteroid- and exercise-induced arthropathy in a horse. *J Am Vet Med Assoc.* 1984;184(3):302–308.

25. Caron JP. Intra-articular injections for joint disease in horses. *Vet Clin North Am Equine Pract.* 2005;21(3):559–573.

26. Trotter GW. Intra-articular corticosteroids. In: McIlwraith CW, Trotter GW, eds. *Joint disease in the horse.* Philadelphia, PA: Saunders; 1996:237–256.

27. Axelrod L. Glucocorticoids. In: Harris WN, Kelley WN, Ruddy S, et al, eds. *Textbook of rheumatology.* 4th ed. Philadelphia, PA: Saunders; 1993:749–796.

28. Laufer S, Greim C, Bertsche T. An in vitro screening assay for the detection of inhibitors of pro-inflammatory cytokine synthesis: a useful tool for the development of new anti-arthritic and disease modifying drugs. *Osteoarthritis Cartilage.* 2002;10(12):961–967.

29. Garvican ER, Vaughan-Thomas A, Redmond C, et al. MMP-mediated collagen breakdown induced by activated protein C in equine cartilage is reduced by corticosteroids. *J Orthop Res.* 2010;28(3):370–378.

30. Foland JW, McIlwraith CW, Trotter GW, et al. Effect of betamethasone and exercise on equine carpal joints with osteochondral fragments. *Vet Surg.* 1994;23(5):369–376.

31. Frisbie DD, Kawcak CE, Trotter GW, et al. Effects of triamcinolone acetonide on an in vivo equine osteochondral fragment exercise model. *Equine Vet J.* 1997;29(5):349–359.

32. Frisbie DD, Kawcak CE, Baxter GM, et al. Effects of 6α-methylprednisolone acetate on an equine osteochondral fragment exercise model. *Am J Vet Res.* 1998;59:1619–1628.

33. Murray RC, Znaor N, Tanner KE, et al. The effect of intra-articular methylprednisolone acetate and exercise on equine carpal subchondral and cancellous bone microhardness. *Equine Vet J.* 2002;34(3):306–310.

34. Carter BG, Bertone AL, Weisbrook SE, et al. Influence of methylprednisolone acetate on osteochondral healing in exercised tarsocrural joints of horses. *Am J Vet Res.* 1996;57(6):914–922.

35. Byron CR, Benson BM, Stewart AA, et al. Effects of methylprednisolone acetate and glucosamine on proteoglycan production by equine chondrocytes in vitro. *Am J Vet Res.* 2008;69(9):1123–1128.

36. Fubini SL, Todhunter RJ, Burton-Wurster N, et al. Corticosteroids alter the differentiated phenotype of articular chondrocytes. *J Orthop Res.* 2001;19(4):688–695.

37. Murphy DJ, Todhunter RJ, Fubini SL, et al. The effects of methylprednisolone on normal and monocyte-conditioned medium-treated articular cartilage from dogs and horses. *Vet Surg.* 2000;29(6):546–557.

38. Galon J, Franchimont D, Hiroi N, et al. Gene profiling reveals unknown enhancing and suppressive actions of glucocorticoids on immune cells. *FASEB J.* 2002;16(1):61–71.

39. Seshadri V, Coyle CH, Chu CR. Lidocaine potentiates the chondrotoxicity of methylprednisolone acetate. *Arthroscopy.* 2009;25(4):337–347.

40. Kristiansen KK, Kold SE. Multivariable analysis of factors outcome of two treatment protocols in 128 cases of horses responded positively to intra-articular analgesia of the distal interphalangeal joint. *Equine Vet J.* 2007;39(2):150–156.

41. Schumacher J, Gillette ER, DeGraves F, et al. The effects of local anesthetic solution in the navicular bursa of horses with lameness caused by distal interphalangeal joint pain. *Equine Vet J.* 2003;35(5):502–505.

42. Kawcak CE, Norrdin RW, Frisbie DD, et al. Effects of osteochondral fragmentation and intra-articular triamcinolone acetonide treatment on subchondral bone in the equine carpus. *Equine Vet J.* 1998;30(1):66–71.

43. Bolt DM, Ishihara A, Weisbrode SE, et al. Effects of triamcinolone acetonide, sodium hyaluronate, amikacin sulfate, and mepivacaine hydrochloride, alone and in combination, on morphology and matrix composition of lipopolysaccharide-challenged and unchallenged equine articular cartilage explants. *Am J Vet Res.* 2008;69(7):861–867.

44. Dechant JE, Baxter GM, Frisbie DD, et al. Effects of dosage titration of methylprednisolone acetate and triamcinolone acetonide on interleukin-l-conditioned equine articular cartilage explants in vitro. *Equine Vet J.* 2003;35(5):444–450.

45. Kay AT, Bolt DM, Ishihara A, et al. Anti-inflammatory and analgesic effects of intra-articular injection of triamcinolone acetonide, mepivacaine hydrochloride, or both on lipopolysaccharide-induced lameness in horses. *Am J Vet Res.* 2008;69(12):1646–1654.

46. Chen CL, Sailor JA, Collier J, et al. Synovial and serum levels of triamcinolone following intra-articular administration of triamcinolone acetonide in the horse. *J Vet Pharmacol Ther.* 1992;15(3):240–246.

47. Caron JP, Genovese RL. Principles and practices of joint disease treatment. In: Ross MW, Dyson SJ, eds. *Diagnostics and management of lameness in the horse.* Philadelphia, PA: Elsevier Science; 2003:746–763.

48. Doyle AJ, Stewart AA, Constable PD, et al. Effects of sodium hyaluronate and methylprednisolone acetate on proteoglycan synthesis in equine articular cartilage explants. *Am J Vet Res.* 2006;66(1):48–53.

49. Yates AC, Stewart AA, Byron CR, et al. Effects of sodium hyaluronate and methylprednisolone acetate on proteoglycan metabolism in equine articular chondrocytes treated with interleukin-1. *Am J Vet Res.* 2006;67(12):1980–1986.

50. Ozturk C, Atamaz F, Hepguler S, et al. The safety and efficacy of intra-articular hyaluronan with/without corticosteroid in knee osteoarthritis: 1 year, single-blind, randomized study. *Rheumatol Int.* 2006;26(4):314–319.

51. Frisbie DD, Kawcak CE, McIlwraith CW, et al. Evaluation of polysulfated glycosaminoglycan or sodium hyaluronan administered intra-articularly for treatment of horses with experimentally induced osteoarthritis. *Am J Vet Res.* 2009;70(2):203–209.

52. de Grauw JC, Visser-Meuer MC, Lashley F, et al. Intraarticular treatment with triamcinolone compared to triamcinolone with hyaluronate: a randomized open-label multicenter clinical trial in 80 lame horses. *Equine Vet J.* 2015. http://dx.doi.org/10.1111/evj.12383.

53. Frisbie DD, Kawcak CE, Werpy NM, et al. Combination of intraarticular (IA) triamcinolone acetonide and polysulfated glycosaminoglycan compared to IA polysulfated glycosaminoglycan or placebo for treatment of osteoarthritis using an equine experimental model. In: *Proc Am Assoc Equine Pract.* 2010;56:25–26.

54. Genovese RL. The use of corticosteroids in racetrack practice. In: *Proc Symposium Effective Use of Corticosteroids in Veterinary Practice.* 1983:56–65.

55. McCluskey MJ, Kavenagh PB. Clinical use of triamcinolone acetonide in the horses (205 cases) and the incidence of glucocorticoid-induced laminitis associated with its use. *Equine Vet Educ.* 2004;16(2):86–89.

56. Dutton H. The corticosteroid laminitis story: 1. Duty of care. *Equine Vet J.* 2007;39(1):5–6.

57. Bailey SR, Elliott J. The corticosteroid laminitis story: 2. Science of if, when and how. *Equine Vet J.* 2007;39(1):7–11.

58. Bathe AP. The corticosteroid laminitis story: 3. The clinician's viewpoint. *Equine Vet J.* 2007;39(1):12–13.

59. Labens R, Mellor DJ, Vaute LC. Retrospective study of the effect of intra-articular treatment of osteoarthritis of the distal tarsal joints in 51 horses. *Vet Rec.* 2007;161(18):611–616.

60. Ferris DJ, Frisbie DD, McIlwraith CW, et al. Current joint therapy usage in equine practice: a survey of veterinarians 2009. *Equine Vet J.* 2011;43(5):530–535.

61. McIlwraith CW. Managing joint disease in the racehorse in the face stricter drug restrictions. In: *Proc Am Assoc Equine Pract.* 2013;59:436–442.

62. Krook L, Maylin GA. Fractures in Thoroughbred horses. *Cornell Vet.* 1988;78(Suppl 11):1–133.

63. Hill TD, Carmichel D, Maylin G, et al. Track conditions and racing injuries in Thoroughbred horses. *Cornell Vet.* 1986;76(4):361–379.

64. Glade MJ, Krook L. Glucocorticoid-induced inhibition of osteolysis in the development of osteopetrosis, osteonecrosis and osteoporosis. *Cornell Vet.* 1982;72(1):76–91.

65. Kawcak CE, McIlwraith CW, Norrdin RW, et al. Clinical effects of exercise on subchondral bone of carpal and metacarpophalangeal joints in horses. *Am J Vet Res.* 2000;61(10):1252–1258.

66. Norrdin RW, Kawcak CW, Capwell BA, et al. Subchondral bone failure in an equine model of overload arthrosis. *Bone.* 1998;22(2):133–139.

67. Whitton RC, Jackson MA, Campbell AJD, et al. Musculoskeletal injury rates in Thoroughbred racehorses following local steroid injection. *Vet J.* 2013;200(1):71–76.

68. Grey RG, Gottlieb NL. Intra-articular corticosteroids. An updated assessment. *Clin Orthop.* 1983;177:235–263.

69. Kendall PH. Triamcinolone hexacetonide: a new corticosteroid for intra-articular therapy. *Ann Phys Med.* 1967;9(2):55–58.

70. Wright JM, Knight C, Heunneyball I. The effect of side chain structures on the biochemical and therapeutic properties of the intra-articular dexamethasone 21-esters. *Clin Exp Rheum.* 1986;4(4):331–339.

71. Autefage A, Alvinerie M, Toutain PL. Synovial fluid and plasma kinetics of methylprednisolone and methylprednisolone acetate in horses following intra-articular administration of methylprednisolone acetate. *Equine Vet J.* 1986;18(3):193–198.

72. Coppoc G. Relationship of the dosage form of a corticosteroid to its therapeutic efficiency. *J Am Vet Assoc.* 1984;185:1098–1101.

73. Derendorf H, Mollmann H, Gruner A, et al. Pharmacokinetics and pharmacodynamics of glucocorticoids suspensions after intra-articular administration. *Clin Pharmacol Ther.* 1986;39(3):313–317.

74. Alvinerie M, Toutain PL. Determination of methylprednisolone and methylprednisolone acetate in synovial fluid using high-performance liquid chromatography. *J Chromatogr.* 1984;309:385–390.

75. Soma LR, Uboh CE, Luo Y, et al. Pharmacokinetics of methyl-prednisolone acetate after intra-articular administration and its effect on endogenous hydrocortisone and cortisone secretion in horses. *Am J Vet Res.* 2006;67(4):654–662.

76. Short CR, Beadle RE. Pharmacology of anti-arthritic drugs. *Vet Clin North Am Small Anim Pract.* 1978;8(3):401–406.

77. Myers SL. Suppression of hyaluronic acid synthesis in synovial organ cultures by corticosteroid suspension. *Arthritis Rheum.* 1985;28(22):1275–1282.

78. Pelletier B, Martel-Pelletier J. Protective effects of corticosteroids on cartilage lesions and osteophyte formation in the Pond-Nuki dog model of osteoarthritis. *Arthritis Rheum.* 1989;32(2):181–193.

79. Serena A, Schumacher J, Schramme MC, et al. Concentration of methylprednisolone in the centrodistal joint after administration of methylprednisolone acetate in the tarso-metatarsal joint. *Equine Vet J.* 2005;37(2):172–174.

80. Lillich JD, Bertone AL, Schmall LM, et al. Plasma, urine and synovial fluid disposition of methylprednisolone acetate and isoflupredone acetate after intra-articular administration in horses. *Am J Vet Res.* 1996;57(2):187–192.

81. Yao Z, Hoffman EP, Ghimbovschi S, et al. Mathematical modeling of corticosteroid pharmacogenomics in rat muscle following acute and chronic methylprednisolone dosing. *Mol Pharm.* 2008;5(2):328–339.

82. Yao Z, Dubois DC, Almon RR, et al. Pharmacokinetics/pharmacodynamic model of corticosterone and lipocytopenia by methylprednisolone in rats. *J Pharm Sciences.* 2008;97(7):2820–2832.

83. Neustadt DH. Intra-articular therapy for rheumatoid synovitis of the knee: effect of the post-injection rest regime. *Clin Rheumatol Pract.* 1985;3:65–68.

84. Chakrabarty K, Pharoah PDP, Scott DGI. A randomized controlled study of post-injection rest following intra-articular steroid therapy for knee synovitis. *Br J Rheumatol.* 1994;33(5):464–468.

85. RMTC White Paper: RMTC position statement on corticosteroids. www.rmtcnet.com/resources/RMTC%20Position%20Paper%20on%20Corticosteroids.pdf; 2013.

86. AAEP White Paper: Clinical guidelines for veterinarians practicing in a pari-mutuel environment. http://m.aaep.org/images/files/AAEPClinicalGuidelinesPariMutuelEnvironment.pdf; 2010.

87. Knych HK, Harrison LM, Casbeer HC, et al. Disposition of methylprednisolone acetate in plasma, urine and synovial fluid following intra-articular administration to exercised Thoroughbred horses. *J Vet Pharmacol Ther.* 2013;37(2):125–132.

88. Menendez MI, Phelps MA, Hothem EA, et al. Pharmacokinetics of methylprednisolone acetate after intra-articular administration and subsequent suppression of endogenous hydrocortisone secretion in exercising horses. *Am J Vet Res.* 2012;73(9):1453–1461.

89. Knych HK, Vidal MA, Casbeer HC, et al. Pharmacokinetics of triamcinolone acetonide following intramuscular and intra-articular administration to exercised Thoroughbred horses. *Equine Vet J.* 2013;45(6):715–720.

90. Soma LR, Uboh CE, You Y, et al. Pharmacokinetics of intra-articular, intravenous, and intramuscular administration of triamcinolone acetonide and its effect on endogenous plasma hydrocortisone and cortisone concentrations in horses. *Am J Vet Res.* 2011;72(9):1234–1242.

13

Hyaluronan

David D. Frisbie

Hyaluronan (HA) (disaccharide composed of D-glucuronic acid and *N*-acetyl-D-glucosamine) is integral to normal joint function. It is a significant molecule in both the synovial fluid and articular cartilage where it provides the backbone of the aggregating proteoglycan aggrecan. It is a molecule made up of repeating units and as such can have various lengths. Based mainly on in vitro work, both the concentration and molecular weight (degree of polymerization) appear to be important in the normal function of HA. To that extent, in disease, the concentration and length of HA are believed to be decreased along with its lubricating properties, leaving the joint underprotected.[1] Although the method of measuring HA molecular weight is not universally agreed upon (the same sample may have numerous estimates of molecular weight depending on the testing method), normal synovial fluid HA is thought to be in the 0.5 to 3.0 million Dalton molecular weight range at a concentration between 0.33 and 1.5 g/L.[2-4] HA is made by either the synoviocytes if destined for synovial fluid or chondrocytes if destined for incorporation into extracellular matrix.[5] When exogenous HA is administered into the joint it has a very short half-life (in the magnitude of hours[6]) and an even shorter half-life when administered intravenously (IV) (in the magnitude of minutes[7]).

One of the functions of HA in the joint is boundary lubrication, at high load and slow speed. Boundary lubrication is dependent on two main molecules: HA and lubricin (proteoglycan 4).[1] The other major function attributed to HA is as a barrier that regulates fluid exchange at the level of the synovial membrane, thus controlling the intraarticular synovial environment.[8]

ROLE OF HYALURONAN IN JOINT DISEASE

The role of HA in diseased joints is to both maintain a lubricating environment and to help minimize the mediators of joint disease such as white blood cells (WBCs), free radicals, and proinflammatory cytokines.[9] The importance of these roles has previously been reviewed in other sections of this text as well as the previous edition of this text.[9] More recently, a direct correlation with the lubricating properties of HA and articular cartilage erosion as well as hemorrhage within the diseased joint has been made.[10] Further, exogenous administration of an HA-containing substance provided a significant improvement, albeit transient, in synovial fluid lubricating properties in diseased joints. It is important to note that this improvement was associated with significantly less hemorrhage and decreased articular cartilage erosion (D.D. Frisbie, unpublished data, 2014).

The use of HA in the treatment of joint disease has been extensively reviewed in the previous edition of this book and the chapter on HA serves as a good resource to the basic science, much of which was conducted before 1996 and does not need to be repeated here. A few key points to revisit are the effect of molecular weight, dose, and frequency of dose.

Molecular Weight and Cross-linking

The effectiveness of HA based on molecular weight is the most controversial aspect of its clinical use and various opinions of the effect of molecular weight have been published.[11] The author's opinion, based on extensive review of the literature, is as follows: There is a critical molecular weight of HA that consistently shows benefit at about 500,000 Daltons or greater.[12] Thus, the use of HA of molecular weight greater than half a million Daltons is recommended. Most commercial products are about 1 to 3 million Daltons; however, some synthetic cross-linked exogenous HA products are on the market. These products have been introduced to provide benefit by so-called viscosupplementation of joints. Briefly, the concept of viscosupplementation refers to the injection of HA or its derivative in an attempt to return the elasticity and viscosity of the synovial fluid to normal or higher levels. Cross-linked HA has been developed as an improvement to other synthetic HAs that are not cross-linked and increase the molecular weight from 1 to 3 million to greater than 6 million Daltons (MDa). Cross-linked HA has a longer retention time in the synovial space and appears to be more resistant to free radicals. Hylan G-F 20 (Synvisc, Genzyme), a cross-linked HA with a molecular mass on average greater than 6 MDa, has demonstrated favorable results in large multicenter human clinical studies, showing similar effectiveness as a nonsteroidal medication.[13-15] An experimental study conducted in the horse failed to show beneficial effects of hylan G-F 20, but it does propose a difference in the equine study (an acute experimental synovitis model) compared with the more chronic OA (in the human trial) as one possible explanation for this outcome.[16] The authors also suggested that the severity of the inflammation in the model may have been too harsh to observe a significant treatment effect. A recent randomized, double-blind, controlled trial in humans (N=426) compared mid to low molecular weight formulations (mid 0.8 to 1.5 million Daltons product to a low 0.5 to 0.7 million Dalton product).[17] This was done in patients with knee OA who were administered 20 to 25 mg of respective molecular weight HA once a week for 3 treatments and then followed for 26 weeks. The midweight product showed statistical superiority, reducing pain by up to 50% for 6 months post-treatment. This brings up the question of the relative costs of the products based on effectiveness, that is, cost/benefit ratio. With lack of substantial proof that the high molecular weight products are clinically superior to the midmolecular weight (1 to 3 million Daltons) and midmolecular weight showing superiority to low molecular weight it seems prudent to recommend midmolecular weight products based on a cost/benefit ratio (Table 13-1) (Figure 13-1).

Dosage of Hyaluronan

Dose titrations of HA have been performed in the horse. Specifically 0, 1, 10, 20, and 40 mg per joint have been evaluated using an equine fracture model of OA.[18] This study demonstrated that a dose of at least 20 mg per joint was needed to demonstrate a clinical improvement in pain measured by force plate analysis. This dose was given in the carpus and thus one should be careful with extrapolating (which the author estimates at 10 to 15 mL) to other joints. The author is unaware of specific dose frequency studies that have been carried out in the horse; rather it appears that equine practitioners rely on studies carried out human patients,[19]

suggesting that at least 3 doses are required (administered 1 week apart) to see significant effects in clinical parameters of pain and effusion.

Symptom-modifying versus Disease-modifying Effects of Hyaluronan

In the treatment of joint disease two main effects are sought: first, symptom-modifying effects, via a symptom-modifying osteoarthritic drug (SMOAD) and second, disease-modifying effect via a disease-modifying osteoarthritic drug (DMOAD). In the human medical field, intraarticular HA is considered a mainstream SMOAD. In support of this statement, the most comprehensive study compiling published human trials

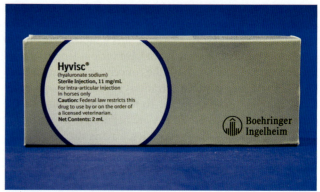

FIGURE 13-1 Hyvisc® is an example of a midmolecular weight HA that is commonly used in clinical cases.

TABLE 13-1	**Partial Listing of Available Hyaluronan Products**						
Product Name	Manufacturer	Concentration	Molecular Weight (Daltons)	How Supplied	Recommended Dose (for Small- to Medium-Size Joints)	Standard Availability	Cost
Hylartin V	Pfizer	10 mg/mL	3.5×10^6	2-mL syringe 20 mg	20 mg	Each	$63.02
MAP-5 (used intraarticularly at this dose)*	Bioniche	10.3 mg/mL (2 mL) 5 mg/mL (10 mL)	7.5×10^5	2-mL vial 10-mL vial	20 mg	10 mL 2 mL	$36.26 $17.58
Legend (Hyonate) Intravenous/ intraarticular use	Bayer	10 mg/mL	3×10^5	4-mL vial	40 mg (IV)	Box of 6 (IV) Box of 6 (IA)	$72.75[†] $42.88[†]
Hyalovet (Hya-lovet 20)	Boehringer	10 mg/mL	$4-7 \times 10^5$	2-mL syringe	20 mg	2 mL	$43.62
HyCoat (used intraarticularly)	Neogen	5 mg/mL	$>1.0 \times 10^6$	10-mL vial	30 mg	10 mL	$34.85
Hyvisc	Boehringer	11 mg/mL	2.1×10^6	2-mL syringe	20 mg	each	$57.65
Gel-50	Bexco Pharma	17 mg/mL	—	3-mL syringe	51 mg	each	$30.22

Availability and costs are as of 2014.
*Not licensed for use in the U.S.
[†]Cost per dose.

demonstrated a 28% to 54% reduction in pain compared with baseline values and a 9% to 32% improvement in function for the 76 trials with up to 18 months of follow-up included.[19] In equine medicine, the level of evidence for SMOAD activity is not as compelling; however, nor are the number of studies or the level of evidence (quality of studies). Both experimental and clinical equine studies have shown SMOAD activity associated with HA administration.[4,20,21] In the author's clinical experience an SMOAD activity of HA alone does exist but is less in comparison to the SMOAD effects of other medications such as corticosteroids.

Demonstration of DMOAD activity of HA has been more elusive than SMOAD activity. There have been two interesting long-term human trials published that have shown DMOAD activity in knee OA. The first study included 79 patients who received either HA (4 courses of 3 injections weekly of HA, high molecular weight product) or standard care but no injections (control group).[22] This study was 24 months long and used magnetic resonance imaging (MRI) outcome parameters of patients with Kellgren-Lawrence grade II through IV disease. Significant beneficial effects were noted in these symptomatic patients treated with HA by preservation of cartilage volume and no significant cartilage loss versus the control population. The second long-term human study had 40-month follow-up and also used 4 courses of treatments (months 0, 7, 14, and 27) with 5 weekly injections at each treatment course of a midmolecular weight product. The results indicated significantly more responders (as defined using the Osteoarthritis Research Society International (OARSI) 2004 criteria[23]; one example would be 50% reduction in pain) versus placebo.[24] This was true at all of the observed time points out to the last 40-month visit. This study offered novel evidence that repeated treatment courses of intraarticular (IA) HA not only improve knee OA symptoms between treatment periods, but also exert a marked carry-over effect for at least 1 year after the last course of treatment. Although it was not possible based on the design of this study to determine if the carry-over effect reflects true OA remission or DMOAD, it does suggest alteration of expected disease course.

A study that obtained articular cartilage biopsies both before and 6 months after the onset of treatment with either 5 weekly injections of a low-molecular weight HA or 3 weekly injections of methylprednisolone acetate (MPA) (40 mg) provided histologic insight into the two treatment regimens.[25] The authors reported "a significant reconstitution of the superficial layer together with an improvement in chondrocyte density and territorial matrix appearance. Furthermore, chondrocytes appeared to have significantly improved based on mitochondria storage functions. Hyaluronan treatment produced results that were significantly superior to those delivered with MPA in almost all the morphometric estimators." A study in the Colorado State University equine OA model, using a midmolecular weight product once a week for 3 injections, demonstrated DMOAD activity. Specifically, a decrease in histologic articular cartilage fibrillation as well as improvements in synovial membrane parameters were noted.[26] Thus, in both well-controlled large

human trials and one experimental study in horses, good evidence for DMOAD action of HA administered weekly for 3+ treatments exists.

Although observing significant benefits over placebo treatment is useful information, the clinician is also aided by studies comparing HA with other medications. This provides a relative potency and/or potential comparisons for various mechanisms of action. With respect to HA the majority of comparisons have been done in human patients and were compared with corticosteroids; these well-conducted studies are worth reviewing for the equine clinician. A Level I-1b (randomized controlled clinical) study compared the use of high-molecular weight HA (3 weekly injections) with a single injection of 2 mL of betamethasone sodium phosphate-betamethasone acetate with a 6-month follow-up period.[27] The primary outcomes were the Western Ontario and McMaster Universities Arthritis Index (WOMAC) and other functional standardized measures. This study did not demonstrate significant differences between treatment groups. A study that assessed a low-molecular weight HA injected weekly for 3 treatments compared with weekly (3 treatments) injection with methylprednisolone acetate (40 mg) demonstrated short-term equivalence (1 week posttreatment).[28] However, at 45 days posttreatment superiority in pain outcome parameters were seen in the HA-treated group. A larger (N=200+) study compared a high-molecular weight product (3 weekly treatments) with triamcinolone hexotonide (single 40-mg injection).[29] Although pain relief was improved faster with the corticosteroid (in 1 to 2 weeks) compared with HA treatment, at 12 and 26 weeks significantly more improvement in the WOMAC scores were seen in the HA versus the corticosteroid treatment group. These findings were also true for both the patient and investigator visual analog pain scale (VAS) at 12 and 26 weeks.

In a survey of equine practitioners the respondents were asked to rate their usage of HA compared with other medications; responses can be found in Table 13-2. In interpreting this table it is important to note a respondent could choose more than one product; that is, the total percent per question does not sum to 100. It is also worth noting that Legend® was a separate response because of the prevalence of its IV versus IA route of administration. As an interesting observation most respondents used a midmolecular weight HA IA.

Combination Therapy with Hyaluronan and Corticosteroids

The use of HA in combination with a corticosteroid is common in equine practice; therefore, some discussion about the evidence for this is warranted. In a survey of equine practitioners, combined use of corticosteroid and HA was reported 59% of the time.[30] In vitro support for this combination therapy also exists. Specifically, the combination of HA (midmolecular weight) and triamcinolone acetonide was shown to have a more beneficial effect on proteoglycan matrix metabolism in the presence of IL-1 stimulation compared with the treatments individually.[31] Further, an interesting in vivo study in the rabbit knee looked at the individual

TABLE 13-2 Treatment of Various Conditions by Product: Total Respondents for the Question was 727				
	HA Products	Adequan	Legend	Polyglycan
Preventative/prophylactic measure in a high-performance horse	IA 184 (25.3)	IM 569 (78.3)	IV 464 (63.8)	IV 134 (18.4)
Chronic case involving "maintenance" or routine injections	IA 376 (51.7)	IM 425 (58.5)	IV 321 (44.2)	IV 105 (14.4)
Chronic case with radiographic evidence of osteoarthritis	IA 408 (56.1)	IM 344 (47.3)	IV 260 (35.8)	IV 86 (11.8)
Postoperative horse returning to training and regular work	IA 307 (42.2)	IM 396 (54.5)	IV 313 (43.1)	IV 90 (12.4)
Acute disease of high motion joints	IA 453 (62.3)	IM 253 (34.8)	IV 233 (32.1)	IV 74 (10.2)
Acute disease of low motion joints	IA 307 (42.2)	IM 325 (44.7)	IV 226 (31.1)	IV 82 (11.3)
Ligament or tendon lesions	IL 114 (15.7)	IM 201 (27.7)	IV 142 (19.5)	IV 59 (8.1)
Tendon sheath applications	IS 303 (41.7)	IM 153 (21.1)	IV 140 (19.3)	IV 52 (7.2)

From Ferris DJ, Frisbie DD, McIlwraith CW, et al.: Current joint therapy usage in equine practice: a survey of veterinarians 2009, Equine Vet J 43:530-535, 2011.
IA, Intraarticular; *IL*, intralesional, *IM*, intramuscular; *IS*, intrasheath; *IV*, intravenous.

and combined use of HA and/or corticosteroids. Results demonstrated a 52% reduction in histologic pathology with HA alone (midmolecular weight product, 1 to 2 million Daltons), a 72% reduction in pathology with corticosteroid alone0 and a 88% reduction in pathology with the combination of corticosteroid and HA.[32] The combination therapy also produced a reduction in lipid peroxidation with the combination therapy, which was not seen with either corticosteroid or HA alone. A group of human patients were followed using the WOMAC pain assessment criteria as well as MRI for a year following treatment with either HA alone or HA with one of the three injections per course containing corticosteroid (triamcinolone acetonide).[33] This study concluded that the combination therapy provided a more rapid improvement in pain, had beneficial effects during the 1-year posttreatment, and showed no signs of deleterious effects on joint structure while managing the knee OA. It is, therefore, the author's opinion that, based on the peer-reviewed literature to date, some synergistic action between the combination therapies may exist and is compelling enough for the routine use of a combination of triamcinolone acetonide and a midmolecular weight HA product.

The Use of Hyaluronan Intravenously

The IV use of HA, specifically Legend, is prevalent in equine practice.[30] In fact the prophylactic use is prevalent as well, despite the product not having a label claim to that effect. In a survey of American Association of Equine Practitioners who used Legend, 82% used the product IV with 63% of its usage aimed at preventative or prophylactic effects. In a well-accepted model of equine OA, IV Legend was shown to significantly improve clinical lameness and synovial membrane histology (specifically vascularity and cellular infiltration) and synovial fluid parameters, such as lower PGE_2 and total protein levels.[34] It is notable that these improvements were seen 42 days following the last of three treatments (40 mg) that were given

1 week apart. The prophylactic properties of IV Legend were also assessed in a 9-month study of racing Quarter horses (N=140).[35] HA-treated horses tended to race longer before requiring the first joint injection and to have a better speed index, higher average number of starts, and more money earned compared with placebo-treated horses. Thus, it provides some level of evidence of benefit of IV HA used prophylactically.

SUMMARY

A significant moderate effect in improving knee pain in human patients lasting 5 to 13 weeks has been demonstrated by numerous clinical reports and confirmed by a systematic review of the literature. In the author's opinion, the equine literature does not contradict these findings. When HA has been combined with corticosteroids beneficial results have been realized, thus giving support for the clinical practice of combination therapies. This, for the author, is 20 to 22 mg of a midmolecular weight HA with 3 to 5 mg of triamcinolone acetonide in a 10 to 15 mL joint as a single injection. Further (2 weekly injections) treatment with HA alone should be considered based on published human clinical trials. Still further, placebo-controlled and anecdotal evidence for prophylactic effect following the IV administration of HA may exist.

REFERENCES

1. Antonacci JM, Schmidt TA, Serventi LA, et al. Effects of equine joint injury on boundary lubrication of articular cartilage by synovial fluid: role of hyaluronan. *Arthritis Rheum.* 2012;64(9):2917–2926.
2. Tulamo RM, Heiskanen T, Salonen M. Concentration and molecular weight distribution of hyaluronate in synovial fluid from clinically normal horses and horses with diseased joints. *Am J Vet Res.* 1994;55(5):710–715.

3. Tew WP. Sodium hyaluronate and the treatment of equine joint disorders. In: *Proceedings Am Assoc Equine Pract*. 1984;30:67–85.

4. Howard RD, McIlwraith CW. Hyaluronan and its use in the treatment of equine joint disease. In: McIlwraith CW, Trotter GW, eds. *Joint disease in the horse*. 1st ed. Philadelphia, PA: Saunders; 1996:257–269.

5. Winter WT, Smith PJ, Arnott S. Hyaluronic acid: structure of a fully extended 3-fold helical sodium salt and comparison with the less extended 4-fold helical forms. *J Mol Biol*. 1975;99(2):219–235.

6. Fraser JR, Kimpton WG, Pierscionek BK, et al. The kinetics of hyaluronan in normal and acutely inflamed synovial joints: observations with experimental arthritis in sheep. *Semin Arthritis Rheum*. 1993;22(6 Suppl 1):9–17.

7. Fraser JR, Laurent TC, Pertoft H, et al. Plasma clearance, tissue distribution and metabolism of hyaluronic acid injected intravenously in the rabbit. *Biochem J*. 1981;200(2):415–424.

8. Kerr HR, Warburton B. Surface rheological properties of hyaluronic acid solutions. *Biorheology*. 1985;22(2):133–144.

9. McIlwraith CW, Trotter GW. In: McIlwraith CW, Trotter GW, eds. *Joint disease in the horse*. 1st ed. Philadelphia, PA: Saunders; 1996:490.

10. Temple-Wong MM, Sah RL, Frisbie DD, et al. Redefining joint therapy. 4th *World Veterinary Orthopaedic Congress*. 2014. abstract.

11. Frisbie DD. Principals of treatment of joint disease, section xii, musculoskeletal system. In: Auer JA, Stick JA, eds. *Equine surgery*. 3rd ed. Saunders; 2005:1055–1073.

12. Smith MM, Ghosh P. The synthesis of hyaluronic acid by human synovial fibroblasts is influenced by the nature of the hyaluronate in the extracellular environment. *Rheumatol Int*. 1987;7(3):113–122.

13. van den Bekerom MPJ, Lamme B, Sermon A, et al. What is the evidence for viscosupplementation in the treatment of patients with hip osteoarthritis? Systematic review of the literature. *Arch Orthop Trauma Surg*. 2008;128(8):815–823.

14. Conrozier T, Jerosch J, Beks P, et al. Prospective, multi-centre, randomized evaluation of the safety and efficacy of five dosing regimens of viscosupplementation with hylan G-F 20 in patients with symptomatic tibio-femoral osteoarthritis: a pilot study. *Arch Orthop Trauma Surg*. 2009;129(3):417–423.

15. Spitzer AI, Bockow BI, Brander VA, et al. Hylan G-F 20 improves hip osteoarthritis: a prospective, randomized study. *Phys Sportsmed*. 2010;38(2):35–47.

16. Peloso JG, Stick JA, Caron JP, et al. Effects of hylan on amphotericin-induced carpal lameness in equids. *Am J Vet Res*. 1993;54(9):1527–1534.

17. Berenbaum F, Grifka J, Cazzaniga S, et al. A randomised, double-blind, controlled trial comparing two intra-articular hyaluronic acid preparations differing by their molecular weight in symptomatic knee osteoarthritis. *Ann Rheum Dis*. 2012;71(9):1454–1460.

18. Auer J, Fackelman G. Treatment of degenerative joint disease of the horse: a review and commentary. *Vet Surg*. 1981;10(2):80–90.

19. Bellamy N, Campbell J, Robinson V, et al. Viscosupplementation for the treatment of osteoarthritis of the knee. *Cochrane Database Syst Rev*. 2006;19(2): CD005321.

20. Auer JA, Fackelman GE, Gingerich DA, et al. Effect of hyaluronic acid in naturally occurring and experimentally induced osteoarthritis. *Am J Vet Res*. 1980;41(4):568–574.

21. Gaustad G, Larsen S. Comparison of polysulphated glycosaminoglycan and sodium hyaluronate with placebo in treatment of traumatic arthritis in horses. *Equine Vet J*. 1995;27(5):356–362.

22. Wang Y, Hall S, Hanna F, et al. Effects of hylan G-F 20 supplementation on cartilage preservation detected by magnetic resonance imaging in osteoarthritis of the knee: a two-year single-blind clinical trial. *BMC Musculoskelet Dis*. 2011;12:195–203.

23. Pham T, van der Heijde D, Altman RD, et al. OMERACT-OARSI initiative: Osteoarthritis Research Society International set of responder criteria for osteoarthritis clinical trials revisited. *Osteoarthritis Cartilage*. 2004;12(5):389–399.

24. Navarro-Sarabia F, Coronel P, Collantes E, et al. A 40-month multicentre, randomised placebo-controlled study to assess the efficacy and carry-over effect of repeated intra-articular injections of hyaluronic acid in knee osteoarthritis: the AMELIA project. *Ann Rheum Dis*. 2011;70(11):1957–1962.

25. Guidolin DD, Ronchetti IP, Lini E, et al. Morphological analysis of articular cartilage biopsies from a randomized, clinical study comparing the effects of 500-730 kDa sodium hyaluronate (Hyalgan) and methylprednisolone acetate on primary osteoarthritis of the knee. *Osteoarthritis Cartilage*. 2001;9(4):371–381.

26. Frisbie DD, Kawcak CE, Werpy NM, et al. Evaluation of polysulfated glycosaminoglycan or sodium hyaluronan administered intra-articularly for treatment of horses with experimentally induced osteoarthritis. *Am J Vet Res*. 2009;70(2):203–209.

27. Leopold SS, Redd BB, Warme WJ, et al. Corticosteroid compared with hyaluronic acid injections for the treatment of osteoarthritis of the knee: a prospective, randomized trial. *J Bone Joint Surg Am*. 2003;85-A(7):1197–1203.

28. Leardini G, Mattara L, Franceschini M, et al. Intra-articular treatment of knee osteoarthritis. A comparative study between hyaluronic acid and 6-methyl prednisolone acetate. *Clin Exp Rheumatol*. 1991;9(4):375–381.

29. Caborn D, Rush J, Lanzer W, et al. A randomized, single-blind comparison of the efficacy and tolerability of hylan G-F 20 and triamcinolone hexacetonide in patients with osteoarthritis of the knee. *J Rheumatol*. 2004;31(2):333–343.

30. Ferris DJ, Frisbie DD, McIlwraith CW, et al. Current joint therapy usage in equine practice: a survey of veterinarians 2009. *Equine Vet J*. 2011;43(5):530–535.

31. Schaefer EC, Stewart AA, Durgam SS, et al. Effects of sodium hyaluronate and triamcinolone acetonide on glucosaminoglycan metabolism in equine articular chondrocytes treated with interleukin-1. *Am J Vet Res*. 2009;70(12):1494–1501.

32. Karakurum G, Karakok M, Tarakcioglu M, et al. Comparative effect of intra-articular administration of hyaluronan and/or cortisone with evaluation of malondialdehyde on degenerative osteoarthritis of the rabbit's knee. *Tohoku J Exp Med*. 2003;199(3):127–134.

33. Ozturk C, Atamaz F, Hepguler S, et al. The safety and efficacy of intraarticular hyaluronan with/without corticosteroid in knee osteoarthritis: 1-year, single-blind, randomized study. *Rheumatol Int*. 2006;26(4):314–319.

34. Kawcak CE, Frisbie DD, McIlwraith CW, et al. Effects of intravenously administered sodium hyaluronate on equine carpal joints with osteochondral fragments under exercise. *Am J Vet Res*. 1997;58(10):1132–1140.

35. McIlwraith CW, Goodman NL, Frisbie DD. Prospective study on the prophylactic value of intravenous hyaluronan in 2-year-old racing Quarter horses. In: *Proc Am Assoc Equine Pract*. 1998;44:269.

14

Polysulfated Glycosaminoglycan (Adequan®)

C. Wayne McIlwraith

Polysulfated glycosaminoglycan (PSGAG) belongs to a group of polysulfated polysaccharides that includes, in addition to PSGAG (Adequan), pentosan polysulfate (discussed elsewhere) and chondroitin sulfate (CS). These drugs are disease-modifying osteoarthritic drugs (DMOADs) and therefore PSGAG has been traditionally used when cartilage damage is presumed present rather than in the treatment of synovitis.[1] However, recent work questions the traditional approach as there is evidence for a significant effect on synovitis (see below). The use of DMOADs is meant to prevent, retard, or reverse the morphologic cartilaginous lesions of osteoarthritis (OA), with the major criterion for inclusion being prevention of cartilage degeneration. The principal GAG in PSGAG is CS and the product is made from an extract of bovine lung and trachea modified by sulfate esterification. Adequan is marketed for both intraarticular (IA) and intramuscular (IM) use (Figure 14-1).

EARLY STUDIES IN IN VITRO AND IN VIVO MODELS

Adequan was reviewed extensively in the first edition of this textbook.[1] One in vitro study demonstrated that PSGAG was the only drug tested (others included phenylbutazone, flunixin meglumine, betamethasone, and hyaluronan [HA]) that inhibited stromelysin (now classified as MMP-3).[2] Three other in vitro studies on the effect of PSGAG on equine cartilage had contradictory results. PSGAG caused increased collagen and GAG synthesis in both articular cartilage explants and cell cultures from normal and osteoarthritic equine cartilage. However,[3] other work found a dose-dependent inhibition of proteoglycan synthesis, little effect on proteoglycan degradation, and no effect on proteoglycan monomer size.[4] Various studies have supported the value of IA PSGAG (250 mg) in equine OA, including a clinical study,[5] a study using a Freund adjuvant-induced OA model,[6] and a carpal synovitis model using sodium monoiodoacetate.[7] In the latter study, there was significant reduction of articular cartilage fibrillation, erosion, less chondrocyte death, and markedly improved GAG staining. However, PSGAG had no benefit in healing preexisting articular cartilage lesions in the latter study[7] or in a different study in ponies.[8]

CLINICAL USE AND MORE RECENT EVIDENCE FOR EFFICACY

I have traditionally recommended the use of IA PSGAG after arthroscopic surgery when there is substantial loss of articular cartilage (most commonly in the carpus). On reflection, we had never demonstrated resolution of articular cartilage damage or enhanced repair of articular cartilage damage but rather identified clinically that there was rapid resolution of synovitis and hemarthrosis, the latter being a common consequence to débridement of articular defects down to subchondral bone. In addition to the clinical observations following IA therapy with PSGAG, examination of the early literature consistently shows benefit with IA use.[5-7] In contrast, although the use of IM Adequan became popular, there is limited evidence for its efficacy and this is discussed below. The IA and IM use will therefore be examined separately.

Intraarticular Use of PSGAG

Earlier in vivo work with the Freund adjuvant model and the monoiodoacetate model has been mentioned above. A more recent study using the Colorado State University (CSU) osteochondral fragment-exercise model compared IA PSGAG with either IA HA or saline; synovial fluid effusion was significantly reduced with PSGAG compared with both saline and HA. The degree of vascularity and subintimal fibrosis of the synovium was significantly reduced with PSGAG treatment compared with controls.[9] Assessing the author's clinical results with this study, it seems that the main value of IA PSGAG appears to be for severe (and acute) synovitis most commonly seen after arthroscopic surgery when there is considerable débridement of bone. However, the UK data sheet for the product expressly states "do not inject into actively inflamed joints. In the presence of active joint inflammation, therapy with a suitable antiinflammatory drug should be given before intraarticular treatment with Adequan." Not only would this seem inappropriate based on work with the CSU equine model but a more recent study suggests that the combination of a corticosteroid (triamcinolone acetonide [TA]) and PSGAG is less effective in the CSU model than either drug alone.[10] It should also be noted that the Frisbie et al. (2009)[9] study provided support for PSGAG still being classifiable as a DMOAD as there was a trend ($P > 0.05$ but < 0.1) for significantly less cartilage

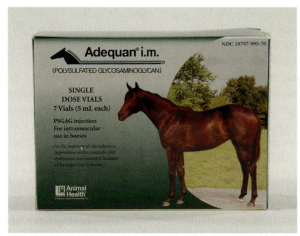

FIGURE 14-1 Intraarticular and intramuscular preparations of Adequan.

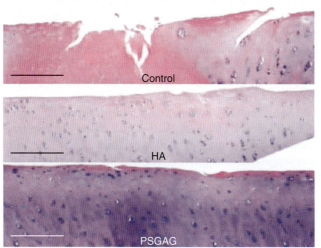

FIGURE 14-2 Photomicrographs of sections of articular cartilage showing cartilage fibrillation in a comparative study in the equine osteochondral fragment model where controlled horses received intraarticular saline, a second group received HA, and PSGAG was administered to the third group. There was significant amelioration of fibrillation with HA and a strong trend with PSGAG.

fibrillation (Figure 14-2). Further, as noted previously in Chapter 11, concurrent testing of IA HA in the same study as testing IA Adequan[11] showed a decrease in synovial effusion with PSGAG compared to HA or saline, a trend for decreased synovial membrane vascularity and subintimal fibrosis with HA, but significantly less cartilage fibrillation with HA (this was a trend with PSGAG).

In an earlier double-blind, placebo-controlled study in 77 Standardbred horses, an IA dose of 250 mg PSGAG was compared with 20 mg of IA HA and 2 mL of saline for three treatments in traumatic arthritis.[12] This study showed that all three treatments were effective in traumatic arthritis but HA and PSGAG were superior (and no difference was detected between the two products). In the survey on current joint therapy usage in equine practice by Ferris et al. (2011), the majority of respondents selected PSGAG (423/674, 62.8%)

as the most frequently used disease-modifying medication, independent of route of administration. However, the majority of respondents who used PSGAG chose to administer it IM (643/764, 84.1%). IM PSGAG was used by 567/727 (78.3%) respondents for prophylactic/preventative treatment. It was also used IM by 425/727 (58.5%) in chronic maintenance cases and by 396/727 (54.5%) in postoperative horses returning to training.[13]

Although more recent data support the value of IA PSGAG, there was a precipitous decline in the use of IA PSGAG starting in the late 1980s and going through the 1990s. Two driving forces were involved in this; the first was demonstration of a slightly increased risk of infection following IA injection of 250 mg of Adequan compared with corticosteroids and HA.[14] However, a companion study found that all risks would be obviated with concurrent IA injection of amikacin sulfate, 125 mg (0.5 mL).[15] The second was development of a 500-mg dose of IM Adequan, which veterinarians chose as a safer alternative. In a survey of 20 practitioners in 2003, 6/7 racehorse veterinarians used intraarticularly administered PSGAG, at least occasionally; whereas, a similar number of nonracehorse veterinarians avoided this practice.[16] In the 2009 survey, the majority of AAEP member respondents selected PSGAG (423/674, 62.8%) as the most frequently used disease-modifying medication, independent of route of administration. However, the majority who used PSGAG chose to administer it IM (643/764, 84.1%).[13] In the meantime IA use of PSGAG remained common in Europe. The multivariable analysis of factors influencing the outcome of two treatment protocols in 128 horses that had responded positively to IA analgesia of the distal interphalangeal joint showed significant positive effects with an IA PSGAG therapy protocol of 3 IA injections approximately 8 days apart.[17] Interestingly, antimicrobial drugs were not administered and no adverse results were reported. However, because of the study suggesting that IA Adequan could potentiate infection[14] and that any risk could be obviated by concurrent IA injection of amikacin,[15] it is the author's recommendation that amikacin should still be used for legal protection.

Intramuscular Use of PSGAG

As noted, the IM administration of PSGAG became popular in the late 1980s and 1990s. However, IM PSGAG (500 mg every 4 days for 7 treatments) produced relatively insignificant effects in horses with sodium monoiodoacetate-induced synovitis.[18] The one significant difference was limited to slightly improved GAG staining in the articular cartilage. In a more recent study using the osteochondral fragment-exercise model in which IM PSGAG was used as a positive control (administered every 4th day for 28 days starting 14 days post-OA induction), decreased GAG levels in the serum 14 days posttreatment was the only significant beneficial effect.[19] In this study, better improvement was seen in horses given extracorporeal shockwave therapy.

In a 1996 survey, PSGAG was considered more effective than HA for the treatment of subacute OA and less effective for idiopathic joint effusion in acute synovitis[20]; however, there is currently only weak evidence to justify IM administration. It has been reported that articular cartilage concentration of PSGAG after IM administration is of a level capable of inhibiting some cartilage-degrading enzymes,[21] but the duration of effective concentration is unclear. A number of articular degradative enzymes were reduced in an in vitro study in other animals, but direct evidence of effectiveness in the horse is lacking.[21,22] Intramuscular PSGAG is principally used as a preventative measure and information from the manufacturer reports that 90% of sales are for such "prophylactic" use. There have been no scientific studies on prophylactic use and the efficacy is difficult to prove or disprove. In the survey published in 2011, the majority of respondents selected PSGAG (Adequan) (423/674, 62.8%) as the most frequently used disease-modifying medication independent of route of administration. However, the majority of respondents who used PSGAG chose to administer it IM (643/764, 84.1%). Most commonly IM PSGAG was used for prophylactic/preventative treatment in 569/727 (78.3%) respondents. It was also used IM by 425/727 (58.5%) in chronic maintenance cases and by 396/727 (54.5%) in postoperative horses starting back into training. Intramuscular PSGAG was the most common medication selected by respondents for treatment of acute disease in low-motion joints (325/727, 44.7%) and the most common treatment used for a tendon or ligament lesion (201/727, 27.7%).[13]

HYALURONAN, SODIUM CHONDROITIN SULFATE, AND *N*-ACETYL-ᴅ-GLUCOSAMINE COMBINATION PRODUCTS

In a previously mentioned survey of equine practitioners, 18% of the respondents indicated that they had used an HA, sodium chondroitin sulfate, and *N*-acetyl-ᴅ-glucosamine combination product (PG) (Polyglycan®) for the treatment of OA.[13] This compounded formulation is not approved by the U.S. Food and Drug Administration, although it is labeled to be administered in the U.S. as a 5-mL dose containing 25 mg of hyaluronic acid sodium salt, 500 mg of sodium chondroitin sulfate, and 500 mg of *N*-acetyl-ᴅ-glucosamine. The products label indicates that it can be used for IA administration as a postsurgical joint lavage.[23] However, despite the IA labeling recommendation, respondents to the survey reported using three routes of administration, namely intravenous (IV) and IM as well as IA (62%, 18%, 22%, respectively).[22]

Despite the reported usage of the product (750,000+ doses had been sold in 2012), there is no Medline-indexed peer review publication on it. At CSU we have recently completed a study to assess the efficacy of the product when administered IA (as directed on the label) in our equine OA model evaluating both clinical signs and/or disease-modifying effects as well as monitoring for any adverse effects. A randomized, blinded, placebo-controlled trial was conducted to assess the clinical, biochemical, and histologic effects of PG administered through an IA route for the treatment of OA. Osteoarthritis was induced in one carpal joint of each of 16 horses. Horses were designated placebo or IA PG treated.[23] All horses

were treated with 125 mg of amikacin sulfate IA and 5 mL of physiologic saline in the middle carpal joint bilaterally on study days 0 (after induction of OA), 7, 14, and 28, except the OA-affected joint of the IA PG horses, which received 5 mL of PG plus 125 mg of amikacin sulfate on similar days. Evaluations included clinical and radiographic examinations, synovial fluid analysis, and gross and histologic examinations as well as histochemical and biochemical analysis. The model induced a similar degree of pathologic changes as reported in other studies.[24] IA treatment of OA-affected joints with PG resulted in a transient 16% improvement in clinical pain (lameness scores) and evidence of improvement trends in bone proliferation radiographically as well as in the degree of full thickness articular cartilage erosion seen grossly when compared with placebo-treated OA joints, although other outcome parameters were not significantly different from those in controls. These findings support potential symptom- and disease-modifying effects of this compound administered IA at the tested dose and frequency. More recent unpublished data examining lubrication function shortly after injection of PG suggest significant improvement in lubrication 4 hours after injection versus saline-injected controls. This provides support for use of the product postsurgically (M.M. Temple-Wong et al., unpublished data).

The product has also been used IV with anecdotal impressions of efficacy. However, testing of IV PG in the chip fragment OA model did not show significant benefit and there was suggestion of negative changes in the bone (D.D. Frisbie et al., unpublished data).

REFERENCES

1. Trotter GW. Polysulfated glycosaminoglycan (Adequan®). In: McIlwraith CW, Trotter GW, eds. *Joint disease in the horse*. Philadelphia, PA: Saunders; 1996:270–280.
2. May SA, Hooke RE, Lees P. The effect of drugs used in the treatment of osteoarthritis on stromelysin (proteoglycanease) of equine synovial cell origin. *Equine Vet J*. 1988;S6:28–32.
3. Glade MJ. Polysulfated glycosaminoglycan accelerates net synthesis of collagen in glycosaminoglycans by arthritic equine cartilage tissues in chondrocytes. *Am J Vet Res*. 1990;51(5):779–785.
4. Caron JP, Eberhart SW, Nachreiner R. Influence of polysulfated glycosaminoglycan on equine articular cartilage in explant culture. *Am J Vet Res*. 1991;52(10):1622–1625.
5. Tew WP. Demonstration by synovial fluid analysis of the efficacy in horses of an investigational drug (L-1016). *J Equine Vet Sci*. 1982;2(2):42–50.
6. White GW, Jones EW, Hamm J, et al. The efficacy of orally administered sulfated glycosaminoglycan in chemically-induced equine synovitis and degenerative joint disease. *J Equine Vet Sci*. 1994;14(7):350–353.
7. Yovich J, Trotter GW, McIlwraith CW, et al. Effects of polysulfated glycosaminoglycan upon chemical and physical defects in equine articular cartilage. *Am J Vet Res*. 1987;48(9):1407–1417.
8. Todhunter RJ, Minor RR, Wootton J, et al. Effects of exercise and polysulfated glycosaminoglycan on repair of articular cartilage defects in the equine carpus. *J Orthop Res*. 1993;11(6):782–795.

9. Frisbie DD, Kawcak CE, McIlwraith CW, et al. Evaluation of polysulfated glycosaminoglycan or sodium hyaluronan administered intra-articularly for treatment of horses with experimentally induced osteoarthritis. *Am J Vet Res.* 2009;70(2):203–209.

10. Frisbie DD, Kawcak CE, Werpy NM, et al. Combination of intraarticular (IA) triamcinolone acetonide and polysulfated glycosaminoglycan compared to IA polysulfated glycosaminoglycan or placebo for treatment of osteoarthritis using an equine experimental model. In: *Proc Am Assoc Equine Pract.* 2010;56:25–26.

11. Frisbie DD, Trotter GW, Powers BE, et al. Arthroscopic subchondral bone plate microfracture technique augments healing of large chondral defects in the radial carpal bone and medial femoral condyle of horses. *Vet Surg.* 1999;28(4):242–255.

12. Gaustad G, Larson S. Comparison of polysulfated glycosaminoglycan and sodium hyaluronate with placebo in treatment of traumatic arthritis in horses. *Equine Vet J.* 1995;27(5):356–362.

13. Ferris DJ, Frisbie DD, McIlwraith CW, et al. Current joint therapy usage in equine practice: a survey of veterinarians 2009. *Equine Vet J.* 2011;43(5):530–535.

14. Gustafson SB, McIlwraith CW, Jones RL. Comparison of the effect of polysulfated glycosaminoglycans, corticosteroids and sodium hyaluronate in the potentiation of a subinfective dose of *Staphylococcus aureus* in the midcarpal joint of horses. *Am J Vet Res.* 1989;50(12):2014–2017.

15. Gustafson SB, McIlwraith CW, Jones RL, et al. Further investigation into the potentiation of infection by intra-articular injection of polysulfated glycosaminoglycan and the effect of filtration and intra-articular amikacin. *Am J Vet Res.* 1989;50(12):2018–2022.

16. Caron JP, Genovese RL. Principles and practices of joint disease treatment. In: Ross MW, Dyson SJ, eds. *Diagnosis and management of lameness in the horse.* Philadelphia, PA: Elsevier; 2003:746–763.

17. Kristiansen KK, Kold SE. Multi-variable analysis of factors influencing outcome of two treatment protocols in 128 cases of horses responding positively to intraarticular analgesia of the distal interphalangeal joint. *Equine Vet J.* 2007;39(2):150–156.

18. Trotter GW, Yovich J, McIlwraith CW, et al. Effects of intramuscular polysulfated glycosaminoglycan on chemical and physical defect in equine articular cartilage. *Can J Vet Res.* 1989;53(2):224–230.

19. Frisbie DD, Kawcak CE, McIlwraith CW. Evaluation of the effect of extracorporeal shockwave treatment on experimentally induced osteoarthritis in middle carpal joints of horses. *Am J Vet Res.* 2009;70(4):449–454.

20. Caron JP, Kaneene JB, Miller R. Results of a survey of equine practitioners on the use and efficacy of polysulfated glycosaminoglycan. *Am J Vet Res.* 1996;209(9):1564–1568.

21. Burba DJ, Collier MA, Default LE, et al. In vivo kinetic study on uptake and distribution of intramuscular titanium-labeled polysulfated glycosaminoglycan in equine body fluid compartments and articular cartilage in an osteochondral defect model. *J Equine Vet Sci.* 1993;13(12):696.

22. Howell DS, Carreno MR, Palletta JP, et al. Articular cartilage breakdown in a lapine model of osteoarthritis: action of glycosaminoglycan polysulfate ester (GAGPS) on proteoglycan enzyme activity, hexuronate, and cell count. *Clin Orthop Relat Res.* 1986;213:69–76.

23. Frisbie DD, McIlwraith CW, Kawcak CE, et al. Evaluation of intra-articular hyaluronan, sodium chondroitin sulfate and N-acetyl-D-glucosamine versus saline (0.9% NaCl) for osteoarthritis using an equine model. *Vet J.* 2013;197(3):824–829.

24. McIlwraith CW, Frisbie DD, Kawcak CE. The horse as a model of naturally occurring osteoarthritis. *Bone Joint Res.* 2012;1(11):297–309.

15

Pentosan Polysulfate

C. Wayne McIlwraith

Although pentosan polysulfate (PPS) as the sodium salt (NaPPS) has been used in Europe for many years as an anti-thrombotic-antilipidemic agent, its potential as a disease-modifying antiarthritic agent has been realized since then.[1] The use of intramuscular (IM) NaPPS in equine joint disease has developed more recently, and its use was initially reviewed by Little and Ghosh in the first edition of this text.[1] A calcium derivative of PPS (CaPPS) has also been developed and can be used IM or orally (this route could offer increased use particularly in small animals). Both NaPPS and CaPPS are semi-synthetic products derived from beech trees. The backbone of PPS, which consists of repeating units of (1-4)-linked β-D-xylano-pyranoses, is isolated from beech-wood hemicellulose (Figure 15-1).

Commercial products available currently include Cartrophen Vet (licensed for use in small animals but not in horses in Australasia and Europe) and more recently Pentosan Equine Injection (250 mg/mL PPS sodium) (Figure 15-2), which is licensed in Australia. It has been shown that peak blood concentrations of PPS occur approximately 2 hours after IM or subcutaneous administration.[2,3]

In the initial review of the potential use of PPS for the treatment of equine joint disease,[1] it was reported that laboratory investigations together with studies using animal models of arthropathy showed that PPS acts on a number of metabolic pathways relevant to the pathogenesis of osteoarthritis (OA). In the same review, multiple modes of action were illustrated (Figure 15-3).[1] These modes of action include preservation of proteoglycan content by promoting the synthesis of large proteoglycans, inhibiting the enzymes responsible for proteoglycan and collagen degradation, and increasing synthesis of tissue inhibitor of metalloproteinase-3 (TIMP-3) by synoviocytes and chondrocytes.[4-6] PPS also has anticoagulant activity and, although the anticoagulant activity is weaker than heparin, it is a more potent fibrinolytic agent and also an inhibitor of thromboxane-induced platelet aggregation.[7] PPS binds to endothelial cells and tissue plasmogen activator and lipoprotein lipase, and super oxide dismutase may be released. Such activities of PPS would be expected to promote mobilization of vascular thrombi and lipids, thereby improving perfusion to tissues.[8] Improvement in the compromised blood flow and the subchondral bone of OA patients that is afforded by PPS could result in improved osteocyte nutrition, as well as a reduction in the pain resulting from vascular hypoperfusion and increased intraosseous pressure attendant with vascular occlusion.[7] Little and Ghosh suggested in 1996 on the basis of these activities that PPS offered considerable potential for the treatment of joint diseases in the horse. The reader is recommended to consult the chapter in the previous edition of this text for further details.[1] This chapter in the second edition will focus principally on more recent studies relative to use of PPS in the horse.

MECHANISMS OF ACTION

In the 1996 review the authors suggested that PPS, unlike nonsteroidal antiinflammatory drugs, does not possess analgesic activity and that to provide symptomatic relief and efficacy a drug must be capable of correcting the pathobiologic imbalances that are present within the respective tissues of OA joints.[1] Based on multiple studies it would appear that PPS could fulfill these requirements. In experimental joint disease in rabbits, oral administration of CaPPS (10 mg/kg, every 7 days) maintained the normal articular cartilage ratio of aggrecan to dermatan sulfate (interpreted by the authors as chondrocytic phenotype).[8] Sodium PPS also stimulates HA synthesis by cultured synoviocytes obtained from both rheumatoid and osteoarthritic human joints.[9] The in vitro effects of NaPPS on HA synthesis were confirmed in a rat air pouch model of inflammation, and increased synthesis of HA was not stimulated by polysulfated glycosaminoglycan (PSGAG).[10]

Several in vivo studies reveal that PPS inhibits various processes that induce degeneration of the articular cartilage matrix. For example, PPS inhibits metalloproteinase 3.[11] There is a suggestion that PPS may modulate receptor-mediated binding of cytokines.[1] In sheep with experimental OA (induced via medial meniscectomy), weekly intraarticular (IA) injections of 25 mg PPS for 4 weeks improved joint function and reduced mean radiographic scores and Mankin histologic scores of articular cartilage damage in the femoral condyle.[12] The simultaneous administration of IGF-1 IA (1 μg) and NaPPS IM (2 mg/kg once weekly from weeks 3 to 6) and IM NaPPS alone significantly reduced the severity of lesions in iatrogenic OA in dogs, but IA IGF-1 and IM PPS combination successfully maintained near-normal levels of active and total neutral MMPs, tissue inhibitor of metalloproteinases (TIMP), as well as hydroxyprotein content.[13] The presence of PPS appeared to decrease the amount of total and active matrix metalloproteinases in the cartilage. The authors

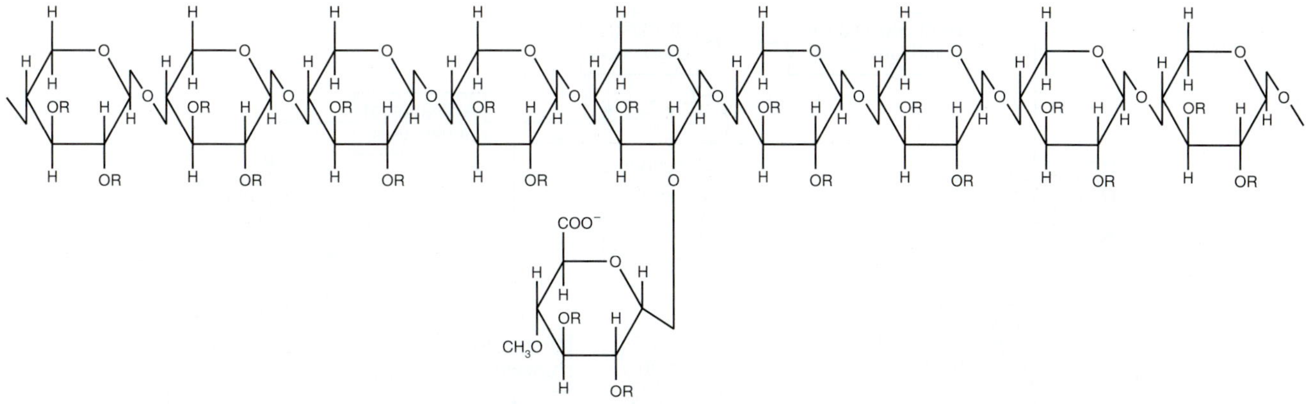

FIGURE 15-1 Pentosan polysulfate (PPS), a polydisperse macromolecule, has an average molecular weight of approximately 5700 Dalton. It is manufactured by sulfation of beech-wood hemicellulose, which consists of (1-4)-linked β-D-xylano-pyranose units with a methylated glucuronyl ring substituted at about every ninth xylano-pyranose ring along the chain (R=H). In PPS, virtually all the hydroxyl groups are esterified (R=SO$_3$ sulfate) to produce a strongly anionic rodlike structure. (Reproduced with permission from Little C., Ghosh P. (1996). Potential use of pentosan polysulfate for the treatment of equine joint disease. In: McIlwraith C.W., Trotter G.W. (Eds.) Joint disease in the horse (p. 282). Philadelphia, PA: Saunders.)

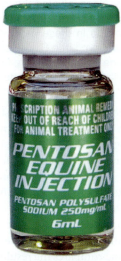

FIGURE 15-2 Pentosan equine injection (pentosan polysulfate sodium 250 mg/mL) as used in the in vivo studies of pentosan polysulfate A 6-mL dose is sufficient for horses at a dose rate of 3 mg/kg. (Courtesy: Ceva Animal Health Pty, Ltd.)

also suggested that PPS reduced enzymatic breakdown of IGF-1 binding protein or receptor, thus allowing IGF-1 to exert its influence.

STUDIES IN HORSES

In Vitro Studies in Horses

Some in vitro studies have been done in horses, including one that revealed that PPS as well as PSGAG stimulate proteoglycan synthesis in chondrocyte monolayer cultures in a concentration-related manner, with maximal effects at a concentration of 10 µg/mL, but neither PSGAG nor PPS exerted significant effects on proteoglycan synthesis in cartilage explants.[14] In another study, it was concluded that it

was improbable that PPS had a substantial effect on gelatinase matrix metalloproteinase activity.[15]

In Vivo Studies in Horses

There are no published reports describing the use of PPS for clinical cases of equine joint disease, but the drug has been used for approximately 20 years in Australia and New Zealand. When administered to racing Thoroughbreds with chronic OA (2 to 3 mg/kg, IM, once weekly for 4 weeks, then as required), PPS treatment improved but did not eliminate clinical signs of joint disease.[1] It has been proposed that because of the vascular effects of the drug, it could decrease the rate of subchondral bone necrosis and sclerosis.[1] A comparison of the lipolytic and anticoagulative properties of heparin and PPS in Thoroughbreds revealed that although there was a comparable lipolytic effect to heparin, including significant increase of plasma-free fatty acids, PPS had much less of an effect on clotting function versus heparin.[16] A study in which single injections of NaPPS at doses of 0, 3 (currently recommended dose for joint problems), 6, and 10 mg/kg were compared revealed a dose-dependent increase in partial prothrombin time.[17] The authors found that the increase was small and remained increased from baseline for 24 hours. They concluded that, on the basis of these findings, doses of PPS up to 3 mg/kg should not be administered to horses within 24 hours of high-stress activities or where there is a risk of physical injury.

The first controlled in vivo study in the horse evaluated IM administered NaPPS for the treatment of experimentally induced OA in horses.[18] The study used the Colorado State University (CSU) equine osteochondral fragment-exercise model that has been used to evaluate multiple treatments in the horse.[19-27] OA was induced arthroscopically in one middle carpal joint of all horses. Nine horses received NaPPS (3 mg/kg, IM) on study days 15, 22, 29, and 36. Nine control horses received the same volume of saline (0.9% NaCl) solution on the same study days. Clinical, radiographic,

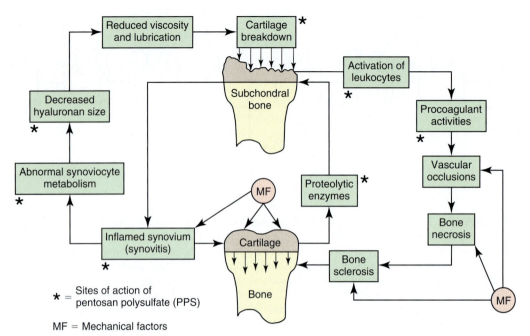

FIGURE 15-3 Interrelationship of pathologic changes in articular cartilage, subchondral bone, joint synovial lining, and synovial fluid that occur in osteoarthritic joints. Once initiated the interdependent pathways can be self-sustaining, leading eventually to complete loss of joint function. Pentosan polysulfate (PPS) has been shown to act at a number of points in these pathways, some of which are identified in this figure. (Reproduced with permission from Little C., Ghosh P. (1996). Potential use of pentosan polysulfate for the treatment of equine joint disease. In: McIlwraith C.W., Trotter G.W. (Eds.) Joint disease in the horse (p. 287). Philadelphia, PA: Saunders.)

gross, histologic, histochemical, and biochemical findings as well as findings of synovial fluid analysis were evaluated. No adverse treatment-related events including any evidence of clotting disturbances were detected. Induced OA caused a substantial increase in lameness, response to flexion, joint effusion, radiographic findings, synovial membrane inflammation, and articular cartilage fibrillation. Articular cartilage fibrillation was significantly reduced by NaPPS ($P = 0.022$), and there was a strong trend ($P = 0.062$) in the mean score of cartilage histology (variables were articular cartilage fibrillation, chondrocyte necrosis, chondrocyte clustering, and focal cell loss, each ranging from 0 to 4) (Figure 15-4). In addition, concentrations of chondroitin sulfate 846 epitope (a synthetic biomarker for chondroitin sulfate synthesis) increased in the synovial fluid of osteoarthritic and nonosteoarthritic joints of treated horses. These results indicated that NaPPS was beneficial in one disease-modifying effect, which provided objective support of NaPPS as a systemic treatment option for OA in horses. Several other variables including lameness, joint flexion, and synovial fluid total protein and chondroitin sulfate 846 epitope concentrations improved but not significantly. Historically, increases in serum and synovial fluid chondroitin sulfate 846 epitope have been interpreted as a reparative response and this would be supported by an increase in synovial fluid chondroitin sulfate 846 epitope concentrations in osteoarthritic versus nonosteoarthritic joints of untreated animals in the present study. The fact that the synovial fluid from both the osteoarthritic and nonosteoarthritic joints of the NaPPS-treated horses had higher chondroitin sulfate 846

epitope concentrations potentially suggests a systemic upregulation of aggrecan synthesis, rather than a simple response to pathologic changes (based on the positive effect in other outcome parameters). The significant decrease in articular cartilage fibrillation supports classification of NaPPS as a disease-modifying osteoarthritic drug (DMOAD). No adverse effects were seen. These results were also consistent with suggestions of Little and Ghosh[1] that, rather than a reduction in signs of lameness, the main effects of the drug were disease-modifying. When one compares the results of IM administration of a recommended dose (3 mg/kg) of PPS in this study to the IM administration of the recommended dose (500 mg) of PSGAG using the same experimental model in a separate study,[23] more favorable outcomes were observed with PPS. In the PSGAG study there was no significant improvement in any outcome variable except for serum GAG concentrations, which were lower at one time point in the PSGAG group compared with the placebo group.

More recently, a second study using the CSU OA model (but conducted in Australia) with an intravenous (IV) combination of sodium PPS, N-acetyl glucosamine (NAG), and HA (Pentosan Gold plus Halo) was carried out.[28] OA was induced arthroscopically in one middle carpal joint as previously described and 8 horses received 3 mg/kg of PPS, 4.8 mg/kg NAG, and 0.12 mg/kg HA IV weekly, and 8 horses received an equivalent volume of IV saline until the completion of the study (day 70). Horses underwent the standardized treadmill exercise program as used in the CSU model. Again, OA caused increases in clinical assessment

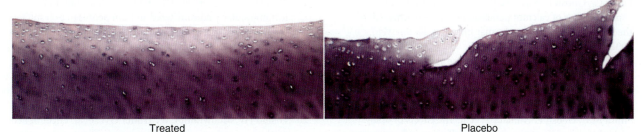

Treated   Placebo

FIGURE 15-4 Photomicrographs of articular cartilage from a placebo-treated middle carpal joint in a horse with experimentally induced osteoarthritis, compared with a NaPPS-treated middle carpal joint in a horse with experimentally induced osteoarthritis. H&E stain; bar = 100 μm. (Reproduced with permission from McIlwraith C.W., Frisbie D.D., Kawcak C.E (2012). Evaluation of intramuscularly administered sodium pentosan polysulfate for treatment of experimentally induced osteoarthritis in horses. Am J Vet Res 73(5), 628-633.)

scores, synovial fluid variables, radiographic, macroscopic, and histologic cartilage scores, synovial fluid and cartilage chondroitin sulfate 846 epitope, and GAG concentration. Total radiographic scores, total macroscopic joint pathology, and microscopic cartilage pathology scores were significantly reduced in horses treated with the combination compared with those in the saline group. Synovial fluid total protein and white blood cell count were higher in OA joints of the combination-treated versus saline-treated horses. In this study the administration of the NaPPS combination drug had no effect on lameness scores, which is consistent with the previous study with NaPPS alone. Although total radiographic scores, total pathology, and macroscopic cartilage scores in OA joints were significantly lower in the treated horses compared with the saline-treated horses, there were no differences in any of the measured histologic and biochemical variables in the articular cartilage or in the synovial membrane histology. DMOAD properties were certainly implied by the changes in the macroscopic parameters, but the DMOAD properties were not as strong as with NaPPS alone.

Relevant to the lack of significant improvement in clinical symptoms in either of the previously mentioned studies, it should be recognized that the degree of lameness in the OA joints is quite low. A clinical study has been done in 39 horses with clinical OA and more obvious lameness (F. Hughes, unpublished data). There were three treatment groups with 13 horses/group: 1) Pentosan Equine once every 5 days for 4 injections (3 mg/kg) (PPS4), 2) Pentosan Equine once every 5 days for 7 injections (3 mg/kg) (PPS7), and 3) Adequan® once every 5 days for 7 injections (500 mg). Lameness was assessed using a 10-cm visual analog scale (VAS) with 0 being no lameness and 10 being non-weight-bearing lameness; in addition, the AAEP score (0-5), flexion/range of motion using VAS with a grade of 0 to 4, and direct measurement of stride length were used. All treatments significantly reduced lameness scores at week 4. Assessments at weeks 2 and 6 demonstrated both pentosan groups significantly reduced lameness scores but Adequan had no significant difference from pretreatment baseline. Horses receiving PPS responded faster than those receiving Adequan (week 2) and horses receiving Adequan tended to regress (become more lame again) after the end of treatments on day 35 (week 6) than those on pentosan who maintained their improvement over the same period. Pentosan-treated groups showed increased stride length at weeks 2, 4, and 6, and the Adequan-treated group showed decreased stride length at weeks 4 and 6. Pentosan treatment groups showed significantly more improvement in stride length than the Adequan group at weeks 2, 4, and 6.

SUMMARY

Anecdotal clinical reports confirm value of PPS, at least with a dose of 3 mg/kg IM once a week for 4 weeks. When the lameness is sufficiently evident, clinical improvement will also be seen but in the controlled study with NaPPS alone there were DMOAD effects, making this product unique to the equine veterinarian. This is the only systemically administered DMOAD reported and each comparison in three studies showed clear superiority to Adequan IM. As discussed in the previous chapter Adequan is a very effective drug IA but has shown less potency in the OA chip fragment model when administered IM. This presumably is a dose effect rather than an insinuation that there is no value in systemic administration.

REFERENCES

1. Little C, Ghosh P. Potential use of pentosan polysulfate for the treatment of equine joint disease. In: McIlwraith CW, Trotter GW, eds. *Joint disease in the horse*. Philadelphia, PA: Saunders; 1996:281–292.
2. MacGregor IR, Dawes J, Paton L, et al. Metabolism of sodium pentosan polysulfate in man – catabolism of the iodinated derivatives. *Thromb Haemost*. 1984;51(3):321–325.
3. Dawes J, Prowse CV, Pepper DS. Absorption of heparin, LMW heparin and SP54 after subcutaneous injection, assessed by competitive binding assay. *Thromb Res*. 1986;44(5):683–693.
4. Ghosh P. The pathobiology of osteoarthritis and the rationale for the use of pentosan polysulfate for its treatment. *Semin Arthritis Rheum*. 1999;28(4):211–267.
5. Ghosh P, Smith M. Osteoarthritis, genetic and molecular mechanisms. *Biogerontology*. 2002;3(1-2):85–88.

6. Fuller CJ, Ghosh P, Barr AR. Plasma and synovial fluid concentrations of calcium pentosan polysulfate achieved in the horse following intramuscular injection. *Equine Vet J.* 2002;34(1):61–64.

7. Ghosh P, Smith M, Wells C. Second line agents in osteoarthritis. In: Dixon JS, Furst DE, eds. *Second line agents in the treatment of rheumatic diseases.* New York, NY: Marcel Dekker; 1992:363–427.

8. Smith MM, Ghosh P, Numata Y, et al. The effects of orally administered calcium pentosan polysulfate on inflammation and cartilage degradation produced in rabbit joints by intraarticular injection of a hyaluronate-polylysine complex. *Arthritis Rheum.* 1994;37(1):125–136.

9. Jimenez SA. The effect of glucosamine on human chondrocyte gene expression. In: *Proc Eur League Against Rheum Symp.* 1996:8–10.

10. Francis DJ, Forrest MJ, Brooks PM, et al. Retardation of articular cartilage degradation by glycosaminoglycan polysulfate, pentosan polysulfate, and DH-40J in the rat air pouch model. *Arthritis Rheum.* 1989;32(5):608–616.

11. Nethery A, Giles I, Jenkins K, et al. The chondroprotective drugs, Arteparon and sodium pentosan polysulfate, increase collagenase activity and inhibit stromelysin activity in vitro. *Biochem Pharmacol.* 1992;44(8):1549–1553.

12. Ghosh P, Armstrong S, Read R, et al. Animal models of early osteoarthritis: their use for the evaluation of potential chondroprotective agents. In: VandenBerg WB, van der Kraan PM, van Lent PLEM, eds. *Joint destruction in arthritis and osteoarthritis.* Austin, Texas: Birkhauser; 1993:195.

13. Rogachefsky RA, Dean DD, Howell DS, et al. Treatment of canine osteoarthritis with insulin-like growth factor (IGF-1) and sodium pentosan polysulfate. *Osteoarthritis Cartilage.* 1993;1(2):105–114.

14. Frean SP, Cambridge H, Lees P. Effects of anti-arthritic drugs on proteoglycan synthesis of equine cartilage. *J Vet Pharmacol Ther.* 2002;25(4):289–298.

15. Clegg PD, Jones MD, Carter SD. The effect of drugs commonly used in the treatment of equine articular disorders on the activity of equine matrix metalloproteinase-2 and 9. *J Vet Pharmacol Ther.* 1998;21(5):406–413.

16. Orme CE, Harris RC. A comparison of the lipolytic and anticoagulant properties of heparin and pentosan polysulfate in the Thoroughbred horse. *Acta Physiol Scand.* 1997;159(2):179–185.

17. Dart AJ, Perkins N, Dowling BA, et al. The effect of three different doses of sodium pentosan polysulfate on haematological and haemostatic variables in adult horses. *Aust Vet J.* 2001;79(9):624–627.

18. McIlwraith CW, Frisbie DD, Kawcak CE. Evaluation of intramuscularly administered sodium pentosan polysulfate for treatment of experimentally induced osteoarthritis in horses. *Am J Vet Res.* 2012;73(5):628–633.

19. Kawcak CE, Frisbie DD, Trotter GW, et al. Effects of intravenous administration of sodium hyaluronate on carpal joints in exercising horses after arthroscopic surgery and osteochondral fragmentation. *Am J Vet Res.* 1997;58(10):1132–1140.

20. Foland JW, McIlwraith CW, Trotter GW, et al. Effect of betamethasone and exercise on equine carpal joints with osteochondral fragments. *Vet Surg.* 1994;23(5):369–376.

21. Frisbie DD, Kawcak CE, Baxter GM, et al. The effects of 6-alpha methylprednisolone acetate on an equine osteochondral fragment exercise model. *Am J Vet Res.* 1998;59(12):1619–1628.

22. Frisbie DD, Kawcak CE, Trotter GW, et al. The effects of triamcinolone acetate on an in vivo equine osteochondral fragment exercise model. *Equine Vet J.* 1997;29(5):349–359.

23. Frisbie DD, Kawcak CE, McIlwraith CW. Evaluation of the effect of extracorporeal shockwave treatment on experimentally induced osteoarthritis in middle carpal joints of horses. *Am J Vet Res.* 2009;70(4):449–454.

24. Frisbie DD, Kawcak CE, McIlwraith CW, et al. Evaluation of polysulfated glycosaminoglycan or sodium hyaluronan administered intra-articularly for treatment of horses with experimentally induced osteoarthritis. *Am J Vet Res.* 2009;70(2):203–209.

25. Frisbie DD, McIlwraith CW, Kawcak CE, et al. Evaluation of topically administered diclofenac liposomal cream for treatment of horses with experimentally induced osteoarthritis. *Am J Vet Res.* 2009;70(2):210–215.

26. Frisbie DD, Kawcak CE, Werpy NM, et al. Clinical, biochemical, and histologic effects of intra-articular administration of autologous conditioned serum in horses with experimentally induced osteoarthritis. *Am J Vet Res.* 2007;68(3):290–296.

27. Frisbie DD, Ghivizzani SC, Robbins PD, et al. Treatment of experimental equine osteoarthritis by an in vivo delivery of equine interleukin-1 receptor antagonist gene. *Gene Ther.* 2002;9(1):12–20.

28. Koenig TJ, Dart AJ, McIlwraith CW, et al. Treatment of experimentally induced osteoarthritis in horses using an intravenous combination of sodium pentosan polysulfate, N-acetyl glucosamine and sodium hyaluronate. *Vet Surg.* 2014;43(5):612–622.

16

Biologic Therapies

David D. Frisbie

Biologic therapy for the treatment of joint disease has blossomed over the last decade. We have reasonable proof-of-principle that some biologic therapies are effective in joint disease, but there is much to learn and to improve/optimize when it comes to biologic therapies in all aspects of medicine including joint therapy. This chapter will outline the current biologic therapies that are being considered in mainstream equine practice and define the composition of the therapy as well as the level of knowledge about applications in the joint, especially those specific to the horse.

AUTOLOGOUS CONDITIONED SERUM

The first report on incubating whole blood with medical-grade glass beads that have undergone processing (coating then washing) to change the surface characteristics was published in 2003,[1] but was purportedly developed in the mid-1990s. It described the production of antiinflammatory cytokines in the absence of significant production of proinflammatory cytokines. These data have not been repeated and have been challenged by some in human[2] as well as horse medicine.[3] Specifically, in the horse we have shown it is important to assess the ratio of antiinflammatory to proinflammatory cytokine production,[3] given clear production of proinflammatory cytokines. In the author's opinion the trade names for autologous conditioned serum (ACS), IRAP® and IRAP II®, are very misleading. It is clear there is significantly more in the ACS than just interleukin (IL)-1 receptor antagonist protein (IRAP). In fact, using differential display electrophoresis and mass spectroscopy identification, the author was able to identify at least 35 different proteins that were differentially regulated (greater than 2×) with the IRAP processing compared with baseline serum (unpublished data). This work, as well as other published results,[1-3] confirms that IRAP is not the only protein in the "soup." Further, it is not definitively known which of the proteins are responsible for the biologic activity. Using equine blood IRAP, IL-10, insulin-like growth factor-1, transforming growth factor-β, tumor necrosis factor (TNF)-α, and IL-1β have all been shown to be significantly upregulated using a commercial ACS kit compared with baseline serum.[3] There is, however, significant evidence for a positive role of IL-1 receptor antagonist in the treatment of equine joint disease and in ACS.[4]

Human Clinical Data for Intraarticular Autologous Conditioned Serum

In a prospective, randomized, patient- and observer-blinded, placebo-controlled trial, ACS was compared with saline or HA alone.[5] The study included 376 human patients with knee OA and had follow-up that extended to 104 weeks with both functional and safety outcomes. The saline and HA injections (1×10^6 Dalton product) were carried out once a week for 3 treatments and the ACS twice a week for 6 treatments. The results indicated that ACS provided significantly superior effects versus those of saline and HA. Further, the adverse events for ACS (23%) were similar to saline (28%) and significantly better than HA (38%). Another randomized controlled study in humans undergoing anterior cruciate ligament (ACL) reconstruction demonstrated a significant improvement in patient-administered outcome (Western Ontario and McMaster Universities Osteoarthritis Index [WOMAC]) in the ACS-(N=31) when compared with placebo-(N=31, saline) treated joints at time points throughout the study; some WOMAC parameters were improved out to 1 year, the length of the study.[6] Further, the short-term reduction in IL-1β was observed at 10 days after treatment in the ACS-treated group compared with controls and enlargement of the bone tunnel (related to the ACL repair) was significantly less in the ACS versus the placebo group. Thus, clinical evidence for the use of ACS in human joint disease does exist.

Equine Intraarticular Autologous Conditioned Serum

The clinical use of ACS in equine patients suffering from joint disease remains anecdotal. However, in the mid 2000s, Thomas Weinberg estimated his clinical usage at over 3000 cases (personal communication). In a published survey of equine practitioners 54% of the 791 respondents indicated they had used ACS and 22% said they used it frequently.[7] The most common reason for ACS use was in corticosteroid-unresponsive joints. Also of interest, more English performance veterinarians were likely to use ACS compared with race or show horse veterinarians in the United States, potentially because of regulatory restrictions. However, racehorse veterinarians in other countries (where the use of corticosteroids is more restricted) are using increasing amounts of ACS.

One Medline-indexed in vivo study assessing ACS in the treatment of experimental equine OA currently exists. This study[8] demonstrated significant improvement in multiple parameters following treatment with ACS versus placebo. The study used a 6-mL treatment once a week for 4 treatments. No adverse events were recorded, and there was a significant improvement in lameness in the ACS-treated versus placebo-treated horses. Treatment with ACS was also able to improve synovial membrane parameters and significantly decrease the degree of gross articular cartilage fibrillation compared with placebo treatment, indicating a disease-modifying property of ACS. Another interesting finding was the continued increased level of presumably endogenous IRAP in the synovial fluid 3 weeks after the first treatment, which remained significantly elevated at the endpoint of the study, 35 days after the last treatment. This suggests a prolonged beneficial effect of ACS treatment. Further research into the clinical benefits still needs to be published; however, positive evidence for the use of intraarticular (IA) ACS exists.

PLATELET-RICH PLASMA

Important Facts about Using Platelet-Rich Plasma

The use of platelet-rich plasma (PRP) in medicine began in 1998 when Marx reported its benefit for healing mandibular defects in humans.[9] Wound healing indications were then published followed by application in tendon and ligamentous injuries and most recently IA applications. Although considerable literature has been published on PRP, this chapter will deal only with issues that relate to the IA application. Having said that, understanding how to define PRP and compare PRP preparations is paramount to its clinical use. In 2012 DeLong et al. proposed a classification system for PRP that nicely outlines the necessary considerations (Figure 16-1). There are three basic factors: the concentration of platelets, the presence of platelet activators, and the level of white blood cells (WBCs) in the preparation.[10] The role of each of these basic factors as well as optimization has not been defined well. It is likely that different disease processes will require different permutations in each of these factors for optimization. However, some general comments can be made.

It is clear that the concentration of PRP is one factor that can be easily compared although the absolute number of platelets can be more elusive. In general, PRP is defined as concentration of platelets that is significantly greater than that in baseline or peripheral blood. From a musculoskeletal point of view, which typically means joint, tendon, and ligament healing, significantly improved results have been seen with preparations that concentrate platelets anywhere from 2× to 3× to 4× to 6×.[10] However, platelet concentrations greater than 6× have been shown to have a negative effect on bone healing, suggesting more is not necessarily better.[11,12] Concentration-dependent deleterious effects have not been published for all tissues.

In general three methods of platelet activation have been reported in the clinical space. The first is endogenous activation; the second is calcium chloride; and the third is thrombin. It has been difficult to quantify the level of platelet activation in situ; however, evidence now exists that platelets are activated when PRP is administered into the joint.[13] In fact, platelets appear to be activated by addition to synovial fluid in vitro.[13] Thus, this is a viable option for activation and additives may not be desired for IA use. Calcium chloride is associated with a low pH solution and has been reported to be associated with significant pain and a burning sensation in people.[10] In an equine study, this did not appear to be the case when the authors compared endogenously activated PRP with that activated with calcium chloride.[14] This group also evaluated bovine thrombin as a method of platelet activation. Thrombin resulted in significant unwanted effects, which included increased synovial fluid total protein and WBC counts as well as effusion, pain on flexion, reluctance to bear weight when the contralateral limb was lifted, and periarticular heat and swelling. Although some of these same symptoms were observed with the endogenously activated PRP and calcium chloride-activated PRP, the magnitude of the change was less for these two activation methods. Based on the changes with

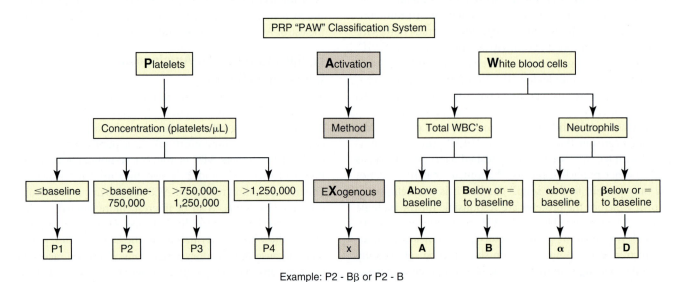

FIGURE 16-1 PRP PAW (platelet-activation white blood cell) classification system. (Reproduced with permission from DeLong J.M., Russell R.P., Mazzocca A.D. (2012). Platelet-rich plasma: the PAW classification system. Arthroscopy 28(7), 998-1009.)

endogenous and calcium chloride activation, the author would consider these two methods of activation as safe. It should be noted that this study operated a PRP system that uses a gravitation filter unit to concentrate the platelets approximately threefold and the WBCs twofold and administered 2.5-mL PRP in the fetlock joint. Thus, different preparation methods or volumes of administration for the PRP preparation most likely would yield different results (Figures 16-2 to 16-4).

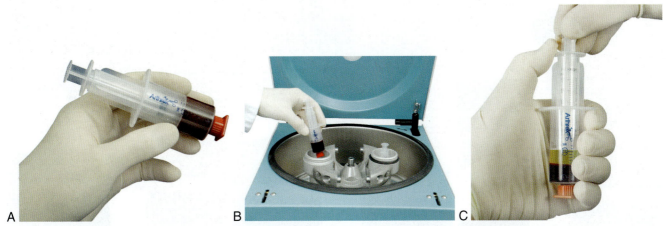

FIGURE 16-2 Different commercially available PRP systems. **(A)** Arthrex ACP™ double syringe system. Blood is drawn into the double syringe, **(B)** centrifuged for 5 minutes where the platelet-containing plasma (ACP) **(C)** is separated from the red blood cells (RBCs). (Images provided by Arthrex.)

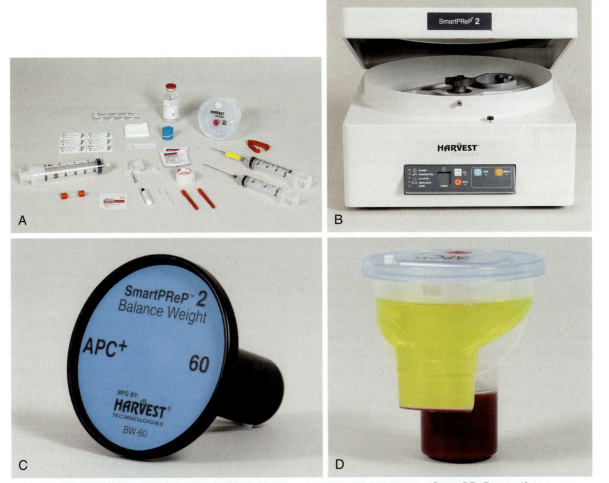

FIGURE 16-3 **(A)** Harvest SmartPReP kit components, **(B)** the Harvest SmartPReP centrifuge; self-decanting and preprogrammed to produce point of care PRP and stem cell concentrate from marrow in 14 minutes, **(C)** 60 mL Balance Weight and illustrating an equine PRP concentrate **(D)**. (Images provided by Terumo BCT.)

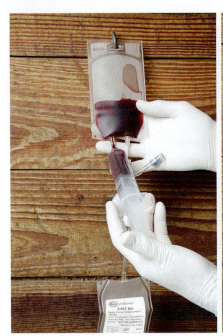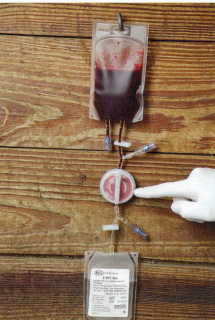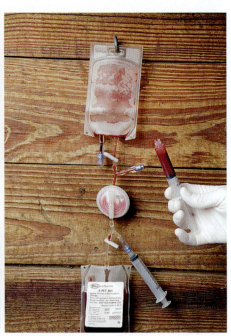

FIGURE 16-4 E-PET (equine platelet enhancement therapy) manufactured by Pall Corp. using gravity and a filter for concentration of platelets and WBC. (Images provided by Pall Animal Health.)

The concentration of WBC that is acceptable or desired in PRP is a hotly debated topic but it in general the literature supports the least number of WBCs being more desirable. Stated another way, studies have shown deleterious effects of high or concentrating WBC where the opposite has not been published, that is, for WBC-poor preparations.[15,16] Clearly, the presence of WBC in PRP can increase the presence of catabolic signaling proteins in vitro[16] and in the author's opinion the concentration of WBC should be avoided. This is further supported by work in our laboratory evaluating the influence of two different preparations (one high-platelet and one low-platelet) on anabolic and catabolic activities in equine cartilage and meniscal explants.[17]

The physical composition of the platelet is also important to understand. Derived from the division or fragmenting of megakaryocytes, platelets are a cellular fragment devoid of a nucleus with a relatively short life span of around 1 week (Figure 16-5A). The platelets contain α granules that, following activation of platelets, are said to degranulate and release presecreted proteins stored inside (Figure 16-5B). The number of proteins cited to be contained within platelets is said to be in excess of 200, and so one must look at PRP as a "soup" of therapeutic factors. Like other such milieus it is important to consider that for any given desired effect such a "soup" will contain good and bad factors; thus a ratio of said factors will ultimately dictate the response in any given situation (Figure 16-5C). The predominant growth factors cited currently in platelets are platelet-derived growth factor (PDGF), transforming growth factor-β (TGF-β), and vascular endothelial growth factor. It is important to understand that platelets synthesize some proteins following activation for about 2 days; these can be proinflammatory or modulatory cytokines such as IL-1,[13,18,19] TNF, and IL-6 as a few examples.[13]

Understanding of the relative importance and interaction of factors released in association with platelets as they relate to musculoskeletal tissues is at a very infantile stage and requires a significant amount of work. This area will undoubtedly be heavily researched and the question "What is in the soup?" should be one clinicians continue to ask.

Human Clinical Data for Intraarticular Platelet-Rich Plasma

By 2014 two systematic reviews had been published on PRP for treating knee OA.[20,21] The first publication in 2013 documents six studies that were assessed as Level I or II, the highest two levels of evidence. Four studies were randomized control trials and two were prospective cohort studies. A total of 653 patient and 727 knees were included in the systematic review. The studies used 2 to 4 injections, a frequency of 1 to 3 weeks, and an injection volume of 3 to 8 mL. The PRP preparation varied in number of centrifugations, concentration of platelets or WBC, and use of an activator. In five of six studies PRP was compared with hyaluronic acid (HA) and with saline in the sixth study. The results indicated a significantly improved functional outcome (WOMAC and International Knee Documentation Committee [IKDC] scores) for a minimum of 24 weeks. Other pain measures did not have significant differences. The overall reported adverse events were "rare" and typically characterized as injection site pain or effusion.[20]

The second systematic review[21] published in 2014 involved 1543 patients. It also reported significant functional improvement after PRP treatment in patients with knee pathology compared with pretreatment or baseline values. Further, the authors noted that the effectiveness of PRP is likely superior to HA with a longer duration of action. They report an overall incidence of adverse events at 9.59%, which was not

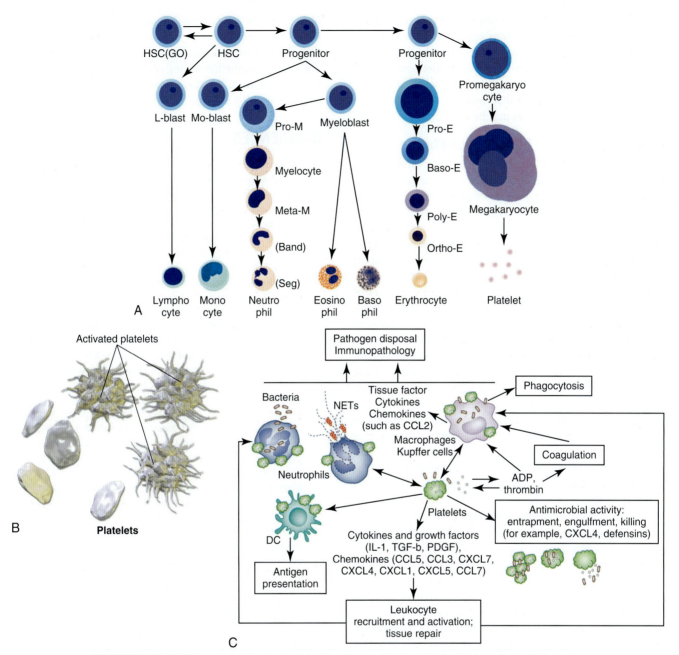

FIGURE 16-5 (A) Schematic diagram of blood cell and platelets outlining the origin of platelets. *Baso-E*, Basophilic erythroblast; *HSC*, hematopoietic stem cell; *L-blast*, lymphoblast, lympho-cyte; *Meta-M*, metamyelocyte, neutrophil, eosinophil, basophil; *Mo-blast*, monoblast, monocyte, myeloblast; *Ortho-E*, orthochromatic erythroblast, erythrocyte, promegakaryocyte, megakaryo-cyte, platelet; *poly-E*, polychromatic erythroblast; *Pro-E*, proerythroblast; *Progenitor*, progenitor cell; *Pro-M*, promyelocyte, myelocyte (© free images by FujiMan Production, Japan). (B) Activated platelets (from Blausen Medical Communications, Inc.). (C) Platelets and leukocytes as partners in innate immunity. (From Mantovani A., Garlanda C. (2013). Platelet-macrophage partnership in innate immunity and inflammation, Nature Immunology 14, 768-770, Figure 1.)

significantly different from HA. They were unable to identify significant discrepancy in effectiveness based on centrifuga-tion methods or activation agents. However, they do note that a single centrifugation and lack of activation overlap with the range of ineffective treatments. Stated another way, the results for the single centrifugation were not as compelling as the double-centrifugation technique. In addition, the number of injections did not indicate a clear dose-response relation-ship but the authors suggest a minimum of three treatments. Lastly, they recommend the use of PRP in milder cases of OA (as opposed to severe) based on their review.[21]

Systematic reviews are important to consider as they sum-marize a large volume of work but sometimes in the processes nuances of individual studies are missed. It is worth noting that one study that compared a single-spin versus a double-spin technique was unable to show significant differences and that more pain and swelling were noted with the double-spin technique.[22] Also, when one versus two injections of PRP were compared no significant differences were detected.[23] The author does not suggest that these are definitive studies but rather that the differences may be subtle.

Equine Intraarticular Platelet-Rich Plasma

Very little published work is available currently on the IA use of PRP in horses. Textor et al. evaluated one commercial product in normal horses using various method of activation followed by IA administration. This group demonstrated that use of either neat (no activator) or $CaCl_2$ to activate the platelets yielded the least clinical reaction (least effusion, response to flexion, and periarticular heat), the best growth factor profile (TGF and PDGF), and the lowest endogenous WBC release into synovial fluid.[14] They used a gravity flow PRP system that is known to concentrate WBC and when cold, that is, 35° F, not concentrate platelets at all. They used a 2.5-mL volume in the fetlock joint. Of interest to clinicians they state "in normal joints, intraarticular PRP induces a mild to moderate inflammatory response in synovial fluid, which lasts ≈ 1 day." These effects are minimized by not using an activator or through the use of $CaCl_2$, which as noted previously can have a less than physiologic pH. Further, they reported that thrombin increased TNF and IL-6 levels compared with no activator or $CaCl_2$.[13] Lastly, they were able to show that platelets became activated by simply being mixed with synovial fluid; thus the addition of exogenous activators may be unnecessary.

To date there have been no Medline-indexed publications, only anecdotal reports, describing the use of PRP in the joint of horses with clinical disease. Bertone et al. described processing of blood using a proprietary system but did not use the term PRP; rather they called the product autologous protein solution (APS).[24] The product concentrates WBCs (12-fold), platelets (1.6-fold), and various proteins (> 3-fold). They described the use of APS in 40 client-owned horses with natural OA. They were able to show significant reduction in lameness at 14 days after treatment and satisfaction based on reported client-assessed parameters at 12 and 52 weeks. The APS had a greater likelihood of benefiting milder cases of OA compared with more severe cases of OA. The concentration of proinflammatory cytokines was not reported and needs to be evaluated along with the effects on disease progression. Where APS fits into the treatment of equine joint disease will need to be explored as will the composition of the "soup."

SUMMARY

The clinical use of either ACS or PRP in equine joints remains anecdotal. There is more published clinical evidence in humans for the use of PRP than in horses. This may in part be because of regulatory factors influencing the ease of PRP versus ACS, where more regulatory hurdles exist in the U.S. with ACS versus PRP. The level of evidence surrounding ACS in horses is greater than that of PRP at the current time. Further, anecdotal concerns have been expressed about the long-term

fibrosis of the joint capsule following the IA use of PRP, which could be consistent with increased levels of TGF-β in PRP (known to be associated with fibrotic joint changes[25]). Thus, although further testing of PRP in equine joint disease is eagerly awaited, the current recommendation would be to use ACS as an IA biologic therapy.

REFERENCES

1. Meijer H, Reinecke J, Becker C, et al. The production of anti-inflammatory cytokines in whole blood by physico-chemical induction. *Inflamm Res.* 2003;52(10):404–407.
2. Rutgers M, Saris DB, Dhert WJ, et al. Cytokine profile of autologous conditioned serum for treatment of osteoarthritis, in vitro effects on cartilage metabolism and intra-articular levels after injection. *Arthritis Res Ther.* 2010;12(3):R114.
3. Hraha TH, Doremus KM, McIlwraith CW, et al. Autologous conditioned serum: the comparative cytokine profiles of two commercial methods (IRAP and IRAP II) using equine blood. *Equine Vet J.* 2011;43(5):516–521.
4. Frisbie DD, Ghivizzani SC, Robbins PD, et al. Treatment of experimental equine osteoarthritis by in vivo delivery of the equine interleukin-1 receptor antagonist gene. *Gene Ther.* 2002;9(1):12–20.
5. Baltzer AW, Moser C, Jansen SA, et al. Autologous conditioned serum (Orthokine) is an effective treatment for knee osteoarthritis. *Osteoarthritis Cartilage.* 2009;17(2):152–160.
6. Darabos N, Haspl M, Moser C, et al. Intraarticular application of autologous conditioned serum (ACS) reduces bone tunnel widening after ACL reconstructive surgery in a randomized controlled trial. *Knee Surg Sports Traumatol Arthrosc.* 2011;19(Suppl 1):S36–46.
7. Ferris DJ, Frisbie DD, McIlwraith CW, et al. Current joint therapy usage in equine practice: a survey of veterinarians 2009. *Equine Vet J.* 2011;43(5):530–535.
8. Frisbie DD, Kawcak CE, Werpy NM, et al. Clinical, biochemical, and histologic effects of intra-articular administration of autologous conditioned serum in horses with experimentally induced osteoarthritis. *Am J Vet Res.* 2007;68(3):297–304.
9. Marx RE, Carlson ER, Eichstaedt RM, et al. Platelet-rich plasma: growth factor enhancement for bone grafts. *Oral Surg Oral Med Oral Pathol Oral Radiol Endod.* 1998;85(6):638–646.
10. DeLong JM, Russell RP, Mazzocca AD. Platelet-rich plasma: the PAW classification system. *Arthroscopy.* 2012;28(7):998–1009.
11. Gruber R, Varga F, Fischer MB, et al. Platelets stimulate proliferation of bone cells: involvement of platelet-derived growth factor, microparticles and membranes. *Clin Oral Impants Res.* 2002;13(5):529–535.
12. Weibrich G, Hansen K, Kleis W, et al. Effect of platelet concentration in platelet-rich plasma on peri-implant bone regeneration. *Bone.* 2004;34(4):665–671.
13. Textor JA, Willits NH, Tablin F. Synovial fluid growth factor and cytokine concentrations after intra-articular injection of a platelet-rich product in horses. *Vet J.* 2013;198(1):217–223.
14. Textor JA, Tablin F. Intra-articular use of a platelet-rich product in normal horses: clinical signs and cytologic responses. *Vet Surg.* 2013;42(5):499–510.
15. Dohan Ehrenfest DM, Rasmusson L, Albrektsson T. Classification of platelet concentrates: from pure platelet-rich plasma (P-PRP) to leucocyte- and platelet-rich fibrin (L-PRF). *Trends Biotechnol.* 2009;27(3):158–167.

16. Sundman EA, Cole BJ, Fortier LA. Growth factor and catabolic cytokine concentrations are influenced by the cellular composition of platelet-rich plasma. *Am J Sports Med.* 2011;39(10):2135–2140.

17. Kisiday JD, McIlwraith CW, Rodkey WR, et al. Effects of platelet-rich plasma composition on anabolic and catabolic activities in equine cartilage and meniscal explants. *Cartilage.* 2012;3(3):245–254.

18. Zimmerman GA, Weyrich AS. Signal-dependent protein synthesis by activated platelets: new pathways to altered phenotype and function. *Arterioscler Thromb Vasc Biol.* 2008;28(3):s17–24.

19. Weyrich AS, Dixon DA, Pabla R, et al. Signal-dependent translation of a regulatory protein, Bcl-3, in activated human platelets. *Proc Natl Acad Sci U S A.* 1998;95(10):5556–5561.

20. Khoshbin A, Leroux T, Wasserstein D, et al. The efficacy of platelet-rich plasma in the treatment of symptomatic knee osteoarthritis: a systematic review with quantitative synthesis. *Arthroscopy.* 2013;29(12):2037–2048.

21. Chang K-V, Hung C-Y, Aliwarga F, et al. Comparative effectiveness of platelet-rich plasma injections for treating knee joint cartilage degenerative pathology: a systematic review and meta-analysis. *Arch Phys Med Rehab.* 2014;95(3):562–575.

22. Filardo G, Kon E, Pereira Ruiz MT, et al. Platelet-rich plasma intra-articular injections for cartilage degeneration and osteoarthritis: single-versus double-spinning approach. *Knee Surg Sports Traumatol Arthrosc.* 2012;20(10):2082–2091.

23. Patel S, Dhillon MS, Aggarwal S, et al. Treatment with platelet-rich plasma is more effective than placebo for knee osteoarthritis: a prospective, double-blind, randomized trial. *Am J Sports Med.* 2013;41(2):356–364.

24. Bertone AL, Ishihara A, Zekas LJ, et al. Evaluation of a single intra-articular injection of autologous protein solution for treatment of osteoarthritis in horses. *Am J Vet Res.* 2014;75(2):141–151.

25. Remst DF, Blom AB, Vitters EL, et al. Gene expression analysis of murine and human osteoarthritis synovium reveals elevation of transforming growth factor β-responsive genes in osteoarthritis-related fibrosis. *Arthritis Rheumatol.* 2014;66(3):647–656.

17

Stem Cells

David D. Frisbie

What defines a "stem cell" is an ever-changing landscape in science as more information is obtained. In general terms stem cells have the ability to self-replicate and differentiate into specific tissue types. In orthopedics we are mainly concerned with mesenchymal stem cells (MSCs). Early isolation of MSCs occurred through adherence to culture plastic monoclonal isolation of self-replicating cells that could differentiate into the various mesenchymal lineages.[1] More recently cell surface markers are being used to describe cell types; however, this method is somewhat incomplete as we do not know all the cell surface markers that exist or the function of each of the receptors. Further definitions and reviews can be found elsewhere.[2] The use of stem cells for treating orthopedic disease has been exponentially growing since 2003 with the number of peer-reviewed and Medline-indexed publications (Figure 17-1) reaching over 250 in 2013. This means the equine practitioner is faced with greater information to help in the best selection of cases in which to use stem cells. This chapter is not an extensive review of stem cells but rather a focused resource on the "best practices" available at the time of this publication. More in-depth discussion can be found elsewhere.[2-4]

CHOICE OF SOURCE FOR MESENCHYMAL STEM CELLS

Although there are many considerations when choosing MSCs for the treatment of joint disease, the first consideration is the tissue source. Multiple studies have been published comparing various tissue sources of MSCs in the horse, and current thought is that bone marrow–derived cells provide the best source for joint-related tissue.[2,5,6] Specific locations and volumes of aspirates have also been assessed and a low-volume (5 mL) aspirate from the ilium has been shown to have significantly better results than other sources as it relates to joint tissues.[5] This is not to say that bone marrow drawn from the sternum or other locations does not produce usable MSCs; rather, the ilium is better when matrix production of the cells is assessed following chondrogenic differentiation (Figures 17-2 and 17-3).

DOSE OF MESENCHYMAL STEM CELLS

Specific studies assessing the dose of MSCs to be used in the equine joint have not been published; however, the range of doses used in studies with successful outcomes has been roughly 10 to 50 million in a 10- to 50-mL joint.[2] A recent double-blind, randomized, placebo-controlled clinical study in human patients with medial meniscectomy suggested 50 million MSCs performed as well if not better long-term than 150 million.[7] The 50 million MSC dose is closer to what the author uses clinically; that is, higher doses are not always better.

TIMING AND NUMBER OF TREATMENTS WITH MESENCHYMAL STEM CELLS

The timing and number of treatments have also yet to be definitively assessed. Based on performance outcomes of clinical studies administering MSCs intraarticularly (IA) as well as studies in tendon injury, significantly better long-term outcomes are seen with delaying MSC treatment past the inflammatory phase of the injury.[8] Most published reports treating joint-related injuries used a single treatment, which has driven the author's clinical use of a single treatment. Other publications focus on these topics in more detail and can be a source of further information.[2,4]

The first Medline-indexed study citing the use of stem cells in equine joints was published in 2007 and assessed the use of stem cells implanted in defects for cartilage resurfacing.[9] The use of stem cells in the joint is a relatively new phenomenon. Although new, equine practitioners have the most experience in veterinary medicine with IA stem cells. The therapeutic use of MSCs in equine joint disease can be broadly divided into three main areas. The first is cartilage resurfacing where the goal is to treat focal defects. The second is diffuse osteoarthritis (OA) where treatment is aimed at both synovial membrane and articular cartilage more globally throughout the joint. Third is the treatment of damaged IA soft tissue structures, such as the meniscus. Each will be discussed separately although it is important to realize disease is often a coalition of all three to varying degrees.

CARTILAGE INJURY/FOCAL RESURFACING

Focal chondral defects are identified in greater than half the arthroscopy procedures carried out in the human knee,[10-12] and similar numbers are seen in clinical cases of equine stifle (knee) arthroscopy.[13] Various strategies have been developed

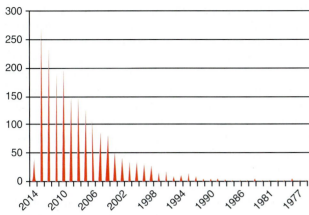

FIGURE 17-1 A frequency table by publication year from a PubMed search on February 11, 2014 using the key words "stem cell" and "joint."

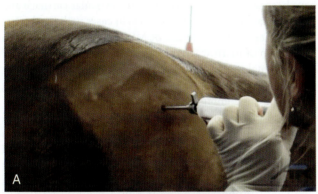

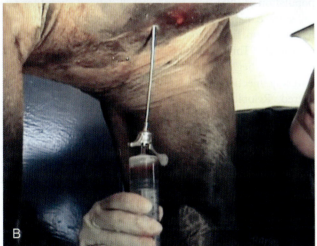

FIGURE 17-2 Bone marrow aspirate from both the ileum (A) and sternum (B).

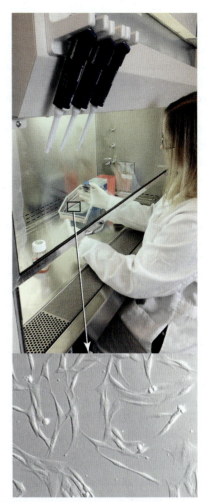

FIGURE 17-3 Images of culture of bone marrow aspirate and expansion of MSCs.

in an attempt to regenerate functional articular cartilage, with mixed results. Two basic strategies exist: MSCs held in a focal defect by a matrix or MSCs injected free into the joint space.

Mesenchymal Stem Cells in a Matrix

Numerous experimental studies using distal femoral condylar defects in laboratory animal models have generally shown an improved reparative response with MSC delivery to the defect

site through the use of a matrix.[14-18] In people, Wakitani et al.[18] also reported a limited number of clinical outcomes following MSC implantation into patellofemoral cartilage lesions. In the first report, bone marrow aspirates were collected from the iliac crest of three patients 3 weeks before the cartilage repair procedure and bone marrow (BM)-derived MSCs were expanded in monolayer culture using autologous serum. The ex vivo-expanded BM MSCs were resuspended in a collagen solution, seeded onto a collagen sheet, implanted in the cartilage defect, and covered with a periosteal or synovial flap, in a procedure somewhat analogous to autologous chondrocyte implantation (ACI). All three patients showed modest clinical improvement at the 6-month reassessment, and the clinical improvements were sustained for 17 to 27 months after implantation. However, assessment of one patient 12 months after the procedure showed incomplete repair of the lesion, and biopsy of another patient 11 months after MSC administration demonstrated predominantly fibrocartilaginous repair. In the second report, the outcomes of 12 femoral condylar lesions treated with MSCs in collagen gel were compared with repair of 12 lesions filled with collagen gel alone.[19] These patients also underwent high tibial osteotomies. The quality of the repair response was monitored via follow-up arthroscopic assessments and needle biopsies of the repair tissue, ranging from 28 to 95 weeks after the initial repair. Although there were no significant clinical differences between the treatment and control groups, histologic examination of the biopsies and arthroscopic appearance of the MSC-treated defects were improved. Although these clinical studies are somewhat anecdotal and the clinical improvements that followed MSC implantation were modest at best, these reports validate the feasibility of MSC implantation in human, and by extension, veterinary patients.

To date, the published literature on focal articular cartilage repair using MSC implantation in the horse is limited to experimental studies. The use of a fibrin scaffold to retain MSCs within cartilage defects has been reported by several groups; however, this technique necessitates that autologous MSCs are prepared before arthroscopy. Because this approach has the disadvantage of being uncertain of the need for MSCs until diagnostic arthroscopy is performed, it has not gained much acceptance. The use of a fibrin matrix to contain or implant the MSCs has also shown very limited success in one equine study. This controlled experimental study using surgically created 15-mm cartilage defects in the lateral trochlear ridge of the distal femur demonstrated no benefit at 8 months despite improvement at 30 days.[9]

Another experimental study evaluated the use of bone marrow autologous concentrate (BMAC) held in the experimental defect with a fibrin glue, and it demonstrated superior results versus microfracture alone in gross, histologic, MRI, and repair tissue biochemistry.[20] Because BMAC is a combination of MSCs and platelet-rich plasma (PRP)/fibrin and this study's design, one cannot assign significant benefit to any of the individual components (i.e., MSC or PRP) but rather to the whole system. Because BMAC contains around 120,000 MSCs, a dose currently considered suboptimal, the role and significance of the cellular (MSC) component has been questioned in this study. In a separate study, a PRP/fibrin control was shown to have significant beneficial results compared with defects not filled with PRP/fibrin,[20] suggesting the results of the Fortier et al. study[21] could be related largely to the PRP and not the MSC components. More in-depth experiments will need to be carried out to definitively answer that question.

MSCs derived from the superficial layer of the articular cartilage (articular cartilage progenitor cells) have shown some promise in healing of focal cartilage defects. The results of this recent study supported the use of autologous articular cartilage progenitor cells based on improved arthroscopic, gross, and histologic outcomes compared with fibrin alone or empty defects.[22] An unexpected finding was the lack of significant benefit when allogeneic articular cartilage progenitor cells were used. In fact, more radiographic pathology was noted in allogeneic-treated defects compared with autologous cells and with most outcome parameters being similar when allogeneic and fibrin alone were compared. Lastly, a study assessing the use of PRP/fibrin with a clinically relevant number of stem cells (10 million) demonstrated surprising results in that significant bone formation in the repair tissue was noted in numerous defects treated with stem cells compared with PRP/fibrin alone.[22] This suggested the use of PRP with a higher number of MSCs (10 million compared with 120,000 in the Fortier et al. study[21]) may yield unwanted results.

With the exception of the autologous articular cartilage progenitor cells, the use of a clinically relevant number of stem cells locked in matrix has not yielded compelling results. Although the mechanisms surrounding these findings have not been clarified, it may be caused in part to a reduced ability of the MSCs to migrate through a matrix, coupled with the matrix inhibiting the important paracrine effects of MSCs.[23,24] Further research in this area is needed. Based on the previous information, the author is not pursuing techniques in which MSCs are contained in a dense matrix or where paracrine effects might be inhibited but rather the injection of the MSCs directly into the joint space.

Direct Intraarticular Injection of Mesenchymal Stem Cells

When MSCs are directly injected into the joint space, cells have been shown to populate both the articular cartilage and the synovial membrane.[25] Clinically, in cases with focal articular cartilage defects the use of MSCs is often coupled with some form of marrow stimulation. A randomized controlled experimental trial in horses[26] as well as two randomized controlled human clinical trials[27,28] demonstrated encouraging results for this combination of techniques.

In the first human study, débridement followed by subchondral drilling was used and patients were treated with either hyaluronan (HA) alone (N=25) or HA plus peripheral blood stem cells (PBSCs). The outcomes were measured using MRI and repair tissue biopsies. In this study, the autologous population of PBSC was somewhat ill-defined except for two cell surface markers; however, based on previous publications by this group, from 2 to 12 million cells were injected at each treatment.[29] This study used 5 weekly injections of HA or HA plus PBSCs beginning 1 week after surgery. A second round of 3 weekly injections at 6 months postsurgery was also administered. Relook arthroscopies with biopsy occurred at 18 months and in the PBSC-treated group a significantly better histologic score and significantly improved MRI morphologic scores were seen versus the control (HA only) group. However, the IKDC scores (knee function score by International Knee Documentation Committee) were not significantly different at 24 months when the 2 groups were compared. In the other human study, cartilage defects were débrided and subjected to subchondral bone microfracture followed by treatment with either HA (N=28) or HA plus bone marrow culture expanded MSCs (approximately 15 million) at 3 weeks postsurgery.[28] All patients received 2 additional HA treatments 1 week apart. The patients were followed for 2 years with significant improvement in IKDC scores as well as two other standardized knee scores (Tegner and Lysholm) in the MSC compared with the HA-only control group. Also, at 1 year the MRI observation of cartilage repair tissue scores was significantly better in the MSC versus the HA control group. Even with some success being shown in one study using a peripheral blood source of stem cells, the use of bone marrow as a source is currently more accepted and has more supporting published studies.

In the experimental equine study, subchondral bone microfracture was performed on focal 1-cm^2 defects of the medial femoral condyle followed by treatment with either HA alone or HA plus 20 million bone marrow-derived culture expanded stem cells.[26] In this study only a single treatment was administered 4 weeks postsurgery. These horses were followed for 12 months and subjected to strenuous exercise on a high-speed treadmill. The horses receiving MSCs had significantly firmer repair tissue at 12 months compared with HA alone and had significantly more aggrecan staining in the repair tissue, suggesting a better matrix being produced by the resident cells of the repair tissue. It appears that in case of focal defects, the results of the direct injection into the joint space coupled with a marrow stimulation technique hold the most promise at this time.

OSTEOARTHRITIS

The treatment of generalized or diffuse OA is a daunting task as the true origin of disease is ill defined. Various factors such as undiagnosed injury, cumulative microinjury, or sequelae secondary to acute injury may all be contributors to progression of diffuse disease. Thus, a single treatment or "silver bullet" is probably unrealistic but nevertheless clinicians treat diffuse OA routinely as it certainly is a source of pain and further deterioration and it warrants discussion here. A 2014 study, which used anterior cruciate ligament transection in rabbits, provides some of the strongest laboratory animal observations.[30] In this study, IA treatment (injection into the joint space) with 1 million bone-derived culture expanded cells occurred 12 weeks after anterior cruciate ligament (ACL) transection surgery with the animals being followed for 20 weeks postsurgery. At the endpoint, treated rabbits had significantly less cartilage degeneration, osteophyte formation, and subchondral sclerosis compared with control animals. Numerous other laboratory animal studies have been published showing significant benefit to MSC administration in models of OA. The evidence from such models has led to, at the time of writing, 11 still-ongoing human clinical trials where MSCs were being used to treat joint OA with the majority of trials focused on the knee.[31] The first human case report to be published on the direct IA administration of stem cells for treatment of general OA dates from 2008 and was based on culturing techniques developed at the Colorado State University (CSU) Orthopaedic Research Center (ORC). The patient was followed up for 24 weeks and had a statistically significant improvement in cartilage and meniscal growth based on longitudinal MRI as well as improved range of motion and visual analog scale pain scores.

In 2009, the first randomized controlled study using IA injection of two different sources of MSCs for treatment of OA was published in the horse.[32] In this study, an adipose-derived product (Vet-Stem), then referred to as stem cells but now defined more correctly as stromal vascular fractions (SVFs) based on the low number of actual stem cells contained in the preparation, was compared with bone marrow-derived culture expanded stem cells. This study demonstrated a superiority of bone-derived culture expanded stem cells to SVF in reducing the prostaglandin E2 levels in synovial fluid (indicative of generalized inflammation) when compared with placebo controls. In addition, the SVFs induced an increase in the potent proinflammatory cytokine tumor necrosis factor alpha (TNF-α). Furthermore, safety was demonstrated for the bone marrow-derived cells based on no significant change in physical parameters such as effusion, heat, and pain following joint flexion or in routine synovial fluid parameters such as white blood cell (WBC) count or total protein (TP). This study used a single treatment (approximately 16 million MSCs) 14 days after disease induction but did not show as compelling results as would later be shown in human and rodent studies treating generalized OA. Furthermore, it is the author's opinion that anecdotal clinical reports have been more supportive of this treatment than were demonstrated by this study. There are potential explanations for this discrepancy between experimental and clinical observations including suboptimal dose, frequency, and/or timing after disease induction. These considerations need to be further investigated.

The issue of a reaction to IA injection of MSCs has been raised in some studies. Specifically, the group at Ohio State University reported moderate IA inflammatory reactions following administration of 15 million MSCs (autologous, allogeneic, or xenogeneic) into normal fetlock joints. The autologous cells were genetically modified and resulted in the least reaction but nucleated cell counts greater than 40,000 cells/μL and TP greater than 4 g/dL were observed.[33] Clinically significant findings were also observed including increases in fetlock circumference, response to range of motion, and soft tissue edema. The group at University of California-Davis also observed significant increases in synovial fluid WBC and TP levels following administration of autologous or allogeneic MSCs that were derived from placenta.[34] In both of the previous studies the allogeneic cells produced a greater response compared with the autologous cells, suggesting further evaluation of IA injection of allogeneic equine MSCs would be appropriate. In clinical cases of IA MSC administration, a 9% occurrence of "flare" was reported.[35] In this study, MSCs were administered with HA, which also reports a 12% flare rate.[36,37] Thus, it was not possible to differentiate the source of the flare since both MSCs and HA were administered concurrently, but one can assume it is not greater than 9%. These data collectively suggest that differences in MSC preparations exist when used IA.

INTRAARTICULAR SOFT TISSUE INJURIES

In equine orthopedics IA administration of MSCs to treat IA soft tissue structures such as the menisci or collateral ligaments has probably received the most attention in part because of early reports and success compared with conventional therapies.

The landmark publication suggesting profound effects following IA MSC therapy was published in 2003.[38] In this study in goats, the ACL was transected in addition to excising the entire medial meniscus leading to a destabilized femorotibial joint. Postoperatively the goats were exercised to induce

OA. Autologous BM MSCs were administered IA (6 million autologous cells), 6 weeks after joint destabilization. The effects of treatment were assessed 6 and 20 weeks after the IA injections. Indices of articular cartilage degeneration and subchondral sclerosis were reduced in the MSC-treated joints at the 6-week assessment, but this protective effect was not as evident at 20 weeks. The remarkable finding was the impressive and rapid regeneration of a "neomeniscus"-like tissue in seven of the nine cell-treated joints (50% to 70% regeneration of the original meniscal volume). The investigators concluded that the decrease in OA seen in the MSC-treated joints was largely secondary to the stabilizing and chondroprotective effects of the regeneration of the meniscus. This was in part because the two MSC-treated cases that did not generate a neomeniscus exhibited early cartilage degeneration as severe as that seen in the control joints. However, the experimental method did not allow clarification regarding whether the MSCs also had a direct effect on articular cartilage and/or progression of OA. A more recent study performed in rabbits with partial (half) medial meniscectomy led to a more in-depth look at the therapeutic effect of IA MSC on the meniscus.[39] In this study, MSCs were obtained from the synovium and 10 million cells implanted 2 weeks postmeniscectomy. The study demonstrated labeled MSCs in the area of the removed meniscus at 14 days after treatment and a significantly greater volume of neomeniscal tissue filling the defect at 4 and 12 weeks after surgery, but by 16 and 24 weeks a similar volume of tissue had filled the control defects. The tissue filling in the control defects was, however, significantly inferior histologically compared with the MSC-treated defects at all time points (4, 12, 16, and 24 weeks). In fact, the histologic scores were approximately 4 times better in the MSC-treated versus the control-treated defects at 24 weeks postsurgery. The histologic OA score on the medial femoral condyle was also significantly improved in the MSC-treated joints (an approximately 5× better ICRS score). In another study using a similar model, MSCs were culture expanded from meniscal tissue and 60 million MSCs were administered at 1 and 2 weeks postmenisectomy.[40] Similar to the previously described studies, significant increase in volume, improvement in histologic character of neomeniscal tissue, decrease in joint OA, and significant improvement in biomechanical properties of the neomeniscal tissue were observed when comparing MSC- with control-treated joints.

In 2014 a randomized, double-blind, controlled study in humans (N=55) undergoing medial meniscectomy and receiving one of three treatments was published.[7] The first treatment group received 50 million allogeneic bone-derived culture expanded MSCs plus HA. The second received 150 million MSCs plus HA, and the last group received HA alone. The meniscal volume was followed using MRI evaluation at 6, 12, and 24 months. The MSC-treated patients had significantly more meniscal volume compared with the controls (> 15%) at 12 and 24 months, and the patients receiving 50 million MSCs performed significantly better than those receiving 150 million MSCs. Further, patients with OA changes who were treated with MSCs had a statistically significant reduction in pain

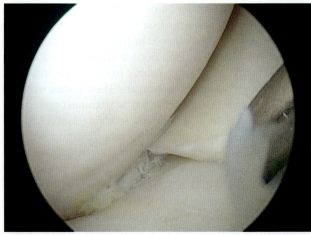

FIGURE 17-4 Arthroscopic pictures demonstrating a mild prolapsed/torn medial meniscus following an acute episode of lameness that was regionalized to the stifle. The horse was treated by meniscectomy and IA stem cells postsurgery and returned to full work 6 months later.

(approximately 2-fold) compared with the HA-alone treated patients; this result was still evident at 2 years after surgery.

Based on the goat and laboratory animal data as well as the Level 1 human clinical trial, it is not surprising we have observed similar significant benefits when using bone-derived culture expanded stem cells to treat equine joints with meniscal damage.[35] Following the beneficial results seen by Murphy et al.,[38] researchers at CSU began treating various clinical cases of joint disease with arthroscopically confirmed soft tissue injury using a combination of HA and autologous bone-derived culture expanded MSCs. The compilation of these cases with long-term follow-up for various joints has been reported.[41] One of these publications focused on cases with stifle disease and more details regarding horses with meniscal injury are available.[35] Specifically, a 6-month follow-up pilot project involving 15 cases was the first study demonstrating promising results (67% returning to full work) following IA treatment with MSCs, and the authors expanded the study into a prospective multicenter trial.[35] In the prospective study horses underwent diagnostic musculoskeletal exams (including IA diagnostic analgesia) followed by diagnostic arthroscopy as well as routine surgical treatment of the stifle problem. These cases had also been refractory to medical treatment. The stifle joints were treated with 15 to 20 million MSCs 3 to 4 weeks after surgery along with HA and the horses were followed for a mean of 24 months. Even with a broad range of IA stifle pathology 76% of the horses went back to work with 43% returning to full work, meaning full expected performance as well as not requiring further IA therapy. Horses that had the primary meniscal injury diagnosed at the time of surgery were significantly more likely to return to work (75%) compared with previous reports where meniscal lesions were treated with surgery alone (Figures 17-4 and 17-5). It is noteworthy that the horses in this study were lamer (2×) than those reported by Walmsley et al.[42] (surgery alone for meniscal lesions). In that study only 6% of the horses with the worst grade of meniscal

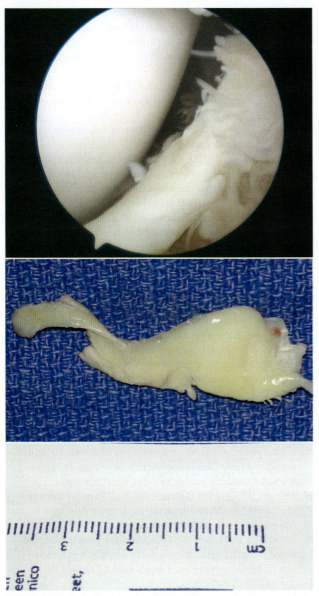

FIGURE 17-5 Arthroscopic view of horse with large meniscal flap (medial meniscus) that was débrided. The joint was subsequently treated with IA stem cells postoperatively and the horse returned to work a year later.

damage (grade 3) were able to go back to full performance and 5 were lame but used for light work; whereas, with surgery plus MSCs in our study 60% of the horses with grade 3 meniscal lesions were able to return to work.

SUMMARY

The vast majority of people in equine orthopedic research are using autologous bone marrow-derived culture expanded stem cells for their IA applications. In cases with focal articular cartilage lesions routine débridement and subchondral bone microfracture followed by treatment using MSCs suspended in HA for more than 4 weeks postsurgery appears to be the treatment of choice. For generalized OA, a preponderance of evidence for effectiveness of IA MSC treatment in horses

does not currently exist but evidence in other species including humans suggests some promise. In cases with IA soft tissue damage, especially the meniscus, it appears that significant long-term improvement with IA MSCs can be realized. In the current environment autologous MSCs are typically injected as a single treatment after the inflammatory phase of healing has occurred. Further research on the option of allogeneic MSCs, as well as optimal dose, frequency, and timing, is expected to be published in the near future, but is currently not available.

REFERENCES

1. Pittenger MF, Mackay AM, Beck SC, et al. Multilineage potential of adult human mesenchymal stem cells. *Science.* 1999;284(5411):143–147.
2. Frisbie DD, Smith RK. Clinical update on the use of mesenchymal stem cells in equine orthopaedics. *Equine Vet J.* 2010;42(1):86–89.
3. Peeters CM, Leijs MJ, Reijman M, et al. Safety of intra-articular cell-therapy with culture-expanded stem cells in humans: a systematic literature review. *Osteoarthritis Cartilage.* 2013;21(10):1465–1473.
4. Stewart MC, Stewart AA. Cell-based therapies in orthopedics. *Vet Clin North Am Equine Pract.* 2011;27(2):233–410.
5. Kisiday JD, Goodrich LR, McIlwraith CW, et al. Effects of equine bone marrow aspirate volume on isolation, proliferation, and differentiation potential of mesenchymal stem cells. *Am J Vet Res.* 2013;74(5):801–807.
6. Vidal MA, Robinson SO, Lopez MJ, et al. Comparison of chondrogenic potential in equine mesenchymal stromal cells derived from adipose tissue and bone marrow. *Vet Surg.* 2008;37(8):713–724.
7. Vangsness Jr CT, Farr II J, Boyd J, et al. Adult human mesenchymal stem cells delivered via intra-articular injection to the knee following partial medial meniscectomy: a randomized, double-blind, controlled study. *J Bone Joint Surg Am.* 2014;96(2):90–98.
8. Smith M, Ravi V, Dart A, et al. The timing of bone-marrow-derived mesenchymal stem cell injection is critical for long-term benefit to infraspinatus tendon in a sheep model. In: *Proc Orthopaedic Research Society Annual Meeting.* 2012; 2012:0161.
9. Wilke MM, Nydam DV, Nixon AJ. Enhanced early chondrogenesis in articular defects following arthroscopic mesenchymal stem cell implantation in an equine model. *J Orthop Res.* 2007;25(7):913–925.
10. Widuchowski W, Widuchowski J, Trzaska T. Articular cartilage defects: study of 25,124 knee arthroscopies. *Knee.* 2007;14(3):177–182.
11. Hjelle K, Solheim E, Strand T, et al. Articular cartilage defects in 1,000 knee arthroscopies. *Arthroscopy.* 2002;18(7):730–734.
12. McNickle AG, Provencher MT, Cole BJ. Overview of existing cartilage repair technology. *Sports Med Arthrosc.* 2008;16(4):196–201.
13. McIlwraith CW, Nixon AJ, Wright IM. Diagnostic and surgical arthroscopy of the femoropatellar and femorotibial joints. In: *Diagnostic and surgical arthroscopy in the horse.* 3rd ed. Edinburgh, UK: Mosby Elsevier; 2005:197–268.
14. Gao X, Wang C, Zhang Y, et al. Repair of large articular cartilage defects with implants of autologous mesenchymal stem cells seeded into β-tricalcium phosphate in a sheep model. *Tissue Eng.* 2004;10(11-12):1818–1829.

15. Guo X, Zheng Q, Yang S, et al. Repair of full-thickness articular cartilage defects by cultured mesenchymal stem cells transfected with the transforming growth factor β1 gene. *Biomed Mater.* 2006;1(4):206–215.
16. Shao XX, Hutmacher DW, Ho ST, et al. Evaluation of a hybrid scaffold/cell construct in repair of high-load-bearing osteochondral defects in rabbits. *Biomaterials.* 2006;27(7):1071–1080.
17. Jung M, Kaszap B, Redöhl A, et al. Enhanced early tissue regeneration after matrix-assisted autologous mesenchymal stem cell transplantation in full thickness chondral defects in a minipig model. *Cell Transplant.* 2009;18(8):923–932.
18. Wakitani S, Nawata M, Tensho K, et al. Repair of articular cartilage defects in the patello-femoral joint with autologous bone marrow mesenchymal cell transplantation: three case reports involving nine defects in five knees. *J Tissue Eng Regen Med.* 2007;1(1):74–79.
19. Wakitani S, Goto T, Pineda SJ, et al. Mesenchymal cell-based repair of large, full-thickness defects of articular cartilage. *J Bone Joint Surg Am.* 1994;76(4):579–592.
20. Goodrich LR, Chen A, Werpy NM, et al. Autologous platelet enhanced fibrin (APEF) scaffold supports in situ repair in the equine model. In: *Proc International Cartilage Repair Society.* 2013.
21. Fortier LA, Potter HG, Rickey EJ, et al. Concentrated bone marrow aspirate improves full-thickness cartilage repair compared with microfracture in the equine model. *J Bone Joint Surg Am.* 2010;92(10):1927–1937.
22. Frisbie DD, McCarthy HE, Archer CW, et al. Evaluation of articular cartilage progenitor cells for the repair of articular defects in an equine model. *J Bone Joint Surg.* 2015. In Press.
23. Hale BW, Goodrich LR, Frisbie DD, et al. Effect of scaffold dilution on migration of mesenchymal stem cells from fibrin hydrogels. *Am J Vet Res.* 2012;73(2):313–318.
24. Leatherman J. Stem cells supporting other stem cells. *Front Genet.* 2013;4:257.
25. Agung M, Ochi M, Yanada S, et al. Mobilization of bone marrow-derived mesenchymal stem cells into the injured tissues after intraarticular injection and their contribution to tissue regeneration. *Knee Surg Sports Traumatol Arthrosc.* 2006;14(12):1307–1314.
26. McIlwraith CW, Frisbie DD, Rodkey WG, et al. Evaluation of intra-articular mesenchymal stem cells to augment healing of microfractured chondral defects. *Arthroscopy.* 2011;27(11):1552–1561.
27. Saw KY, Anz A, Siew-Yoke Jee C, et al. Articular cartilage regeneration with autologous peripheral blood stem cells versus hyaluronic acid: a randomized controlled trial. *Arthroscopy.* 2013;29(4):684–694.
28. Wong KL, Lee KB, Tai BC, et al. Injectable cultured bone marrow-derived mesenchymal stem cells in varus knees with cartilage defects undergoing high tibial osteotomy: a prospective, randomized controlled clinical trial with 2 years' follow-up. *Arthroscopy.* 2013;29(12):2020–2028.
29. Saw KY, Anz A, Merican S, et al. Articular cartilage regeneration with autologous peripheral blood progenitor cells and hyaluronic acid after arthroscopic subchondral drilling: a report of 5 cases with histology. *Arthroscopy.* 2011;27(4):493–506.
30. Singh A, Goel SC, Gupta KK, et al. The role of stem cells in osteoarthritis: an experimental study in rabbits. *Bone Joint Res.* 2014;3(2):32–37.
31. Barry F, Murphy M. Mesenchymal stem cells in joint disease and repair. *Nat Rev Rheumatol.* 2013;9:584–594.
32. Frisbie DD, Kisiday JD, Kawcak CE, et al. Evaluation of adipose-derived stromal vascular fraction or bone marrow-derived mesenchymal stem cells for treatment of osteoarthritis. *J Orthop Res.* 2009;27(12):1675–1680.
33. Pigott JH, Ishihara A, Wellman ML, et al. Inflammatory effects of autologous, genetically modified autologous, allogeneic, and xenogeneic mesenchymal stem cells after intra-articular injection in horses. *Vet Comp Orthop Traumatol.* 2013;26(6):453–460.
34. Carrade DD, Owens SD, Galuppo LD, et al. Clinicopathologic findings following intra-articular injection of autologous and allogeneic placentally derived equine mesenchymal stem cells in horses. *Cytotherapy.* 2011;13(4):419–430.
35. Ferris DJ, Frisbie DD, Kisiday JD, et al. Clinical outcome after intra-articular administration of bone marrow derived mesenchymal stem cells in 33 horses with stifle injury. *Vet Surg.* 2014;43(3):255–265.
36. Boehringer Ingelheim. Hyvisc (hyaluronate sodium) Unleash High Performance. www.bi-vetmedica.com/main/equine/joint_health_portfolio/hyvisc.html.
37. Zoetis. Hylartin V (sodium hyaluronate injection) Hylartin V provides serious joint therapy with heavyweight protection. www.zoetisus.com/products/horses/hylartin-v.aspx.
38. Murphy JM, Fink DJ, Hunziker EB, et al. Stem cell therapy in a caprine model of osteoarthritis. *Arthritis Rheum.* 2003;48(12):3464–3474.
39. Hatsushika D, Muneta T, Horie M, et al. Intraarticular injection of synovial stem cells promotes meniscal regeneration in a rabbit massive meniscal defect model. *J Orthop Res.* 2013;31(9):1354–1359.
40. Shen W, Chen J, Zhu T, et al. Osteoarthritis prevention through meniscal regeneration induced by intra-articular injection of meniscus stem cells. *Stem Cells Dev.* 2013;22(14):2071–2082.
41. Ferris DJ, Frisbie DD, Kisiday JD, et al. Clinical follow-up of horses treated with bone marrow derived mesenchymal stem cells for musculoskeletal lesions. *Proc Am Assoc Equine Pract.* 2009;55:59–60.
42. Walmsley JP. Meniscal tears in horses: an evaluation of clinical signs and arthroscopic treatment of 80 cases. *Equine Vet J.* 2003;35(4):402–406.

18

Physical Rehabilitation

Kevin K. Haussler and Melissa R. King

REHABILITATION ISSUES IN JOINT DISEASE

Pain management and optimized physical function are two key goals in osteoarthritis (OA) treatment and rehabilitation. In humans, appropriate treatment options for OA include intraarticular (IA) medication, exercise, strength training, and weight management.[1] In horses, IA medications and nonsteroidal antiinflammatory drugs (NSAIDs) are often considered first-tier treatment approaches for OA management; however, these medications vary in their ability to abate clinical signs and alter underlying disease processes.[2] Equine practitioners may also be faced with reducing the use of NSAIDs that have less favorable long-term safety profiles needed for management of chronic lameness issues. Recent evidence in humans investigating novel pain management strategies and physical rehabilitation of both acute and chronic joint injuries suggests that surgical or medical management alone may not always be adequate for return to full athletic function or optimization of performance. Similar rehabilitation approaches have been subsequently developed for use in horses; however, there is currently limited controlled literature to support their efficacy in clinical practice. Continued research and the objective assessment of physical modalities such as cryotherapy, stretching exercising, and muscle strengthening may provide additional insights into addressing specific mechanisms of joint injury and healing.

Shorter-term goals of OA management should incorporate graduated methods of pain reduction, limiting adverse effects of acute and chronic joint inflammation, restoring joint flexibility and stability, and finally maximizing strength and coordination of the affected limb or spinal region.[3] The intent of this phase of rehabilitation is to reduce clinical signs, halt harmful disease processes, and mitigate disabilities that hamper the initiation of joint motion and basic exercises. In humans and dogs, it is proposed that the alleviation of joint pain or inflammation alone without addressing critical sensory-motor control mechanisms and enhancing the biomechanical environment of the affected joint may contribute to injury recurrence or suboptimal outcomes for return to full athletic function.[4] Excessive loading of articular structures can exacerbate clinical signs and disease progression by creating an unfavorable balance between the breakdown and repair of affected tissues.[5] Long-term treatment plans include the return to previous levels of activity, optimization of performance, and prevention or recurrence of joint disease

and injury. Therapeutic exercises are applied on an individual basis to restore normal joint biomechanics, or if not possible because of permanent joint disease, then to minimize the frequency and amplitudes of excessive joint loading. The lifelong goal for managing joint disease is to restore or establish suitable joint biomechanics and improve the functional capacity required for each individual patient.

The appropriate application of physical modalities requires the identification of specific rehabilitation issues that are limiting return to function or performance optimization in each patient. Choosing specific modalities to form a tailored treatment plan for an individual patient then follows. Unfortunately, possibly because of lack of sufficient knowledge, training, or facilities, some practitioners may treat all affected patients, irrespective of the type, severity, or location of a disease (e.g., superficial digital flexor tendinitis), with a single treatment modality such as underwater treadmill exercise at the same water level, duration, and treadmill speed without any semblance of physical assessment or individualized treatment plans. This type of approach puts the modality (or paying for the newly acquired rehabilitation equipment) first in the clinical decision-making process and the patient's specific rehabilitation needs or issues secondary. This chapter is outlined according to specific rehabilitation issues that are typically addressed in the progression from acute, subacute, and chronic stages of tissue healing and restoration of joint function. Under each phase of rehabilitation physical modalities that are most likely to have clinical effects for that specific rehabilitation issue are listed. However, most modalities have several proposed mechanisms of action, and a single physical modality might be indicated for several specific rehabilitation issues.

PAIN AND INFLAMMATION

Pain and inflammation are two of the primary disease processes limiting joint function after acute injury. Conservative methods used to address pain and inflammation include applying topical cooling agents (i.e., cryotherapy) and external compression to limit swelling and joint effusion in affected tissues.[6] Additional modalities that use unique physical properties for intended therapeutic effects include electrical stimulation, vibrational therapy, electromagnetic waves, and mechanical or ultrasound waves. Numerous physical modalities have been developed and evaluated for use in pain management in human OA patients.[7,8] Similar levels of evidence do not yet exist for the rehabilitation of joint pain and inflammation in horses

Cryotherapy

Mechanisms of Action

The therapeutic effects of cold therapy are generated through reducing tissue temperatures to 10° to 15° C.[9] The application of cold to an osteoarthritic joint may serve as a neurologic counterirritant by bombarding central pain pathways with painful cold impulses, decreasing nerve conduction velocities in local sensory neurons, and activating descending inhibitory pathways.[10] Local mechanisms of action include decreased tissue metabolism and apoptosis, reduced enzymatic activity and inflammatory mediators (e.g., interleukins, TNF-α).[11] Cold also produces peripheral vasoconstriction and decreased soft-tissue perfusion (up to 80%), which can reduce edema formation and swelling at the site of tissue injury.[12] Increased capillary permeability allows extravasation of plasma, protein, and inflammatory mediators, which stimulate local nociceptors and prolong local inflammatory processes.[13] Tissue cooling is associated with increased tensile properties in ligaments and increased muscle stiffness, which may provide a protective mechanism for acutely injured periarticular tissues via increased joint stiffness.[14]

Clinical Indications

Topically applied cold is widely used in horses with the goal of decreasing acute soft-tissue pain, swelling, and inflammation. Cold therapies can penetrate up to 1 to 4 cm in depth, depending on local circulation and adipose tissue thickness.[15] Human studies have documented the analgesic benefits of cryotherapy for treating synovial articulations perioperatively and during bouts of rheumatoid arthritis.[16,17] In horses, a single report has described the use of cryotherapy to treat lipopolysaccharide-induced synovitis; it concluded that twice-daily treatment for 2 hours was not effective for controlling inflammation.[18] In dogs, local ice bath immersion significantly lowers IA stifle temperatures; however, similar IA studies have not been reported in horses.[19] Cryotherapy research in horses has been currently limited to applications within the distal limbs and focused primarily on inflammatory responses associated with laminitis.[20]

Clinical Applications

Cold therapy can be delivered through the application of ice-water immersion, ice slurries, cold packs, circulating cold water wraps (with or without added compression), and ice massage. Cold immersion using a slurry of crushed ice and water is the most effective method to cool the distal limb in horses (Figure 18-1).[20] The ice-water mixture can be applied using either a tall, vinyl wader boot or a 5-L fluid bag attached firmly around the affected limb segment.[21] Using 5-L fluid bags for cryotherapy may provide a readily available, practical, and efficient application method, especially if multiple limbs are affected.[21] Ice slurries need to be replenished every hour during cryotherapy, which may not always be convenient.

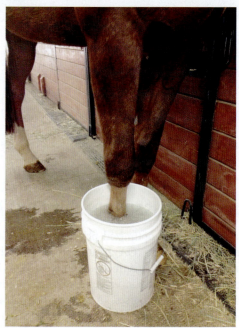

FIGURE 18-1 A horse undergoing ice water immersion of the right distal forelimb with the goal of providing pain relief and reducing inflammation.

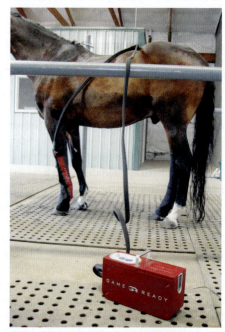

FIGURE 18-2 Application of a circulating ice water and compression unit to the distal forelimb with the goal of reducing joint effusion.

Subsequently, circulating cryotherapy units have been commercially developed to provide a continuous supply of ice water and consistent temperature within a wrap designed to fit specific limb segments (Figure 18-2). In both humans and dogs, circulating cryotherapy and intermittent compression provide a significant reduction in pain, swelling, and lameness and an increase in joint range of motion after orthopedic surgery.[14,22] Unfortunately, the circulating cryotherapy wraps may not exactly match the limb segment contours in individual horses

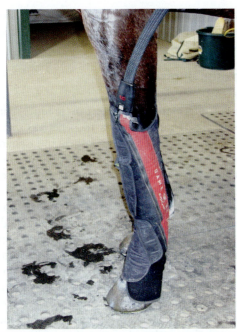

FIGURE 18-3 A commercially available cryocuff applied to the distal forelimb. Conformation of the fetlock and pastern regions may vary between horses, which may prevent adequate skin contact in some horses.

(Figure 18-3). Therefore, tissue cooling is often less effective with circulating cryotherapy units compared with ice water immersion, where cold liquid is always in continuous contact with the skin surface.[19] Using a cold water hose or frozen gel packs positioned in a leg wrap or boot are the least effective methods for applying cryotherapy in horses because of the inability to significantly lower tissue temperatures.[21,23]

Dosage

There is no standardization of the optimal dosage (i.e., duration, frequency) or ideal temperatures required for cold therapy of specific disease conditions in horses.[9] A general recommendation suggests that cryotherapy should be applied for 15 to 20 minutes every 2 to 3 hours during the first 48 hours after acute injury to provide maximal cooling effects at deeper tissue depths.[24] In dogs, 15 minutes of ice water immersion caused a 20° C decrease in IA stifle temperatures.[19] Similar IA measurements have not been reported in horses, but are likely applicable to joints of the distal limb because of the lack of overlying adipose or muscular tissue.[9] The ability to safely achieve low tissue temperatures for extended periods of time (i.e., continuously up to 48 hours) has been reported in several studies investigating equine laminitis.[20,25] Cryotherapy may be indicated for up to 10 to 14 days postinjury, depending on the severity and type of injury. A general rule of thumb for monitoring the need for continued cryotherapy is that the affected tissue should return to normal regional tissue temperatures and no longer has any signs of heat and swelling.

Adverse Effects

Temperatures below 10° C may precipitate tissue damage.[24] However, specific complications from the use of cryotherapy in horses (e.g., ischemia, frostbite) have not been reported in the veterinary literature. Reflex and motor function can be impaired for up to 30 minutes after the application of cold therapy, which can render the patient more susceptible to injury if excess activity is resumed immediately after treatment.

In summary, cryotherapy provides a low-cost, easy, well-tolerated method of cooling tissues, with minimal adverse effects. The topical application of cold can be used to effectively decrease temperatures within skin, tendons, ligaments, and IA tissues.

Heat Therapy
Mechanisms of Action

The topical application of heat with the goal of inducing a therapeutic effect is termed heat therapy or induced hyperthermia. Depending on the stage and severity of OA, heat application can have both beneficial and detrimental effects.[26] Physiologic effects occur at tissue temperatures of 40° to 45° C; whereas, temperatures above 45° C may cause thermal injury and tissue damage. The local application of heat produces increased soft-tissue extensibility, decreased pain, and muscle hypertonicity and induces general relaxation.[27] Pain relief is thought to occur via direct reduction of the painful stimulus and altered metabolic activity of neural receptors[26] Mechanisms of action for thermal therapies are likely linked to the depth of penetration and the method used for heating. Superficial heating sources usually penetrate the skin and subcutaneous tissue up to a depth of 1 to 2 cm, which may be appropriate for some OA-affected joints in animals. Deep thermal modalities (e.g., therapeutic ultrasound) can rapidly increase tissue temperatures by more than 4° C at 3- to 5-cm tissue depths.[14]

Clinical Applications

Heat therapy is generally contraindicated for episodes of acute inflammation as increased joint temperatures increase pro-inflammatory cytokines and tissue-degrading enzymes.[10,28] In humans, superficial heat is often used to decrease pain and stiffness and to improve tissue extensibility and joint range of motion in osteoarthritic patients.[14] Methods of applying superficial heat in horses include topical hot packs or compresses, circulating warm water heating wraps, warm water hosing, and warm water baths.[23] Chemical hot packs are activated by squeezing the contents and an exothermic reaction provides a heating source for a short duration. However, after activation the hot pack may exceed 45° C and could induce thermal injury to the skin surface. In addition, hot packs provide minimal deep tissue heating.[23] In dogs, the application of a 47° C hot compress for 10 minutes significantly increased tissue temperature of the lumbar region at 0.5-, 1.0-, and 1.5-cm depths without causing adverse tissue effects.[26] However, increasing the duration of application time from 10 to 20 minutes in this study did not result in significantly warmer tissue temperatures at any of the measured tissue depths. Kaneps reported that subcutaneous and deep tissue temperatures in horses never exceeded the therapeutic threshold of 41° C with the use of hot water hosing or hot packs (Figure 18-4).[23] Using warm water delivered by a hose is also difficult to maintain a uniform applied temperature within the distal limbs; when surface temperatures exceeded 45° C, the horse stomped its foot, indicating a pain response.[23] Other types of superficial heating sources include clay heating packs, gel packs, and other highly conductive materials that can be heated in a microwave and applied to the patient. In humans, heat therapy has been shown to be an effective adjunct to stretching techniques and is the recommended treatment of choice for enhancing joint range of motion in both clinical and sport settings.[14] To date, there are no studies that demonstrate clinical effectiveness for using superficial heating modalities in horses.

Shortwave Diathermy

Hyperthermia can also be applied via specifically designed mechanical devices (e.g., shortwave diathermy or therapeutic ultrasound). Shortwave diathermy uses microwave energy to therapeutically heat deep tissues and has been reported to improve pain, muscle strength, and physical function in human patients affected by knee OA with benefits maintained for at least 12 months.[29] Shortwave diathermy has been reported to reduce synovial thickness, inflammation, and pain in OA patients.[30] However, the exact mechanisms of action and effects of the metabolism and repair of the articular cartilage in OA are largely unknown.[27] Heating of articulations by microwave sources is reported to increase expression of heat shock protein 70 (Hsp 70) in chondrocytes, which enhances cartilage matrix metabolism and inhibits chondrocyte apoptosis.[27] The use of shortwave diathermy in OA rehabilitation has not been reported in animals; most likely because of the

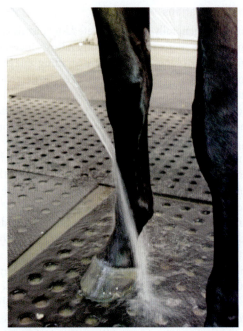

FIGURE 18-4 The application of warm water therapy via a garden hose to the distal forelimb with the goal of providing pain relief and increased tissue extensibility.

inability of veterinary patients to verbally report tissue heating thresholds and the increased risk for iatrogenic tissue damage.[31]

Therapeutic Ultrasound
Mechanisms of Action

Therapeutic ultrasound machines can produce pulsed or continuous ultrasound emissions to penetrate soft tissues up to a 5-cm depth. Pulsed or intermittent ultrasound waves have nonthermal therapeutic effects that include increased cell metabolism and increased phagocytic activity of macrophages.[32] Continuous therapeutic ultrasound waves have deep thermal effects on tissues, which include increased tissue blood flow, enzyme activity, collagen synthesis and extensibility; and decreased pain.[33] Tissues with high protein or collagen content or tissue interphases (e.g., periosteum or entheses) readily absorb sound waves, which results in energy transfer to the surrounding tissues and a localized increase in tissue temperature. In humans, target temperatures for heating tissues range from 40° to 45° C, which stimulates increased rates of metabolism without inducing thermal burns or tissue injury.[14]

Clinical Applications

In general, pulsed therapeutic ultrasound is used in acute inflammatory conditions where deep heating is contraindicated, and continuous ultrasound is indicated in chronic conditions when deep heating would be beneficial in reducing pain, increasing muscle relaxation, and improving soft-tissue extensibility. In humans, therapeutic ultrasound has been widely used for muscle and ligament strains, tendinopathies, OA, joint contracture, calcific tendonitis, superficial and chronic wounds, and chronic pain syndromes.[33] In horses, temperature changes in both tendon and muscle have been reported during therapeutic ultrasound application.[34] The superficial digital flexor tendon can be heated to a therapeutic temperature using treatment intensities of 1.0 W/cm^2 and 1.5 W/cm^2. A nontherapeutic increase in epaxial musculature temperature of 1.3° C was reported at a depth of 1.0 cm, 0.7° C at 4.0 cm, and 0.7° C at an 8-cm tissue depth using an ultrasound frequency of 3.3 MHz and an intensity of 1.5 W/cm^2.[34] Although tissue temperature changes have been reported in horses, there are currently no studies that demonstrate the clinical efficacy of therapeutic ultrasound.

Dosage

In human medicine, there are no established clinical guidelines for optimal dosages of superficial or deep heating modalities for the treatment of OA. The intensity and duration of heat stimulation used for hyperthermia are empirically determined.[27] The ultrasound dosage to a given area is determined by machine settings, relative collagen content of the underlying tissues, size of the treatment area relative to size of the treatment head, and how rapidly the sound head is moved over the treatment area. In veterinary medicine, the application of therapeutic ultrasound is largely influenced by the absorption of sound waves by the hair coat.[35] Attenuation of sound waves, even by the short hair coat of a clipped horse, is expected to decrease thermal effects in underlying tissues. The hair coat must be clipped to the skin for adequate transmission of the sound waves to occur.[35]

Low-intensity Pulsed Ultrasound

Low-intensity pulsed ultrasound (LIPUS) has been reported to increase type II collagen synthesis in articular cartilage, thereby producing chondroprotective effects in a rat OA model.[36] In rabbits, LIPUS application promotes cartilage repair through the downregulation of MMP-13, ERK1/2, and p38.[37] LIPUS was also found to decrease TGF-β production and attenuate the severity and progression of cartilage degeneration in a guinea pig model of human OA.[38] As expected, there was a greater treatment effect in early stages of cartilage degeneration, rather than in later stages. Based on current rodent studies, LIPUS does show promise for use in treating OA in horses; however, clinical studies need to be done to determine safety and efficacy for specific clinical applications.

Extracorporeal Shock Wave Therapy

Extracorporeal shock wave therapy (ESWT) uses electrically or mechanically produced shock waves or sound waves to provide pain relief and to stimulate tissue healing.[39] The primary treatment effect is caused by direct mechanical force; however, the precise mechanism of action of ESWT on articular tissues is not well defined.[40] Shock waves do create transient pressure disturbances, which localize at soft- and hard-tissue interphases. ESWT is becoming increasingly used in equine practice to relieve pain and treat musculoskeletal disorders (Figure 18-5).[41] In rat OA models, ESWT has shown chondroprotective effects associated with improvement in subchondral bone remodeling and articular cartilage parameters.[42] In rabbits, ESWT is reported to significantly reduce the progression of OA possibly because of decreased nitrous oxide

levels within the synovial fluid and decreased chondrocyte apoptosis.[43] In dogs, there are mixed results in treating stifle lameness[40] and hip OA[44] using force platform gait analysis and goniometry outcome parameters. In horses, ESWT has been reported to increase levels of serum biomarkers that are indicative of bone remodeling.[45] In horses with experimentally induced OA, ESWT is reported to significantly decrease lameness, but no disease-modifying effects were evident in results for synovial fluid, synovial membranes, or cartilage.[46] In horses with naturally occurring lameness, ESWT produced an acute improvement in lameness severity that lasted for 2 days.[47] Further studies are needed to determine whether ESWT should be recommended at an early or later stage of OA for pain management or combined with conventional therapies that more directly address specific disease processes.[43] There are fewer treatment variables associated with ESWT, compared with other physical modalities, but there are reported differences in the methods of generating and directing shock waves (e.g., focused versus radial), energy intensities, number of shock waves applied, and specific tissues and disease processes treated. No adverse treatment-related events have been reported from using ESWT in horses.

Low-level Laser Therapy

Low-level laser therapy and infrared light therapy use nonthermal light waves to reduce pain and disability, although the exact mechanism of action is poorly understood (Figure 18-6).[48] Low-level laser therapy is thought to have an analgesic effect as well as biomodulatory effects related to photochemical reactions within cells.[49] As with other physical modalities, the exact light wavelength, dosage, and treatment frequency needed for optimal treatment of select musculoskeletal diseases are largely unknown. However, the real perceived limitation in using

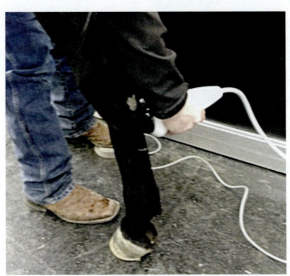

FIGURE 18-5 The application of extracorporeal shock wave therapy to the proximal suspensory ligament region with the goal of proving pain relief and inducing insertional microtrauma and accelerated healing.

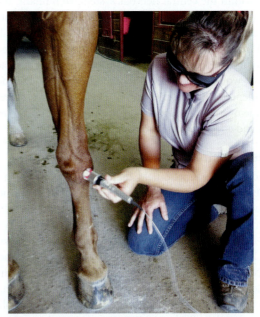

FIGURE 18-6 The application of low-level laser therapy to the carpal region with the goal of reducing joint pain and inflammation.

low-level laser therapy effectively is related to issues of tissue reflectance, penetration, and absorption. Evolutionary, mammals have developed melanin, thick epidermal tissues, and hair coats to help provide some level of protection from harsh environmental factors, such as skin damage caused by ultraviolet light. These protective mechanisms create a substantial barrier for the penetration of any applied light therapy.[50] The exact penetration depth of laser light into human tissue remains unspecified. Similar uncertainty regarding penetration depth arises in treating animals.[50] The depth of tissue penetration and physiologic effects of low-level laser therapy are likely dependent on the light wavelengths used, which are often within the red to near infrared spectrum (600 to 1000 nm). Additional treatment parameters include continuous or pulsed light source, light source power (in mW or W), beam irradiance (10 mW/cm^2 to 5 W/cm^2), duration of treatment per site, tissue or site treated (e.g., open or closed wound), and calculated delivered dosage (Joules/treatment site). Lower dosages of laser therapy have been reported to be as effective as higher dosages for reducing pain and improving joint range of motion.[48] The presence of hair coats and dirt do reduce laser light penetration through the digital flexor tendon region in horses.[50] Low-level laser therapy combined with exercise is reported to be effective in pain relief, joint range of motion, muscular strength, and quality of life in human OA patients.[51] To date, similar work has not been reported in horses.

Transcutaneous Electrical Nerve Stimulation

Transcutaneous electrical nerve stimulation (TENS) uses electric current applied via surface electrodes to preferentially stimulate cutaneous nerves and is used primarily for pain management (Figure 18-7). The mechanism of pain relief is thought to be through the stimulation of inhibitory interneurons at the spinal cord level or the release of endogenous endorphins within the central nervous system. In humans, there is moderate evidence to support TENS as an effective treatment for managing OA pain.[52] The value of incorporating TENS into a treatment plan may be that it can provide some level of temporary pain relief that allows the patient to perform activities that would otherwise be too painful.[53] Although there is no evidence of the effectiveness of TENS in horses, there may be some overlap in the mechanisms of action, clinical indications, and effects reported for electroacupuncture.[54]

Pulsed Electromagnetic Field Therapy

Pulsed electromagnetic field therapy (PEMF) uses an electrically generated magnetic field that is placed around the whole body or adjacent to a body segment of interest (Figure 18-8). The induced magnetic field produces secondary electrical currents within biological tissues, which can be visualized clinically as muscle contractions when applied to horses. Devices that produce PEMFs vary by a number of important features including frequency, waveform, strength, and types of stimulators. In humans, there are many published reviews on the efficacy of PEMF for providing pain relief and improved function in OA.[55-57] In a guinea pig model of OA, PEMFs applied at 75 Hz produced significantly more

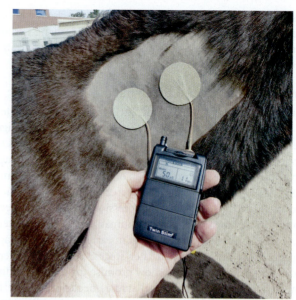

FIGURE 18-7 The application of transcutaneous electrical nerve stimulation to the lateral cervical region with the goal of pain relief within the affected dermatome.

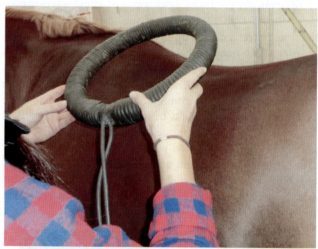

FIGURE 18-8 The application of pulsed electromagnetic field therapy to the wither region with the goal of providing pain relief. The circular coil is held at an appropriate distance from the body to initiate comfortable muscle stimulation and induce contractions.

beneficial effects on histologic measures of cartilage thickness and fibrillation score, compared with 37 Hz.[58] In horses, initial reports of PEMF use were for treating nonunion fractures and stimulating bone healing.[59,60] Currently, there are no reports of PEMF use in treating naturally occurring joint disease in horses. However, in ponies with amphotericin B-induced carpal synovitis, the effect of PEMF on arthritic and nonarthritic joints was measured by comparing synovial fluid parameters, the degree and duration of lameness, carpal joint range of motion, and carpal circumference.[61] In treated ponies, there were significant reductions in the severity and duration of lameness, carpal swelling, and severity of gross pathologic and radiographic changes. It was concluded that

PEMF produced significant beneficial articular effects, and no adverse treatment effects were noted.[61]

Transcutaneous Drug Delivery

In human physical therapy, drug formulations have been delivered transcutaneously via both electrical charges and ultrasound waves in an effort to noninvasively (i.e., no percutaneous injections) deliver therapeutic doses of pain or antiinflammatory medications to superficial and articular tissues.[62] Phonophoresis involves the use of ultrasound waves to mechanically deliver pharmaceuticals transdermally. Phonophoresis of hydrocortisone is a common treatment for a wide variety of soft-tissue as well as IA musculoskeletal disorders. In dogs, IA hydrocortisone levels obtained with phonophoresis are extremely low, compared with those obtained with IA injection.[63] Iontophoresis uses the electrical charge characteristics of drug molecules to drive them into tissues by repulsion from a positive or negative surface electrode. Iontophoresis has been shown to improve temporomandibular joint disorders and knee OA in human studies.[64] In two separate equine studies, dexamethasone sodium phosphate delivery via iontophoresis did not result in detectable concentrations within the synovial fluid or local vasculature.[65,66] Therefore, using current drug formations and application techniques, it does not appear that phonophoresis or iontophoresis are appropriate for use in horses for managing OA or other joint diseases.

PROPRIOCEPTION AND JOINT INSTABILITY

Proprioceptive Acuity

The proprioceptive system is intimately involved in both sensing joint position (i.e., afferent pathways) and contributing to motor activities associated with joint movement (i.e., efferent pathways). There are many different types of mechanoreceptors within skin, fascia, muscles, ligaments, and joint capsules that are capable of feeding proprioceptive information to higher brain centers, with muscle afferent neurons likely being the most important contributor.[67] Muscle spindle and Golgi tendon apparatus receptors provide constant afferent signaling about musculotendinous function and play a critical role in motor control issues and proprioceptive performance. Proprioceptive performance in various tasks including passive movement detection, joint angle reproduction, standing balance, posture, and gait all require the central integration of tactile, proprioceptive, vestibular, and visual information.[68] Interactions between nociceptive and proprioceptive signaling are not fully understood; however, nociceptive and proprioceptive mechanisms likely influence each other within the spinal cord or in peripheral tissues.[69] In humans, proprioceptive acuity has been associated with the presence and severity of OA pain.[70]

Joints are richly innervated with a variety of sensory nerve fibers that convey information to the central nervous system about forces exerted on articular tissues by both low and high threshold mechanical stimuli.[71] High threshold nociceptive afferents terminate primarily in the synovium and periosteum and normally respond only to movement of a joint beyond its working limits.[71] Following joint damage, the mechanical sensitivity of articular nociceptors is altered by physical changes caused by joint effusion and edema that alter local forces and by inflammatory mediators released within the damaged tissue that sensitize articular nociceptive nerve endings.[71] Inflammatory changes in the synovium of osteoarthritic joints are associated with a severe destruction of the capillary and neuronal network that is present in normal synovium.[72] Therefore, the number of mechanoreceptors and free nerve endings within osteoarthritic joint tissues is decreased.[67] Depletion of the density of nerve fibers within the joint capsule and the loss of normally innervated vasculature may have variable consequences on synovial physiology and health of the intracapsular environment.[72]

Active Muscular Contributions

The proprioceptive system is responsible for general monitoring of joint movement and limb position sense, but a more specific function involves sophisticated tailoring of muscle activity to increase joint stability and to protect joint structures from damaging loads.[73] Components of motor control, such as muscle recruitment and coordination and amplitudes of muscle activation, are strongly influenced by afferent proprioceptive signaling from periarticular and IA structures.[4] In humans, altered timing or amplitudes of muscle contractions contribute to uncoordinated movement, which can play a critical role in joint instability and progression of OA. Increased muscular cocontractions are often a compensatory strategy to improve joint stabilization and to protect passive soft-tissue structures; however, higher amplitudes and durations of muscle cocontraction can further increase joint compressive forces and hasten the progression of OA.[74] Therefore, improving muscular strength may be more important than joint position sense in mediating the risk for OA.[75] In humans, knee extensor strength is decreased in OA patients, which emphasizes the need for the development of muscle strengthening exercises within rehabilitation programs.[76] Studies of equine muscle have primarily focused on issues related to exercise physiology and myopathies; however, little to no research has been initiated on the role of muscle activation in joint function and performance as it relates to joint injury and rehabilitation.[4]

Proprioception and Osteoarthritis

Impaired proprioceptive accuracy is reported to be a risk factor for progression of both pain and functional limitations in human OA patients.[77] Altered posture and gait have been clearly demonstrated in various animal models of OA.[67] Joint pain and injury is often coupled with decreased proprioception and altered joint neurophysiology, which results in poor postural control, abnormal joint and limb movement patterns, and increased gait variability.[78] Highly complex neuromuscular integration is required to attempt to maintain coordination and balance with any change in speed or direction. Muscle weakness and incoordination can produce substantial negative effects on joint function, especially at faster gaits, rapid transitions, and high rates of joint loading.[74,75] If these neuromuscular and biomechanical aberrations are not addressed in some fashion, then the articular cartilage will be exposed to continued abnormal and excessive joint forces, which can speed the development and severity of OA.[79]

A generalized proprioceptive deficit appears to be associated with OA; however, this deficit could be caused by the loss of receptors, altered muscle function, or subsequent joint instability.[80] In humans, patients with unilateral knee OA may have impaired proprioceptive accuracy in both knees.[77] The unaffected limb becomes the dominant limb and plays a decisive role in balancing.[78] Similar compensatory stance and gait alterations would be expected in horses with single or multiple joint injuries, which would help to form the neurologic basis needed for increased understanding and management of adaptive and maladaptive limb and axial skeleton movement patterns in these patients. In humans, proprioceptive deficits and abnormal muscle function have been noted immediately and for up to 2 years after partial meniscectomy, which indicates the critical nature of restoring muscle function and proprioception.[81] Similar investigations have not yet been done in horses with meniscal injuries, but it is likely that comparable neurologic deficits occur in both the short and long terms. Individualized exercise programs are reported to be effective in improving proprioceptive accuracy in human osteoarthritic patients.[77] In horses, proprioceptive acuity and active muscular contributions to joint stability deserve attention and further investigation, because these two factors are likely modifiable by exercise interventions.

Joint Instability and Osteoarthritis

The proprioceptive system is actively involved in joint stabilization during static postures, protection against excessive movements, and coordination of joint and limb movements.[77] Muscles, tendons, and collateral ligaments all provide major structural components to joint stability. However, mechanoreceptors and free nerve endings located within joint capsules, ligaments, and muscles also play critical functional roles in nociception and maintaining the proprioception needed during stance and locomotion.[67] Afferent and efferent neuromuscular feedback systems function to help maintain posture and coordination of movement in an effort to prevent injuries. Deficits in both the afferent pathways (i.e., proprioceptive acuity) and muscular effectors (i.e., muscle activation) can produce substantial adverse effects on muscle strength and joint stability.[82] There are numerous physical therapy approaches for addressing proprioception and joint instability, and they can be generally categorized into afferent effects (i.e., sensory) and efferent effects (i.e., motor). A few of these specific forms of physical modalities that can be used to influence proprioception and joint stability related to OA management are discussed here.

External Joint Support

The application of external joint support via compression bandages or support wraps has long been a mainstay of managing acute joint injuries and providing joint stability in horses (Figure 18-9).[83,84] However, the exact biomechanical

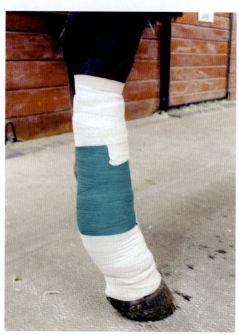

FIGURE 18-9 The application of distal limb bandages with the goal of providing soft tissue compression.

or neurologic mechanisms by which bandages, compression wraps, and other forms of external compression affect proprioception and joint stability are largely unknown.

Kinesio® Tape

Kinesio Tex tape is an adhesive elastic tape designed for use in treating sports injuries and a variety of other musculoskeletal disorders in humans. Manufacturers claim that it supports injured muscles and joints and helps to relieve pain and edema by lifting the skin and allowing improved blood and lymph flow.[85] A review of the current human literature suggests that Kinesio Tape may have a small beneficial role in improving cutaneous proprioception, strength, and joint range of motion, but further studies are needed to confirm these findings.[85] Kinesio Tape has shown effects on underlying muscle activity, but it is unclear whether these changes are beneficial or harmful in the management and prevention of specific human sports injuries. Equine Kinesio Tape certification courses have been initiated; however, the current level of evidence for use in treating musculoskeletal disorders is largely anecdotal, but promising results have been seen in select clinical patients (Figure 18-10).

Athletic Taping

Athletic taping is used frequently by human athletes to stabilize or strengthen soft-tissue structures, but evidence supporting any changes in joint kinematics or clinical effectiveness in managing joint instability or disease in horses is limited. The support capacity of any commercially available bandage to withstand the forces applied during normal equine locomotion has been questioned.[84] Athletic taping of the fetlock has been reported to decrease fetlock flexion during the swing phase from a baseline of 157° ± 4° to 172° ± 4°, which

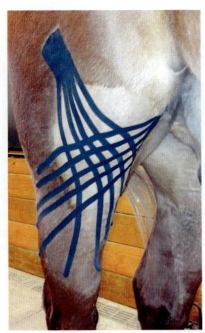

FIGURE 18-10 The application of Kinesio Tex tape to the stifle region in a horse with a trauma-induced seroma with the goal of reducing soft-tissue swelling.

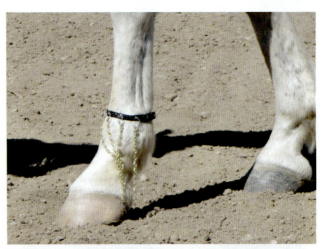

FIGURE 18-11 The application of a tactile stimulation device to the fetlock region with the goal of inducing proprioceptive stimulation and increased joint flexion.

is most likely because of a mechanical restriction of joint flexion during a non-weight-bearing phase of gait.[83] Taping does not alter forelimb kinematics during stance, likely because of the inability to withstand high forces associated with limb weight-bearing. However, peak vertical forces are significantly reduced, which is hypothesized to be caused by enhanced proprioceptive stimulation from the applied tape.[83] In human OA patients, elastic bandages can reduce knee pain and improve static postural sway, but these effects may be dependent on the size and tension of applied bandage.[86] In horses, adverse effects of any external joint support include an increased risk of pressure-induced ischemia and subsequent necrosis (i.e., bandage sores), which can be caused by inconsistent application and tension (range 8 to 19 N/cm^2) or by poor bandage material characteristics.[84]

Support Boots

Support boots are thought to reduce tension within the superficial digital flexor tendon and are frequently recommended for horses convalescing after tendonitis, but evidence of their effectiveness is often limited. Support boots are effective in reducing maximum fetlock extension angles, which may be indicated for OA management and rehabilitation of digital flexor tendon and suspensory ligament injuries.[87] Additionally, a delay in the onset of maximal fetlock extension within the stride cycle may be relevant in reducing or modifying joint and flexor tendon forces. In vitro biomechanical testing of a three-layered bandage, contoured palmar splint, and a carbon fiber exercise boot all produced decreased fetlock joint extension.[88] In humans, knee bracing is an effective option for providing pain relief and reducing muscle cocontractions while diminishing perceived joint instability. Compression wraps or

bandages are easily applied and well tolerated in horses; however, orthotics or braces similar to those in dogs or humans for gross joint and ligament instability are not likely to be well tolerated because of excessive point loading of the orthotic on local soft tissues and the increased risk of pressure sores.

Proprioceptive Exercises

Tactile Stimulation

In humans and small animals, proprioceptive training can be accomplished by using wobble boards or obstacle courses to help reestablish altered articular reflexes and afferent and efferent neurologic pathways. With some imagination, similar proprioceptive devices and exercises have been developed and applied to horses.[3] A lightweight bracelet that provides tactile stimulation to the horse's pastern and coronet region has been developed and tested (Figure 18-11).[89] The application of ankle weights can also alter hoof flight and joint kinematics (Figure 18-12).[90] Peak hoof height increased from baseline (5 ± 1 cm) to intermediate for tactile stimulators (14 ± 7 cm) and highest for limb weights plus tactile stimulators (24 ± 13 cm).[90] Stimulators on the hind pasterns are also associated with increased hind limb joint flexion and increased positive work performed by the hip and tarsal musculature.[91] However, there is often a habituation to the proprioceptive devices and limb weights where they induce the greatest effects initially, followed by a rapid decrease in altered limb kinematics.[89] Different types of pastern stimulators can increase joint flexion and may be appropriate for rehabilitation of specific hind limb gait deficits, such as toe dragging and a shortened stride (Figure 18-13). However, longer durations or repeated applications may be more effective for strength training purposes.[89]

Ground Poles

Walking and trotting over ground poles and cavaletti both in-hand and while ridden are frequently used to improve proprioception and joint ranges of motion (Figure 18-14). Peak heights of the fore and hind hooves increase progressively

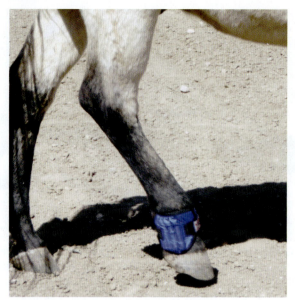

FIGURE 18-12 The application of an ankle weight to the hind fetlock region with the goal of increasing strength and joint flexion.

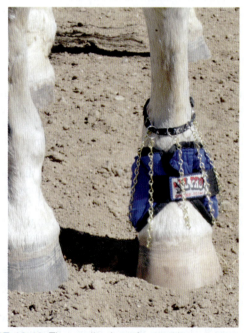

FIGURE 18-13 The application of an ankle weight combined with a tactile stimulation device to the fetlock region with the goal of increasing both strength and proprioceptive stimulation.

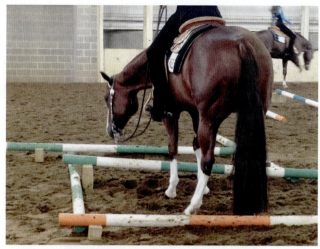

FIGURE 18-14 A horse walking through a series of ground poles with the goal of moving through the obstacle without stepping on or moving the poles.

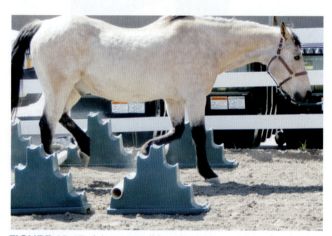

FIGURE 18-15 A horse walking through a series of cavalettis with the goal of increasing joint range of motion and improving motor control and limb coordination.

from baseline (fore: 14 ± 4 cm; hind: 11 ± 2 cm) to low poles (fore: 31 ± 5 cm; hind: 25 ± 4 cm) and to high poles (fore: 41 ± 4 cm; hind: 33 ± 4 cm).[92] Peak forelimb braking ground reaction forces and vertical and braking impulses in the supporting fore and hind limbs also increase when trotting over low (11 cm) and high (20 cm) poles as the limbs are lifted higher during the swing phase to clear the poles.[93] The overall increase in hoof height is caused by increases in entire limb flexion rather than by raising the body higher during the suspension phases of the stride.[92] Increased joint flexion during the swing phase indicates that trotting over poles is effective for activating and strengthening the flexor musculature. Unlike the use of proprioceptive stimulation devices in which the effects decrease over time because of habituation, horses are required to continually elevate the hooves to ensure clearance whenever ground poles or cavaletti are present (Figure 18-15).[92] The need to raise the limbs sufficiently to clear the poles and to place the hooves accurately requires coordination of visual, proprioceptive, and balance information, which may be useful in the rehabilitation of neurologic cases.

Agility Training

In humans, agility and perturbation training has been shown to be effective in decreasing cruciate ligament injuries and improving treatment of joint instability by improving knee joint kinematics and reducing muscle cocontractions.[94] Agility and perturbation training programs may also assist osteoarthritic patients in returning to higher levels of physical activity with less pain and instability following rehabilitation.[95] In humans, these interventions consist of education, stretching, strengthening, plyometrics, and sports-specific agility drills. Similar exercise programs need to be developed and validated in horses with OA. A better understanding of proprioceptive awareness and motor control mechanisms as they relate to joint disease is vitally important in identifying modifiable risk factors and applying preventative measures for development of improved medical, surgical ,and rehabilitative treatment strategies.[4]

Neuromuscular Electrical Stimulation

In humans, knee OA is associated with quadriceps atrophy and weakness; therefore, muscle strengthening is an important aspect of the rehabilitation process.[96] The often proposed clinical indication for neuromuscular electrical stimulation is that it can aid in maintaining muscle development and reinitiating neuromuscular control during the early recovery phase when the patient is unwilling or unable to produce an effective voluntary contraction. Since joint pain and weakness often make it difficult to participate in conventional muscle-strengthening exercises, the elicitation of muscle contraction using electric impulses may provide an alternative approach to initiate muscle contractions and subsequent joint stability. Unfortunately, there is inconsistent evidence in the human literature that neuromuscular electrical stimulation has a significant impact on measures of musculoskeletal pain, function, and muscle strength.[97] This may be caused in part by having no standardized protocols and no validated treatment programs because of large variations in methodology that include treatment parameters, the frequency and duration of treatment, the disease stage and severity, and patient selection. Electrical stimulation is often used in conjunction with an exercise program and is rarely used as a sole treatment modality; therefore, the specific clinical effects associated with neuromuscular electrical stimulation can often be masked.

Neuromuscular electrical stimulation appears to offset the changes in muscle structure and function in OA and following arthroscopic meniscectomy in humans.[98] Neuromuscular electrical stimulation is used clinically to generate contractions of a targeted muscle with up to 80% to 90% of maximum voluntary isometric contraction. Several human studies have demonstrated strength gains using neuromuscular electrical stimulation versus untreated controls, and comparable gains to subjects participating in voluntary exercise programs,[96] However, it is unclear if the role of electric stimulation in improving muscle function is actually related to increased muscle strength, improved voluntary contractions, restored motor control, or possibly proprioceptive activation within injured or atrophied myofascial tissues.[99] The combination of electrical stimulation and exercise has been reported to be effective in alleviating pain and improving voluntary activation in human OA patients, but it did not enhance muscle strength or functional performance.[100] In humans, adding biofeedback training and encouraging several attempts to maximally contract the affected muscle yields greater volitional activation (thus less activation failure) and to helps to speed up the rehabilitation process.[99] Similar biofeedback

training can be attempted in horses as they are asked to perform specific limb movements (e.g., lateral weight shifting) in conjunction with intermittent electrical muscle stimulation of the limb extensor musculature with the goal of activating muscle contractions during functional body movements. The forced contraction and possible discomfort induced by electrical or magnetic muscle stimulation can cause significant apprehension in some horses; therefore, the therapist must be cautious and very familiar with the application of this modality and possible adverse responses.

Vibration Therapy

Whole body vibration involves the application of low-frequency, low-amplitude mechanical stimulation for therapeutic proposes. Vibration therapy was initially developed to prevent astronauts from losing bone and muscle mass while in space. More recently vibrational therapy has been used to influence proprioceptive acuity and to initiate cyclic muscle activation and contraction. All musculoskeletal tissues respond favorably to a range of applied mechanical forces; however, it is often the absence (i.e., reduced gravity or immobilization) or the excessive loading of tissues that leads to tissue injury and degeneration. The effects of cyclic mechanical loading have been evaluated on various tissue types and vibrational therapy may provide a potent countermeasure against the effects of disuse and joint immobilization and assist in tissue healing.[101] Vibration has long been used as a method to induce muscle relaxation and overall well-being. Vibration therapy has more recently been used for neuromuscular reeducation where postural muscles make rapid and constant adjustments to the applied vibrational forces. As with other physical modalities, there are no established standards on the optimal frequency, amplitudes or types of vibration needed for focused rehabilitation of articular cartilage, subchondral bone, ligaments, or muscle pain and hypertonicity.

Anecdotally, whole body vibration has been applied to horses with various claims of effectiveness; however, there are no current studies on the specific effects of vibration on the rehabilitation of musculoskeletal tissues or OA. One equine study has assessed the acute effects of vibrational therapy on clinical and hematologic parameters.[102] After 10 minutes of exposure to 15 to 21 Hz of whole body vibration, there were minimal to no changes in the measured parameters or signs of discomfort in the horses.[102] In humans, whole body vibration has had positive effects on pain relief, proprioception, and muscle strength in OA patients.[103,104] It has been proposed that adding vibration to routine exercise programs may provide added benefits over exercise alone in preventing the onset and progression of OA; however, there is limited evidence that vibration adds significant benefits in patients with risk factors for OA.[105] Whole body or local vibration exercise appears to be a safe method for rehabilitation, but additional studies are needed to assess efficacy in equine patients for stimulating proprioceptive awareness and motor control mechanisms responsible for joint stability and movement patterns.

JOINT STIFFNESS

Joint stiffness can be caused by pain-related limitations in joint mobility and secondary muscle guarding or joint capsule fibrosis associated with chronic soft-tissue inflammation and increased collagen cross-linking. Decreased joint range of motion can contribute to reduced functional capabilities and an increased prevalence of maladaptive gait strategies, both of which can contribute to the clinical progression of OA.[106] Rehabilitation methods used to directly address joint stiffness include the application of heat, stretching exercises, therapeutic massage, joint mobilization, and spinal manipulation. Passive and active joint range-of-motion and stretching exercises are important in decreasing joint effusion, soft-tissue swelling, and overall stiffness. In acute inflammatory conditions, pretreatment with antiinflammatories may help to reduce pain and inflammation associated with an increase in joint mobilization or stretching exercises.

Heat Therapy

There is good evidence that heat therapy immediately increases joint range of motion.[14] Heat is thought to increase the viscoelastic properties of collagenous tissues (i.e., decrease stiffness) and to increase muscle relaxation and extensibility in preparation for physical activity or rehabilitation.[26] There is further evidence that heat improves the therapeutic effects of stretching beginning after a single treatment session with cumulative effects when repeated over a period of days or months.[107] Heat therapy may also increase a patient's stretch tolerance because of sensory stimulation and analgesia. Heating muscles causes decreased muscle spindle activity and increased Golgi tendon organ firing via both alpha and gamma motor neuron pathways.[14] These neurologic effects manifest as reduced muscle guarding and increased muscle relaxation.

Stretching Exercises

As a warm-up to exercise, slow and gentle stretching of the affected joint and adjacent musculature is recommended (Figure 18-16). Passive and active stretching techniques have therapeutic effects on periarticular structures of osteoarthritic joints. Slow, gentle stretches are an effective means to increase tissue extensibility and to restore normal joint function and movement.[108] Passive stretching exercises are defined as the practitioner applying soft-tissue or end-range of joint motion static stretches without any patient participation (i.e., passive). Passive stretches are effective in animals, provided that complete patient relaxation is attained.[3] Periarticular connective and muscles have been implicated as a primary source of osteoarthritic pain, compared with articular surfaces or subchondral bone.[109] Manually applied passive joint movements and active range-of-motion exercises appear to reduce connective tissue restrictions, which results in increased joint mobility and pain relief.[110]

Active stretching exercises are defined as the patient doing the stretching by themselves, which is challenging to accomplish in horses; however, active stretching of the axial skeleton can be induced with food treats or other training techniques

(e.g., clicker training).[3] Active stretching of the appendicular articulations can be accomplished by supported protraction and retraction in the unweighted limb as the horse gradually extends the limb and attempts to bear weight (Figure 18-17). Active weighted limb stretching exercises can be done while the horse is standing with the toe placed on a small elevated surface to induce stretch in the digital flexor tendons. Active stretching is preferred in later rehabilitation stages for managing joint stiffness as both sensory and motor pathways of the proprioceptive-motor control systems are activated as a transition to return to function and athletic performance. In contrast, passive stretching exercises primarily focus on stimulating joint and muscle proprioceptors in an effort to decrease pain and increase joint mobility without active muscle contractions.

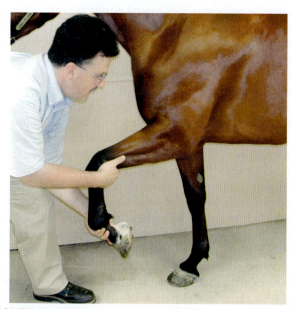

FIGURE 18-16 Passive stretching of the upper forelimb with the goal of increasing triceps muscle extensibility and shoulder joint extension.

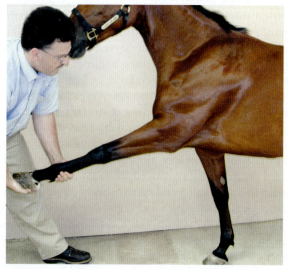

FIGURE 18-17 Active-assisted stretching of the entire forelimb with the goal of increasing neuromuscular activation and forelimb protraction.

Manual Therapies

Manual therapy techniques can be applied in different dosages in terms of force, amplitude, rate, repetition and duration.[111] Unfortunately, most manual therapy studies describe the type of technique used and applied dosage based solely on individual clinical presentations. Therefore, there is minimal research into the optimal dosage required to produce a specific treatment effect.[112] Muscles adjacent to or acting across osteoarthritic joints are often hypertonic and painful because of prolonged cocontractions and limb splinting. Therapeutic massage involves manipulation of soft tissues with the goal of inducing muscle relaxation, increasing soft-tissue extensibility, and reducing pain and joint stiffness.[113] Regular massage can help to decrease pain and improve flexibility (Figure 18-18). Mobilization is a skilled passive movement applied to a joint or related soft tissue at varying amplitudes and depths of penetration.[109] The purpose of soft-tissue or joint mobilization is to focus on the evaluation of structures that produce pain or limit function. Passive joint mobilization is indicated for modulating pain, increasing joint motion, and improving cartilage nutrition (Figure 18-19).[114] Chiropractic treatment produces increased joint motion and reduced pain via both mechanical and neurologic mechanisms.[115] In an effort to relieve the pain or stiffness, many animals with OA compensate by shifting their center of gravity or altering locomotion, which may increase stress in other articulations and precipitate secondary OA in those joints. Chiropractic care may help to reduce or prevent secondary mechanical stresses and improve overall joint function. Manual therapy appears to be a safe intervention as increased clinical signs are typically the only adverse events reported.[111]

NEUROMUSCULAR CONTROL

Muscle atrophy, altered muscle timing, reduced amplitudes of muscle activation, and compensatory muscle hypertonicity and guarding can all contribute to poor neuromuscular control and an increased risk for joint reinjury in osteoarthritic patients.[116] The neurophysiologic abnormalities associated with poor motor control may be addressed with proprioceptive, balance, and coordination retraining exercises (Figure 18-20).[67,81] Joint capsule, tendon, muscle, and ligament proprioceptors provide the afferent information needed for motor control; whereas, the alpha and gamma motor neurons provide efferent signaling to provide appropriate timing and amplitudes of muscle activation required for both fine and gross body movements.[116] In humans, quadriceps muscle dysfunction is a common consequence of knee joint injury and disease.[117] However, joint pain and effusion are equally potent in inhibiting muscle activation and coordination.[118] Altered feedback from joint damage or edema may negatively affect dynamic joint stabilization, thereby increasing the patient's susceptibility to further soft-tissue injury and progression of OA.[119] More subtle changes can be associated with altered timing and amplitudes of muscle contraction or cocontractions of agonist-antagonist

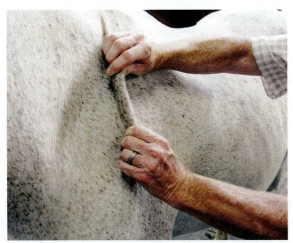

FIGURE 18-18 Skin and superficial fascia mobilization over the lateral scapular region with the goal of increasing tissue extensibility and reducing fascial restrictions or fibrosis.

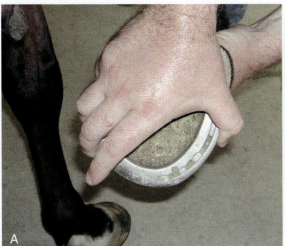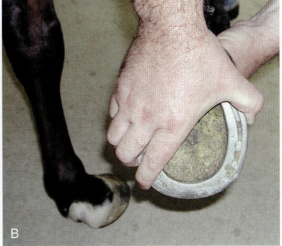

FIGURE 18-19 Induced (**A**) internal and (**B**) external hoof rotation during joint mobilization of the pastern and coffin joints with the goal of increasing accessory joint movements within the distal forelimb.

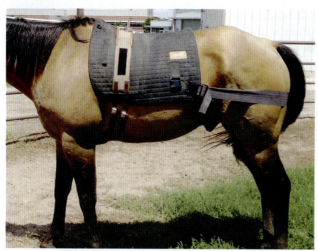

FIGURE 18-20 A horse with a saddle pad with an attached wide elastic band (Equicore) that spans the caudal thigh region with the goal of increasing pelvic limb protraction and improving core stability of the pelvic region.

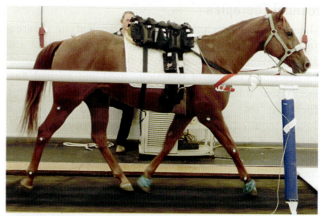

FIGURE 18-21 A horse undergoing treadmill exercise while wearing a weighted saddle with the goal of increasing musculoskeletal and cardiovascular fitness during the transition to ridden exercise.

muscle pairs in an effort to increase muscle guarding and prevent painful joint motion. Increased joint flexion angles and decreased muscle moments provide a mechanical explanation for the effect of joint effusion on muscle activation in osteoarthritic patients.[118]

Muscle Atrophy

The treatment focus for specifically addressing muscle atrophy associated with chronic lameness and joint disease is to minimize the clinical effects of muscle weakness and fatigue. In humans, knee OA is associated with quadriceps muscle atrophy and weakness, so muscle strengthening is an important component of the rehabilitation process.[96] Since pain and joint stiffness often make it difficult to use conventional strength exercises, neuromuscular electrical stimulation may be an alternative approach for use in osteoarthritic patients to help support muscle strengthening and neuromotor control. Electrical stimulation has been reported to increase quadriceps muscle thickness and knee extensor torque, as well as decrease joint pain, stiffness, and functional limitation.[100] Similar work needs to be done in horses to assess the effects of muscle strengthening on clinical signs and disease progression in OA.

Muscle Timing

Osteoarthritis can also produce alterations in muscle timing, which lead to altered gait patterns, cocontraction of agonist and antagonist muscle groups, and possibly stumbling or tripping. Human osteoarthritic patients demonstrate reduced walking speed, shorter stride lengths, and a prolonged stance phase, compared with control subjects.[120] Abnormal, excessive, and repetitive joint loading all together create a cumulative load, which is a critical factor in the pathogenesis of OA.[121] Some of these kinematics and kinetics abnormalities can persist for long periods of time.[122] Altered kinematics and kinetics during loading acceptance are associated with prolonged quadriceps and hamstring

muscular cocontractions during stance.[122] Altered muscle activation may interfere with normal joint load distribution and facilitate OA progression.[123] Therapeutic interventions should focus not only on quadriceps strengthening but also on improving muscle balance acting across the knee.[123] Quadriceps muscle strengthening exercises are often recommended for horses with intermittent upward fixation of the patella; however, muscle timing and agonist-antagonist balance may be equally important rehabilitation issues to consider.[124] Therapeutic exercises need to focus on addressing issues of improving motor control and restoring reflexes and agility with the overall goal of training muscles when to fire and shut off appropriately for a specific functional activity or athletic demand (Figure 18-21).[3]

Muscle Strength

Reduced amplitudes of muscle activation reflect a decrease in the strength of muscle contraction, which can lead to joint instability, reduced joint ranges of motion, and decreased performance or impulsion.[120] Quadriceps weakness is common in human patients with knee OA and has been attributed to impaired voluntary muscle activation.[99] Greater quadriceps strength has been found to reduce the risk for symptomatic knee OA and joint space narrowing.[125] However, it is not clear if increased quadriceps muscle strength relates to greater muscle mass or improved muscle activation patterns.[126] Recent evidence suggests that thigh muscle mass does not appear to offer protection against incident or worsening knee OA.[125] Therefore, rehabilitation efforts should focus on improving neuromuscular activation, rather than muscle mass.[126] Providing adequate instruction and feedback helps human subjects to maximally contract a target muscle and produce greater volitional activation.[99] Similar muscle strengthening exercises need to be developed and validated in horses with OA. Some of these exercises might include ground pole or cavaletti work to strengthen muscle activation during joint loading; stretching and passive joint range-of-motion exercises to improve joint mobility and stability; and plyometric or impulsion training with small jumps or rapid changes in direction.

Muscle Guarding

Compensatory muscle hypertonicity and guarding is a natural response to muscle weakness or joint pain and contributes to reduced functional capabilities. Muscle activation patterns greatly influence the rate, amplitudes. and patterns of joint loading.[4] Emerging evidence supports a critical role for joint kinematics and muscle activation patterns in the development and progression of OA.[127] Osteoarthritic patients may also use different motor control or biomechanical strategies to execute the same walking tasks.[128] Future work should integrate measures of abnormal joint loading with assessments of the total exposure to loading during physical activity to better link biomechanics with clinical outcomes in OA research.[127] In horses, flexibility exercises such as stretching, joint mobilization, and chiropractic care may provide options for addressing muscle hypertonicity and improving functional capabilities in affected patients.[108] Exercise programs should be individualized for each patient and modified according to clinical signs of pain or inflammation.[3] Low-impact exercise such as in-hand walking at a comfortable pace and duration are preferred over vigorous or uncontrolled activities. A controlled exercise program should include frequent short bouts of daily light-to-moderate exercise, which are interspersed with rest and recovery periods. Excessive or uncontrolled exercises that require jumping or sudden starts and stops should be discouraged.

ENDURANCE AND STRENGTH

Reduced performance, general deconditioning, and fatigue are common clinical signs in patients with OA. Appropriate muscle strengthening and development are critical to maintaining joint function, as muscles aid in shock absorption, regulate the rate of limb loading, and optimize force transmission across joints during stance and locomotion.[81] Numerous human clinical trials have substantiated the effectiveness of exercise therapy in reducing pain and improving function in osteoarthritic patients.[129] The ideal exercise program should provide clinical relief of osteoarthritic signs without causing increased discomfort or accelerating underlying disease processes.[109]

The initial phase of any exercise program should focus on proper technique and gradually increases repetitions or intensity to minimize risk of reinjury and to expand endurance capabilities. Rehabilitative programs also need to incorporate neuromuscular control exercises to restore muscle timing and coordination.[4] The second phase of rehabilitation then incorporates more strength training with increased joint loading, intensity, duration, and frequency. Underwater treadmill exercise may be an excellent method to increase both endurance and strength although providing reduced weight bearing in affected joints.[130] Additional forms of exercise to improve musculoskeletal strength and endurance include ankle weights for limb strength, sea walkers, or softer ground surfaces for increased resistance or effort required for walking, mechanical walkers (i.e., Eurociser), and application of a weighted surcingle or saddle for trunk stability and strength (Figure 18-22).[3] Muscle-enhancing interventions focused on

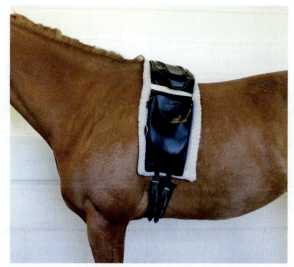

FIGURE 18-22 A horse with a weighted surcingle with the goal of increasing girth or saddle pressure without a rider.

the affected limb and adjacent axial skeleton should be considered for long-term OA management to improve muscle activity and overall musculoskeletal function.

The systemic benefits of exercise are generally accepted; however, a working knowledge of underlying molecular, cellular, and tissue responses to exercise is important in the development of targeted and specific rehabilitation protocols.[131] Chondrocytes and the extracellular matrix respond to local changes in mechanical loading and hydrostatic pressure.[132] Articular cartilage regions under higher load have increased aggrecan content and more robust collagen networks than do unloaded areas. Similarly, in vivo models demonstrate decreased matrix synthesis and cartilage thinning in immobilized limbs; whereas, the contralateral weight-bearing side exhibits increased glycosaminoglycan synthesis and the overall content of cartilage matrix.[133] Mechanical loading can affect matrix homeostasis by interacting with inflammatory and catabolic signaling pathways.

Under normal conditions, the cartilage extracellular matrix continuously undergoes remodeling and a homeostatic balance exists between inflammatory mediators and inhibitors.[134] Moderate activity can act as an antiinflammatory signal by suppressing IL-1, MMP, and cyclooxygenase-2 with a rapid and sustained reduction of these inflammatory mediators and a concomitant upregulation of IL-10, which has an antiinflammatory role. Conversely, intense exercise can enhance IL-1 and MMP expression and matrix catabolism.[135]

Exercise prescription must be patient-specific and within the tolerance levels of the individual. The surface on which horses exercise should limit impact and torque; turf or shallow arena sand or synthetic surfaces are preferable to hard surfaces or deep sand.[136,137] In humans, clinical evaluation suggests that "one-size-fits all" exercise regimens are largely ineffective, and evidence suggests that individualized and properly targeted exercise programs typically provide improved outcomes. Once identified, optimal loading patterns that have the potential to stimulate repair of tissues should be incorporated into

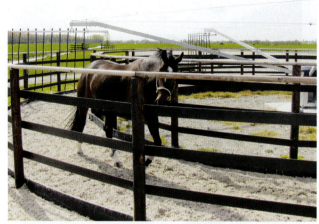

FIGURE 18-23 A horse undergoing walking exercise in a mechanical walker with the goal of gradually increasing tissue remodeling and musculoskeletal fitness.

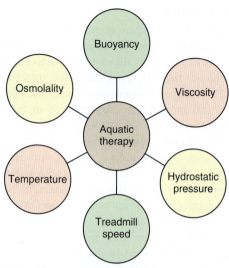

FIGURE 18-24 The factors that influence the clinical application and effectiveness of aquatic therapies.

exercise-based therapies (Figure 18-23). In general, continuous static compression is shown to downregulate proteoglycan synthesis in a dose-dependent manner.[138] Similarly, impact loading in which a supraphysiologic load is applied as a single bout or repetitive attacks is another harmful stimulus for cartilage tissue and is shown to stimulate degenerative changes both in vitro and in vivo. However, when the cartilage is subject to compression followed by release, synthesis of extracellular matrix and proteoglycans is induced, particularly when the earlier compression is supraphysiologic and inhibitory.

Greater specificity in designing exercise-based therapies requires identifying the mechanisms responsible for both beneficial and traumatic effects. Although the potential for beneficial effects of mechanical loading has been observed, a threshold effect has been demonstrated, with dependence on frequencies, magnitudes, and durations. The protective effects of moderate exercise and its positive impact on increasing cartilaginous synthesis and glycosaminoglycans content are well documented in various animal studies. Going above acceptable loading parameters increases matrix breakdown, as is evident in numerous in vitro studies and in animal studies.[132]

USE OF AQUATIC THERAPIES IN MANAGING JOINT DISEASE

Physical rehabilitation is an effective treatment option for managing primary musculoskeletal injuries, as well as reducing or limiting harmful compensatory gait abnormalities in humans.[139] Rehabilitation programs designed to address OA and musculoskeletal injuries often incorporate some form of aquatic exercise. Exercising in water provides an effective medium for increasing joint mobility, promoting normal motor patterns, increasing muscle activation and reducing the incidence of secondary musculoskeletal injuries caused by primary joint pathology.[140] Humans with lower extremity OA show a significant increase in limb-loading parameters, improved joint range of motion, and a significant reduction in the severity of balance deficits following aquatic exercise.[141]

The enhancements in muscle strength and function associated with aquatic exercise also significantly improve proprioceptive deficits, poor motor control, and abnormal locomotor characteristics typically found in osteoarthritic adults.[142] Although aquatic therapy is widely used in rehabilitation programs for humans, there are few investigations into the benefits of this form of exercise for equine patients. We now turn attention to the different mechanisms of action of aquatic therapy and its potential use in the clinical management of equine musculoskeletal injuries.

Mechanisms of Action

Therapeutic aquatic interventions can be used to address sensory and motor disturbances associated with musculoskeletal injuries in an effort to achieve functional restoration of full athletic performance. Aquatic therapies, such as underwater treadmill exercise and swimming, have been reported in humans to increase cardiovascular endurance, improve muscle strength and timing, decrease limb edema, improve joint range of motion, decrease pain, and reduce mechanical stresses applied to the limb.[143] Exercising in water provides a medium in which the mechanisms of increased buoyancy, hydrostatic pressure, and viscosity, along with the ability to alter both temperature and osmolality, can be applied in different combinations to play an important role in individualized musculoskeletal rehabilitation (Figure 18-24). The increased resistance and buoyancy inherent in aquatic exercise increases joint stability and reduces weight-bearing stresses on muscles and joints.[144-146] Immersion of the distal limb causes circumferential compression, which increases proportionately with water depth. The increased extravascular hydrostatic pressure promotes circulation and reduces edema.[143] Hydrotherapy can also aid in decreasing pain through temperature effects. Immersion in warm water causes vasodilation, increased circulation, and decreased muscle spasms[147]; whereas, cold water acts to reduce inflammation by restricting blood flow and reducing the accumulation of inflammatory mediators.[148] Aquatic conditions with higher solute concentrations

TABLE 18-1	Summary of the Mechanisms of Actions and the Reported Therapeutic Effects of Aquatic Therapy
Aquatic Therapy Variables	**Therapeutic Effects**
Buoyancy	• Reduced weight-bearing stresses on joint and soft-tissue structures • Improved joint range of motion
Viscosity	• Increased muscle activity • Enhanced neuromuscular control
Hydrostatic pressure	• Reduced edema • Increased joint range of motion • Decreased pain
Temperature	• Increased soft-tissue perfusion and lymphatic drainage (warm) • Reduced blood flow and decreases inflammation and pain (cold)
Osmolality	• Improved mechanical nociceptive thresholds • Reduced edema

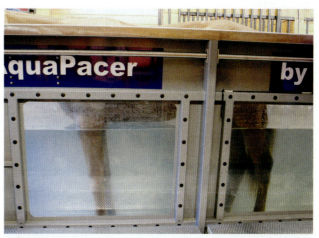

FIGURE 18-25 A horse standing in an above-ground underwater treadmill that provides the ability to readily alter the water level within the unit with the goal of providing individualized exercise and joint-specific rehabilitation.

provide an osmotic effect, which can ultimately reduce edema and decrease pain.[149] Aquatic therapy is a versatile treatment modality capable of producing a wide variety of therapeutic effects and therefore is considered an effective method for the rehabilitation of individuals with musculoskeletal injuries, OA, or postsurgical repair (Table 18-1).[150]

Buoyancy

In the context of aquatic therapy, buoyancy is defined as a lifting force that acts to reduce axial loading of the joints by minimizing vertical ground reaction forces (Figure 18-25). Underwater force platform analysis of human subjects demonstrate a significant reduction in vertical ground reaction forces during walking,[141] which is inversely correlated with the depth of water immersion. Humans walking at a slow pace in water at the level of the manubrium have a 75% reduction in weight bearing, but only a 25% reduction in weight bearing when walking in water at level of the pelvis.[151] Walking at a fast pace in water at the level of the manubrium decreased impact forces by ⅓ to ½ of body weight compared with walking on land.[145] In horses, water at the level of the tuber coxae produces a 75% reduction in body weight, although water at elbow height has a 10% to 15% reduction in weight bearing.[152] Increased buoyancy reduces the effects of weight-bearing stress placed on joints and the surrounding soft-tissue structures, which helps to reduce pain and inflammation associated with impact-loading exercises. Underwater kinematic analysis in humans has also demonstrated that increased buoyancy improves joint range of motion. Humans with lower extremity OA show increased limb flexion while walking in water versus relatively decreased joint range of motion when walking on land.[153] The buoyancy effects of aquatic therapy can produce both kinetic and kinematic effects that

are directly applicable to the clinical management of musculoskeletal morbidities in horses.

Viscosity

The viscosity of water is about 800 times greater than that of air. Therefore, the increased effort needed to move through water requires increased muscle activation, which improves muscle strength, motor control, and joint stability.[141] Electromyographic analysis during underwater exercise in human patients demonstrates increased activation of the agonist muscles during concentric contractions.[153] Increased agonist muscle activity is required to accelerate the limb in the direction of movement. However, during the same concentric contraction a reduced coactivation of the antagonist muscle group occurred.[153] Concentric muscle contractions during land locomotion cause the antagonist muscles to become activated to help decelerate the limb segments in preparation for foot contact. However, when exercising in water the increased resistance applied in the direction of motion requires minimal muscular braking of the limb segments.[153] Humans with knee OA routinely demonstrate an inhibition of the quadriceps muscle group and a corresponding increase in the activity of the antagonist hamstring muscle group. The increased activation of the hamstring muscles is a normal compensatory mechanism that helps to stabilize the knee and to attenuate joint loading forces during locomotion.[154] Patients with quadriceps inhibition also demonstrate increased impulsive loading of the limb, which leads to excessive or abnormal loading of articular structures and progression of OA.[155] The increased resistance to limb movement provided by aquatic therapy reactivates the agonist muscles and reduces cocontraction of paired antagonist muscles, which enhances neuromuscular control and the coordination of muscle activity (Figure 18-26). These mechanisms are important contributors to the functional restoration of muscle function and motor control in the rehabilitation of OA.

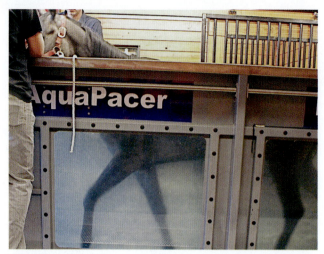

FIGURE 18-26 A horse walking on an above-ground underwater treadmill with the water level above the point of the shoulder with the goal of increasing muscular effort and strengthening during limb protraction.

Hydrostatic Pressure

Hydrostatic pressure facilitates an increase in neuromuscular function by stimulating cutaneous sensory nerves and joint mechanoreceptors. Joint mechanoreceptors are responsible for 1) signaling joint position and movement, 2) aiding in the control of both timing and direction of joint movement, 3) initiating reflexive muscular responses that maintain joint stability, and 4) playing a primary role in joint nociception.[156] These specialized receptors function both as proprioceptors and modifiers of muscle activity to increase joint stability and to protect joint structures from excessive or abnormal loading.[73] Under normal circumstances, stretching of the joint capsule and surrounding ligaments causes increased activation of the joint mechanoreceptors, which synapse onto the gamma-motor neuron within the ventral horn of the spinal cord. The increased afferent signaling from the joint mechanoreceptors induces fine adjustments in muscle tension to counteract the induced tissue strain, which subsequently increases joint stability.[73] Reflex mechanisms mediated by joint receptors help to protect an injured joint from further damage via either inhibition or activation of muscular guarding in response to joint pain.[157] The joint mechanoreceptors also register mechanical deformation of the joint capsule and changes in IA pressure during joint loading. The increase in IA pressure associated with joint effusion and synovitis causes reflex afferent excitation of 1b interneurons located within the ventral horn of the spinal cord, which results in inhibition of the muscles that act on that joint.[158]

Afferent excitation of joint mechanoreceptors induced by increased IA pressure may be dampened by the effects of increased hydrostatic pressure when the limb is immersed in water.[143] The reduced inhibition of the spinal cord 1b interneurons causes increased activation of the alpha motor neurons, which produces increased muscle activation and tone. In addition, the immersion of the distal limb in water applies a circumferential compression of equal magnitude increasing extravascular hydrostatic pressure, which in turn promotes venous return and lymphatic drainage. The improved venous and lymphatic circulation reduces edema and decreases soft-tissue swelling that ultimately increases joint range of motion and decreases pain.[143] Reduced soft-tissue swelling and joint effusion may further improve synaptic information from the joint mechanoreceptors and reestablish neuromuscular control critical for optimal joint motion and athletic activity.

Temperature Effects

The thermodynamic properties of water provide markedly different therapeutic effects depending on temperature. Full body immersion in water at a temperature of 32° C produces a central redistribution of blood volume caused by pronounced peripheral vasoconstriction.[147] Reduced blood flow to the extremities decreases tissue metabolism and provides an analgesic effect by decreasing nerve conduction[148] Conversely, warm water immersion at 36° C causes vasodilation, which reduces peripheral vascular resistance and increases tissue perfusion.[147] Increased soft-tissue perfusion may aid in dissipating inflammatory mediators associated with local inflammation and pain.[143] Water temperature during aquatic exercise may also play an important role in nociception by acting on local thermal receptors, as well as increasing the release of endogenous opioids.[159] Horses that stood in warm (38° to 40° C) spring water for 15 minutes demonstrated an increase in parasympathetic nervous system activity, indicating that immersion in warm spring water may have a relaxing effect that aids in decreasing pain, muscle spasms, and improves healing.[160] The physiologic effects of cold and warm water on vascular tone and tissue metabolism provide a useful tool to address the different inflammatory stages of musculoskeletal injury.

Osmotic Pressure

Exercising in water with higher solute concentrations has been reported to have antiinflammatory, osmotic, and analgesic effects (Figure 18-27).[149] In humans, a 2-week course of daily exercise in mineral water demonstrated increased mechanical nociceptive thresholds (i.e., reduced pain) over the medial aspect of osteoarthritic femorotibial joints.[161] Similarly, humans with fibromyalgia report significant improvements in pain scores lasting up to 3 months following exercise in a sulphur pool.[162] Horses diagnosed with distal limb injuries stood in hypertonic (20 g/L sodium chloride, 30 g/L magnesium sulphate) cold water baths (5° to 9° C) for 10 minutes, 3 days a week for 4 weeks.[163] These horses demonstrated both clinical and ultrasonographic healing of digital flexor tendon and suspensory ligament lesions.[163] Visual improvements in the degree of soft-tissue swelling were also demonstrated within 8 days of the initiation of hypertonic cold water therapy.[163] In horses, tendonitis and desmitis monitored ultrasonographically demonstrated reduced peritendinous and periligamentous edema, decreased inflammatory infiltration, and improved collagen fiber alignment after the 4 weeks of hypertonic cold water therapy.[163] The added mineral components in water provide an increased osmotic effect, which

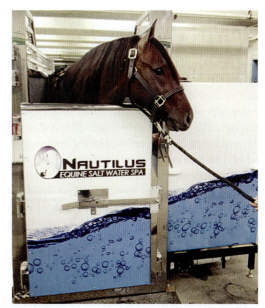

FIGURE 18-27 A horse standing in a salt water unit that provides osmotic, temperature (i.e., cold), and hydrostatic effects with the goal of reducing tissue inflammation and soft-tissue swelling or joint effusion. (Courtesy of Nautilus Equine Therapy Spa, LLC.)

reduces soft-tissue inflammation and swelling, decreases pain, and ultimately improves joint range of motion. These osmotic effects can play an important role in managing soft-tissue changes associated with musculoskeletal injury in horses.

Efficacy of Aquatic Therapy
Aquatic Therapy for Human Patients

Aquatic therapy is a commonly prescribed postoperative form of rehabilitation after various joint surgeries and for the management of human OA.[149] The therapeutic effects of water are particularly useful for management of disabled patients with significant joint pain associated with weight bearing and land exercise. Patients undergoing arthroscopic surgery and joint replacement are also commonly referred for aquatic therapy. Aquatic exercise decreases weight-bearing stresses applied to the operated joint, which provides earlier and more intensive rehabilitation without risk of increasing pain or overloading injured tissues.[164] Human patients undergoing surgical reconstruction of their anterior cruciate ligament demonstrated improved knee range of motion and quadriceps muscle strength following aquatic therapy, compared with traditional clinic-based rehabilitation programs.[165] Two weeks after total hip joint replacement, patients participating in aquatic therapy also demonstrated significant gains in hip abduction strength, versus standard physical therapy programs.[166]

Few randomized, clinical trials have assessed aquatic therapy for the nonsurgical management of patients with knee or hip OA. Patients with knee or hip OA undergoing a 6-week program of aquatic therapy showed improved physical function, increased muscle strength, and a significant reduction in pain, versus no intervention.[167,168] Land-based rehabilitation in OA patients produced higher pain scores before

and following a functional timed walking test, compared with aquatic therapy patients.[169] Aquatic therapy appears to be beneficial in the management of clinical signs associated with OA (i.e., symptom modifying); however, controlled, randomized studies are too few to determine if aquatic therapy reduces the progression of cartilage degradation (i.e., disease modifying).

Aquatic Therapy in Dogs

Several aquatic therapy studies in dogs have demonstrated significant improvements in joint range of motion. Aquatic therapy postcranial cruciate ligament reconstruction produces significant increases in joint range of motion, not only in the operated stifle, but also in the nonoperated stifle.[170] A similar canine study demonstrated normalization of pelvic limb biomechanics with no significant differences in peak vertical force or vertical impulse between the repaired and contralateral limb at 6-month follow up.[171] Kinematic analysis of dogs walking on an underwater treadmill demonstrated that joint flexion is maximized when the depth of the water is maintained above the joint of interest.[172] Thigh circumference and stifle joint range of motion assessed in cranial cruciate ligament-deficient dogs after tibial plateau osteotomy showed that underwater treadmill exercise significantly improved these two parameters, compared with cage rest and controlled walking.[173] Six weeks after surgery, there was no difference in thigh circumference or joint range of motion between the affected and unaffected limbs in the aquatic therapy group. In contrast, the cage rest and controlled walking group had continued progression of joint stiffness and atrophy of the thigh musculature.[173]

Aquatic Therapy in Horses

Although aquatic therapy is widely used in rehabilitation programs, there are few investigations into the benefits of this form of exercise for equine patients. Equine investigations involving aquatic therapy focus mainly on the horse's physiologic responses to exercising in water.[174-176] Swim training programs provide improvements in cardiovascular function, reductions in musculoskeletal injury (e.g., tendonitis) and increases in fast-twitch, high-oxidative muscle fibers, which reflect improved aerobic capacity.[177,178] Fine-wire electromyography has been used to measure increased muscle activation of the thoracic limb musculature during pool swimming exercise, compared with ground walking.[179] More recently, changes in stride parameters have been assessed while horses walked in various depths of water.[180] Underwater treadmill exercise with water at the level of the ulna produced increased stride lengths and reduced stride frequencies, compared with walking in water at the level of the pastern joint.[180] A similar study assessed the influence of water depth on distal limb joint range of motion.[181] The varied depths of water (from <1 cm water height to the level of the stifle joint) significantly influenced the fetlock, carpal, and tarsal joint range of motion.[181] Results of this study demonstrate that water at varying depths promotes joint specific increases in ranges of motion, therefore providing the ability to adapt therapeutic protocols to target certain joints. The efficacy of underwater treadmill exercise to diminish the progression of experimentally induced carpal OA was studied at the Colorado State University, Equine Orthopaedic Research Center.[182] This project was undertaken to provide an objective assessment of the pathologic characteristics associated with OA and the potential clinical and disease-modifying effects of aquatic therapy. Underwater treadmill exercise was able to reestablish baseline levels of passive carpal flexion, returning the carpal joint to full range of motion. In addition, horses exercised on the underwater treadmill demonstrated evenly distributed thoracic limb axial loading, symmetrical timing of select thoracic limb musculature, and significant improvements in static balance control under various stance conditions. The improvement in clinical signs of OA in the aquatic therapy group was further supported by evidence of disease-modifying effects at the histologic level. Underwater treadmill exercise reduced joint capsule fibrosis and decreased the degree of inflammatory infiltrate present in the synovial membrane. Results from this study indicate that underwater treadmill exercise is a viable therapeutic option in managing OA in horses, which is fundamental to providing evidence-based support for equine aquatic therapy.[182]

Treatment Variables

Equine aquatic therapy primarily involves the use of underwater treadmills (above-ground or in-ground units), swimming pools (circular or straight), aqua walkers, and standing salt water spas or whirlpools. The in-ground underwater treadmills by design have the capacity to hold a greater amount of water and thus provide more buoyancy in comparison to the above-ground units (Figure 18-28). The above-ground

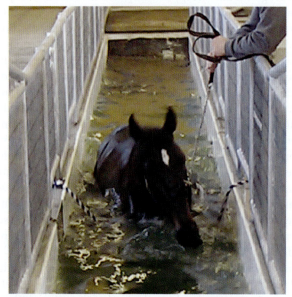

FIGURE 18-28 A horse walking on a below-ground underwater treadmill with the water level at the tuber coxa with the goal of increasing buoyancy and reducing limb impact although increasing cardiovascular fitness and strengthening in preparation for ridden exercise.

underwater treadmill units are able to change the depth of water between each patient, allowing for targeted rehabilitation protocols designed to improve joint range of motion. Both underwater treadmill units can come installed with hydrojets creating additional turbulent fluid flow, which increases the resistance of limb movement through the water-enhancing muscle strength and timing. In addition, underwater treadmill units have the ability to vary treadmill speed, water temperature, and solute concentration. Horses frequently require a period of 3 to 5 days to become acclimated and trained to exercise in the underwater treadmill units.

The aqua walkers are mechanical walkers fitted within a circular pool that contains a consistent depth of water. The diameter of the aqua walker dictates how many horses can be exercised at a time; most systems are able to exercise six to eight horses simultaneously. Horses are not completely buoyant and are separated from each other by dividers creating an individual "pen" for each horse. The depth of the water is dictated by the system design; some have just a shallow trough with water maintained no higher than the fetlock joint, although others maintain the water height at the level of the stifle joint. The speed of system is controlled; however, unlike the underwater treadmills, the horse may not walk at the consistent speed set by the unit. Some horses choose to slow down and then rush forward as the divider approaches them from behind only to slow down again once they catch up to the divider in front of them. Similar to the underwater treadmill units the aqua walkers are able to vary the water temperature and solute concentration.

Swimming horses typically require linear or circular-shaped pools with ramps installed for ease of entry and exit. Equine pools should be designed so that handlers on each side of the horse's head can walk alongside during each exercise session. To ensure complete buoyancy the water depth should be more than 12 feet deep. Linear pools may decrease cardiorespiratory stress as the horse is allowed to recover upon exiting while being walked back to the entry point.[183] Conversely, continuous lap swimming in circular pools does not allow for cardiorespiratory recovery until completion of the exercise session. Horses are not natural swimmers and often use their thoracic limbs to maintain balance while the pelvic limbs are primarily used for propulsion. The explosive nature of the pelvic limb propulsion often results in extreme ranges of motion through the hip, stifle, and hock joints. In addition, upon entry into the water, horses often adopt a posture that results in cervical, thoracolumbar, and pelvic extension. In the authors' opinion swimming horses with thoracolumbar, sacroiliac, hip, stifle, and hock injuries should be approached with caution.

Treatment Protocol Considerations

Aquatic therapy rehabilitation protocols should be developed to meet the needs of each individual patient following a complete assessment and understanding of the desired long term-goals for athletic performance. Not only should the injury and physical conditions be considered, but understanding the temperament, behavioral response to water exposure, and previous history of aquatic therapy is crucial to developing a solid therapeutic plan. The development and progression of an aquatic therapy program should involve three main components: intensity, duration, and frequency of applied therapy. The depth of water, turbulence, and speed of walking can influence intensity of exercise on the underwater treadmill. It is difficult to control intensity while swimming, as most horses are allowed to select a self-determined pace. However, some linear pools can provide a higher intensity workload by having horses swim against a current. The initial duration of treatment is greatly influenced by the nature of the injury, body condition, preinjury and postinjury fitness level, and presence of muscle weakness or atrophy. Initially horses may only be able to exercise for 5 minutes in the first week of therapy. The goal is to be able to increase the duration of walking by 5-minute increments weekly until 20 minutes is reached. Similarly, swimming sessions may involve only being able to swim 1 or 2 laps initially (5 to 8 minutes), working up to swimming (continuously for a circular pool) for a total of 9 to 12 laps. The frequency of treatment is often dictated by the horse's response to the rehabilitation program. Typically the more intensive the exercise program, the faster the return to function as long as the horse is not overloaded and is given time to adapt and strengthen.[184] The majority of underwater treadmill protocols are designed for daily aquatic therapy, 5 days a week. Swimming protocols range from 3 times a week to 15-minute sessions 3 times a week combined with 5-minute sessions twice a week. It is critical to remember when progressing within a rehabilitation program that only one aspect of the protocol should be changed at a time. If intensity and duration are changed simultaneously, then these changes may be too much too soon.

Precautions

Swimming horses with respiratory disease should be avoided as the increase in hydrostatic pressure will influence lung volume, preventing adequate ventilation.[175] Aquatic therapy should also be avoided if the horse has any of the following conditions:

- Unhealed surgical incisions
- Open, infected, draining wounds
- Upper pelvic limb lameness
- Thoracolumbar pain/injury
- Acute joint inflammation
- Acute myositis
- Elevated temperature
- Fearful or panicky
- Cardiovascular compromise

Monitoring Procedures

Monitoring recovery heart rates is a useful tool in recognizing when a horse can progress in the rehabilitation program. Heart rates and recovery rates can be monitored before, during, and immediately following exercise to quantify the level of intensity. The heart rate during aquatic therapy should not exceed 200 beats per minute and the time required for the heart rate to decrease to 60 beats per minute should be less than 10 minutes. Rehabilitation therapeutic protocols should not increase in intensity if target heart rate is exceeded or if there is an extended recovery period.

The ability to quantitatively assess injury regression is crucial to monitoring the efficacy of therapeutic interventions. Evidence-based practice requires the use of valid, reliable, and sensitive tools to monitor treatment effectiveness. Pressure algometry, goniometry, and limb circumference are reliable and objective methods of determining pain, joint range of motion, swelling, and muscle mass and are often used to assess articular responses to physical therapy.[185] Horses should be evaluated daily before each aquatic therapy session for any palpable musculoskeletal defects in the affected limb and for any alterations in the degree of lameness. If appropriate, ultrasonography should be repeated at monthly intervals to assist in adjusting the protocol.

Aquatic therapy incorporates several different mechanisms of action, all of which have particular benefit in the management of equine musculoskeletal disorders. The current human and veterinary literature suggests that aquatic therapy has beneficial effects on several OA-related morbidities, such as pain reduction and increased joint range of motion. Well-designed, controlled clinical trials using aquatic therapy are needed in horses to determine dosage effects (e.g., water level, duration, and speed) and to assess clinical changes in soft-tissue swelling, joint stability, and motor control patterns associated with adaptive and maladaptive compensatory gait alterations. The diverse physical characteristics of aquatic therapy provide unique approaches to individualized rehabilitation of OA and secondary musculoskeletal issues in horses.

SUMMARY

Numerous rehabilitative approaches are available to manage specific clinical aspects of OA; however, no single form of therapy is superior or highly efficacious in all phases of joint injury and healing. The individual patient is best served by identification of the primary rehabilitative issues that limit mobility or performance at that point in time based on physical examination, gait analysis, diagnostic imaging, and functional assessments of neuromuscular capabilities. Once a specific diagnosis or rehabilitation issue (i.e., pain, proprioception, flexibility, endurance, or strength) has been defined, focused treatment options can be applied and response to therapy monitored as individual rehabilitation issues resolve and others become clinically relevant (Box 18-1). There is a growing body of evidence that rehabilitation programs that focus on reducing pain, maintaining or improving proprioceptive acuity and strength, and enhancing joint stability through neuromuscular training may have the potential to improve function and alter the progression of OA in horses.

BOX 18-1 General Guidelines for Osteoarthritis Management

The goals for osteoarthritis rehabilitation include reducing pain, increasing joint mobility, improving muscle strength and coordination, and optimizing the overall functional status within individual patients.

Pain Management

Osteoarthritis is characterized as a chronic, degenerative disease process with bouts of acute pain or inflammation. Therefore, periodic nonsteroid antiinflammatory drugs (NSAIDs) combined with cryotherapy of similar pain management strategies are needed for long-term pain relief in affected horses. Owners and trainers should develop a routine for regularly assessing affected joints for the presence of heat and swelling or increased lameness or stiffness. Management of minor flare-ups of pain or inflammation is preferable to ignoring clinical signs until a severe or debilitating lameness is present.

Joint Stability and Balance

Optimizing joint stability and proprioception are key issues in preventing reinjury of affected osteoarthritic joints. A seemingly minor misstep or stumble can aggravate or precipitate new injuries in adjacent tissues or compensatory structures. Maintaining good joint and body awareness with periodic proprioceptive exercises helps to protect affected joints and minimize progression of osteoarthritis. Core stability is also important for axial skeleton osteoarthritis as epaxial muscle atrophy and subsequent neck or trunk weakness predispose affected joints to increased biomechanical instability and risk of re-injury. Monitoring footing and ground surfaces is important is minimize stumbling or poor foot placement, which can exacerbate joint instability.

Flexibility

Joint mobility or flexibility is needed for any type of activity or form of locomotion. Daily stretching or joint mobilization exercises may help to restore joint motion in the short term; however, continuous exposure to low-grades of joint movement (e.g., pasture turnout) are typically the easiest and best way to maintain long-term joint flexibility. Stall confinement should be minimized as this limits natural movements and the freedom to move affected joints and supporting soft tissues through normal ranges of motion.

Muscular Fitness

Muscular fitness refers to strength and endurance needed to perform activities of daily living and any athletic endeavors. Appropriate muscle timing and amplitudes of contraction are needed to maintain free and fluid joint motion and to minimize biomechanical stresses applied to affected articulations. Appropriate types and intensities of strength training within individual patients are needed to help retain and build muscle mass and motor control.

Controlled Exercise

Individualized types and intensities of aerobic exercise are needed to maintain physical and mental fitness in affected horses. Exercise or training programs should include consistent levels of exercise that are appropriate for the individual horse and the severity and location of osteoarthritis. Walking on a straight line on even ground is the most basic level of controlled exercise in osteoarthritic patients. Increasing the speed or duration of exercise is appropriate as long as joint pain or stiffness is not aggravated during riding. Circling or working on inclines or uneven ground surfaces may be acceptable for some horses. Exercise should be discontinued at any sign of discomfort or fatigue, as these may increase the risk for joint instability. Be realistic about the amount and type of exercise an individual horse can participate in.

Rest and Recovery

Prolonged periods of high-intensity exercise or rapid movements can aggravate osteoarthritis. Appropriate levels of rest are needed after intense exercise to allow body systems and local tissues to respond and recover. Adequate warm-up activities or stretching may help to prepare joints and adjacent tissues for increased loading and use. Participating in different types of exercise (e.g., cross training) may help to limit local tissue stress associated with cyclic or repetitive activities. Monitoring the horse's willingness and ability to perform exercise or specific movements is critical for long-term management of affected horses.

Environmental Modifications

Environmental modifications for patients with osteoarthritis may include avoiding cold, damp weather and providing a warm, dry, indoor shelter. Stall size and bedding should minimize any difficulties associated with rising or lying down. Herd dynamics need to be monitored so that affected horses are not overly pursued or bullied by other horses with higher social status. Smooth and consistent ground surfaces provide good footing and reduce the risk for missteps and aberrant joint loading. Removing any obstacles or required steps may be needed for severely affected patients. The use of a hay net or elevated water source may be useful for horses with cervical spine osteoarthritis. Conversely, feeding off the ground or in a pasture setting may help to increase neck flexibility and muscle development in affected horses. Weight loss may be indicated in obese patients with lower limb osteoarthritis to reduce joint loading conditions.

REFERENCES

1. McAlindon TE, Bannuru RR, Sullivan MC, et al. OARSI guidelines for the non-surgical management of knee osteoarthritis. *Osteoarthritis Cartilage.* 2014;22(3):363–388.
2. McIlwraith CW. The use of intra-articular corticosteroids in the horse: what is known on a scientific basis? *Equine Vet J.* 2010;42(6):563–571.
3. Paulekas R, Haussler KK. Principles and practice of therapeutic exercise for horses. *J Equine Vet Sci.* 2009;29(12):870–893.
4. Adrian CP, Haussler KK, Kawcak C, et al. The role of muscle activation in cruciate disease. *Vet Surg.* 2013;42(7):765–773.
5. Bockstahler BA, Vobornik A, Muller M, et al. Compensatory load redistribution in naturally occurring osteoarthritis of the elbow joint and induced weight-bearing lameness of the forelimbs compared with clinically sound dogs. *Vet J.* 2009;180(2):202–212.
6. Porter M. Equine rehabilitation therapy for joint disease. *Vet Clin North Am Equine Pract.* 2005;21(3):599–607.

7. Davis AM. Osteoarthritis year in review: rehabilitation and outcomes. *Osteoarthritis Cartilage*. 2012;20(3):201–206.

8. Walsh NE, Hurley MV. Evidence based guidelines and current practice for physiotherapy management of knee osteoarthritis. *Musculoskeletal Care*. 2009;7(1):45–56.

9. Petrov R, MacDonald MH, Tesch AM, et al. Influence of topically applied cold treatment on core temperature and cell viability in equine superficial digital flexor tendons. *Am J Vet Res*. 2003;64(7):835–844.

10. Sluka KA, Christy MR, Peterson WL, et al. Reduction of pain-related behaviors with either cold or heat treatment in an animal model of acute arthritis. *Arch Phys Med Rehabil*. 1999;80(3):313–317.

11. Algafly AA, George KP. The effect of cryotherapy on nerve conduction velocity, pain threshold and pain tolerance. *Br J Sports Med*. 2007;41(6):365–369. discussion 369.

12. Worster AA, Gaughan EM, Hoskinson JJ, et al. Effects of external thermal manipulation on laminar temperature and perfusion scintigraphy of the equine digit. *N Z Vet J*. 2000;48(4):111–116.

13. Rexing J, Dunning D, Siegel AM, et al. Effects of cold compression, bandaging, and microcurrent electrical therapy after cranial cruciate ligament repair in dogs. *Vet Surg*. 2010;39(1):54–58.

14. Bleakley CM, Costello JT. Do thermal agents affect range of movement and mechanical properties in soft tissues? A systematic review. *Arch Phys Med Rehabil*. 2012;94(1):149–163.

15. Brosseau L, Rahman P, Toupin-April K, et al. A systematic critical appraisal for non-pharmacological management of osteoarthritis using the Appraisal of Guidelines Research and Evaluation II Instrument. *PLoS One*. 2014;9: e82986.

16. Sanchez-Inchausti G, Vaquero-Martin J, Vidal-Fernandez C. Effect of arthroscopy and continuous cryotherapy on the intra-articular temperature of the knee. *Arthroscopy*. 2005;21(5):552–556.

17. Guillot X, Tordi N, Mourot L, et al. Cryotherapy in inflammatory rheumatic diseases: a systematic review. *Expert Rev Clin Immunol*. 2013;10(2):281–294.

18. Hassan K, MacDonald M, Petrov R, et al. Investigation of the effects of local cryotherapy on intra-articular temperature and experimentally induced synovitis in horses. *Proceedings 21st Annual Meeting Association of Equine Sports Medicine*. 2001; 2001:70–72.

19. Bocobo C, Fast A, Kingery W, et al. The effect of ice on intra-articular temperature in the knee of the dog. *Am J Phys Med Rehabil*. 1991;70(4):181–185.

20. Pollitt CC, van Eps AW. Prolonged, continuous distal limb cryotherapy in the horse. *Equine Vet J*. 2004;36(3):216–220.

21. Reesink HL, Divers TJ, Bookbinder LC, et al. Measurement of digital laminar and venous temperatures as a means of comparing three methods of topically applied cold treatment for digits of horses. *Am J Vet Res*. 2012;73(6):860–866.

22. Drygas KA, McClure SR, Goring RL, et al. Effect of cold compression therapy on postoperative pain, swelling, range of motion, and lameness after tibial plateau leveling osteotomy in dogs. *J Am Vet Med Assoc*. 2011;238(10):1284–1291.

23. Kaneps AJ. Tissue temperature response to hot and cold therapy in the metacarpal region of a horse. *Proc Am Assoc Equine Practitioners*. 2000;46:208–213.

24. Millard RP, Towle-Millard HA, Rankin DC, et al. Effect of cold compress application on tissue temperature in healthy dogs. *Am J Vet Res*. 2013;74(3):443–447.

25. van Eps AW, Pollitt CC. Equine laminitis: cryotherapy reduces the severity of the acute lesion. *Equine Vet J*. 2004;36(3):255–260.

26. Millard RP, Towle-Millard HA, Rankin DC, et al. Effect of warm compress application on tissue temperature in healthy dogs. *Am J Vet Res*. 2013;74(3):448–451.

27. Takahashi KA, Tonomura H, Arai Y, et al. Hyperthermia for the treatment of articular cartilage with osteoarthritis. *Int J Hyperthermia*. 2009;25(8):661–667.

28. Hosaka Y, Ozoe S, Kirisawa R, et al. Effect of heat on synthesis of gelatinases and pro-inflammatory cytokines in equine tendinocytes. *Biomed Res*. 2006;27(5):233–241.

29. Rabini A, Piazzini DB, Tancredi G, et al. Deep heating therapy via microwave diathermy relieves pain and improves physical function in patients with knee osteoarthritis: a double-blind randomized clinical trial. *Eur J Phys Rehabil Med*. 2012;48(4):549–559.

30. Jan MH, Chai HM, Wang CL, et al. Effects of repetitive shortwave diathermy for reducing synovitis in patients with knee osteoarthritis: an ultrasonographic study. *Phys Ther*. 2006;86(2):236–244.

31. Lideo L, Milan R. Ultrasound monitoring of shortwave diathermic treatment of gastrocnemius strain in a dog. *J Ultrasound*. 2014;16(4):231–234.

32. Tascioglu F, Kuzgun S, Armagan O, et al. Short-term effectiveness of ultrasound therapy in knee osteoarthritis. *J Int Med Res*. 2010;38(4):1233–1242.

33. Rutjes AW, Nuesch E, Sterchi R, et al. Therapeutic ultrasound for osteoarthritis of the knee or hip. *Cochrane Database Syst Rev*. 2010;(1). CD003132.

34. Montgomery L, Elliott SB, Adair HS. Muscle and tendon heating rates with therapeutic ultrasound in horses. *Vet Surg*. 2013;42(3):243–249.

35. Steiss JE, Adams CC. Effect of coat on rate of temperature increase in muscle during ultrasound treatment of dogs. *Am J Vet Res*. 1999;60(1):76–80.

36. Naito K, Watari T, Muta T, et al. Low-intensity pulsed ultrasound (LIPUS) increases the articular cartilage type II collagen in a rat osteoarthritis model. *J Orthop Res*. 2009;28(3):361–369.

37. Li X, Li J, Cheng K, et al. Effect of low-intensity pulsed ultrasound on MMP-13 and MAPKs signaling pathway in rabbit knee osteoarthritis. *Cell Biochem Biophys*. 2011;61(2):427–434.

38. Gurkan I, Ranganathan A, Yang X, et al. Modification of osteoarthritis in the guinea pig with pulsed low-intensity ultrasound treatment. *Osteoarthritis Cartilage*. 2010; 18(5):724–733.

39. McClure SR, Sonea IM, Evans RB, et al. Evaluation of analgesia resulting from extracorporeal shock wave therapy and radial pressure wave therapy in the limbs of horses and sheep. *Am J Vet Res*. 2005;66(10):1702–1708.

40. Dahlberg J, Fitch G, Evans RB, et al. The evaluation of extracorporeal shockwave therapy in naturally occurring osteoarthritis of the stifle joint in dogs. *Vet Comp Orthop Traumatol*. 2005;18(3):147–152.

41. Bolt DM, Burba DJ, Hubert JD, et al. Evaluation of cutaneous analgesia after non-focused extracorporeal shock wave application over the 3rd metacarpal bone in horses. *Can J Vet Res*. 2004;68(4):288–292.

42. Wang CJ, Hsu SL, Weng LH, et al. Extracorporeal shockwave therapy shows a number of treatment related chondroprotective effect in osteoarthritis of the knee in rats. *BMC Musculoskelet Disord.* 2013;14:44.

43. Zhao Z, Ji H, Jing R, et al. Extracorporeal shock-wave therapy reduces progression of knee osteoarthritis in rabbits by reducing nitric oxide level and chondrocyte apoptosis. *Arch Orthop Trauma Surg.* 2012;132(11):1547–1553.

44. Mueller M, Bockstahler B, Skalicky M, et al. Effects of radial shockwave therapy on the limb function of dogs with hip osteoarthritis. *Vet Rec.* 2007;160(22):762–765.

45. Kawcak CE, Frisbie DD, McIlwraith CW. Effects of extracorporeal shock wave therapy and polysulfated glycosaminoglycan treatment on subchondral bone, serum biomarkers, and synovial fluid biomarkers in horses with induced osteoarthritis. *Am J Vet Res.* 2011;72(6):772–779.

46. Frisbie DD, Kawcak CE, McIlwraith CW. Evaluation of the effect of extracorporeal shock wave treatment on experimentally induced osteoarthritis in middle carpal joints of horses. *Am J Vet Res.* 2009;70(4):449–454.

47. Dahlberg JA, McClure SR, Evans RB, et al. Force platform evaluation of lameness severity following extracorporeal shock wave therapy in horses with unilateral forelimb lameness. *J Am Vet Med Assoc.* 2006;229(1):100–103.

48. Brosseau L, Welch V, Wells G, et al. Low level laser therapy (classes I, II and III) for treating osteoarthritis. *Cochrane Database Syst Rev.* 2004;(3): CD002046.

49. Hegedus B, Viharos L, Gervain M, et al. The effect of low-level laser in knee osteoarthritis: a double-blind, randomized, placebo-controlled trial. *Photomed Laser Surg.* 2009;27(4):577–584.

50. Ryan T, Smith R. An investigation into the depth of penetration of low level laser therapy through the equine tendon in vivo. *Ir Vet J.* 2007;60(5):295–299.

51. Alfredo PP, Bjordal JM, Dreyer SH, et al. Efficacy of low level laser therapy associated with exercises in knee osteoarthritis: a randomized double-blind study. *Clin Rehabil.* 2011;26(6):523–533.

52. Law PP, Cheing GL, Tsui AY. Does transcutaneous electrical nerve stimulation improve the physical performance of people with knee osteoarthritis? *J Clin Rheumatol.* 2004;10(6):295–299.

53. Pietrosimone BG, Saliba SA, Hart JM, et al. Effects of transcutaneous electrical nerve stimulation and therapeutic exercise on quadriceps activation in people with tibiofemoral osteoarthritis. *J Orthop Sports Phys Ther.* 2011;41(4):4–12.

54. Shmalberg J, Xie H. The clinical application of equine acupuncture. *J Equine Vet Sci.* 2009;29(10):645–652.

55. Ryang We S, Koog YH, Jeong KI, et al. Effects of pulsed electromagnetic field on knee osteoarthritis: a systematic review. *Rheumatology (Oxford).* 2012;52(5):815–824.

56. Vavken P, Arrich F, Schuhfried O, et al. Effectiveness of pulsed electromagnetic field therapy in the management of osteoarthritis of the knee: a meta-analysis of randomized controlled trials. *J Rehabil Med.* 2009;41(6):406–411.

57. Nelson FR, Zvirbulis R, Pilla AA. Non-invasive electromagnetic field therapy produces rapid and substantial pain reduction in early knee osteoarthritis: a randomized double-blind pilot study. *Rheumatol Int.* 2012;33(8):2169–2173.

58. Veronesi F, Torricelli P, Giavaresi G, et al. In vivo effect of two different pulsed electromagnetic field frequencies on osteoarthritis. *J Orthop Res.* 2014;32(5):677–685.

59. Kold SE, Hickman J, Meisen F. Preliminary study of quantitative aspects and the effect of pulsed electromagnetic field treatment on the incorporation of equine cancellous bone grafts. *Equine Vet J.* 1987;19(2):120–124.

60. Cane V, Botti P, Soana S. Pulsed magnetic fields improve osteoblast activity during the repair of an experimental osseous defect. *J Orthop Res.* 1993;11(5):664–670.

61. Crawford WH, Houge JC, Neirby DT, et al. Pulsed radio frequency therapy of experimentally induced arthritis in ponies. *Can J Vet Res.* 1991;55(1):76–85.

62. Akinbo SR, Aiyejusunle CB, Akinyemi OA, et al. Comparison of the therapeutic efficacy of phonophoresis and iontophoresis using dexamethasone sodium phosphate in the management of patients with knee osteoarthritis. *Niger Postgrad Med J.* 2007;14(3):190–194.

63. Muir WS, Magee FP, Longo JA, et al. Comparison of ultrasonically applied vs. intra-articular injected hydrocortisone levels in canine knees. *Orthop Rev.* 1990;19(4):351–356.

64. Rosenstein ED. Topical agents in the treatment of rheumatic disorders. *Rheum Dis Clin North Am.* 1999;25(4):899–918.

65. Kaneps AJ, Craig AM, Walker KC, et al. Iontophoretic administration of dexamethasone into the tarsocrural joint in horses. *Am J Vet Res.* 2002;63(1):11–14.

66. Blackford J, Doherty TJ, Ferslew KE, et al. Iontophoresis of dexamethosone-phosphate into the equine tibiotarsal joint. *J Vet Pharmacol Ther.* 2000;23(4):229–236.

67. Moraes MR, Cavalcante ML, Leite JA, et al. The characteristics of the mechanoreceptors of the hip with arthrosis. *J Orthop Surg Res.* 2011;6:58.

68. Kars HJ, Hijmans JM, Geertzen JH, et al. The effect of reduced somatosensation on standing balance: a systematic review. *J Diabetes Sci Technol.* 2009;3(4):931–943.

69. Wu Q, Henry JL. Functional changes in muscle afferent neurones in an osteoarthritis model: implications for impaired proprioceptive performance. *PLoS One.* 2012;7: e36854.

70. Felson DT, Gross KD, Nevitt MC, et al. The effects of impaired joint position sense on the development and progression of pain and structural damage in knee osteoarthritis. *Arthritis Rheum.* 2009;61(8):1070–1076.

71. Grubb BD. Activation of sensory neurons in the arthritic joint. *Novartis Found Symp.* 2004;260:28–36. discussion 36-48, 100-104, 277–279.

72. Eitner A, Pester J, Nietzsche S, et al. The innervation of synovium of human osteoarthritic joints in comparison with normal rat and sheep synovium. *Osteoarthritis Cartilage.* 2013;21(9):1383–1391.

73. Salo P. The role of joint innervation in the pathogenesis of arthritis. *Can J Surg.* 1999;42(2):91–100.

74. Knarr BA, Zeni Jr JA, Higginson JS. Comparison of electromyography and joint moment as indicators of co-contraction. *J Electromyogr Kinesiol.* 2012;22(4):607–611.

75. Segal NA, Glass NA, Felson DT, et al. Effect of quadriceps strength and proprioception on risk for knee osteoarthritis. *Med Sci Sports Exerc.* 2010;42(11):2081–2088.

76. Ling SM, Conwit RA, Talbot L, et al. Electromyographic patterns suggest changes in motor unit physiology associated with early osteoarthritis of the knee. *Osteoarthritis Cartilage.* 2007;15(10):1134–1140.

77. Knoop J, Steultjens MP, van der Leeden M, et al. Proprioception in knee osteoarthritis: a narrative review. *Osteoarthritis Cartilage.* 2011;19(4):381–388.

78. Kiss RM. Effect of degree of knee osteoarthritis on balancing capacity after sudden perturbation. *J Electromyogr Kinesiol.* 2012;22(4):575–581.

79. Lund H, Juul-Kristensen B, Hansen K, et al. Movement detection impaired in patients with knee osteoarthritis compared to healthy controls: a cross-sectional case-control study. *J Musculoskelet Neuronal Interact.* 2008;8(4):391–400.

80. Hewitt BA, Refshauge KM, Kilbreath SL. Kinesthesia at the knee: the effect of osteoarthritis and bandage application. *Arthritis Rheum.* 2002;47(5):479–483.

81. Malliou P, Gioftsidou A, Pafis G, et al. Proprioception and functional deficits of partial meniscectomized knees. *Eur J Phys Rehabil Med.* 2012;48(2):231–236.

82. Chang AH, Lee SJ, Zhao H, et al. Impaired varus-valgus proprioception and neuromuscular stabilization in medial knee osteoarthritis. *J Biomech.* 2013;47(2):360–366.

83. Ramon T, Prades M, Armengou L, et al. Effects of athletic taping of the fetlock on distal limb mechanics. *Equine Vet J.* 2004;36(8):764–768.

84. Morlock M, Nassutt R, Bonin V. The influence of bandage characteristics and inter-individual application variations on underneath bandage pressures. *Clin Biomech (Bristol, Avon).* 1997;12(3):S10.

85. Williams S, Whatman C, Hume PA, et al. Kinesio taping in treatment and prevention of sports injuries: a meta-analysis of the evidence for its effectiveness. *Sports Med.* 2011;42(2):153–164.

86. Hassan BS, Mockett S, Doherty M. Influence of elastic bandage on knee pain, proprioception, and postural sway in subjects with knee osteoarthritis. *Ann Rheum Dis.* 2002;61(1):24–28.

87. Kicker CJ, Peham C, Girtler D, et al. Influence of support boots on fetlock joint angle of the forelimb of the horse at walk and trot. *Equine Vet J.* 2004;36(8):769–771.

88. Smith RK, McGuigan MP, Hyde JT, et al. In vitro evaluation of nonrigid support systems for the equine metacarpophalangeal joint. *Equine Vet J.* 2002;34(7):726–731.

89. Clayton HM, White AD, Kaiser LJ, et al. Short-term habituation of equine limb kinematics to tactile stimulation of the coronet. *Vet Comp Orthop Traumatol.* 2008;21(3):211–214.

90. Clayton HM, Lavagnino M, Kaiser LJ, et al. Evaluation of biomechanical effects of four stimulation devices placed on the hind feet of trotting horses. *Am J Vet Res.* 2011;72(11):1489–1495.

91. Clayton HM, White AD, Kaiser LJ, et al. Hindlimb response to tactile stimulation of the pastern and coronet. *Equine Vet J.* 2010;42(3):227–233.

92. Brown S, Stubbs NC, Kaiser LJ, et al. Swing phase kinematics of horses trotting over poles. *Equine Vet J.* 2015;47(1):107–112.

93. Clayton HM, Stubbs NC, Lavagnino M. Stance phase kinematics and kinetics of horses trotting over poles. *Equine Vet J.* 2015;47(1):113–118.

94. Mandelbaum BR, Silvers HJ, Watanabe DS, et al. Effectiveness of a neuromuscular and proprioceptive training program in preventing anterior cruciate ligament injuries in female athletes: 2-year follow-up. *Am J Sports Med.* 2005;33(7):1003–1010.

95. Fitzgerald GK, Childs JD, Ridge TM, et al. Agility and perturbation training for a physically active individual with knee osteoarthritis. *Phys Ther.* 2002;82(4):372–382.

96. Vaz MA, Baroni BM, Geremia JM, et al. Neuromuscular electrical stimulation (NMES) reduces structural and functional losses of quadriceps muscle and improves health status in patients with knee osteoarthritis. *J Orthop Res.* 2012;31(4):511–516.

97. Giggins O, Fullen B, Coughlan G. Neuromuscular electrical stimulation in the treatment of knee osteoarthritis: a systematic review and meta-analysis. *Clin Rehabil.* 2012;26(10):867–881.

98. Akkaya N, Ardic F, Ozgen M, et al. Efficacy of electromyographic biofeedback and electrical stimulation following arthroscopic partial meniscectomy: a randomized controlled trial. *Clin Rehabil.* 2011;26(3):224–236.

99. Lewek MD, Rudolph KS, Snyder-Mackler L. Quadriceps femoris muscle weakness and activation failure in patients with symptomatic knee osteoarthritis. *J Orthop Res.* 2004;22(1):110–115.

100. Elboim-Gabyzon M, Rozen N, Laufer Y. Does neuromuscular electrical stimulation enhance the effectiveness of an exercise programme in subjects with knee osteoarthritis? A randomized controlled trial. *Clin Rehabil.* 2012;27(3):246–257.

101. Liphardt AM, Mundermann A, Koo S, et al. Vibration training intervention to maintain cartilage thickness and serum concentrations of cartilage oligometric matrix protein (COMP) during immobilization. *Osteoarthritis Cartilage.* 2009;17(12):1598–1603.

102. Carstanjen B, Balali M, Gajewski Z, et al. Short-term whole body vibration exercise in adult healthy horses. *Pol J Vet Sci.* 2013;16(2):403–405.

103. Trans T, Aaboe J, Henriksen M, et al. Effect of whole body vibration exercise on muscle strength and proprioception in females with knee osteoarthritis. *Knee.* 2009;16(4):256–261.

104. Park YG, Kwon BS, Park JW, et al. Therapeutic effect of whole body vibration on chronic knee osteoarthritis. *Ann Rehabil Med.* 2013;37(4):505–515.

105. Segal NA, Glass NA, Shakoor N, et al. Vibration platform training in women at risk for symptomatic knee osteoarthritis. *PM R.* 2012;5(3):201–209. quiz 209.

106. van Harreveld PD, Lillich JD, Kawcak CE, et al. Effects of immobilization followed by remobilization on mineral density, histomorphometric features, and formation of the bones of the metacarpophalangeal joint in horses. *Am J Vet Res.* 2002;63(2):276–281.

107. Nakano J, Yamabayashi C, Scott A, et al. The effect of heat applied with stretch to increase range of motion: a systematic review. *Phys Ther Sport.* 2012;13(3):180–188.

108. Frick A. Stretching exercises for horses: are they effective? *J Equine Vet Sci.* 2010;30(1):50–59.

109. Deyle GD, Henderson NE, Matekel RL, et al. Effectiveness of manual physical therapy and exercise in osteoarthritis of the knee. A randomized, controlled trial. *Ann Intern Med.* 2000;132(3):173–181.

110. Corey SM, Vizzard MA, Bouffard NA, et al. Stretching of the back improves gait, mechanical sensitivity and connective tissue inflammation in a rodent model. *PLoS One.* 2012;7(1): e29831.

111. French HP, Brennan A, White B, et al. Manual therapy for osteoarthritis of the hip or knee - a systematic review. *Man Ther.* 2011;16(2):109–117.

112. Haussler KK, Hill AE, Puttlitz CM, et al. Effects of vertebral mobilization and manipulation on kinematics of the thoracolumbar region. *Am J Vet Res.* 2007;68(5):508–516.

113. Scott M, Swenson LA. Evaluating the benefits of equine massage therapy: a review of the evidence and current practices. *J Equine Vet Sci.* 2009;29(9):687–697.

114. Haussler KK. The role of manual therapies in equine pain management. *Vet Clin North Am Equine Pract.* 2010;26(3):579–601.

115. Haussler KK. Review of manual therapy techniques in equine practice. *J Equine Vet Sci.* 2009;29(12):849–869.

116. Hubbard TJ, Hicks-Little C, Cordova M. Mechanical and sensorimotor implications with ankle osteoarthritis. *Arch Phys Med Rehabil.* 2009;90(7):1136–1141.

117. Palmieri-Smith RM, Villwock M, Downie B, et al. Pain and effusion and quadriceps activation and strength. *J Athl Train.* 2013;48(2):186–191.

118. Rutherford DJ, Hubley-Kozey CL, Stanish WD. Knee effusion affects knee mechanics and muscle activity during gait in individuals with knee osteoarthritis. *Osteoarthritis Cartilage.* 2012;20(9):974–981.

119. Hopkins JT, Palmieri R. Effects of ankle joint effusion on lower leg function. *Clin J Sport Med.* 2004;14(1):1–7.

120. Al-Zahrani KS, Bakheit AM. A study of the gait characteristics of patients with chronic osteoarthritis of the knee. *Disabil Rehabil.* 2002;24(5):275–280.

121. Liikavainio T, Isolehto J, Helminen HJ, et al. Loading and gait symmetry during level and stair walking in asymptomatic subjects with knee osteoarthritis: importance of quadriceps femoris in reducing impact force during heel strike? *Knee.* 2007;14(3):231–238.

122. Benedetti MG, Catani F, Bilotta TW, et al. Muscle activation pattern and gait biomechanics after total knee replacement. *Clin Biomech (Bristol, Avon).* 2003;18(9):871–876.

123. Hortobagyi T, Westerkamp L, Beam S, et al. Altered hamstring-quadriceps muscle balance in patients with knee osteoarthritis. *Clin Biomech (Bristol, Avon).* 2005;20(1):97–104.

124. Dumoulin M, Pille F, Desmet P, et al. Upward fixation of the patella in the horse. A retrospective study. *Vet Comp Orthop Traumatol.* 2007;20(2):119–125.

125. Segal NA, Findlay C, Wang K, et al. The longitudinal relationship between thigh muscle mass and the development of knee osteoarthritis. *Osteoarthritis Cartilage.* 2012;20(12):1534–1540.

126. Pietrosimone BG, Saliba SA. Changes in voluntary quadriceps activation predict changes in quadriceps strength after therapeutic exercise in patients with knee osteoarthritis. *Knee.* 2012;19(6):939–943.

127. Maly MR. Abnormal and cumulative loading in knee osteoarthritis. *Curr Opin Rheumatol.* 2008;20(5):547–552.

128. Liikavainio T, Bragge T, Hakkarainen M, et al. Gait and muscle activation changes in men with knee osteoarthritis. *Knee.* 2009;17(1):69–76.

129. Bijlsma JW, Knahr K. Strategies for the prevention and management of osteoarthritis of the hip and knee. *Best Pract Res Clin Rheumatol.* 2007;21(1):59–76.

130. King MR, Haussler KK, Kawcak CE, et al. Mechanisms of aquatic therapy and its potential use in managing equine osteoarthritis. *Equine Veter Education.* 2013;25(4):204–209.

131. Luria A, Chu CR. Articular cartilage changes in maturing athletes: new targets for joint rejuvenation. *Sports Health.* 2014;6(1):18–30.

132. Grodzinsky AJ, Levenston ME, Jin M, et al. Cartilage tissue remodeling in response to mechanical forces. *Annu Rev Biomed Eng.* 2000;2:691–713.

133. van Harreveld PD, Lillich JD, Kawcak CE, et al. Clinical evaluation of the effects of immobilization followed by remobilization and exercise on the metacarpophalangeal joint in horses. *Am J Vet Res.* 2002;63(2):282–288.

134. Brama PA, Tekoppele JM, Bank RA, et al. Influence of different exercise levels and age on the biochemical characteristics of immature equine articular cartilage. *Equine Vet J.* 1999;(Suppl 31):55–61.

135. Cappelli K, Felicetti M, Capomaccio S, et al. Exercise-induced up-regulation of MMP-1 and IL-8 genes in endurance horses. *BMC Physiol.* 2009;9:12.

136. Crevier-Denoix N, Robin D, Pourcelot P, et al. Ground reaction force and kinematic analysis of limb loading on two different beach sand tracks in harness trotters. *Equine Vet J.* 2011;(Suppl 38):544–551.

137. Setterbo JJ, Garcia TC, Campbell IP, et al. Hoof accelerations and ground reaction forces of Thoroughbred racehorses measured on dirt, synthetic, and turf track surfaces. *Am J Vet Res.* 2009;70(10):1220–1229.

138. Thambyah A, Zhao JY, Bevill SL, et al. Macro-, micro- and ultrastructural investigation of how degeneration influences the response of cartilage to loading. *J Mech Behav Biomed Mater.* 2011;5(1):206–215.

139. Hurley M. The effects of joint damage on muscle function, proprioception and rehabilitation. *Manual Therapy.* 1997;2(1):11.

140. Prins J, Cutner D. Aquatic therapy in the rehabilitation of athletic injuries. *Clin Sports Med.* 1999;18(2):447–461.

141. Miyoshi T, Shirota T, Yamamoto S-I, et al. Effect of the walking speed to the lower limb joint angular displacements, joint moments and ground reaction forces during walking in water. *Disabil Rehabil.* 2004;26(12):724–732.

142. Messier S, Royer T, Craven T, et al. Long-term exercise and its effect on balance in older, osteoarthritic adults: results from the Fitness, Arthritis, and Seniors Trial (FAST). *J Am Geriatr Soc.* 2000;48(2):131–138.

143. Kamioka H, Tsutanji K, Okuizumi H, et al. Effectiveness of aquatic exercise and balneotherapy: a summary of systematic reviews based on randomized controlled trials of water immersion therapies. *J Epidemiol.* 2010;20(1):2–12.

144. Evans B, Cureton K, Purvis J. Metabolic and circulatory responses to walking and jogging in water. *Res Q.* 1978;49(4):442–449.

145. Nakazawa K, Yano H, Miyashita M. Ground reaction forces during walking in water. *Med Sci Aquatic Sports.* 1994:28–34.

146. Hinman R, Heywood S, Day A. Aquatic physical therapy for hip and knee osteoarthritis: results of a single-blind randomized controlled trial. *Physical Therapy.* 2007;87(1):32–43.

147. Yamazaki F, Endo Y, Torii R, et al. Continuous monitoring of change in hemodilution during water immersion in humans: effect of water temperature. *Aviation, Space. Environ Med.* 2000;71(6):632–639.

148. Buchner H, Schildboeck U. Physiotherapy applied to the horse: a review. *Equine Vet J.* 2006;38(6):574–580.

149. Bender T, Karagulle Z, Balint GP, et al. Hydrotherapy, balneotherapy, and spa treatment in pain management. *Rheumatol Int.* 2005;25(3):220–224.

150. Masumoto K, Takasugi S, Hotto N, et al. Electromyographic analysis on walking in water in healthy humans. *J Physiol Anthropol Appl Human Sci.* 2004;23(4):119–127.

151. Harrison R, Hilman M. Loading of the lower limb when walking partially immersed: implications for clinical practice. *Physiotherapy.* 1992;78(3):164–166.

152. McClintock SA, Hutchins DR, Brownlow MA. Determination of weight reduction in horses in floatation tanks. *Equine Vet J.* 1987;19(1):70–71.

153. Poyhonen T, Keskinen K, Kyrolainen H, et al. Neuromuscular function during therapeutic knee exercise underwater and on dry land. *Arch Phys Med Rehabil.* 2001;82(10):1446–1452.

154. Dixon J, Howe T. Quadriceps force generation in patients with osteoarthritis of the knee and asymptomatic participants during patellar tendon reflex reactions: an exploratory cross-sectional study. *BMC Musculoskeletal Disorders.* 2005;6:1–6.

155. Brandt KD. Neuromuscular aspects of osteoarthritis: a perspective. *Novartis Found Symp.* 2004;260:49–58. discussion 58-63, 100-104, 277–279.

156. Newton R. Joint receptor contributions to reflexive and kinesthetic responses. *Phys Ther.* 1982;62(1):22–29.

157. Iles J, Stokes M, Young A. Reflex actions of knee joint afferents during contraction of the human quadriceps. *Clin Physiol.* 1990;10(5):489–500.

158. Hopkins J, Ingersoll C, Krause B, et al. Effect of knee joint effusion on quadriceps and soleus motoneuron pool excitability. *Med Sports Sci Sports Exercise.* 2001;33(1):123–126.

159. Coruzzi P, Ravanetti C, Musiari L, et al. Circulating opioid peptides during water immersion in normal man. *Clin Sci (Lond).* 1988;74(2):133–136.

160. Kato T, Ohmura H, Hiraga A, et al. Changes in heart rate variability in horses during immersion in warm springwater. *Am J Vet Res.* 2003;64(12):1482–1485.

161. Yurtkuran M, Yurtkuran M, Alp A, et al. Balneotherapy and tap water therapy in the treatment of knee osteoarthritis. *Rheumatol Int.* 2006;27(1):19–27.

162. McVeigh J, McGaughey H, Hall M, et al. The effectiveness of hydrotherapy in the management of fibromyalgia syndrome: a systematic review. *Rheumatol Int.* 2008;29(2):119–130.

163. Hunt E. Response of twenty-seven horses with lower leg injuries to cold spa bath hydrotherapy. *J Equine Vet Sci.* 2001;21(4):188–193.

164. Kim Y-S, Park J, Shim J. Effects of aquatic backward locomotion exercise and progressive resistance exercise on lumbar extension strength in patients who have undergone lumbar diskectomy. *Arch Phys Med Rehabil.* 2010;91(2):208–214.

165. Silva L, Valim V, Pessanha A, et al. Hydrotherapy versus conventional land-based exercise for the management of patients with osteoarthritis of the knee: a randomized clinical trial. *Phys Ther.* 2008;88(1):12–21.

166. Rahmann A, Brauer S, Nitz J. A specific inpatient aquatic physiotherapy program improves strength after total hip or knee replacement surgery: a randomized controlled trial. *Arch Phys Med Rehabil.* 2009;90(5):745–755.

167. Bartels EM, Lund H, Hagen KB, et al. Aquatic exercise for the treatment of knee and hip osteoarthritis. *Cochrane Database Syst Rev.* 2007;(4): CD005523.

168. Hinman RS, Heywood SE, Day AR. Aquatic physical therapy for hip and knee osteoarthritis: results of a single-blind randomized controlled trial. *Phys Ther.* 2007;87(1):32–43.

169. Bartels E, Lund H, Hagen K, et al. Aquatic exercise for the treatment of knee and hip osteoarthritis. *Cochrane Collaboration.* 2009:1–35.

170. Marsolais GS, McLean S, Derrick T, et al. Kinematic analysis of the hind limb during swimming and walking in healthy dogs and dogs with surgically corrected cranial cruciate ligament rupture. *J Am Vet Med Assoc.* 2003;222(6):739–743.

171. Marsolais GS, Dvorak G, Conzemius MG. Effects of postoperative rehabilitation on limb function after cranial cruciate ligament repair in dogs. *J Am Vet Med Assoc.* 2002;220(9):1325–1330.

172. Jackson A, Millis D, Stevens M, et al. *Joint kinematics during underwater treadmill activity.* Knoxville, TN, 191. Second International Symposium on Rehabilitation and Physical Therapy in Veterinary Medicine 2002; 2002.

173. Monk ML, Preston CA, McGowan CM. Effects of early intensive postoperative physiotherapy on limb function after tibial plateau leveling osteotomy in dogs with deficiency of the cranial cruciate ligament. *Am J Vet Res.* 2006;67(3):529–536.

174. Voss B, Mohr E, Krzywanek H. Effects of aqua-treadmill exercise on selected blood parameters and on heart-rate variability of horses. *J Vet Med Assoc Physiol Pathol Clin Med.* 2002;49(3):137–143.

175. Hobo S, Yosjida K, Yoshihara T. Characteristics of respiratory function during swimming exercise in Thoroughbreds. *J Vet Med Sci.* 1998;60(6):687–689.

176. Nankervis KJ, Williams RJ. Heart rate responses during acclimation of horses to water treadmill exercise. *Equine Vet J.* 2006;36(Suppl):110–112.

177. Misumi K, Sakamoto H, Shimizu R. Changes in skeletal muscle composition in response to swimming training for young horses. *J Vet Med Sci.* 1995;57(5):959–961.

178. Misumi K, Sakamoto H, Shimizu R. The validity of swimming training for two-year-old thoroughbreds. *J Vet Med Sci.* 1994;56(2):217–222.

179. Tokuriki M, Ohtsuki R, Kai M, et al. EMG activity of the muscles of the neck and forelimbs during different forms of locomotion. *Equine Vet J.* 1999;30(Suppl):231–234.

180. Scott R, Nankervis K, Stringer C, et al. The effect of water height on stride frequency, stride length and heart rate during water treadmill exercise. *Equine Vet J.* 2010;38(Suppl):662–664.

181. Mendez-Angulo JL, Firshman AM, Groschen DM, et al. Effect of water depth on amount of flexion and extension of joints of the distal aspects of the limbs in healthy horses walking on an underwater treadmill. *Am J Vet Res.* 2013;74(4):557–566.

182. King M, Haussler K, Kawcak C, et al. Effect of underwater treadmill exercise on postural sway in horses with experimentally induced carpal osteoarthritis. *Am J Vet Res.* 2013;74:971–982.

183. Bromiley MW. *Equine injury, therapy and rehabilitation.* 3rd ed. Ames, IA: Blackwell Publishing; 2007.

184. McGowan CM, Stubbs NC, Jull GA. Equine physiotherapy: a comparative view of the science underlying the profession. *Equine Vet J.* 2007;39(1):90–94.

185. Gajdosik R, Bohannon R. Clinical measurement of range of motion. *Phys Ther.* 1987;67(12):1867–1872.

19

Use of Oral Joint Supplements in Equine Joint Disease*

C. Wayne McIlwraith

Osteoarthritis (OA) is the single most common cause of lameness in horses.[1] In one survey, approximately 60% of lameness problems in horses were related to OA.[2] Similarly OA is the most common form of human arthritis, affecting at least 20 million Americans, and its prevalence is expected to double over the next two decades.[3,4] OA involves a complex interaction of biologic and pathologic processes highlighted by eventual degradation of articular cartilage.[5,6] With the horse population in the United States currently estimated to be 7.3 million,[7] this means millions of horses have this debilitating musculoskeletal condition. Multiple conventional therapies are available for treating OA with the goal of preventing further degradation although restoring function.[6,8]

Oral joint supplements (OJSs) are a common choice of clients and have been perceived as a benign treatment for OA in horses.[8] The high prevalence of OA in combination with the lack of a definitive cure for OA has probably contributed to the popularity of OJSs among owners, veterinarians, and trainers. These supplements, according to recent market surveys, are the most popular type of nutritional supplements for horses and account for approximately ⅓ (34%) of all equine supplement sales and ½ of all pet supplements sold in the U.S. for equine consumption; it is estimated that 49% of all horse owners purchase and administer some form of dietary supplement for their horses (Packaged Facts 2008).[9] In a study of feeding practices in 3-day event horses, the authors found that horses were supplemented with an average of four different oral products daily including electrolytes, plain salt, and OJSs.[10]

INDICATIONS FOR ORAL JOINT SUPPLEMENTS

OJSs are fed to horses for one of two purposes: to treat lame horses and make chronically unsound horses sound or to prevent/delay the development of joint problems. The first instance is flawed because often the source of lameness is never diagnosed when the owner or trainer elects to use supplements without consulting a veterinarian. The second premise is hard to disprove but is the basis for high use of both licensed drugs such as intramuscular Adequan® and intravenous Legend® as well as OJSs.

The critical components of articular cartilage are type II collagen fibrils (which provide a structural framework) and extracellular matrix, which consists of aggrecan molecules and water (Figure 19-1). The aggrecan molecule consists of aggregations of proteoglycan molecules on a hyaluronan (HA) backbone. The proteoglycan molecule, in turn, consists of a protein backbone with CS and keratan sulfate side chains. These carry negative charges and, because of repulsion of each other as well as attraction of water, provide the compressive resistance to the articular cartilage.[6] Maintenance of these molecules is critical and some OJSs provide potential building blocks for these molecules. The osteoarthritic process is associated with multiple deleterious mediators released from inflamed synovial membrane or induced by trauma that initiate a cascade of degradation in the articular cartilage. Interleukin-1 (IL-1) is considered a major cytokine initiating this cascade, and this can influence other cells to cause increased release of metalloproteinases, aggrecanase, and prostaglandin E2 (PGE2). Although this negative process can be influenced by certain OJSs in vitro (Figure 19-2), there is less certainty about their effects in vivo after undergoing digestion.

In 2005 OJS sales reached more than $1 billion for companion animals, and that number was expected to double in the next 3 years. There are more than 100 equine OJS products currently on the market in the U.S. and such products are used worldwide. This is a disturbing trend for an industry that, for the most part, is unregulated by the U.S. Food and Drug Administration (FDA) or other governing bodies, and has a weak in vivo scientific basis.[11]

TERMINOLOGY AND REGULATORY ISSUES IN THE USE OF ORAL JOINT SUPPLEMENTS (A U.S. PERSPECTIVE)

The term nutraceutical was adopted in veterinary medicine from the medical profession and refers to compounds that

*The author wishes to acknowledge that most of this information in this chapter was previously published in McIlwraith C.W. (2013). Oral joint supplements in the management of osteoarthritis. In: Geor R.J., Harris P.A., Coenen M. (Eds.). Equine applied and clinical nutrition (pp. 549-557). Saunders-Elsevier.

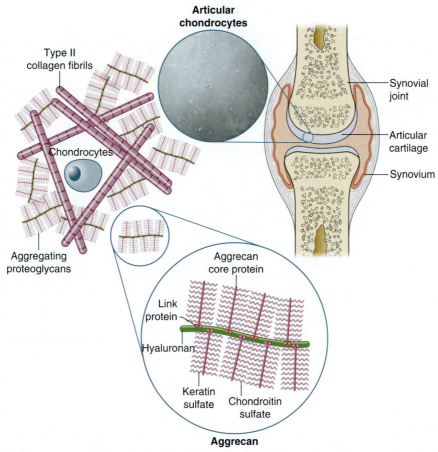

FIGURE 19-1 A schematic depiction of articular cartilage. The left panel shows the major components including chondrocytes, type II collagen fibrils, and aggregating proteoglycans (aggrecans). The aggrecan structure is shown in the bottom panel. (Reproduced with permission from McIlwraith C.W. (2013). Oral joint supplements in the management of osteoarthritis. In: Geor R.J., Harris P.A., Coenen M. (Eds.). Equine applied and clinical nutrition (pp. 549-557). Saunders-Elsevier.)

are neither nutrients nor pharmaceuticals by combining the words "nutrients" (nourishing food or food component) with "pharmaceuticals" (medical drug).[12] The nutraceutical category comprises a broad list of products including nutrients, dietary supplements, functional foods, and phytochemicals (including herbs) that are not recognized by the U.S. FDA as food or drugs and are intended for the treatment or prevention of disease. The difference between a feed and a nutraceutical is that a nutraceutical is unlikely to have an established nutritive value. Feeds are required to have nutritive value and are accountable, by labeling, for these values. OJSs fall between foods and drugs and have advantages over either because they are not required to list ingredients or nutrient profiles as required for feeds, and in many cases, intend to treat or prevent disease without first undergoing proper drug approval.[12]

A supplement was initially defined legally by the Federal Food, Drug and Cosmetic Act, but this was amended in 1994 by the Dietary Supplement Health Education Act (DSHEA). Technically, the DSHEA only covers human products and defines a dietary supplement as a product intended to

supplement the diet and contains at least one or more of the following: a vitamin; a mineral; an herb or other botanical; an amino acid; a dietary substance for use to supplement the diet by increasing intakes; or a concentrate, metabolite, constituent, extract, or combination of any of the previously mentioned ingredients.[13] The jurisdiction of veterinary products is primarily the responsibility of the North American Veterinary Nutraceutical Council (NAVNC), which was formed in 1996 to promote and enhance the further quality, safety, and long-term effectiveness of nutraceuticals used in veterinary medicine.[8] The NAVNC has defined a veterinary nutraceutical as a "non-drug substance that is produced in a purified or extracted form and administered orally to provide agents required for normal bone and body structure and function with the intent of improving the health and well-being of animals."[14]

The DSHEA allows manufacturers to make claims with regard to health, structure, function, and nutrient content of a nutraceutical. The Center for Veterinary Medicine allows products to be marketed as nutraceuticals provided they do not claim to treat, cure, or mitigate disease[8]; hence, the

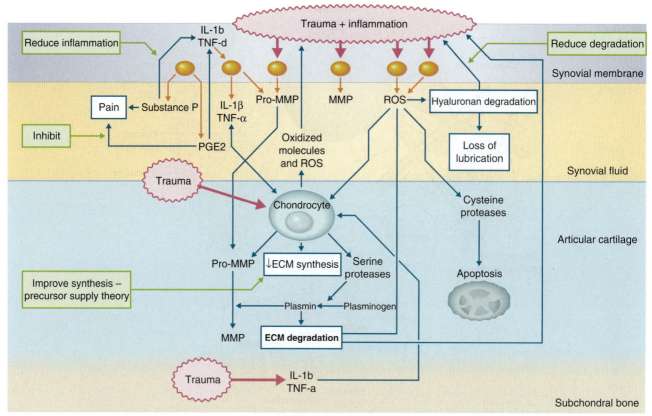

FIGURE 19-2 A schematic outlining the mechanisms for development of osteoarthritis and the possible mechanisms of action for oral joint supplements in mitigating these processes. (Reproduced with permission from McIlwraith C.W. (2013). Oral joint supplements in the management of osteoarthritis. In: Geor R.J., Harris P.A., Coenen M. (Eds.). Equine applied and clinical nutrition (pp. 549-557). Saunders-Elsevier.)

common practice in advertising of improving joint "health." The FDA perceives veterinary nutraceuticals as unapproved drugs, even though they are not labeled or marketed as drugs. The FDA does not regulate these products unless they become unsafe or have labels that claim a drug use; therefore, there is no requirement to prove safety or efficacy of a nutraceutical. It is the author's opinion that there are two principal issues involved with this regulation: (1) The issue is sufficiently low on the FDA radar screen that there is very little attention paid to it and (2) there is hardly an incentive for a nutraceutical manufacturer to prove efficacy, as such research costs money and a negative result could hurt sales.[13]

Manufacturers do not have to register themselves or their supplements with the FDA. In general a manufacturer has to comply with the FDA Ingredient Recognition Program, which entails applying for complete ingredient definitions as described by not-for-profit organization of state and federal feed regulators, the Association of American Feed Control Officials.[13] There are no requirements of Good Manufacturing Practices for manufacturers to guarantee high-quality and batch-to-batch consistency,[11] and because there is no postproduction monitoring of veterinary nutritional supplements, a myriad of poor-quality supplements are available.[15]

TYPES OF ORAL JOINT SUPPLEMENTS

The majority of joint supplements include glucosamine (GU) and/or chondroitin sulfate (CS) along with other added ingredients. Historically, the first products available for the horse included a CS product from bovine trachea and a complex of glycosaminoglycans and other nutrients from the sea mussel *Perna canaliculus*. GU is an amino monosaccharide; it is the principal component of O-linked and N-linked glycosaminoglycans and is produced in the body by the addition of amino groups to glucose. This molecule is subsequently acetylated to acetyl GU. Hyaluronan (HA), keratan sulfate, and heparan sulfate are composed in part of repeating units of acetyl GU. CS consists of alternating disaccharide units of glucuronic acid and sulfated *N*-acetyl galactosamine molecules and is a principal glycosaminoglycan of aggregating proteoglycan (aggrecan).

Many OJSs have GU and CS as principal components. They may contain additional ingredients including manganese, vitamin C, hyaluronan (hyaluronic acid or HA), polyunsaturated fatty acids (PUFAs), rare earth mineral supplements, unsaponified avocado soy (ASU), extract of green-lipped mussel *(Perna canaliculus),* cetylmyristoleate, methylsulfonylmethane, and various herbs. With the exception of the latter two (which have no good equine documentation available), these various products will be discussed below.

Glucosamine and/or Chondroitin Sulfate
Mechanisms of Action and In Vitro Studies

In vitro studies have investigated the effects of GU and CS, individually or in combination, but of course, differ greatly in the source of products, as well as dosages used, study conditions, and responses measured.[16] GU and/or CS are thought to counteract cartilage degradation[17-28] by inhibiting degradative enzymes such as collagenase and aggrecanase[22,24,26,29,30] and intermediary mediators such as nitric oxide, PGE2, and nuclear factor kappa B.[18,19,24,26,28,31-36] Synthesis of extracellular matrix components is thought to be stimulated in the presence of GU and/or CS[23,27,31,37-39] by provision of substrate, which may be deficient through dilution or hypermetabolic states[39]; upregulation of gene expression[20,40]; stimulation of cellular receptors and cellular signaling mechanisms, such as CD44 involved in positive feedback[31,41,42]; and inhibition of negative intermediary messengers, such as nuclear factor kappa B, nitric oxide, and PGE2.[18,19,24,26,34,35-37]

The precursor supply theory is the most popular explanation regarding the apparent beneficial effects of GU in OA.[43] In this theory, GU supplies excess basic building blocks for the synthesis of cartilage glycosaminoglycans (GAG)[18,44,45] and/or bypasses rate-limiting steps in GAG synthesis.[8,18] In addition, these structure-modifying agents appear to counteract inflammation primarily through their inhibition of intermediate messengers, such as nuclear factor kappa B, nitric oxide, and PGE2,[18,19,24,26,28,31,34-36] that mediate inflammatory responses, in addition to their previously described antianabolic and procatabolic effects. However, these structure-modifying agents have not been found to directly inhibit cyclooxygenase (COX) enzymes, in contrast to many antiarthritic medications.[46] CS has also been shown to affect cell-based inflammatory events by inhibiting chemotaxis, reducing phagocytosis and lysozyme release, and protecting cell membranes from free radical injury.[47]

Dosages used to determine the effects of GU and CS on cartilage metabolism in in vitro studies have varied from physiologic (μg/mL) to pharmacologic (mg/mL) concentrations.[16] Depending on the study, beneficial effects have been reported for dosages as low as 10 μg/mL to as high as 25 mg/mL. Some studies have compared combination treatments to GU or CS alone.[20,21,24,27] Combinations of GU and CS were considered to be the most effective in these studies,[20,21,24,27] and although synergy was suggested by some authors,[21] the effect tended to be additive and not synergistic.[16]

The effects of varying doses of GU and CS alone and in combination on cartilage metabolism in normal and recombinant IL-1α-conditioned equine articular cartilage have been evaluated in the author's laboratory using equine cartilage explants.[27] Articular cartilage explants were allocated randomly to treatment with 4 doses of GU, CS, or GU + CS in the absence of IL-1 (normal explants) and in the presence of 40 mg/mL recombinant IL-1α (Gibco-Light Technologies) (IL-1-conditioned explants). The patented joint supplements used were SCHG49GU and TRH122 low-molecular-weight sodium (Nutramax Laboratories). The treatment groups investigated for both normal and IL-1-conditioned explants were: treatment without GU or CS; four GU concentrations, 12.5, 25, 125, and 250 μg/mL; four CS concentrations, 12.5, 25, 125, and 250 μg/mL; and four GU + CS concentrations 12.5, 25, 125, and 250 μg/mL each of GU and CS (in a 1:1 ratio by concentration). There was no significant negative effect of GU, CS, or GU + CS on normal cartilage explant metabolism. In normal (no IL-1) explants, the most substantial effects observed with the GU, CS, and GU + CS treatments were in reducing GAG degradation, without evidence for an advantage of GU + CS versus GU or CS alone. On the other hand, the highest dosage of GU + CS was more effective than all other treatments in reducing GAG degradation in IL-1-conditioned explants. The ability of GU and CS to protect against cartilage matrix degradation in osteoarthritic and stimulated chondrocytes in cartilage explants has been observed in other in vitro studies.[17-24,32] The higher doses of test ingredients (125 and 250 μg/mL) tended to be more effective than the lower doses,[27] and these dosage ranges were within the ranges of other in vitro studies. High dosages of GU such as 6.5 and 25 mg/mL have been shown to have detrimental effects on cartilage metabolism and chondrocyte viability in studies using bovine articular cartilage explants.[48]

In summary, purported mechanisms explaining the role for GU in OA are (1) provision of substrate for synthesis of cartilage glycosaminoglycans (precursor supply theory) and (2) mediation of inflammatory responses. CS is thought to counteract cartilage inflammatory responses. In addition, there is in vitro evidence that GU and CS protect against cartilage matrix degradation.

Bioavailability and Pharmacokinetics

The obvious flaw with in vitro studies of oral OJSs is that products are tested before undergoing any modification through digestion and absorption. In a relatively recent study a simulated digestion protocol with ultrafiltration was applied before testing the potential antiinflammatory and chondroprotective properties of New Zealand green-lipped mussel, abalone, and shark cartilage.[49] The authors showed that shark cartilage and New Zealand green-lipped mussel significantly inhibited IL-1-induced PGE2 synthesis and IL-1-induced GAG release and abalone was an effective inhibitor of IL-1 induced NO production. This model proved useful for evaluating dietary nutraceuticals in vitro when the components were predigested before testing.

The efficacy of orally administered GU and/or CS depends on the absorption of an oral dose to a sufficient extent to attain therapeutic blood and tissue levels. Studies have also suggested that GU and CS exhibit a high degree of trophism for articular cartilage,[33,47] which means that blood levels may not equate to tissue levels. However, in the absence of good in vivo efficacy studies in the horse, oral bioavailability provides an important means of extrapolating results from in vitro studies to the in vivo setting by providing some prediction of fluid and tissue concentrations for GU and CS after oral dosing.

In horses, the oral absorption of 8.0- and 16.9-kDa molecular weight CS was compared because in vitro studies suggested that the molecular weight of CS was negatively associated with its permeability across the gastrointestinal tract.[50] The oral bioavailability of 8.0-kDa CS was 32% versus 22% with 16.9-kDa CS.[51,52] The oral bioavailability of GU hydrochloride in horses was found to be 2.5% to 5.9% with a large volume of distribution, which indicates very poor absorption from the intestinal tract, but extensive tissue uptake.[44,52] Although serum levels of 4.5 to 6.5 μg/mL for disaccharide fractions of CS[51,52] and 10.6 μg/mL for GU[52] were attained, the dose was 5 to 10 times the typical labeled dose of GU to achieve these levels. Laverty et al. showed that maximum levels of GU serum reached 6 μM (about 1 μg/mL) in the serum and about 0.3 to 0.7 μM in the synovial fluid after clinically suggested doses of GU hydrochloride were administered orally.[44] GU concentrations in the synovial fluid also appeared to be relatively stable over time (remaining elevated at 0.1 to 0.7 μM 12 hours after dosing) in that study[44] and Dechant and Baxter suggested that this could indicate minimal use of GU by articular tissues.[16] Based on these bioavailability studies, it could be concluded that CS has increased potential for efficacy because of greater oral absorption.[51,52] However, the CS bioavailability study could be disputed because the assays measured disaccharide fractions of CS, which are not known to be biologically active.[16]

Claims have been made by suppliers and medical authorities that GU sulfate is superior to GU hydrochloride, but this rationale has been questioned.[53] In a study of eight female horses, GU sulfate and GU hydrochloride were administered at doses of 20 mg/kg by either intravenous or nasogastric intubation and plasma samples were collected. Glucosamine was assayed by liquid chromatography electrospray ionization-tandem mass spectrometry (LCESI/MS/MS). Synovial fluid concentrations of GU were significantly higher at 1 and 6 hours following oral treatment with GU sulfate versus GU hydrochloride. Twelve hours following oral administration, GU levels in the plasma and the synovial fluid were still significantly higher than baseline GU sulfate preparation but not for the hydrochloride preparation. The conclusion was that higher synovial fluid concentrations of GU were achieved with GU sulfate, but whether or not this difference translated into a therapeutic effect on the joint tissues remains to be elucidated.[54] In a follow-up study, the same research group demonstrated that joint inflammation (induced with *Escherichia coli* lipopolysaccharide) increases GU levels obtained in synovial fluid following oral administration of GU hydrochloride up to fourfold higher than in clinically normal joints, suggesting the possibility of an enhanced effect (as synovitis is important in the pathobiology of equine OA).[55] On the other hand, the maximal GU levels attainable in the synovial fluid in the presence of inflammation based on these studies will likely be in the range of 1 to 18 μM for both horses and humans, and most in vitro studies showing benefits with GU used considerably higher concentrations.[55]

In summary, there is some controversy over which substances should be measured in studies on the bioavailability and pharmacokinetics of GU and CS. In general, the bioavailability of GU and CS appears to be low. In addition, molecular size of active ingredient, dose, and joint inflammatory status may influence delivery to the target site of action.

Clinical Trials and Experimental Studies
Horses
Clinical trials and in vivo experimental studies in horses are limited and results are variable. This was highlighted in a recent review of 15 in vivo studies in the equine literature in which the authors signaled an encouraging trend: manufacturers of these products are investing in research, but most do not meet a quality standard that provided sufficient confidence in the results reported.[56] Consequently, the overall level of evidence for in vivo demonstration of efficacy is weak. Administration of Cosequin® in horses with OA in the distal interphalangeal, metacarpophalangeal, tarsometatarsal, or carpal joints resulted in improvement in lameness grade, flexion test grade, and stride length within 2 weeks; however, no further improvement in lameness grade and no significant changes in other variables were seen after 4 weeks.[57] Twenty-five horses were in the study and there was no placebo group. It has been pointed out by others that the lack of continued improvement may be attributable to the return of most of the horses to exercise and competition after an initial 2 weeks of treatment. Return to previously obtainable performance levels and continuation in a competition career are necessary for a treatment to be considered successful, as well as fulfilling the expectation of the owners of the affected horses.[58]

Results of other studies using Cosequin have reported no beneficial effects in a chemically induced model of OA,[59] but it should be recognized that the model is hardly representative of clinical OA. Administration of another product containing GU, glutamic acid, glycine, and glucuronic acid (Chondrosulf) showed results in improvement in vertical ground reaction force and reduction of gait asymmetry in cases of OA of the distal intertarsal or tarsometatarsal joints. In another clinical study, an oral supplement containing 1.2 g GU sodium sulfate, 1.2 g GU potassium sulfate, 1.2 g GU hydrochloride, 300 mg N-acetyl-D-GU, and 1.2 g of CS per dose (together with 300 mg of ascorbate and 100 mg of manganese) was given for 2 years to 8 horses.[60] The frequency of distal tarsal joint injection decreased from a mean of 1.7 injections/year before supplementation to 0.85 injections/year with supplementation; there was also a notable drop in the injection frequency after 5 to 8 months of supplementation, which was seen as an indication of efficacy.[60] However, this study was neither controlled nor blinded and relied on the subjective evaluation of lameness (diagnosis of distal tarsal pain/tarsitis by flexion palpation, radiographic, and intraarticular anesthesia) by a single veterinarian and trainer.

A recent placebo-controlled study investigating the effect of 3 months of oral supplementation with a compound containing GU, CS, and methyl sulfonyl methane in a group of geriatric horses (age 29 ± 4 years) used kinematic outcome criteria (primary: stride length; secondary: carpal flexion, fore fetlock extension, and tarsal range of motion). No effect of the supplement on these gait parameters could be demonstrated, leading to the conclusion that the use of a GU/CS/methyl sulfonyl methane supplement to improve stiff gait in geriatric horses could not be supported because of the lack of a sizeable effect.[61]

Humans

Numerous clinical studies have been done with human OA patients. The Glucosamine/chondroitin Arthritis Intervention Trial (GAIT) is the best known and was a multicenter trial that assigned 1583 patients to randomly receive 1500 mg of GU, 1200 mg of CS, both GU and CS, 200 mg of celecoxib (Celebrex®), or placebo for 24 weeks. Patients randomized to celecoxib had significant improvement in knee pain compared with those randomized to placebo. No statistically significant improvement in knee pain versus placebo was seen among patients randomized to dietary supplements, although a subset of patients with moderate to severe knee pain at entry who received the combination of GU and CS seemed to experience some improvement and patients taking CS were found to have statistically significant decrease in knee joint swelling.[62] A major limitation of the study noted by the authors was the high rate of response to placebo (60%) and the relatively mild degree of OA among the participants. A posthoc analysis was then undertaken to further assess the observation that patients receiving CS compared with patients who received placebo had improvement in joint swelling.[63] The results of this analysis suggested that patients with Kellgren and Lawrence grade II radiographic changes were substantially more responsive to CS than those with Kellgren and Lawrence grade III changes. Also, improvement was more likely to occur in the CS-treated patients with lower WOMAC (Western Ontario and McMaster Universities Arthritis Index) Function and Stiffness Scores, and a numerical trend was seen also in patients with lower WOMAC Pain Scores.

In another study as part of the GAIT study, progressive loss of joint space width (JSW) in patients with knee OA who satisfied radiographic criteria (Kellgren/Lawrence grade II or III and JSW of at least 2 mm at baseline) was studied. The mean JSW loss at 2 years in knees with OA in the placebo group, adjusted for design and clinical factors, was 0.166 mm. No statistically significant difference in mean JSW loss was observed in any treatment group versus the placebo group. There was a trend towards improvement in the grade II knees. The authors concluded that the power of the study was diminished by the limited sample size, variance of JSW treatment, and smaller than expected loss of JSW.[64]

Wandel and colleagues performed a metaanalysis of studies examining the effect of GU, CS, or both on joint pain and on radiologic progression of disease in OA of the hip or knee.[65] Ten trials involving a total of 3803 patients were included. It was concluded that, compared with placebo, GU, CS, and their combination do not reduce joint pain or have an impact on narrowing of joint space, and the authors recommended that use of GU and CS for treatment of hip or knee OA should be discouraged.

Valid conclusions regarding the efficacy of OJSs in horses are not possible because of a lack of well-designed studies.

Metaanalysis of data from human studies indicates that GU, CS, or GU/CS does not reduce joint pain or other clinical signs of OA.

Despite this, some more positive studies have been published recently. In a review article in 2013 it was reported that CS exerts an in vitro beneficial effect on the metabolism of different cell lines including chondrocytes, synoviocytes, and cells from the subchondral bone, all involved in OA, and clinical trials have reported a beneficial effect on pain and function.[66] In addition, the structure-modifying effects of CS were analyzed in recent metaanalyses. A small but significant reduction in the rate of decline in joint space has been demonstrated in knee OA. The authors also pointed out that the CS quality of several nutraceuticals was poor and it is critical that pharmaceutical-grade CS is used rather than food supplements in the treatment of OA.[66]

More recently it has been reported that there is a convergent body of evidence that GU sulfate given at a daily oral dose of 1500 mg is able to significantly reduce the symptoms of OA in people. There are two independent studies showing a reduction in joint space narrowing in patients with mild to moderate knee OA, and this translates into a 50% reduction in the incidence of OA-related surgery of the lower limbs during a 5-year period following the withdrawal of treatment.[67] Specifically, 106 patients on placebo had a mean joint space loss after 3 years of -0.31 mm (95% confidence interval [CI] -0.48 to -0.13); there was no significant joint space loss in the 106 patients on GU sulfate (-0.06 mm; -0.22 to 0.09).[68] In a second study, in patients with mild to moderate OA and average JSWs of slightly less than 4 mm, progressive joint space narrowing with placebo was -0.19 mm (95% CI -0.29 to -0.09 mm); there was no change in the GU sulfate-treated group (0.04 mm; 95% CI -0.06 to 0.14) ($P = 0.001$).[69]

Despite this, Towheed et al. recently updated the Cochrane Review of available data with the intent of investigating what might predicate differences in GU trial results.[70] An analysis restricted to the eight studies that reported adequate allocation concealment showed no benefit of GU for pain and WOMAC function. Collectively, however, the pooled data from 20 eligible studies favored GU over placebo with a 28% improvement in pain relief and a 21% improvement in function according to the Lequesne index.[70] It should be noted that there are a number of positive studies since publication of this study. There was also a difference in the quality of GU preparations, and specific higher quality GU had superior results.[71] In a clinical review of CS in OA, it was classified as a symptomatic, slow-acting drug for the treatment of OA (SYSADOA), and it was noted that two pivotal studies provided evidence that oral CS does have structure-modifying effects in knee OA patients.[72]

Positive effects have also been seen with ASUs in clinical OA.[73]

Product Quality and Purity

Because of a lack of regulation and oversight, OJS product quality can vary considerably. One study compared labeled claims with laboratory analysis for GU and CS content and found that the measured composition varied significantly (0% to 115% from labeled claims).[50] Oke et al. analyzed 23 commercially available equine OJSs containing GU, as well as 1 positive (GU hydrochloride) and 3 negative controls.[15] The range of GU free base compared to the amount expected in each product based on the label claim was 0% to 221.2% with a median of 99.0% and 106%, respectively. Of the 23 products included in the study, 9 (39.1%) contained less GU than claimed by the manufacturer and 4 (17.4%) had less than 30% of the expected amount of GU.[15] Of the 23 products, only 5 OJSs achieved the recommended dosage (approximately 10 g/GU/day) suggested by the study of Laverty et al.[44]

Sasha's Blend

Sasha's Blend (New Zealand green-lipped mussel, shark cartilage, abalone, and *Biota orientalis* lipid extract) is a proprietary mixture of bioactive lipids obtained from New Zealand green-lipped mussel *(Perna canaliculus),* abalone *(Haliotis* sp.), shark cartilage *(Galeorhinus galeus),* and a lipid extract from *Biota orientalis* (Sasha's EQ Powder). Raw ingredients are manufactured in New Zealand with the four constituents artificially digested in vitro, and an extract of each simulated digest has been evaluated by use of a cartilage explant model of inflammation.[49] Each constituent has been shown to exert unique effects on the formation of rh-IL-1β-induced PGE2, GAG, and chondrocyte viability in equine cartilage explants. More recently the product has been tested in 22 healthy horses. Twelve horses were fed 0, 15, 45, or 75 g of Sasha's Equine Powder (SEQ) (3 horses per treatment) daily for 84 days. Ten other horses received 0 or 15 g of SEQ per day (5 horses per treatment) for 29 days (beginning day −14). One middle carpal joint in each horse was injected twice with IL-1β (10 and 100 ng on day 0 and 1, respectively) and the contralateral joint similarly injected with saline (0.9% NaCl solution). In this study, administration of the SEQ (up to 75 g/day) to horses for 84 days did not induce any adverse effects.[74] Synovial fluid PGE2, GAG, protein concentration, and leukocyte count increased after intraarticular injection of IL-1β (versus saline injection) in horses that received no SEQ, but in horses that were fed SEQ intraarticular IL-1β injections did not induce significant increases in synovial fluid PGE2 and GAG concentrations. These results suggested that SEQ could be useful in preventing inflammation associated with synovitis and OA in horses.

Hyaluronan (Hyaluronic Acid)

Intraarticular HA has been used in the horse for many years.[75] Oral HA formulated for the horse has been available for about 8 years, and anecdotal reports have suggested that its use has been effective in treating lameness associated with synovial effusion and OA. Hyaluronan has been shown to be absorbed by rats and beagles when administered orally,[76] but there are no published data from equine studies. Other GAG products such as chondroitin, dermatan, and heparan sulfates have also been shown to be absorbed orally in rats and man.[77-80]

A double-blind controlled study has been reported in 48 yearlings, which were operated arthroscopically for unilateral or bilateral osteochondritis dissecans of the tarsus (yearlings were included only if they had mild or no synovial effusion presurgery).[81] Twenty-four of the yearlings (27 joints) were treated with 100 mg of HA orally for 30 days postoperatively and 24 (30 joints) with placebo orally for 30 days. Thirty days after arthroscopic surgery, a blinded examiner scored the effusion of the dorsomedial tarsocrural joint individually using a scale of 0 to 5 (0 = no effusion, 1 = barely palpable, 2 = palpable effusion [without plantar effusion], 3 = golf ball size effusion with plantar effusion, 4 = tennis ball size effusion with plantar effusion, 5 = greater than tennis ball size effusion with plantar effusion). The mean 30-day effusion score of the HA-treated group (27 joints) was 0.7 although that of the placebo group (30 joints) was 2.05 ($P \leq 0.0001$). Similar results were noted when comparing active treatment versus placebo for each lesion location, as well as for lesion size. This author feels the results speak for themselves; however, the mechanism of action is certainly less obvious. In a recently conducted survey using the Colorado State University (CSU) osteochondral fragment model, there was a significant reduction in the PGE2 levels of the OA joints in horses treated with oral HA compared with both the OA joints of the placebo-treated horses (D.D. Frisbie, C.W. McIlwraith, and C. Kawcak unpublished data).

Extract of Green-lipped Mussel *(Perna canaliculus)*

As mentioned previously, one of the first products made available for the horse was a complex of glycosaminoglycans and other nutrients from the sea mussel *Perna canaliculus.* Since then clinical trials have demonstrated the efficacy of lyophilized products from *Perna canaliculus* (LPPC) in treating osteoarthritic conditions in man and dogs[82-84] and more recently in horses.[85] In vitro data show that LPPC has a range of antiinflammatory activities including inhibition of tumor necrosis factor-α, COX-2 expression, PGE2, phospholipase A2 (PLA2), oxygen radical absorbance capacity (ORAC), antioxidant capacity, lipolytic, and fibrinolytic activities.[86,87]

A randomized, double-blind, placebo-controlled study on the efficacy of a unique extract of green-lipped mussel *(Perna canaliculus)* in horses with chronic fetlock lameness attributed to OA was recently reported. This study was performed in New Zealand and data were analyzed from 26 horses with primary fetlock lameness in a multicenter trial. The study design was a partial crossover with a washout period and consisted of 19 horses treated with LPPC and 20 with placebo. Horses were dosed orally with 25 mg/kg/day LPPC or placebo for 56 days. Efficacy was evaluated by clinical assessment of lameness, passive flexion, pain, swelling, and heat in the affected joint.[85] Relationships between variables were analyzed using an ordinal logistic model with random effects for horse and X treatment according to a modified-intention-to-treat analysis. Clinical evaluation of horses with a fetlock lameness treated with LPPC showed a significant reduction in severity of lameness ($P < 0.001$), improved response to joint flexion ($P < 0.001$) and reduced joint pain ($P = 0.014$) when compared with horses treated with placebo. It was concluded that LPPC significantly alleviated the severity of lameness and joint pain and improved response to joint flexion in horses with lameness attributable to OA in the fetlock.

Avocado Soy Unsaponified

ASU extracts are produced by extracting the oils from avocados and soybeans, collecting the unsaponifiable fractions (i.e., the oil that remains after hydrolysis and does not form soaps) and combining these in various ratios. This product has been reported to be beneficial in randomized, placebo-controlled human trials.[88-90] In vitro studies have displayed anabolic, anticatabolic, and antiinflammatory effects on human chondrocytes. ASU increased the basal synthesis of aggrecan and reversed the IL-1β-induced reduction of aggrecan synthesis by human chondrocytes in alginate beads.[91] It also decreased the spontaneous and IL-1β-induced production of matrix metalloproteinase (MMP)-3, IL-6 and -8, and PGE2, although it weakly reversed the IL-1-induced inhibition of tissue inhibitor of metalloproteinase-1 TIMP-1 production.[91,92]

In a blinded, placebo-controlled study using the CSU osteochondral chip fragment model, horses were randomly assigned to two groups with the ASU extract group receiving the supplement mixed with molasses although the placebo group only received molasses from days 0 to 70. The ASU supplementation did not have a significant effect on pain or lameness, but there was a significant reduction in the degree of macroscopic cartilage erosion and synovial hemorrhage scores in the ASU- versus placebo-treated joints, as well as a significant decrease in intimal hyperplasia (inflammation) in the synovial membrane. There was also a decrease in the cartilage disease score.[93] A significant decrease in cartilage disease indicates that this product could be classified as a disease-modifying osteoarthritic drug. Although the improvements were modest, they were more significant than those seen with other products including parenteral polysulfated GAG, intravenous HA, and oral HA products tested using the same model of equine OA, at least at the level of articular cartilage change. Unfortunately, the ASU extract product used in the CSU equine study cannot be made available in the U.S. At present the only ASU product available in North America is sold in combination with GU and CS (Cosequin ASU™). Considerable in vitro work has been done with this product, but, as yet, no in vivo efficacy has been reported.

Polyunsaturated Fatty Acids

Polyunsaturated fatty acids (PUFAs), at sufficiently high intakes as found in oily fish and fish oils, decrease production of inflammatory cytokines, arachidonic acid-derived eicosanoids (prostaglandins, thromboxanes, leukotrienes, and other oxidized derivatives), and other inflammatory agents such as reactive oxygen species and adhesion molecules.[94] Omega-3 (n-3) PUFAs contain α-linolenic acid that is desaturated in the body to produce eicosapentaenoic acid and docosahexaenoic acid analogs of arachidonic acid.[8] There is some evidence that n-3 PUFA can be beneficial in humans[95] and dogs[96,97] with OA, and in vitro studies have demonstrated positive outcomes.[98,99] An in vivo study in a spontaneous

guinea pig model showed that dietary n-3 PUFAs reduced disease in OA-prone animals.[100]

Although there is currently no evidence of efficacy in the horse, the potential for usefulness of PUFAs in equine OA has led to it being incorporated into some OJSs.

Cetyl Myristoleate

Cetyl myristoleate (CM) is another fatty acid that is being used in equine joint supplements. CM is an ester of cis-9-tetradecenoic acid (myristoleic acid) and 1-hexadecanol (cetyl alcohol) and is a 14-carbon monounsaturated omega-5 fatty acid.[8] CM may act by inhibition of the 5-lipooxygenase pathway, which is responsible for the metabolism of leukotrienes, potent inflammatory mediators, from the arachidonic acid cascade.[101] Studies in adjuvant-induced arthritis and collagen-induced arthritis in rats have demonstrated that CM can confer protection and reduce severity of the disease, respectively.[102,103] A study in human knee OA has been reported where CM showed improvement in knee flexion and function.[104]

A product containing CM, GU hydrochloride, methylsulfonylmethane, and hydrolyzed collagen (Myristol™) was investigated in a blind, controlled clinical trial with 39 horses. Each horse was scored using American Association of Equine Practitioners (AAEP) guidelines for lameness, as well as a 0- to 10-cm visual analog scale (VAS) for lameness at walk, lameness at trot, response to joint flexion, lameness after flexion, and quality of life.[105] Horses were assessed on day 0, 14, 28, and 42 days after treatment. A responder was defined as improving 1 grade on the AAEP Lameness Scale or 2 cm on the VAS. The Myristol treatment group improved significantly more than the placebo group in AAEP lameness score, lameness at walk, response to joint flexion, lameness after flexion, and quality of life.

SUMMARY

Use of OJSs in horses is prevalent worldwide. Although data from in vitro studies suggest mitigation of joint disease, evidence regarding the in vivo efficacy of OJSs is still limited, in part because of a lack of well-designed clinical trials. However, more recently, results from randomized, placebo controlled studies have begun to emerge.[84]

REFERENCES

1. Clegg P, Booth R. Drugs used to treat osteoarthritis in the horse. *Practice*. 2000;22:594–603.
2. Caron JP, Genovese RL. Principals and practices of joint disease treatment. In: Ross MW, Dyson S, eds. *Diagnosis and management of lameness in the horse*. Philadelphia, PA: Saunders; 2003:746–764.
3. Helmick CG, Felson DT, Lawrence RC, et al. For the National Arthritis Data Workgroup. Estimates for the prevalence of arthritis and other rheumatic diseases on the United States. Part I. *Arthritis Rheum*. 2008;58(1):15–25.
4. Lawrence RC, Felson DT, Helmick CG, et al. For the National Arthritis Data Workgroup. Estimates for the prevalence of arthritis and other rheumatic diseases on the United States. Part II. *Arthritis Rheum*. 2008;58(1):26–35.

5. McIlwraith CW. General pathobiology of the joint in response to injury. In: McIlwraith CW, Trotter GW, eds. *Joint disease in the horse*. Philadelphia, PA: Saunders; 1996:40–70.

6. McIlwraith CW. From arthroscopy to gene therapy—30 years of looking in joints. Frank Milne Lecture. *Proc Am Assoc Equine Pract*. 2005;51:65–113.

7. American Veterinary Medical Association. US Pet Ownership and Demographic Sourcebook. Center for info. 2012. management staff.

8. Trumble TN. The use of nutraceuticals for osteoarthritis in horses. *North Am Vet Clin Equine Pract*. 2005;21(3):575–597.

9. Packaged Facts, Publishing Division of MarketResearch.com, Inc; February 2008. www.packagedfacts.com/pet-supplements-market-c1641

10. Burk AO, Williams CA. Feeding management practices and supplement use in top-level event horses. *Comp Exercise Physiol*. 2008;5(2):5–93.

11. Oke SL, McIlwraith CW. Review of the potential indications and contraindications for equine oral health supplements. *Proc Am Assoc Equine Pract*. 2008;54:261–267.

12. Duren S. Oral joint supplements. Panacea or expensive fad? *Adv Equine Nutr*. 2005;3:77–83.

13. McIlwraith CW. Licensed medications, 'generic' medications, compounding and nutraceuticals—what is scientifically validated, where do we encounter scientific mistruth, where are we legally? *Proc Am Assoc Equine Pract*. 2004;50:459–475.

14. Booth DM. Balancing fact and fiction of novel ingredients: definitions, regulations and evaluations. *Vet Clin North Am Pract*. 2004;34(1):7–38.

15. Oke SL, Aghazadeh-Habashi A, Weese JS, et al. Evaluation of glucosamine levels in commercial equine oral supplements for joints. *Equine Vet J*. 2006;38(1):93–95.

16. Dechant JE, Baxter GM. Glucosamine and chondroitin sulfate as structure modifying agents in horses. *Equine Vet Educ*. 2007;19(2):90–96.

17. Sandy JD, Garnett D, Thompson V, et al. Chondrocyte-mediated catabolism of aggrecan: aggrecanase dependent cleavage induced by interleukin-l or retinoic acid can be inhibited by glucosamine. *Biochem J*. 1998;335(Pt 1):59–66.

18. Fenton JJ, Chlebek-Brown KA, Peters TL, et al. Glucosamine HCl reduces equine articular degeneration in explant cultures. *Osteoarthritis Cartilage*. 2000;8(4):258–265.

19. Fenton JJ, Chlebek-Brown KA, Caron JP, et al. Effect of glucosamine on interleukin-1-conditioned articular cartilage. *Equine Vet J Suppl*. 2002;34:219–223.

20. Grande D, O'Grady C, Garone E, et al. Chondroprotective and gene expression effects of nutritional supplements on articular cartilage. *Osteoarthritis Cartilage*. 2000;8(Suppl B):534–535.

21. Lippiello L, Woodward J, Karpman R, et al. In vivo chondroprotection and metabolic synergy of glucosamine and chondroitin sulfate. *Clin Orthop Rel Res*. 2000;381:229–240.

22. Lippiello L, Sung Han M, Henderson T. Protective effect of the chondroprotective agent Cosequin DS on bovine articular cartilage exposed in vitro to non-steroidal anti-inflammatory agents. *Vet Ther*. 2002;3(2):128–135.

23. Nerucci E, Fioravanti A, Cicero MR, et al. Effects of chondroitin sulfate and interleukin-l, on human chondrocyte cultures exposed to pressurization: a biochemical and morphological study. *Osteoarthritis Cartilage*. 2001;8(4):279–287.

24. Orth MW, Peters TL, Hawkins JL. Inhibition of articular cartilage degradation by glucosamine-HCl and chondroitin sulfate. *Equine Vet J Suppl*. 2002;34:224–229.

25. Ilic MZ, Martinac B, Handley CJ. Effects of long-term exposure to glucosamine and mannosamine on aggrecan degradation in articular cartilage. *Osteoarthritis Cartilage*. 2003;11(8):613–622.

26. Mello DM, Nielson BD, Peters TL, et al. Comparison of inhibitory effects of glucosamine and mannosamine on bovine articular cartilage degeneration in vitro. *Am J Vet Res*. 2004;65:1440–1445.

27. Dechant JE, Baxter GM, Frisbie DD, et al. Effects of glucosamine hydrochloride and chondroitin sulfate, alone an in combination, on normal and interleukin-l conditioned equine articular cartilage explant metabolism. *Equine Vet J*. 2005;37(3):227–231.

28. Neil KM, Orth MW, Coussens PM, et al. Effects of glucosamine and chondroitin sulfate on mediators of osteoarthritis in cultured equine chondrocytes stimulated by use of recombinant equine interleukin-l. *Am J Vet Res*. 2005:1861–1869.

29. Wright IM. Oral supplements in the treatment and prevention of joint diseases: a review of their potential application to the horse. *Equine Vet Educ*. 2001;13(3):135–139.

30. Chan P-S, Caron JP, Orth MW. Effect of glucosamine and chondroitin sulfate on regulation of gene expression of proteolytic enzymes and their inhibitors in interleukin-1-challenged bovine articular cartilage explants. *Am J Vet Res*. 2005;66(11):1870–1876.

31. Bassleer CT, Combal JP, Bougaret S, et al. Effects of chondroitin sulfate and interleukin-1 beta on human articular chondrocytes cultivated in clusters. *Osteoarthritis Cartilage*. 1998;6(3):196–204.

32. Byron CR, Orth MW, Venta PJ, et al. Influence of glucosamine on matrix metalloproteinase expression and activity in lipopolysaccharide-stimulated equine chondrocytes. *Am J Vet Res*. 2003;64(6):666–671.

33. Dodge GR, Regatte RR, Hall JO. The fate of oral glucosamine traced by BC-labeling in the dog. *Osteoarthritis Cartilage*. 2005;9(Suppl B):541.

34. Largo R, Alvarez-Soria MA, Diez-Ortego I, et al. Glucosamine inhibits IL-1-induced NFkB activation in human osteoarthritic chondrocytes. *Osteoarthritis Cartilage*. 2003;11(4):290–298.

35. Nakamura H, Shibakawa A, Tanaka M, et al. Effects of glucosamine hydrochloride on the production of prostaglandin E2, nitric oxide and metalloproteinases by chondrocytes and synoviocytes in osteoarthritis. *Clin Exp Rheumatol*. 2004;22:293–299.

36. Schlueter AE, Orth MW. Further studies on the ability of glucosamine and chondroitin sulfate to regulate catabolic mediators in vitro. *Equine Vet J*. 2004;36(7):634–636.

37. Bassleer CT, Rovati L, Franchimont P. Stimulation of proteoglycan production by glucosamine sulfate in chondrocytes isolated from human osteoarthritic articular cartilage in vitro. *Osteoarthritis Cartilage*. 1998;6(6):427–434.

38. Noyszewski EA, Wroblewski K, Dodge GR, et al. Preferential incorporation of glucosamine into the galactosamine moieties of chondroitin sulfates in articular cartilage explants. *Arthritis Rheum*. 2001;44(5):1089–1095.

39. Lippiello L. Glucosamine and chondroitin sulfate: biological response modifiers of chondrocytes under simulated conditions of joint stress. *Osteoarthritis Cartilage*. 2003;11(5):335–342.

40. Dodge GR, Jimenez SA. Glucosamine sulfate modulates the levels of aggrecan and matrix metalloproteinase-3 synthesized by cultured human osteoarthritis articular chondrocytes. *Osteoarthritis Cartilage*. 2003;11(6):424–432.

41. Esford LE, Maiti A, Bader SA. Analysis of CD44 interactions with hyaluronan in murine L cell fibroblasts deficient in glycosaminoglycan synthesis: a role for chondroitin sulfate. *J Cell Sci.* 1998;111(Pt 7):1021–1029.

42. Platt D. The role of disease-modifying agents glucosamine and chondroitin sulfate in the management of equine degenerative joint disease. *Equine Vet Educ.* 2001;13:206–215.

43. Oke SL, Weese JS. Review of glucosamine-containing oral joint supplements: are they effective in the horse? *Proc Am Assoc Equine Pract.* 2006;52:574–579.

44. Laverty S, Sandy JD, Celeste T, et al. Synovial fluid levels and serum pharmacokinetics in a large animal model following treatment with oral glycosaminoglycan at clinically relevant doses. *Arthritis Rheum.* 2005;52(1):181–191.

45. Kelly GS. The role of glucosamine sulfate and chondroitin sulfates in the treatment of degenerative joint disease. *Alt Med Rev.* 1998;3(1):27–39.

46. Seaver B, Smith JR. Inhibition of COX isoforms by nutraceuticals. *J Herb Pharmacother.* 2004;4(2):11–18.

47. Ronca E, Palmieri L, Panicucci P, et al. Anti-inflammatory activity of chondroitin sulfate. *Osteoarthritis Cartilage.* 1998;6(Suppl A):14–21.

48. De Mattei M, Plati A, Pasello M, et al. High doses of glucosamine HCl have detrimental effects on bovine articular cartilage explants cultured in vivo. *Osteoarthritis Cartilage.* 2002;10(10):816–825.

49. Pearson W, Orth MW, Karrow NA, et al. Anti-inflammatory and chondroprotective effects of nutraceuticals from Sasha's Blend in a cartilage explant model of inflammation. *Mol Nutr Food Res.* 2007;51(8):1020–1030.

50. Adebowale AO, Cox DS, Linang I, et al. Analysis of glucosamine and chondroitin sulfate content in marketed products and CACO-2 permeability of chondroitin sulfate raw materials. *J Am Nutraceuticals Assoc.* 2000;3:37–44.

51. Eddington ND, Du J, White N. Evidence of the oral absorption of chondroitin sulfate as determined by total disaccharide content after oral and intravenous administration to horses. *Proc Am Assoc Equine Pract.* 2001;47:326–328.

52. Du J, White N, Eddington ND. The bioavailability and pharmacokinetics of glucosamine hydrochloride and chondroitin sulfate after oral, intravenous single dose administration in the horse. *Bio Pharm Drug Dispos.* 2004;25(3):109–116.

53. Block JA, Oegema TR, Sande JT, et al. The effects of oral glucosamine on joint health: is a change of research approach needed? *Osteoarthritis Cartilage.* 2010;18(1):5–11.

54. Meulyzer M, Vachon P, Beaudry F. Comparison of pharmacokinetics of glucosamine in synovial fluid levels following administration of glucosamine sulfate or glucosamine hydrochloride. *Osteoarthritis Cartilage.* 2008;16(9):973–979.

55. Meulyzer M, Vachon P, Beaudry F, et al. Joint inflammation increases glucosamine levels attained in synovial fluid following oral administration of glucosamine hydrochloride. *Osteoarthritis Cartilage.* 2009;17(2):228–234.

56. Pearson W, Lindinger M. Low quality of evidence of glucosamine-based nutraceuticals in equine joint disease: review of in vivo studies. *Equine Vet J.* 2009;41(7):706–712.

57. Hanson R, Malley LR, Huff GK, et al. Oral treatment with a glucosamine-chondroitin sulfate compound for degenerative joint disease in horses: 25 cases. *Equine Pract.* 1997;19(9):16–22.

58. Neil KM, Caron JP, Orth MW. The role of glucosamine and chondroitin sulfate in treatment for and prevention of osteoarthritis in animals. *J Am Vet Med Assoc.* 2005;226(7):1079–1088.

59. White GW, Jones EW, Hamm J. The efficacy of orally administrated sulfated glycosaminoglycan in chemically induced equine synovitis and degenerative joint disease. *J Equine Vet Sci.* 1994;14(7):350–353.

60. Rogers MR. The effect of oral glucosamine and chondroitin sulfate supplementation on frequency of intra-articular therapy of the horse tarsus. *Intern J Appl Res Vet Med.* 2006;4(2):155–162.

61. Higler MH, Brommer H, L'Ami JJ, et al. The effects of three-month oral supplementation with a nutraceutical and exercise on the locomotor pattern of aged horses. *Equine Vet J.* 2013;46(5):611–617.

62. Clegg DO, Reda DJ, Harris CL, et al. Glucosamine, chondroitin sulfate, and the two in combination for painful knee arthritis. *N Engl J Med.* 2006;354(8):795–808.

63. Hochberg MC, Clegg DO. Potential effects of chondroitin sulfate on joint swelling: a GAIT report. *Osteoarthritis Cartilage.* 2008;16(Suppl 3):S22–S24.

64. Sawitzke ED, Shi H, Finco MF, et al. The effect of glucosamine and/or chondroitin sulfate on the progression of knee osteoarthritis. *Arthritis Rheum.* 2008;58(10):3183–3193.

65. Wandel S, Juni P, Tendal B, et al. Effects of glucosamine, chondroitin, or placebo in patients with osteoarthritis of hip or knee: network meta-analysis. *BMJ.* 2010;341: c4675.

66. Hochberg MC, Chevalier X, Henrotin Y, et al. Symptom and structure modification in osteoarthritis with pharmaceutical-grade chondroitin sulfate: what's the evidence? *Curr Med Res Opin.* 2013;29(3):259–267.

67. Reginster J-Y, Neuprez A, Lecart M-P, et al. Role of glucosamine in the treatment of osteoarthritis. *Rheum Int.* 2012;32(10):2959–2967.

68. Reginster J-Y, Deroisy R, Rovati LC, et al. Long-term effect of glucosamine sulfate in osteoarthritis progression: a randomized, placebo-controlled clinical trial. *Lancet.* 2001;357(9252):251–256.

69. Pavelka K, Gatterova J, Olejarova O, et al. Glucosamine sulfate use and delay of progression of knee osteoarthritis. *Arch Intern Med.* 2002;162(18):2113–2123.

70. Towheed TE, Maxwell L, Anastassiades TP, et al. Glucosamine therapy for treating osteoarthritis. *Cochrane Database Syst Rev.* 2005;(1). CD002946.

71. McAlindon TE, Biggee BA. Nutritional factors in osteoarthritis: recent developments. *Curr Opin Rheum.* 2005;17(5):647–652.

72. Uebelhart D. Clinical review of chondroitin sulfate in osteoarthritis. *Osteoarthritis Cartilage.* 2008;16(Suppl 3):S19–S21.

73. Ragle RL, Sawitzke AD. Nutraceuticals in the management of osteoarthritis. A critical review. *Drugs Aging.* 2012;29(9):717–731.

74. Pearson W, Orth MW, Lindinger MI. Evaluation of inflammatory responses induced via intraarticular injection of interleukin-1 in horses receiving a dietary nutraceutical and assessment of the clinical effects of long-term nutraceutical administration. *Am J Vet Res.* 2009;70(7):848–861.

75. Howard RD, McIlwraith CW. Hyaluronan and its use in the treatment of equine joint disease. In: McIlwraith CW, Trotter GW, eds. *Joint disease in the horse.* Philadelphia, PA: Saunders; 2006:257–269.

76. Schauss AG, Balogh L, Polyak A, et al. Absorption, distribution and excretion of 99 mTechnetium labeled hyaluronan after single oral doses in rats and beagle dogs. *FASEB J Abstract.* 2004;129:4.

77. Silvestro L, Lanza R, Otti E, et al. Human pharmacokinetics of glycosaminoglycan using deuterium-labeled and unlabeled substances: evidence for oral absorption. *Semin Thromb Hemost.* 1994;20(3):281–292.

78. Dawes J, Hodson BA, Pepper DS. The absorption, clearance and metabolic fate of dermatan sulfate administered to man—studies using a radio iodinated derivative. *Thromb Hemost.* 1989;62(3):945–949.

79. Dawes J, McLaren M, Forbes C, et al. The pharmacokinetics of dermatan sulfate MF701 in healthy human volunteers. *Br J Coin Pharmacol.* 1991;32(3):361–366.

80. Salartash K, Gonze MD, Leone-Bay A, et al. Oral low-molecular weight heparin and delivery agent prevents jugular venous thrombosis in the rat. *J Vasc Surg.* 1999;30(3):526–531.

81. Bergin BJ, Pierce SW, Bramlage LR, et al. Oral hyaluronan gel reduces post-operative tarsocrural effusion in the yearling Thoroughbred. Clinical evidence. *Equine Vet J.* 2006;38(4):375–378.

82. Audeval B, Bouchacourt P. Double-blind placebo-controlled study of the mussel Perna canaliculus (New Zealand green-lipped mussel) in gonoarthrosis (arthritis of the knee). *La Gazette Medicale.* 1986;93:111–115.

83. Kendall RV, Lawson JW, Hurley LA. New research and a clinical report on the use of Perna canaliculus in the management of arthritis. *Townsend Letter for Doctors & Patients.* 2000:99–111.

84. Pollard B, Guilford WG, Ankenbauer-Perkins KL, et al. Clinical efficacy and tolerance of an extract of green-lipped mussel (Perna canaliculus) in dogs presumptively diagnosed with degenerative joint disease. *N Z Vet J.* 2006;54(3):114–118.

85. Cayzer J, Hedderley D, Gray S. A randomised, double-blinded, placebo-controlled study on the efficacy of a unique extract of green-lipped mussel (Perna canaliculus) in horses with chronic fetlock lameness attributed to osteoarthritis. *Equine Vet J.* 2012;44(4):393–398.

86. Rainsford KD, Whitehouse MW. Gastroprotective and anti-inflammatory properties of green lipped mussel (Perna canaliculus) preparation. *Arzneim Forsch/Drug Res.* 1980;30(12):2128–2132.

87. Cheras PA, Stevenson L, Myers SP. Vascular mechanisms in osteoarthritis: rationale for treatment with a marine-based complementary medicine. *Osteoarthritis Cartilage.* 2005;13:S95.

88. Appelboom T, Schuermans J, Berbruggen G, et al. Symptom modifying effects of avocado/soybean unsaponifiables (ASU) in knee osteoarthritis. A double-blind, prospective placebo controlled study. *Scand J Rheumatol.* 2001;30(4):242–247.

89. Maheu E, Maziers B, Valat JP, et al. Symptomatic efficacy of avocado/soy bean unsaponifiables in the treatment of osteoarthritis of the knee and hip. A prospective, randomized, double-blind, placebo-controlled, multi-center clinical trial with a 6 month treatment period and a 2 month follow-up to demonstrate a persistent effect. *Arthritis Rheum.* 1998;41:81–91.

90. Blotman F, Maheu E, Wulwik A, et al. Efficacy and safety of avocado/soy bean unsaponifiables in the treatment of osteoarthritis of the knee and hips. A prospective, multi-center, 3-month randomized, double-blind, placebo-controlled trial. *Rev Rheum Engl Ed.* 1997;64(12):825–834.

91. Henrotin YE, Sanchez C, Deberg MA, et al. Avocado/soy bean unsaponifiables increase aggrecan synthesis and reduce catabolic and pro-inflammatory mediator production by human osteoarthritic chondrocytes. *J Rheumatol.* 2003;30(8):1825–1834.

92. Henrotin YE, Labasse AH, Jaspar JM, et al. Effects of the avocado/soy bean unsaponifiable mixtures on metalloproteinases, cytokines and prostaglandin E2 production by human articular chondrocytes. *Clin Rheumatol.* 1998;17(1):31–39.

93. Kawcak CE, Frisbie DD, McIlwraith CW, et al. Evaluation of avocado and soybean unsaponifiable extracts for treatment of horses with experimentally induced osteoarthritis using an equine model. *Am J Vet Res.* 2007;68(6):598–604.

94. Calder PC. N-3 polyunsaturated fatty acids, inflammation, and inflammatory diseases. *Am J Clin Nutrition.* 2006;83(6):S1505–S1519.

95. Gruenwald J, Petzold E, Busch R, et al. Effect of glucosamine sulfate with or without omega-3 fatty acids in patients with osteoarthritis. *Adv Ther.* 2009;26(9):858–871.

96. Roush JK, Cross AR, Renberg WC, et al. A multicenter study of the effect of dietary supplementation with fish oil omega-3 fatty acids on carprofen dosage in dogs with osteoarthritis. *J Am Vet Med Assoc.* 2010;236(5):535–539.

97. Fritsh D, Allen TA, Dodd CE, et al. Dose-titration effects of fish oil in osteoarthritic dogs. *J Vet Intern Med.* 2010;24:1020–1026.

98. Hurst S, Zainal Z, Caterson B, et al. Dietary fatty acids in arthritis. *Prostaglandins Leukot Essent Fatty Acids.* 2010;82(4-6):315–318.

99. Zainal Z, Longman AJ, Hurst S, et al. Relative efficacies of omega-3 polyunsaturated fatty acids in reducing expression of key proteins in a model system for studying osteoarthritis. *Osteoarthritis Cartilage.* 2009;17(7):896–905.

100. Knott L, Avery NC, Hollander AP, et al. Regulation of osteoarthritis by omega-2 (N-3) polyunsaturated fatty acids in a naturally occurring model of disease. *Osteoarthritis Cartilage.* 2011;19(9):1150–1157.

101. Bonnet C, Bertin P, Cook-Moreau J, et al. Lipooxygenase products in expression of 5-lipooxygenase and 5-lipooxygenase-activating protein in human cultured synovial cells. *Prostaglandins.* 1995;50(3):127–135.

102. Diehl HW, May EL. Cetyl myristoleate isolated from Swiss albino mice: an apparent protective agent against adjuvant arthritis in rats. *J Pharm Sci.* 1994;83(3):296–299.

103. Hunter Jr KW, Galt RA, Stehouwer JS, et al. Synthesis of cetyl myristoleate and evaluation of its therapeutic efficacy in a murine model of collagen-induced arthritis. *Pharmacol Res.* 2003;47(1):43–47.

104. Hesslink Jr R, Armstrong III D, Nagendran MV, et al. Cetylated fatty acids improve knee functions in patients with osteoarthritis. *J Rheumatol.* 2002;29(8):1708–1712.

105. Keegan KG, Hughes. F, Lane T, et al. Effects of an oral nutraceutical on clinical aspects of joint disease in a blinded, controlled clinical trial: 39 horses. *Proc Am Assoc Equine Pract.* 2007;53:252–255.

20

Distal Limb

David D. Frisbie, Natasha M. Werpy, Christopher E. Kawcak, and Myra F. Barrett

DISTAL INTERPHALANGEAL JOINT

David D. Frisbie, Natasha Werpy

The distal interphalangeal (DIP) joint is an anatomically complex area of the horse and regionalizing pain to the area is challenging at best because of this complexity. It is not uncommon to have bilateral disease with either acute or chronic onset. Although synovial distention is easily palpated digitally, it is not specific for primary DIP lesions; rather it is an inflammation of the joint that may be primary to a DIP lesion or secondary to a lesion in an adjacent structure(s). Perineural anesthesia of the palmar nerves at the level of the proximal sesamoids bones is typically required to desensitize the joint region, and intraarticular (IA) analgesia of the DIP joint is not specific to pain limited to the IA space and can desensitize adjacent structures. Thus, the analgesic blocking pattern must be interpreted in conjunction with imaging as well as clinical signs to provide a list of differential diagnoses. In the authors' experience an increase in lameness after a static flexion of the distal limb is often encountered in DIP pathology but differentiating a response that is from the DIP versus the proximal interphalangeal or fetlock joint is difficult. The response and duration of response to treatment of the DIP joint often help the authors determine primary or secondary lesions. Specifically, lack of response suggests that the DIP is not the primary lesion, as does a shortened duration of response, that is, 2 to 6 weeks of improvement. Improvements in imaging including the increased availability of magnetic resonance imaging (MRI) have made vast improvements in our understanding of disease processes including treating clinical pain in this region.

Radiographic Evaluation

The standard radiographic views for a foot study typically suffice for evaluating the DIP joint and include a lateromedial, dorsoproximal-palmarodistal oblique (D60Pr-PaDiO), palmaroproximal-palmarodistal oblique (Pa45Pr-PaDiO) projection (skyline), and the horizontal dorsopalmar view.

Oblique and flexed views can be considered depending on the case presentation. Proper foot preparation is required to produce a diagnostic radiographic study. Cleaning and packing of the feet and in some cases removal of the shoes are an essential part of the process.

Oblique dorsopalmar views highlighting the collateral ligament insertions on the distal phalanx and the palmar processes should be considered when it is not possible to remove the shoes. Correct positioning of all of the views is important to ensure a study of diagnostic quality will be produced. However, the skyline view is the most challenging; small degrees of obliquity on this view can markedly impact the appearance of the navicular bone. A clearly defined joint space between the dorsal or articular surface of the navicular bone and the palmar surface of the middle phalanx is an important anatomic landmark that indicates this radiographic view is properly positioned. Before assessing a radiographic study for abnormalities, the image quality should be evaluated as this can directly impact interpretation.

Nuclear Scintigraphy

It has been one author's (NW) experience that horses can have lameness that is localized to the foot/DIP region with negative findings on radiography, ultrasound, and MRI; however, there is marked increased radiopharmaceutical uptake in one or several bones of the foot (Figure 20-1) that is considered to be clinically relevant. Although this is not a frequent occurrence, it should be considered when other imaging modalities do not yield a diagnosis. Conversely, nuclear scintigraphy can yield a false-negative result especially in instances of injury and/or defects affecting the articular cartilage and/or subchondral bone of the DIP joint. In certain horses with DIP joint injury, there are no associated trabecular bone abnormalities radiographically accompanying either articular cartilage or subchondral bone defects (Figure 20-2). The lack of associated trabecular bone abnormalities seems to translate into no increase in bone turnover, even in the face of marked joint injury, resulting in a negative nuclear scintigraphy examination. Therefore, negative results from a nuclear scintigraphy examination do not

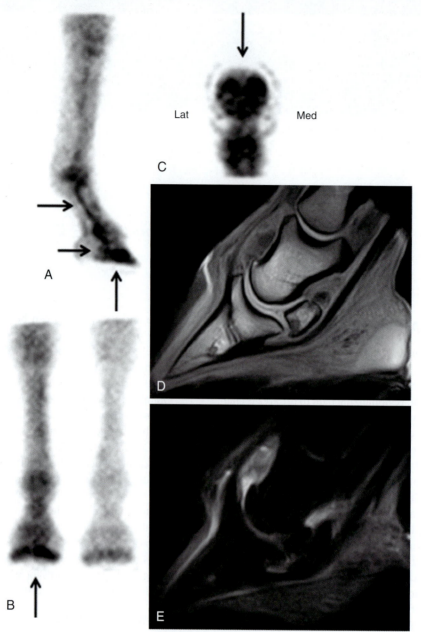

FIGURE 20-1 Nuclear scintigraphy (A, B, C), T1-weighted gradient echo (D), and short tau inversion recovery (STIR) (E) sagittal magnetic resonance (MR) images from a horse with a grade 3 lameness localized to the right fore distal limb with perineural analgesia of the palmar digital nerves. Initially, a radiographic study was performed with no significant abnormalities identified. Magnetic resonance imaging (MRI) was then performed with abnormalities identified that did not correlate with the degree of lameness. Following repeat blocking with the same response to perineural analgesia of the palmar digital nerves, nuclear scintigraphy was performed. On bone phase images, there was marked increased radiopharmaceutical uptake (arrows) in the distal phalanx and in the palmar aspect of the middle and distal phalanges. In addition, there was uptake in the sesamoid bones. This pattern has been identified in cases with lameness localized to the distal limb following MRI examination using both high-field and low-field MRI systems with subsequent increased radiopharmaceutical uptake on nuclear scintigraphy examination. The uptake is considered clinically relevant despite the lack of structural abnormalities on the MR images, based on an author's opinion (NW).

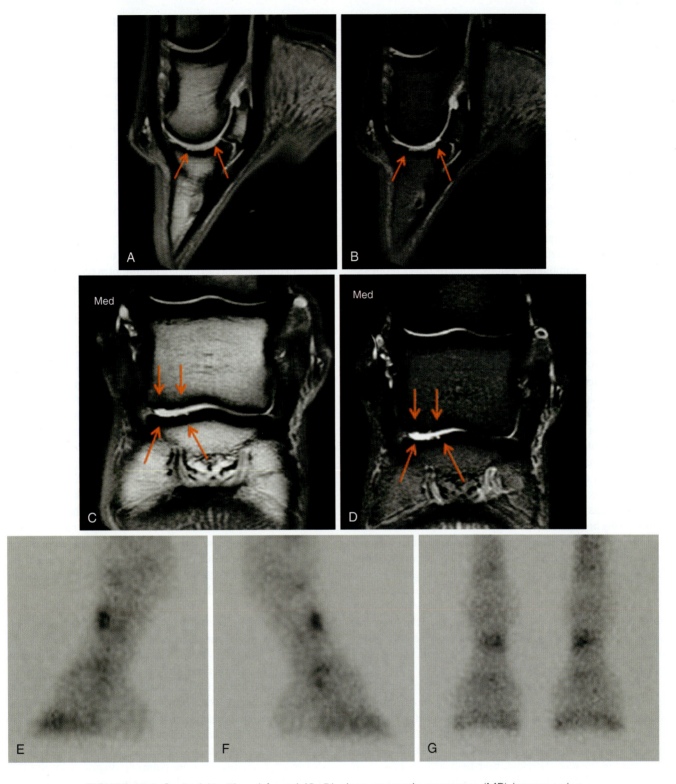

FIGURE 20-2 Sagittal (A, B) and frontal (C, D) plane magnetic resonance (MR) images using proton density (A, C) and short tau inversion recovery (STIR) (B, D) sequences and corresponding nuclear scintigraphy (E, F, G) images from an upper level jumper with chronic lameness varying between grade 2 and 3, localized to the distal interphalangeal (DIP) joint with intraarticular analgesia. Extensive damage to the articular surfaces is present, characterized by the articular cartilage loss (arrows) in the medial aspect of the DIP joint with multiple shallow subchondral bone defects (arrows), affecting both the middle and distal phalanges with no adjacent trabecular bone reaction. No adjacent sclerosis in the trabecular bone or fluid within the subchondral or trabecular bone deep to the defects is present. Therefore no abnormalities would be present on radiographic or nuclear scintigraphy examination. Marked articular cartilage loss with or without associated subchondral bone loss and no trabecular bone reaction occur in the DIP joint more frequently than in other joints, which tend to demonstrate adjacent trabecular bone abnormalities when there is clinically relevant articular cartilage loss. Therefore, this type of joint injury will require a modality that can specifically image articular cartilage to achieve a diagnosis.

preclude clinically relevant DIP joint disease. Furthermore, small or subtle osseous lesions, depending on their location, may not be evident on scintigraphic examination.

Ultrasound

Ultrasound of the foot can be used to evaluate the dorsal and palmar periarticular margins of the DIP joint, associated soft tissue structures, and the proximal aspect of the collateral ligaments. The dorsal aspect of the DIP joint and the collateral ligaments are most frequently evaluated using a linear probe. Evaluation of the palmar aspect of the foot requires a microconvex probe because of the skin contour and a wider far field of view, allowing visibility of the pertinent anatomy in the suprasesamoidean and potentially sesamoidean regions. A microconvex probe can increase the visibility of the proximal aspect of the collateral ligaments of the DIP joint. The extent of the collateral ligaments that is visible is dependent of the foot conformation, specifically the relationship between the position or height of the coronary band relative to the collateral ligaments as well as the skin surface contour. The periople is the distal extent of the window for imaging collateral ligaments; a distally oriented probe placed on the periople identifies the distal extent of the ligament that can be evaluated with ultrasound. However, it is important to recognize that this probe placement may not produce echogenic fibers in the ligament, depending on the ligament fiber orientation at this level. Therefore, assessment of size, shape, and margins may be all that is possible at this level using this technique. Use of a microconvex probe, although necessary for certain regions of the foot, has less detail or resolution compared with a linear probe; using both probes when applicable can provide the most information possible as each probe contributes different types of diagnostic information. The pie-shaped image produced by a convex probe (micro or macro) provides a more global picture of the anatomy versus a linear probe, especially at greater depths. For a less experienced ultrasonographer, this image can be helpful in identifying anatomy and getting oriented to the structures in the image. Once the anatomy in the region is identified using a convex probe, a linear probe can be used for increased detail and better assessment of the structures.

The joint capsule, presence, and nature of synovial proliferation and enthesophyte formation, as well as effusion and periarticular proliferation, can be well assessed with ultrasound of the DIP joint. The joint recess, periarticular margins, and collateral ligaments are superficially located on the dorsal aspect of the foot. Although near-field artifacts have been minimized with technical advances in ultrasound, a standoff pad will be necessary in some horses to image the dorsal aspect of the foot. Standoff pads result in artifact and decreased beam penetration and should only be used when necessary. They aid not only in the assessment of superficially located structures, but also allow visibility of skin contour. Assessing the contour of the skin surface can be helpful, especially with subtle injury. In certain cases, focal, mild swelling can be more evident with ultrasound using a standoff pad that will highlight the skin contour than with palpation. In addition, confirmation of a palpable abnormality can be achieved with evaluation of the skin contour, and the ultrasound exam can then focus on identifying the source of the swelling. Standoff artifact is often

reduced by increased probe pressure. However, increased probe pressure can obscure subtle abnormalities and displace effusion leading to an underestimating of lesion severity. Therefore, variable amounts of pressure should be used in the same area to gain all the information possible.

Soft tissue and osseous abnormalities affecting the collateral ligaments of the DIP joint can be identified with ultrasound. The curvature of the collateral ligaments as well as the ligament anatomy with multiple fiber bundles should be considered when performing an ultrasound examination of these ligaments. Because of the ligament curvature and variable fiber pattern, multiple beam angles will be required to create echogenicity within the ligament. The orientation of different fiber bundles within the ligament can create a nonuniform echo pattern at the various probe angles. All the normal fibers within the ligament should be echogenic when the ultrasound beam is perpendicular to their longitudinal axis. However, because of both the ligament curvature and the different fiber bundles, it may not be possible to create uniform echogenicity in all the ligament fibers with a single probe position. Within the short distance at the level of the coronary band, where the collateral ligaments can be visualized, two to three different probe positions with a range of ultrasound beam orientations created by changing the probe angle are often required to create echogenicity within all of the ligament fibers. Soft tissue swelling at the level of the coronary band, which can be present with collateral ligament injury, changes the skin contour, making ultrasound examination technically easier. In cases with no swelling, the skin surface can be concave, making it more difficult to position the probe properly. As with any anatomic region, ultrasound is more sensitive to superficial bone surface abnormalities than radiographs. Assessment for osseous proliferation and/or resorption at the collateral ligaments attachments on the middle phalanx can be readily performed with ultrasound.

The palmar approach to the foot can be used to evaluate the proximopalmar recess of the DIP joint and periarticular margins. The synovial membranes of the proximopalmar recess of the DIP joint, the dorsodistal aspect of the digital sheath, and the proximal recess of the navicular bone come together proximal to the navicular bone and are sometimes referred to as the T-ligament. The synovial membrane separating these recesses changes position in response to fluid distribution within each of the individual synovial recesses (Figure 20-3). Therefore, it is important to recognize that this synovial membrane or T-ligament can be palmarly displaced by the DIP joint effusion and dorsally displaced by navicular bursal effusion. Effusion within these recesses is quite easily visualized using the palmar approach to the foot. However, because the effect of effusion on the position of the synovial membrane or T-ligament in the palmar aspect of the foot, a single midline longitudinal (midsagittal image) may not be adequate to distinguish the source of increased fluid on the palmar aspect of the foot. Fully defining the peripheral margins and extent of the various synovial membranes on the palmar aspect of the foot is necessary to correctly determine the origin of increased fluid in this region. This is also true when imaging slightly more proximally, directed at the proximal extent of the navicular bursa. The distal extent of the dorsal recess of the digital

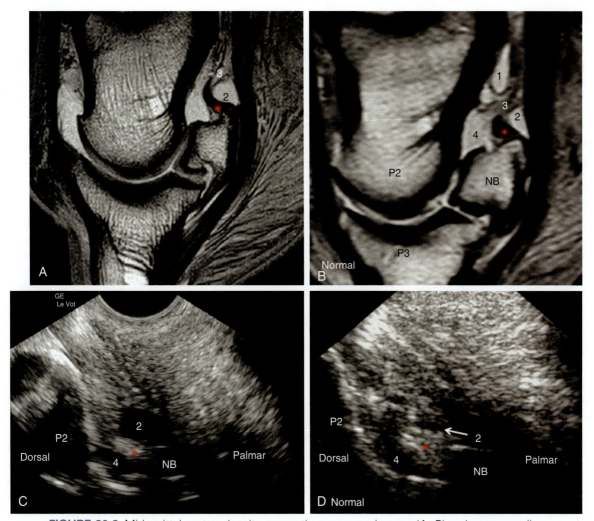

FIGURE 20-3 Midsagittal proton density magnetic resonance images (**A, B**) and corresponding longitudinal midline ultrasound images (**C, D**) at the level of the supersesamoidean region from two horses. One horse with normal anatomy in this region (**B, D**) is compared with a horse with moderate effusion (**A, C**) in the navicular bursa (**2**) that results in dorsal displacement of the collateral sesamoidean ligament (asterisk) and the T-ligament (**3**). The T-ligament can be displaced dorsally with increased fluid in the navicular bursa and palmarly with increased fluid in the distal interphalangeal joint (**4**). The dorsal distal recess of the digital sheath (**1**) is visible proximal to the T-ligament and can also influence its position with effusion.

sheath becomes visible at this level and is continuous with the synovial membrane separating the proximal palmar recess of the DIP joint from the navicular bursa (see Figure 20-3).

Advanced Imaging (Magnetic Resonance Imaging and Computed Tomography)

The hoof capsule greatly limits ultrasound access to the structures in the foot, and radiographic and nuclear scintigraphy examinations have marked limitations for certain types of injury, making advanced imaging essential for the diagnosis of many abnormalities within the hoof capsule. Advanced imaging, such as computed tomography (CT) and MRI, provides multiplanar images with high resolution and no superimposition of structures. MRI has superior soft tissue detail and can detect the presence of osseous fluid, which can occur with many types of joint injury. In addition, the presence of osseous fluid can impact both treatment and prognosis,

making it an important component of the diagnosis. CT has superior bone detail, and contrast CT can provide information that cannot be identified with standard imaging modalities. CT lacks soft tissue detail compared with MRI. If there is particular interest in the vascular patterns or tissue permeability of an injury, MRI can be the modality of choice, especially if vascular imaging is not included in the current MRI software and/or intravascular contrast is not routinely used as part of the usual MRI protocol. Although CT arthrography can be used to identify articular cartilage defects, currently available methods do not readily allow identification of diffuse degenerative injury or intrasubstance tears of the articular cartilage. MRI can detect changes in signal pattern consistent with diffuse injury. Clinical sequences can be maximized to evaluate the articular cartilage and specialized techniques, such as T1ρ, T2 mapping, and gadolinium contrast, have been developed for cartilage imaging and are aimed at detecting articular cartilage degeneration before morphologic change. In contrast to CT, MRI cannot distinguish well between osseous proliferation at soft tissue interfaces, such as enthesophyte formation at joint capsule and collateral ligaments, or within soft tissues in many cases. Although this is somewhat sequence-selection-dependent, CT is superior for identification of these types of abnormalities.

PATHOLOGIC CHANGE IN THE DISTAL INTERPHALANGEAL JOINT

Osteochondrosis/Developmental Orthopedic Disease

Osteochondral fragments in the dorsal aspect of the joint and in the proximopalmar recess are both possible manifestations of osteochondrosis.[1] However, other causes for these fragments remain possible; they include trauma resulting in a fracture fragment, endochondral ossification of a loose cartilage fragment, and a separate center of ossification when associated with the extensor process. The radiographic diagnosis of osteochondral fragments is quite straightforward and the adjacent subchondral bone margins should be closely scrutinized for any abnormalities. It is recognized that fragments in the dorsal aspect of the DIP joint can be found without recognizable clinical pain; conversely, pain can range from moderate to severe. Response to IA DIP anesthesia or to IA treatment of the joint is often necessary to confirm the relevance of such fragments. As previously noted, IA DIP anesthesia has been certainly recognized to diffuse and desensitize structures beyond the joint capsule, making clinical interpretation more challenging. Although a substantial range of fragment size exists, most are amenable to arthroscopic removal, which is described elsewhere.[2] The results of arthroscopic removal are favorable; there is one report documenting 87% return to athletic function.[3] Large fragments were historically removed through arthrotomies and have been reported to carry a poorer prognosis (57%),[4] although arthroscopic removal has been associated with an improved outcome of these large fragments (75%).[5] The latter has been the authors' experience with the use of motorized equipment. Palmar or plantar fragmentation can also be observed and when associated with clinical pain arthroscopic removal is likewise recommended.[2]

Osseous cystlike lesions can be identified in the DIP joint, more frequently affecting the distal phalanx than the middle phalanx. A focal lucency, in certain cases bordered by sclerosis, can be identified radiographically. Nuclear scintigraphy can be used to determine if the surrounding bone is active, which is not necessarily a direct indicator of clinical relevance. MRI can be used to characterize the contents of the osseous cystlike lesion as well as the presence, absence, and/or condition of the overlying articular cartilage/communication with the joint space and any trabecular bone reaction such as fluid or sclerosis. CT arthrography can be used to evaluate the superficial margin and thickness of the articular cartilage and trabecular bone sclerosis, as well as joint communication. This technique will obviously lack any fluid detection associated with the cyst contents and the surrounding bone and will be unable to aid in any detection of intrasubstance changes within the articular

cartilage. These are all components that help determine clinical relevance. Treatment with IA medication can provide clinical relief to some cases and is typically the first-line treatment. Autologous conditioned serum and polysulfated glycosaminoglycan are used in refractory cases that are not amenable to surgery. Cystic lesion in the coffin bone can be centrally located, making arthroscopic and/or surgical access (through the hoof capsule) challenging. In one report of young horses with arthroscopically accessible lesions, 90% had a successful outcome; however, reports of cyst débridement through the hoof capsule are described and the long-term prognosis is less clear.[6]

Osteoarthritis

Osteoarthritis (OA) and associated abnormalities of the DIP joint have a wide range of imaging presentations. Once radiographic evidence of marked OA is present, the management of horses at a high level of athletic performance can be challenging. As in many joints, early detection of joint disease may allow earlier intervention and management to have a greater impact on sustaining athletic performance. Synovitis is one of the early signs of joint disease and variable degrees of synovial proliferation and synovial membrane thickening can be well identified with ultrasound and MRI. In addition, joint capsule thickening as a result of capsulitis versus joint capsule scarring indicating chronicity can be well distinguished with these modalities. Digital radiography, with an appropriate window and level, can demonstrate soft tissue swelling associated with the dorsal recess of the DIP joint by evaluating the skin contour on the lateromedial view. CT images using a soft tissue window will reveal skin contour and can provide information about joint capsule thickening and synovial proliferation versus effusion, and contrast arthrography will further characterize these findings, although intravascular contrast can highlight inflammation of the synovial membrane and/or synovial proliferation. Enthesophyte formation at joint capsule attachments will be evident on radiographs, ultrasound, MRI, and CT. Ultrasound will be limited to the joint capsule attachments, which can be visualized proximal to the coronary band.

In assessing the DIP joint, the size and contour of the periarticular margins are evaluated. There is normal anatomic variation in the shape and size of the distal phalanx extensor process, and this should not be confused with periarticular osteophyte formation (Figure 20-4). Although periarticular osteophyte formation is most easily recognized on the dorsal joint margins, the palmar or plantar margins should be closely evaluated. This is important because osteophyte formation can be present on the palmar or plantar margins of the joint and the dorsal aspect can be unaffected. Periarticular osteophyte formation can be detected using radiographs, ultrasound, MRI, and CT, similar to enthesophyte formation. However, ultrasound will be limited to the periarticular margins, which can be visualized proximal to the coronary band. The visibility of periarticular osteophytes with the different imaging modalities is dependent on their size and location. Superimposition of periarticular margins on radiographs can obscure the visibility of osteophytes. MRI has limitations when evaluating periarticular margins, and sequence selection plays an important role in the visibility of these areas (Figure 20-5).

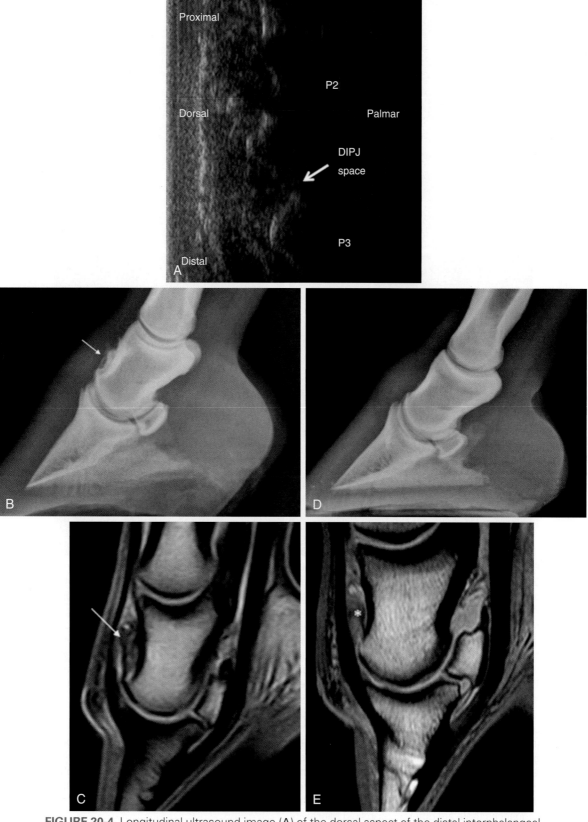

FIGURE 20-4 Longitudinal ultrasound image (**A**) of the dorsal aspect of the distal interphalangeal joint with corresponding lateral radiograph (**B**) and sagittal proton density magnetic resonance (MR) image (**C**) from a horse with osseous proliferation (arrow) on the dorsal aspect of the middle and distal phalanges. Lateral radiograph (**D**) and sagittal proton density magnetic resonance imaging (MRI) (**E**) of a horse with synovial proliferation (*) in the dorsal recess of the distal interphalangeal joint. The osseous proliferation is easily identified on the ultrasound and radiograph images. However, when comparing the MR images, the signal intensity of osseous and synovial proliferation is similar, making it difficult to distinguish them on MR images.

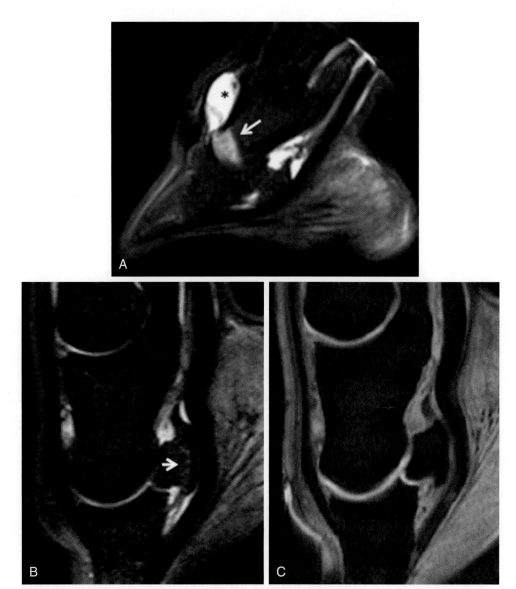

FIGURE 20-5 **(A)** Short tau inversion recovery (STIR) magnetic resonance (MR) image from an upper level jumping horse with moderate trabecular bone fluid (arrow) in the dorsal distal aspect of the middle phalanx associated with acute lameness following an event. In addition, moderate effusion (*) is present in the distal interphalangeal joint. The dorsal distal aspect of the middle phalanx is a predilection site for bone contusion following athletic performance, which leads to the presence of fluid in this region. However, this fluid extends along the subchondral bone margin, which is always cause for concern related to damage to the articular surfaces. Damage to the articular cartilage or subchondral bone can occur at the same time as the bone contusion as a result of athletic trauma. The fluid from the bone contusion may be visible on initial magnetic resonance imaging (MRI); however, the subchondral bone and articular cartilage damage may not.

In the author's (NW) experience, a large percentage of horses with dorsal distal P2 fluid and no other detectable abnormalities may return to work following rest and resolution of fluid, which takes from 30 days to 6 months, depending on severity. However, a certain number of these horses go on to develop pronounced joint disease. The joint disease is characterized by articular cartilage and/or subchondral bone loss, as well as periarticular osteophyte development and enthesophyte formation at joint capsule attachments associated with development of chronic lameness. STIR or fat-suppressed images are critical for the identification of osseous fluid. Within the available MRI sequences there are differences in fluid sensitivity.

Proton density **(B)** and T1-gradient echo **(C)** sagittal MR images, both with fat suppression. There is a difference in fluid sensitivity between these sequences as evidenced by the presence of mild fluid (arrow) in the palmar aspect of the navicular bone adjacent to the flexor surface in the proton density image **(B)**. This fluid is not appreciable in the T1-weighted gradient echo image **(C)** because of the decreased sensitivity to fluid. These images have the same slice thickness with the remaining sequence parameters maximized for clinical imaging.

Thus, the combination of radiographs and MRI is quite beneficial as these modalities offset each other's advantages and disadvantages.

Damage or loss of articular surfaces of the DIP joint, as well as subchondral bone loss, has significant implications to the long-term athletic career of performance horses and is the source of pain in most breeds and disciplines. A wide variety of manifestations of articular surface damage can occur in the DIP joint. Articular cartilage damage or loss resulting in joint space narrowing of the DIP joint does not typically become radiographically evident until severe changes have occurred. Further, large areas of full thickness articular cartilage defects can be present in the DIP joint with a radiographically normal joint space width. It often requires other imaging modalities to diagnosis early articular cartilage and subtle subchondral bone loss.

Because of the challenges of articular cartilage imaging, MRI system selection becomes a critical factor if specific concerns about the articular cartilage of the DIP joint are on the differential diagnosis. Low-field imaging is quite prevalent in equine veterinary medicine and produces diagnostic-quality images that allow the diagnosis of numerous types of injuries in the foot that cannot be identified with standard imaging modalities (radiographs and ultrasound). At this time, however, low-field MR systems do not provide consistently reliable imaging of the articular cartilage. Although it has been reported that surgically created defects in the joint could be identified using a low-field system,[7] several factors in this study did not recreate imaging issues in clinical patients. Therefore, in one of the author's (NW) opinion, the results are not directly applicable to clinical imaging at this time. Because of the limitation and difficulty in detecting articular cartilage defects in the DIP, the authors prefer to use the highest field magnet available in challenging cases involving the foot. It has been one author's experience (DDF) that even using a 1.5-T magnet can miss articular cartilage lesions subsequently identified on a 3-T scan of the same horse.

Other considerations associated with DIP cartilage pathology can occur without subchondral bone loss, trabecular bone abnormalities, or periarticular osteophyte formation (see Figure 20-2). Such cases often have no radiographic evidence of DIP osteoarthritis and negative nuclear scintigraphy examinations. These horses typically have pronounced synovitis if the joint has not been recently treated. Advanced imaging with a high-field magnet, preferably 3 T, is required for a definitive diagnosis in these cases.

Although articular cartilage loss can be seen in isolation in the DIP joint, it is frequently accompanied by subchondral bone loss. Subchondral bone loss or focal subchondral bone defects can be encountered in the DIP joint without associated trabecular bone abnormalities. As the damage to the subchondral bone worsens, it will be become radiographically evident. If trabecular bone sclerosis is present adjacent to the subchondral bone loss, this is an important radiographic finding. As more MRI studies are done and horses followed sequentially, it appears that early detection of fluid and subtle

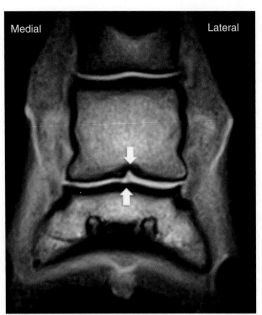

FIGURE 20-6 Frontal plane T1-weighted gradient echo magnetic resonance (MR) image of a front foot. A V-shaped subchondral bone depression is present in the distal aspect of the middle phalanx on midline with minimal sclerosis and no fluid on fat-suppressed images. On the opposing surface of distal phalanx there is a shallow subchondral bone depression with no trabecular bone reaction. These subchondral bone depressions can be seen in symptomatic and asymptomatic horses with lameness localized to the distal interphalangeal joint. Assessment of the articular cartilage and adjacent trabecular bone is a critical part of determining the clinical relevance of these depressions. Articular cartilage assessment will be limited with low-field magnetic resonance imaging (MRI) examinations. In the author's (NW) experience, cases with trabecular bone reaction and articular cartilage disruption are considered more clinically relevant. Disruption of the articular cartilage can allow synovial fluid to extend into the depression and may lead to development of pathologic change. Bilateral or unilateral symmetry when comparing fore and hindlimbs is also a consideration in regard to clinical relevance.

changes in the subchondral bone may precede formation of subchondral bone cysts.

Also of interest are cases with trabecular bone fluid along the subchondral bone margin when no additional findings are present (Figure 20-6). In many cases MRI reexamination and additional imaging modalities are necessary to fully understand the significance of this finding. The presence of increased radiopharmaceutical uptake as a result of osseous fluid is variable, perhaps relating both to the stage of the injury and the bone response. Therefore, a negative nuclear scintigraphy examination does not preclude the presence of osseous fluid. It has been the experience of one author (DDF) that, historically, rest and/or treatment with bisphosphonates has resolved clinical lameness in these cases but scientific evidence is lacking. More recently, regional perfusion with mesenchymal stem cells (MSCs) in conjunction with rest has also yielded good results anecdotally. A subchondral bone depression can be seen in the sagittal ridge of the distal

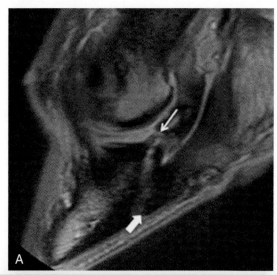

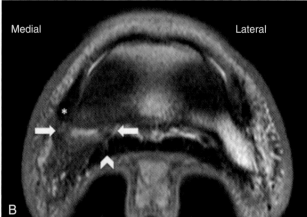

FIGURE 20-7 Sagittal and transverse proton density magnetic resonance images from two horses with distal phalanx fractures. In the sagittal image (A), the fracture line extends from the solar margin of the bone (block arrow) through the palmar aspect of the articular surface and continues into the impar ligament (line arrow) splitting it into dorsal and palmar halves. In the transverse image (B), the medial extent of the fracture line (block arrow) extends through the palmar margin of the medial fossa of the distal phalanx with associated medial collateral ligament enlargement (*) and palmar margin fraying of the ligament. The lateral extent of the fracture line (block arrow) extends through the attachment of the deep digital flexor tendon on the axial margin of the palmar process with a focal split (chevron) in the lateral lobe of the deep digital flexor tendon.

phalanx, both unilaterally and bilaterally (Figure 20-7). In certain horses there is a depression in the opposing surface of the distal phalanx. Various sizes and shapes occur in these depressions when comparing different horses and the right and left forelimbs of the same horse. Several theories have been proposed for this finding from developmental orthopedic disease (DOD), especially when the depressions are bilateral, to normal anatomic variation. In one author's (NW) opinion the midline sagittal ridge depressions are more likely to be clinically relevant when the overlying articular cartilage is abnormal on MRI.

Fracture of the Distal Phalanx

Fractures involving the distal phalanx can present with surprisingly subtle clinical signs, presumably because of stabilization provided by the hoof capsule. Some degree of hoof tester sensitivity is often noted as in response to distal limb flexion. Perineural anesthesia at the level of the sesamoid bones is typically required to abolish the lameness with articular fractures.

Radiographic diagnosis of a fracture requires the x-ray beam to be tangential to the fracture line, which can be challenging. Numerous oblique views can be required to identify a fracture line. The visibility of the fracture line is increased by performing the radiograph study 7 to 10 days following the onset of lameness because of resorption and resultant widening of the fracture line. Packing and frog cleft artifacts can create linear lucent lines superimposed over the distal phalanx, and they should not be confused with a fracture. Assessing whether or not the fracture is articular is important in determining a management plan and prognosis, as articular fractures can lead to development of OA and permanent joint disease. It should be noted that this type of fracture often heals with a fibrous union and will, even in a healed state, be radiographically evident without clinical pain.

Nuclear scintigraphy is useful in that increased radiopharmaceutical uptake may indicate the presence of a fracture, providing the examination occurs at a point where osteoclastic activity has increased, indicative of marked bone turnover. CT will demonstrate fractures without any superimposition of bone and 3-dimensional reconstructions are helpful to visualize the fracture in a format that more closely represents the anatomy.

Horses with marked lameness and no radiographic diagnosis often present for advanced imaging to achieve a diagnosis. Therefore, distal phalanx fractures are sometimes diagnosed with advanced imaging. Use of MRI in these cases allows diagnosis of the fracture and reveals any osseous inflammation and associated soft tissue injury. Depending on the orientation of the fracture, soft tissue structures and their osseous attachments can be affected, providing valuable information for management (Figure 20-8). The collateral ligaments of the DIP joints and their insertions on the fossa of the distal phalanx can be affected, which is more pertinent relative to the topic of joint disease. However, any soft tissue structure that is attached to the distal phalanx, including the deep digital flexor tendon and impar ligament, may be impacted by a fracture. Therefore, advanced imaging may have advantages over radiographs in more clearly delineating all the abnormalities associated with a fracture.

Advanced imaging can also provide beneficial information when evaluating nonacute fractures and their clinical significance. However, in cases where the articular surface is affected, the clinical significance is rarely debatable. The ability to assess fluid and more clearly evaluate sclerosis and the appearance of the fracture line is extremely helpful in cases of nonacute fracture where clinical significance is of question. Other sources of articular surface discontinuity, such as

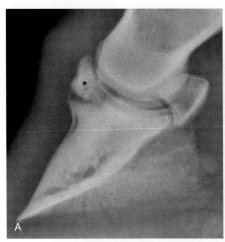
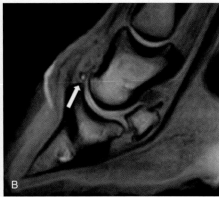
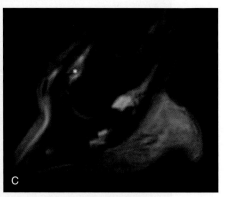

FIGURE 20-8 Lateral radiograph (**A**) of a horse with a distal phalanx extensor process fragment (*) involving a large area of the articular surface, which will lead to distal interphalangeal joint disease and affect the long-term athletic performance of this horse. Contrast with the T1-weighted gradient echo (**B**) and short tau inversion recovery (STIR) (**C**) magnetic resonance images with a small distal phalanx extensor process fragment (block arrow on **B**) with no obvious articular component and no osseous fluid as evidenced by low-signal intensity on STIR images (**C**). However, there is thickening of the distal interphalangeal joint capsule and synovial proliferation (*), indicating some degree of chronic joint inflammation (**C**).

navicular fracture, bipartite or tripartite navicular bones, and middle phalanx fracture (covered in the pastern section), will contribute to the development of OA.

Distal articular phalanx fractures are usually treated by either conservative management with supportive shoes (rim shoe or shoe with multiple clips), which is often reserved for younger horses and less displaced fractures, or lag screw fixation (the reader is directed to more detailed text).[8] Some degree of secondary OA is expected with articular fractures of the distal phalanx and appropriate IA therapy should also be in the long-term plan for the horse.

Fragmentation of the extensor process is frequently encountered with fragments of various sizes (Figure 20-9). Assessment of the articular component, if any, and any associated osseous or joint reaction is important in determining the clinical relevance of this finding. Both radiographs and ultrasound can provide information about extensor process fracture.

Periarticular Soft Tissues

The periarticular soft tissue structures of interest include the joint capsule, as previously described relative to synovitis, and the collateral ligaments. Soft tissue and osseous abnormalities can affect the collateral ligaments of the DIP joint. Often, more than one imaging modality is required for complete characterization of the lesions. Radiographs can demonstrate osseous abnormalities at the attachments of the collateral ligaments on the middle and distal phalanges (Figure 20-10). As with all soft tissue attachments, a variety of abnormalities can be encountered that will affect which specific imaging modality best demonstrates the lesion. Lysis or resorption, proliferation or enthesophyte formation, and osseous cystlike lesions can all occur at the collateral ligament attachments on the

middle and distal phalanges, and they may be accompanied by trabecular bone fluid, sclerosis, or both.

Collateral ligament injury (medial and/or lateral) is one of the more common periarticular soft tissue injuries of the DIP joint. It is often in the forelimbs and can be bilateral. Diagnosis in the field can be challenging, and the injury may often present as a failed IA DIP joint treatment. Diagnostic anesthesia of the affected side at the level of the sesamoid typically results in significant (>80%) improvement in the lameness, which is often more pronounced with the affected side on the outside of a circle. Also, the history often has periods of relative soundness followed by significant, acute increase in clinical pain. Uneven ground seems to exacerbate the clinical lameness. In one author's (DDF) experience, the use of blocks (2 to 3 cm high), placed either medial or lateral to load the DIP joint unevenly, is of little definitive use in diagnosis of collateral ligament injury. Further, IA anesthesia usually improves but does not abolish the lameness, probably in relation to the amount of extracapsular ligament involvement.

Radiographs can easily demonstrate moderate or greater osseous abnormalities at the attachments of the collateral ligaments of the DIP joints. More subtle abnormalities can be identified radiographically. However, close scrutiny of the eminences of the middle phalanx and the fossae of the distal phalanx is required for diagnosis. Nuclear scintigraphy can be helpful in demonstrating regions of abnormality associated with the collateral ligaments. However, other osseous abnormalities can occur in close proximity. Therefore, increased radiopharmaceutical uptake in this region will often have several differential diagnoses that will be further delineated with additional imaging and correlation with case presentation. The attachments of the collateral ligaments should be evaluated for enthesophyte formation, resorption, and osseous

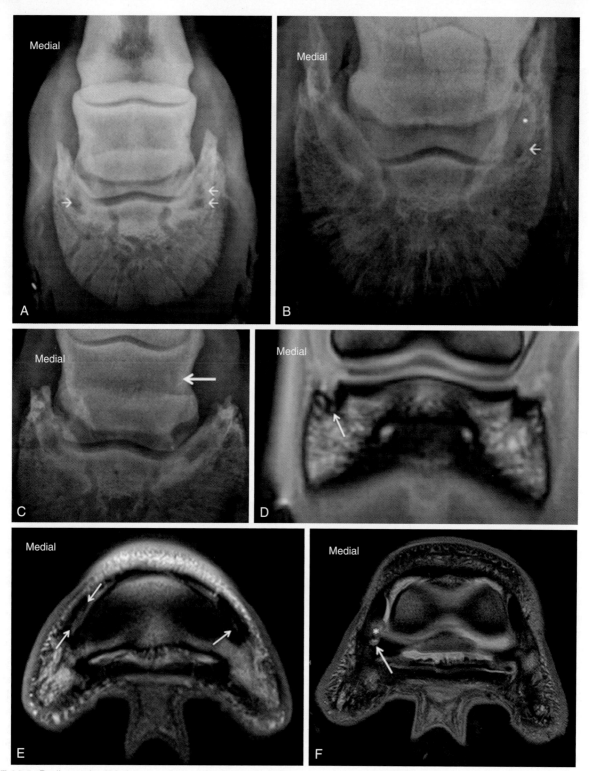

FIGURE 20-9 Radiographs (60 degrees dorsopalmar view) of a front foot from three different horses (**A, B, C**) with osseous cystlike lesions (arrows) at the insertion (**A, B**) and origin (**C**) of the collateral ligaments of the distal interphalangeal joint. These lesions are frequently bordered by sclerosis and can have a large area of sclerosis as seen in **B** (*). An osseous cystlike lesion at the level of the middle phalanx associated with the collateral ligament origin should be visible ultrasonographically if it extends to the peripheral surface or if the bone density is decreased enough that it can be penetrated by the sound beam. Fiber abnormalities within the collateral ligaments at the level of the coronary band or proximal to it can be well identified. However, the true distal extent of the lesion may not be appreciated with this modality. Similarly, collateral ligament injuries associated with insertional lesions (**A, B**) are very difficult to impossible to visualize on ultrasound if the fiber disruption begins well below the coronary band. Magnetic resonance imaging (MRI) is required for the diagnosis of collateral ligament injuries at this level. Frontal plane T1 gradient echo MRI image (**D**) of fore foot of a horse with a small osseous cystlike lesion at the insertion of the collateral ligament of the distal interphalangeal joint. This lesion is similar to a previously described radiographic image (**B**). However, this osseous cystlike lesion does not have a sclerotic border.

Transverse proton density MRI images (**E, F**) from two different horses with osseous cystlike lesions of the distal phalanx and axial fiber disruption affecting the collateral ligament of the distal interphalangeal joint. The horse in image (**E**) has moderate axial fiber disruption (arrows) of the medial collateral ligament and focal moderate palmar axial fiber disruption (arrow) of the lateral collateral ligament. The horse in image (**F**) has moderate palmar axial fiber disruption (arrow) affecting the medial collateral ligament extending into the fibrous attachment (*) to the collateral cartilage. Medial is on the left in the transverse images.

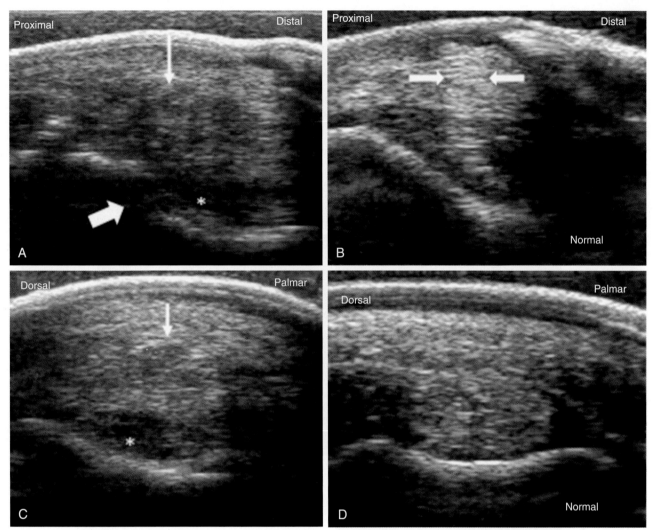

FIGURE 20-10 Ultrasound images of the attachment of the collateral ligament of the distal interphalangeal joint at the level of the middle phalanx from a horse with injury to the collateral ligament (A, C) as compared to a normal ligament (B, D). The abnormal collateral ligament (A, C) is moderately enlarged (line arrow) with an area of focal fiber disruption (*) surrounded by diffuse fiber abnormality as compared to the normal image (B, D). There is resorption and enthesophyte formation of the fossa of the middle phalanx at the attachment of the collateral ligament characterized by an irregular bone margin (block arrow on A). The periople is outlined (block arrows on B) in the normal image. The periople can aid in imaging of the collateral ligament because it provides a window with less absorption of the ultrasound beam, allowing greater visibility of the ligament as evidenced by the linear hyperechoic region on the longitudinal image of the normal horse.

The longitudinal images (A, C) are oriented with proximal on the left and distal on the right. The transverse images (B, D) are oriented with dorsal on the left and palmar on the right.

cystlike lesions. These lesions are more frequently encountered at the insertion on the distal phalanx. However, they can occur on the middle phalanx and are best visualized on the horizontal and oblique dorsopalmar projections. Ultrasound demonstrates osseous abnormalities at the attachment of the collateral ligaments on the middle phalanx, providing they extend to the surface.

Ultrasound can be used to image the proximal one-fourth to one-third of the collateral ligaments of the DIP joint, depending on the foot conformation and position of the coronary band relative to the joint. Fiber disruption can be identified as decreased echogenicity that becomes more pronounced as the severity of the injury increases, and it should have decreased echogenicity regardless of beam angle (Figure 20-11). Moderate severe injury can have associated periligament swelling and/or edema, and fibrosis of this region can occur with chronic injury.

There are certainly limitations to ultrasound of the collateral ligaments of the DIP joint, not only based on the limited viewing window, but also on the range of abnormalities. Subtle changes may require advanced imaging for a diagnosis, of which MRI (especially high field) will be superior for identification of subtle, diffuse fiber abnormalities. In addition, diagnosis of any osseous fluid component will require

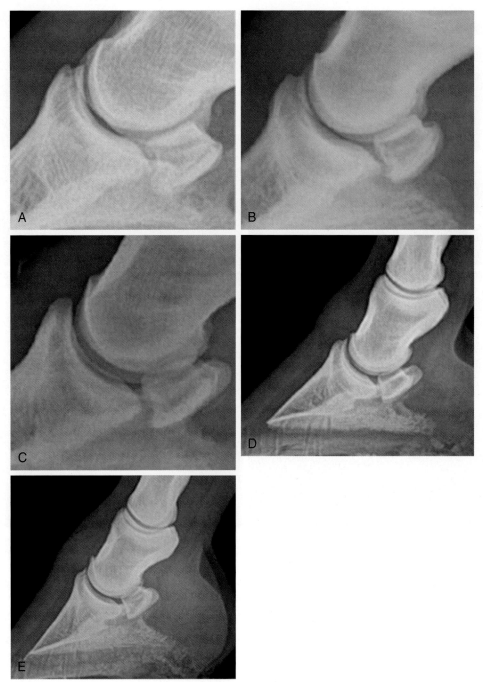

FIGURE 20-11 Normal anatomic variation of the extensor process of the distal phalanx on lateral to medial radiographs (**A** through **D**) compared with distal interphalangeal joint arthrosis (**E**) with periarticular osteophyte formation. The extensor process can have multiple different shapes with or without a focal notch in the proximal aspect, adjacent to the periarticular margin. Images **D** and **E** are the right and left forelimbs of a horse with a normal extensor process (**D**) and an extensor process that is abnormally shaped because of periarticular osteophyte formation (**E**). Comparison to the opposite limb is beneficial to aid in determination of normal anatomic variation versus periarticular osteophyte formation. In addition, ultrasound of the dorsal recess of the distal interphalangeal joint could be used to evaluate the periarticular margins as well as the joint recesses for effusion and joint capsule thickening, further indication of joint inflammation.

MRI. Axial margin fiber disruption is a common collateral ligament injury, most often occurring at the level of the joint and distal phalanx. CT arthrography can demonstrate this injury well, as the region of axial margin fiber disruption is often occupied by the collateral recess of the DIP joint leading to an abnormal contrast distribution. Using a soft tissue window when evaluating these studies will aid in the diagnosis of more subtle and diffuse fiber abnormalities within the collateral ligaments but not to the degree that can be achieved with MRI.

It is important to recognize that interpretation of collateral ligament injury on MRI is quite challenging for numerous reasons. The different fiber bundles create a mixed signal pattern. Therefore, on MRI, normal collateral ligaments are not a solid shade of gray or black but a mixture. The ligaments are subject to magic angle effect, which in the author's (NW) opinion means that the signal pattern is often not the same when comparing the medial and lateral ligaments of a limb or when comparing the ligaments between limbs. This is in contention to reports by Dyson. Several factors must be considered when evaluating the collateral ligaments of the DIP joint on MR images. Adequate time spent understanding the anatomy, effects of sequence selection, and result of magic angle effect is required to avoid misinterpretation of the images.

Treatment of collateral ligament injury can be challenging and usually requires a decreased exercise protocol and/or stall rest for 2 to 6 months depending on degree of injury and response to treatment. Exercise is typically increased using straight lines and large circles as long as the patient is not showing clinical signs of pain. In the author's practice (DDF), the first line of therapy for collateral ligament damage is shockwave therapy: 200 to 400 pulses over the injured area. If clinical improvement is seen, the treatment is repeated until soundness is achieved or improvement ceases. If shockwave is refractory or if there is moderate to severe damage, intralesional treatment with bone-derived culture-expanded MSCs is used. Typically, 1 to 5 million MSCs are injected into the lesion based on either ultrasound guidance or radiographic positioning (diagnosis is typically via MRI in these cases) if the distal extent of the ligament is involved. Adjunctively the DIP joint is treated with 10 million MSCs with 20 mg of hyaluronic acid and 10 to 20 million MSCs administered via regional limb perfusion (total volume of 20 mL with a tourniquet in place for 20 to 30 minutes). As mentioned, MSC treatment is typically reserved for the refractory or moderate to severe cases but follow-up of 42 cases (B. Hague, personal communication, 2014), 21 of which had greater than 6 months' follow-up, resulted in 65% of the horses returning to their intended use without requiring further treatment for collateral ligament injury. In one study looking at the overall return to full athletic function following collateral ligament injury independent of treatment, 33 (47.8%) of 69 horses were considered successful (S. Dyson, unpublished data, 1980 to 2002). It is assumed that the patient population of the latter study was more diverse and had cases ranging from slight to severe. When osseous involvement is present, surgical intervention has been described but in the author's experience (DDF) this is not necessary. When joint instability or when radiographic OA is present, a more guarded prognosis should be expected.

PROXIMAL INTERPHALANGEAL JOINT

Christopher E. Kawcak, Myra F. Barrett

Anatomy

The proximal interphalangeal (PIP) joint, commonly referred to as the pastern joint, is susceptible to injury because of its small cross-sectional area (which tolerates a large vertical load) and the relative lack of soft tissue covering around the joint. It is a joint of relatively low motion and yet undergoes pathologic processes that are typical of high-motion joints. Many tendons and ligaments surround the joint; however, unlike most joints there is a smaller area around the joint at which synovial effusion can be appreciated. Many disease processes can occur in the PIP joint. Synovitis, capsulitis, osteochondral fragmentation, osteochondral fracture, and subchondral cystic lesions are common. Because of its distal location and relative lack of soft tissue covering, the PIP joint is also susceptible to laceration and contamination.

Accurate characterization of pain in the PIP joint can be difficult. The joint is located next to the area where a palmar digital nerve block is performed and the joint can often be desensitized with this block. There is some documentation that a palmar digital nerve block performed just proximal to the collateral cartilages of the foot is unlikely to block the PIP joint. Variability does exist, and there is a chance that a horse with PIP joint pain can improve with a palmar digital nerve block. IA administration of mepivacaine is usually the best technique for confirming pain in the joint; however, the block is usually performed in the palmar/plantar aspect of the joint near the neurovascular bundle, and extravasation of mepivacaine can occur, thus confusing the blocking pattern. Although a large number of pathologic processes in the PIP joint can be diagnosed with radiographs, ultrasound and volumetric imaging techniques are often needed to confirm or better characterize the disease process.

Imaging Parameters

Imaging of the PIP joint is often included in foot studies, as the images generally overlap. However, when the PIP joint is of specific interest, the best radiographic evaluation will include images specifically centered on the pastern joint.

Similarly, although the PIP joint is often included in high-field MRI of the equine foot, the MRI parameters can be modified when the PIP joint is of specific interest. For example, on proton density fat-saturated sequences (PDFS), it is not uncommon for there to be incomplete fat saturation of the more proximal portion of the scan and decreased resolution of the PIP joint, caused by changes in anatomic thickness from the hoof to the pastern region. This can be accounted for by either centering the PIP joint in the isocenter of the magnet or applying Play-Doh® to the palmar aspect of the pastern. Using Play-Doh creates a more uniform thickness and improves resolution of the PIP joint. CT evaluation more readily includes all of the anatomy and takes less time to acquire images than MRI. However, if a horse has asymmetry of the pastern, separate reconstructed images may sometimes be necessary for symmetric evaluation of the foot versus the pastern.

Ultrasound evaluation of the pastern varies. A "pastern" ultrasound is often confined to the soft tissue structures on the palmar aspect of the limb. However, a complete evaluation of the PIP joint should not only include the palmar structures, but also the entire periarticular margin, joint capsule, and collateral ligaments.

Osteoarthritis

Radiographically, OA in the PIP joint is generally first recognized by periarticular osteophyte formation. Osteophytosis of the dorsal proximal aspect of the middle phalanx is a common finding and is of variable clinical significance. Although osteophyte formation can be an early indicator of OA, small osteophytes in the absence of other indicators of joint disease, particularly in the hindlimb, can be an incidental or a relatively minor finding. The mechanism of OA in high-load, low-motion joints is different from that in high-motion joints.[9,10] In turn, the way in which OA is manifested radiographically in low-motion joints is somewhat different from high-motion joints. In low-motion joints, there is often greater periarticular osseous proliferation. With progressive joint disease, osteophytes increase in size, and there is increased periarticular new bone formation on the dorsal aspect of the joint. Often with more chronic disease, proliferative bone can be found

extending along the dorsal distal third of the proximal phalanx and proximal aspect of the middle phalanx, secondary to chronic synovitis and joint capsule enthesopathy (Figure 20-12A). Care must be taken when interpreting dorsopalmar/plantar (DP) radiographs with significant dorsal bone proliferation, as the superimposed bone can create a heterogeneous appearance that can give the false appearance of subchondral bone erosions, or mask true erosive or subchondral cystic lesion, or both (Figure 20-12B). Proliferative bone will also form on the medial and lateral aspects of the joint. Osteophyte formation can also occur on the palmar proximal aspect of the middle phalanx. The palmar distal diaphysis and metaphysis of the proximal phalanx can develop a scooped appearance caused by bone resorption secondary to chronic synovitis; in more severe cases, this can be seen on the dorsal aspect of the joint as well.

In addition to exhibiting greater proliferative bone, low-motion joints have a greater tendency to develop subchondral bone lysis secondary to OA than do high-motion joints. Thus, chronic advanced OA of the PIP joint can be manifested by focal or multifocal areas of subchondral lysis. This can found anywhere in the joint but is often most easily detected radiographically on the horizontal or 30° DP view. It is typically associated with adjacent subchondral bone sclerosis. Comparison of the symmetry of the subchondral bone on the medial and lateral halves of the joint can improve detection of more subtle subchondral sclerosis and lysis. The subchondral bone should be symmetric in thickness on the corresponding medial and lateral portions of the joint, and the articular margin should be well defined throughout the joint. By directly

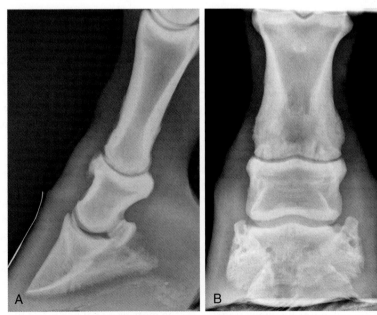

FIGURE 20-12 (**A**) Lateral view. Advanced osteoarthritic changes of the proximal interphalangeal (PIP) joint with marked osseous proliferation on the dorsal proximal aspect of the middle phalanx and scooped and undulating contour of the distal dorsal aspect of the proximal phalanx secondary to chronic synovitis. There is an ill-defined lucency in the palmar subchondral bone of the proximal phalanx. (**B**) Heterogeneous appearance of the proximal interphalangeal (PIP) joint space because of superimposition of the dorsal osseous proliferation.

comparing medial and lateral aspects of the joint, subtle differences are more readily identified.

Radiographic joint space narrowing of the PIP joint provides strong evidence of diffuse thinning or loss of articular cartilage. The width of the PIP joint should normally be thinner than the DIP and wider than the fetlock joint. A horizontal or 30 degrees DP radiograph that includes all three joints is the ideal image to assess the width of the PIP joint radiographically (Figure 20-13). Narrowing can occur on only one side of the joint or diffusely throughout. Joint space narrowing is typically accompanied by significant subchondral bone sclerosis and periarticular remodeling (Figure 20-14).

The use of MRI vastly enhances early detection of subchondral bone lysis and sclerosis as well as early articular cartilage loss in the absence of secondary osseous change.[11,12] Additionally, MRI allows for evaluation of abnormal osseous fluid signal (often referred to as bone marrow edema) in the subchondral bone, which can accompany cartilage damage.[13] Increased fluid in the subchondral bone of the PIP joint can also be seen as a precursor to more extensive subchondral lysis and subchondral cystic lesions that can develop when joint disease progresses.

Subchondral cystic lesions of the PIP joint are generally reported to occur in conjunction with advanced OA. However, the description of the changes seen in conjunction with advanced OA is a radiographic diagnosis. With the use of MRI and CT, subchondral cystic lesions can be detected before radiographic evidence of either a cystic lesion or OA changes. Both MRI and CT are more sensitive to detection of early subchondral cystic lesions than radiography, although the presence of fluid signal in the lesion on MRI can aid in detection of subtle lesions (Figure 20-15). Radiographically, subchondral cystic lesions in the PIP joint are often difficult to detect until there is more extensive bone damage and surrounding sclerosis. With chronicity and increasing severity and size of subchondral cystic lesions, the surrounding subchondral trabecular bone becomes progressively more sclerotic, enhancing the detection of bone abnormalities radiographically (Figure 20-16).

MRI is reportedly more sensitive at detecting osteophytes than radiography,[11] although small periarticular osteophytes can still be difficult to detect with MRI.[12] Including a T1 gradient echo (GRE) sequence can help to improve detection

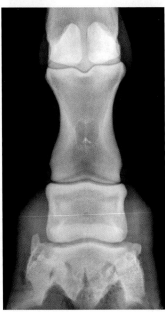

FIGURE 20-13 Horizontal dorsopalmar projection (DP) radiograph demonstrating the normal differences in width between the fetlock joint, proximal interphalangeal (PIP) joint, and distal interphalangeal (DIP) joint.

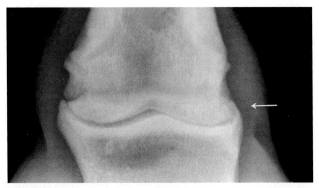

FIGURE 20-14 Cropped horizontal dorsopalmar projection (DP) radiograph showing marked diffuse narrowing of the medial aspect of the proximal interphalangeal joint (arrow) with marked bone sclerosis. There is also moderate narrowing, subchondral bone irregularity, and lysis of the lateral aspect of the joint. Periarticular remodeling is present medially and laterally.

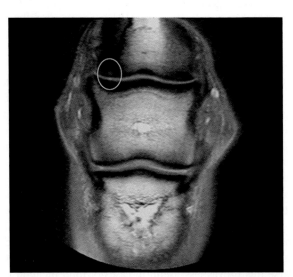

FIGURE 20-15 Dorsal plane proton density (PD)-weighted magnetic resonance image of the proximal interphalangeal joint. There is moderate subchondral sclerosis of the distal medial aspect of the proximal phalanx with a subtle area of subchondral lysis and focal cartilage loss (circle). Radiographs were within normal limits. The patient's lameness was resolved with intraarticular analgesia of the proximal interphalangeal (PIP) joint.

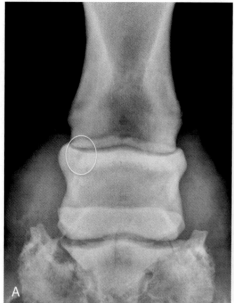
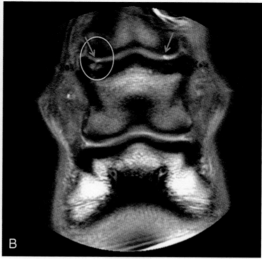

FIGURE 20-16 (A) D30P 30 degree dorsopalmar radiograph of the proximal interphalangeal joint. A focal lucency with surrounding subchondral bone sclerosis is in the proximal medial aspect of the middle phalanx. (B) Corresponding magnetic resonance image. Dorsal plane PD image. The corresponding subchondral osseous cystic lesions are noted as well as cartilage defects on both the medial and lateral aspect of the joint (arrows).

of osteophytes and other osseous proliferation because of increased contrast between soft tissues and bone when compared with PD and T2 fast spin echo (FSE) sequences. Ultrasound is also more sensitive in the detection of osseous proliferation, bone erosions, and osteophyte formation than radiography and even sometimes MRI.[14,15]

Ultrasonography is also a good means with which to assess joint capsule thickness, effusion, and synovial proliferation. In cases when a radiograph or MRI is equivocal, follow-up scanning with ultrasound is often useful to further investigate periarticular bone change, and it can improve interpretation of findings from other modalities.

CT provides excellent bone detail and will allow for detection of earlier subchondral bone erosions and osteophyte formation than radiography. Although CT is more limited in the evaluation of cartilage, contrast arthrography will improve evaluation of cartilage, however still not to a level that is commensurate with MRI.

Scintigraphic evaluation of OA of the PIP joint can be challenging because there are variable degrees of normal uptake in this joint depending on the patient's sport and level of activity. In particular, sport horses tend to exhibit more uptake, which is often incidental. Evaluating symmetry can help in identifying more mild changes in uptake, but of course this proves less useful in cases of mild bilateral OA. Radiography or other imaging is recommended to further evaluate areas of increased radiopharmaceutical uptake; bear in mind, however, that a normal radiograph does not exclude the presence of disease. Intraarticular analgesia can also be performed in cases in which there is scintigraphic uptake to confirm or deny this as a source of lameness.

The cause of insidious, progressive OA in the PIP joint is unknown. Unlike many other joints in the distal limb, this is a

low-motion joint. Repetitive trauma, especially in athletes, is thought to play a role and there is strong subjective evidence that subtle conformational abnormalities may predispose the horse to abnormal stresses within the PIP joint. As an example, both base-narrow and base-wide horses, whether toed in or toed out, are thought to be predisposed to OA of the PIP joint, although this is not definitive.[16] Asynchronous loading of the joint is thought to be the cause in horses with these conformations. Horses with upright pastern conformation are also thought to be predisposed to OA in the PIP joint. Horses that undergo significant loading of the hindlimbs, especially if twisting and turning are involved, are thought to be predisposed as well. Injury to the pastern area caused by external trauma may also predispose the joint not only to fracture and luxation but also to consequential OA in the future. Trauma, whether caused by internal stresses or external forces, may also cause bruising and edema within the subchondral bone, which can lead to joint pain.

Horses with pain in the PIP joint, which lack significant abnormalities on imaging, can often be treated effectively through a combination of IA medication and extracorporeal shockwave therapy. It appears that joint capsule disease is common in the PIP joint; therefore, extracorporeal shockwave therapy may help mitigate the pain that may arise from the joint capsule insertion in the bone. Topical antiinflammatory medication may also be useful, and some clinicians have advocated the administration of medication through regional venous profusion. Hoof and pastern conformations should be characterized using radiography and any abnormalities corrected so as to obtain optimum loading of the joint.

For advanced cases of OA of the PIP joint in which medical therapy is no longer effective, arthrodesis of the PIP joint is a viable option with the possibility of the horse returning to athletic use. Numerous surgical techniques have been advocated for arthrodesis of the PIP joint.

Facilitated ankylosis (without surgery) of the PIP joint has been advocated. Caston et al. have shown that in 34 horses, 50% were sound and 38% were improved after IA ethanol injection for facilitated ankylosis.[17] For this procedure, horses were sedated and an abaxial nerve block was performed. A palmar/plantar needle approach was used with the limb non-weight-bearing and radiographs and/or contrast materials were used to confirm needle placement; 70% ethyl alcohol was injected until the joint was felt to be pressurized. Stall rest was not recommended and the horses were either turned out or ridden if deemed comfortable enough. Horses with persistent lameness were reevaluated and reinjected 1 month after initial therapy.[17]

Laser-facilitated arthrodesis has also been used to a limited extent. A diode laser was used across the joint followed by three parallel 5.5-mm screws in lag fashion applied through stab incisions.[18] Five of six horses were sound and returned to intended use with this technique. This limited approach is thought to be less expensive and less painful than the standard open technique.

Surgical arthrodesis of the pastern is the most commonly used technique. The open approach, regardless of the implants used, best guarantees removal of articular cartilage, forage of subchondral bone, and complete reduction of the joint. Although several techniques are used, the authors prefer a single small dorsal plate with lateral and medial 5.5-mm transarticular screws placed in lag fashion. With this technique, horses need to be cast-immobilized for only 2 weeks and prognosis for return to soundness is good. Implant removal is not necessary, and those with hindlimb arthrodesis carry an excellent prognosis and those with forelimb arthrodesis carry a very good prognosis.[19]

Juvenile Subchondral Osseous Cystic Lesions

Subchondral osseous cystic lesions can be seen in both young horses with minimal or no evidence of OA and in mature horses with more advanced joint disease.[20,21] In young horses, these subchondral cystic lesions are easily detected radiographically on both lateral and DP views. As previously mentioned, they occur most frequently unilaterally in the distal condyle of the proximal phalanx and are most common in hindlimbs.[22] These cystic lesions can regress if seen originally in horses under 1 year of age; however, they have also been reported to develop in juvenile horses that have had normal radiographs at 6 months of age.[22] Typically, single cysts are of minimal clinical significance and often considered incidental. Multiple cysts seen in very young horses often occur in conjunction with osteoarthritic changes and are more likely to be associated with lameness.[21,23]

Subchondral cystic lesions of the PIP joint typically occur in younger horses, and often thickening in the pastern is appreciated. Lameness may or may not be present but the swelling around the pastern area necessitates further diagnostic work up. On occasion, lesions may be seen on routine presale radiographs of horses that may show no swelling or clinical signs of disease. Small cystic lesions on yearling films have been known to resolve or cause few problems, although many can manifest into clinically relevant disease. Subchondral cystic lesions are difficult to treat arthroscopically; in most cases a pastern arthrodesis is performed because it typically carries a good prognosis, especially in a young horse.

Collateral Ligament Desmopathy

Damage to the collateral ligaments of the PIP joint is not seen with nearly the frequency as desmopathy of the collateral ligaments of the DIP joint. Collateral ligament injury in the PIP joint is usually secondary to acute trauma. Avulsions can occur and more frequently affect the proximal attachment of the ligament. Radiographic indications of a collateral ligament injury include osseous irregularity or avulsion fragmentation at the site of the attachment of the collateral ligaments in the collateral fossa of proximal phalanx and adjacent soft tissue swelling. In more chronic cases, secondary osteoarthritic changes are often noted. Because of the tightness of the pastern joint capsule and the presence of other supporting ligaments (palmar axial and abaxial ligaments and medial and lateral portions of the collateral sesamoidean ligaments), stressed views to try to demonstrate joint instability are often unrewarding (Figure 20-17).

Ultrasound examination of the collateral ligaments of the PIP joint is readily performed. Occasionally the insertion of the ligament on the middle phalanx can be difficult to visualize in horses with short pasterns or with high or ossified ungual cartilages. The medial and lateral portions of the collateral sesamoidean ligament lie very close and just dorsal to the collateral ligaments and sometimes can be difficult to fully differentiate, both on ultrasound and MRI. Ultrasonographically, a damaged ligament will appear hypoechoic and thickened, with loss of normal fiber pattern. Avulsion fragments can be present. Adjacent soft tissue thickening is quite common. On MRI the ligament will typically demonstrate increased signal and diffuse thickening, although in some chronic cases the ligament will be low signal and thickened because of fibrosis.

Desmopathy of the collateral ligaments can sometimes occur in conjunction with injury to the collateral ligaments of the DIP joint.[24] In general this tends to be less severe than the damage seen secondary to trauma, and the clinical significance is uncertain. This is often best appreciated with MRI, although less subtle cases can also be detected with ultrasound.

PIP Joint Luxation

Luxation of the PIP joint is not uncommon and damage can occur to the joint capsule, collateral ligaments, and any of the tendons and ligaments around the joint. Luxation can occur most commonly in the dorsal direction and occasionally in the palmar/plantar direction.

Horses that undergo complete luxation are usually non-weight-bearing or at the very least lame at the walk and significant swelling is seen around the joint. Horses that undergo subluxation of the PIP joint may have less severe lameness and the lameness may not be apparent until the joint is flexed or manipulated.

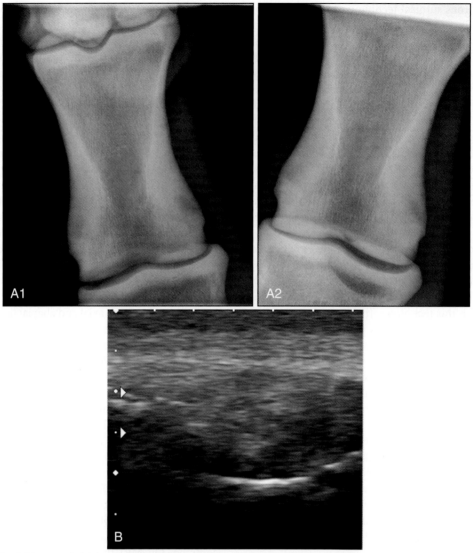

FIGURE 20-17 (A) Medial and lateral stressed view radiographs of the proximal interphalangeal (PIP) joint. There is no significant difference in joint space widening. (B) Ultrasound image of the lateral collateral ligament of the PIP joint. There is diffuse marked disruption of fibers and loss of normal echogenicity, consistent with severe damage to the lateral collateral ligament.

Diagnosis is confirmed using radiography. In some cases of subtle subluxation, stress views are needed to document the changes in the joint. In addition, characterization of soft tissue disease around the joint should be made using ultrasonography and/or volumetric imaging techniques such as MRI or CT.

Complete luxation of the PIP joint should be immediately treated through proper stabilization techniques of the lower limb. This would include use of a lower limb bandage with a dorsal splint that goes from toe to carpus. Any wounds should be addressed and contamination of the PIP joint or surrounding synovial structures such as the digital sheath should be confirmed. Surgical arthrodesis of the PIP joint is usually required to allow for horses to become athletically useful; however, the prognosis is not only dependent on the ability to stabilize the joint but also on the severity of soft tissue injury around the joint. Hence, soft tissue disease should be characterized to provide an accurate prognosis to the owner.

Osteochondral Fracture

Fractures of the first and second phalanx, in variable configurations can influence the PIP joint. Simple, uniaxial palmar/plantar eminence fractures can occur or one or both pastern bones could be shattered. The cause of these fractures may be either acutely traumatic in nature or because of repetitive loading and twisting, as is common in some disciplines of use.

Clinical signs of horses with osteochondral fracture in the PIP joint can vary from subtle to severe. Horses with uniaxial palmar/plantar eminence fractures may be relatively comfortable at the walk and yet show lameness at a trot. Horses with comminuted P2 or P1 fractures are non-weight-bearing with significant swelling and easily identifiable instability of the lower limb.

Radiographic imaging is usually sufficient to identify and characterize fractures, although CT is sometimes useful for presurgical planning to assist in repair.

Horses identified with osteochondral fracture of the PIP joint usually require immediate stabilization for transport and ultimate treatment. This includes the use of a lower limb splint, in which a PVC splint is applied over a lower limb bandage from the toe to the carpus/tarsus. The ultimate treatment of osteochondral fractures usually involves reduction and stabilization of the fracture in addition to arthrodesis. Although small fractures have been stabilized through lag screw fixation, in most instances arthrodesis is also performed since the likelihood of OA is high. Securing the eminence fractures into the arthrodesis construct is controversial. This author (CK) prefers to secure those pieces into the repair to enhance stability and prevent further abnormal stress to the ligaments and tendons in the palmar/plantar aspect of the joint. A single plate with two transarticular screws or two plates can be used depending on the surgeon's preference.

Comminuted fractures of the second phalanx can be repaired using internal fixation. In these cases two plates are necessary to stabilize the distal fragments and fuse the joint. External coaptation is necessary and the length of coaptation depends on the severity of the comminution and the stability of the repair. In most cases of comminuted fracture, the fractures will extend into the DIP joint. It is difficult if not impossible to realign and stabilize fracture lines within the DIP and this concern must be addressed when rendering a prognosis for repair of these fractures. Although most comminuted fractures can now be repaired using plates, on occasion an external fixator is needed in which transfixation pin casts are used because of the severity of comminution.

Fractures of the first phalanx emanating from the proximal aspect are quite common but progression into the distal aspect of the first phalanx and into PIP joint is relatively uncommon. The most concern with these fractures centers around the metacarpophalangeal and metatarsophalangeal joints. Rarely is the PIP joint of limitation to the prognosis, mainly because this area can be adequately reduced and stabilized using lag screws.

REFERENCES

1. Dyson SJ. The distal phalanx and distal interphalangeal joint. In: Ross MW, Dyson SJ, eds. *Diagnosis and management of lameness in the horse*. St. Louis, MO: Elsevier/Saunders; 2nd ed 2011:349–366.
2. McIlwraith CW, Nixon AJ, Wright IM. Arthroscopic surgery of the distal and proximal interphalangeal joints. In: McIlwraith CW, Nixon AJ, Wright IM, eds. *Diagnostic and surgical arthroscopy in the horse*. 4th ed. London, Elsevier; 2015:316–365.
3. Boening KJ. Arthroscopic surgery of the distal and proximal interphalangeal joints. *Clin Tech Equine Pract*. 2002;1(4):218–225.
4. Dechant JE, Trotter GW, Stashak TS, et al. Removal of large fragments of the extensor process of the distal phalanx via arthrotomy in horses: 14 cases (1992-1998). *J Am Vet Med Assoc*. 2000;217(9):1351–1355.
5. Ter Braake F. Arthroscopic removal of large fragments of the extensor process of the distal phalanx in 4 horses. *Equine Vet Educ*. 2005;17(2):101–105.
6. Story MR, Bramlage LR. Arthroscopic debridement of subchondral bone cysts in the distal phalanx of 11 horses (1994-2000). *Equine Vet J*. 2004;36(4):356–360.
7. Olive J. Distal interphalangeal articular cartilage assessment using low-field magnetic resonance imaging. *Vet Radiol Ultrasound*. 2010;51(3):259–266.
8. Watkins JP. Fractures of the middle phalanx. In: Nixon AJ, ed. *Equine fracture repair*. Philadelphia, PA: Saunders; 1996:129–145.
9. McIlwraith CW, Vachon A. Review of pathogenesis and treatment of degenerative joint disease. *Equine Vet J Suppl*. 1988;(6):3–11.
10. Kidd JA, Fuller C, Barr ARS. Osteoarthritis in the horse. *Equine Vet Educ*. 2001;13(3):160–168.
11. Conaghan PG, Felson D, Gold G, et al. MRI and non-cartilaginous structures in knee osteoarthritis. *Osteoarthritis Cartilage*. 2006;14(Suppl A):A87–A94.
12. Kornaat PR, Ceulemans RYT, Kroon HM, et al. MRI assessment of knee osteoarthritis: Knee Osteoarthritis Scoring System (KOSS)—inter-observer and intra-observer reproducibility of a compartment-based scoring system. *Skeletal Radiol*. 2005;34:95–102.
13. Link TM, Steinbach LS, Ghosh S, et al. Osteoarthritis: MR imaging findings in different stages of disease and correlation with clinical findings. *Radiology*. 2003;226(2):373–381.
14. Mathiessen A, Haugen IK, Slatkowsky-Christensen B, et al. Ultrasonographic assessment of osteophytes in 127 patients with hand osteoarthritis: exploring reliability and associations with MRI, radiographs and clinical joint. *Ann Rheum Dis*. 2013;72(1):51–56.
15. Wakefield RJ, Gibbon WW, Conaghan PG, et al. The value of sonography in the detection of bone erosions in patients with rheumatoid arthritis: a comparison with conventional radiography. *Arthritis Rheum*. 2000;43(12):2762–2770.
16. Baxter GM, Stashak TS. In: Baxter GM, ed. *Adam's and Stashak's lameness in horses*. 6th ed. London, UK: Blackwell Publishing; 2011:559.
17. Caston S, McClure S, Beug J, et al. Retrospective evaluation of facilitated pastern ankylosis using intra-articular ethanol injections: 34 cases (2006-2012). *Equine Vet J*. 2013;45(4):442–447.
18. Watts AE, Fortier LA, Nixon AJ, et al. A technique for laser facilitated equine pastern arthrodesis using parallel screws inserted in lag fashion. *Vet Surg*. 2010;39(2):244–253.
19. Knox PM, Watkins JP. Proximal interphalangeal joint arthrodesis using a combination plate-screw technique in 53 horses (1994-2003). *Equine Vet J*. 2006;38(6):538–542.
20. McIlwraith CW. Subchondral cystic lesions in the horse—the indications, methods and results of surgery. *Equine Vet Educ*. 1990;2(2):75–80.
21. Denoix JM, Jeffcott LB, McIlwraith CW, et al. A review of terminology for equine juvenile osteochondral conditions (JOCC) based on anatomical and functional considerations. *Vet J*. 2013;197(1):29–35.
22. Jacquet S, Robert C, Valette JP, et al. Evolution of radiological findings detected in the limbs of 321 young horses between the ages of 6 and 18 months. *Vet J*. 2013;197(1):58–64.
23. Sherlock C, Mair T. Osseous cyst-like lesions/subchondral bone cysts of the phalanges. *Equine Vet Educ*. 2011;23(4):191–204.
24. Murray R, Dyson S. The foot and pastern. In: Murray RC, ed. *Equine MRI*. Oxford, UK: Wiley-Blackwell; 2010:271–314.

21

Fetlock

Christopher E. Kawcak and Myra F. Barrett

ANATOMY

The fetlock joint (metacarpophalangeal/metatarsophalangeal joint) is a high motion joint with a small cross-sectional area and little soft tissue covering, which makes it predisposed to injury. When the ground reaction and muscle forces are taken into consideration, this joint undergoes five to seven times its body weight in stress. The joint is composed of the first phalanx, a pair of proximal sesamoid bones, and the distal aspect of the third metacarpus or metatarsus. There are two principal articulating surfaces, the first phalanx-metacarpus/metatarsus articulation and the proximal sesamoid bone-metacarpus/metatarsus articulation. These articulations function in unison to provide support to the metacarpophalangeal/metatarsophalangeal joint without true axial weight-bearing support. The support mechanism comes from the suspensory apparatus, which allows the joint to function normally.

Several disease processes can occur within the fetlock joint. Most of the injuries with athletic use are caused by repetitive loading, usually at the proximal sesamoid bone-metacarpus/metatarsus articulation. The suspensory apparatus is intimately involved with normal functioning of the fetlock joint and injury to this structure can result in significant fetlock joint disease. Although injuries in the fetlock joint are typical of most joint injuries (synovitis, capsulitis, osteochondral fragmentation, osteochondral fracture, luxation etc.), most injuries in the fetlock joint are caused by chronic fatigue injuries from repetitive loading of the joint that occur because of exercise. Therefore, this allows an opportunity to detect many of these injuries before physical damage occurs within the joint.

The fetlock joint is sensitive to injury and as such often manifests clinical signs that are often outwardly apparent. Synovial effusion is easily detectable in the dorsal and palmar/plantar aspects of the joint because of the easily palpable joint capsule in these locations. The fetlock joint has a large range of motion, which can be reduced with disease and can be painful during flexion. Because of limited soft tissue covering, synovial effusion, joint capsule thickening, tendon and ligament swelling, and soft tissue swelling are easily detected in this area. Disease of the subchondral bone in the fetlock joint is common; however, the clinical signs of this problem are usually not apparent unless the intra-articular environment is involved. Significant subchondral bone damage in the form of severe sclerosis, edema, bruising, or microdamage can occur, yet with little to no outward signs of joint effusion or swelling. In these cases, advanced diagnostic imaging such as nuclear scintigraphy or volumetric imaging using computed tomography (CT) or magnetic resonance imaging (MRI) are needed to best characterize the disease process. From a clinical standpoint, lameness due to subchondral bone disease may be apparent but usually will not improve with intraarticular analgesia. A low four-point nerve block or a lateral palmar/plantar nerve block is needed to alleviate the pain associated with such damage. Another complex characteristic of diagnosing fetlock joint disease is because of unusual blocking patterns. It is not uncommon for lesions in the proximal first phalanx joint surface to improve with a palmar digital nerve block. In addition, some lower limb lesions can be inadvertently blocked with intraarticular administration of mepivacaine, which may extravasate from the joint around the palmar/plantar nerves at the level of the fetlock joint. Therefore, care must be taken in interpreting these blocks as they could lead at times to misdiagnosis.

Osteochondral Fragmentation

The most common sites for osteochondral fragmentation to occur in the fetlock joint are on the proximal dorsal aspect of the first phalanx, the proximal palmar/plantar aspect of the first phalanx, and the proximal sesamoid bones.[1] Fragmentation can occur on the distal third metacarpal condyles; however, they are unusual in nature and are usually a response to some form of acute trauma. Osteochondral fragmentation in the fetlock joint is common in racehorses, especially Thoroughbreds; however, they can be seen in young horses and in these cases may be a manifestation of developmental orthopedic disease.[1-4]

Osteochondral fragmentation in the fetlock joint usually causes lameness and synovial effusion. However, some dorsal and palmar/plantar osteochondral fragments of the first phalanx in young horses do not induce clinical signs, but are detected on routine survey radiographs used for sale.

Diagnosis

Diagnosis of osteochondral fragmentation in the fetlock joint is routinely confirmed using radiography. For osteochondral fragmentation of the proximal sesamoid bones, ultrasound may be needed to characterize any associated lesions in suspensory ligament branches. More advanced diagnostic imaging such as nuclear scintigraphy or volumetric imaging is used to better characterize some cases of disease associated with fragmentation.

Treatment

Although joints with osteochondral fragmentation can be treated conservatively, definitive therapy is accomplished through arthroscopic removal of fragmentation.[1-4] The techniques for arthroscopic removal of fragmentation in the fetlock joint have been described[1] and will not be reviewed here. However, a consistent determinant of prognosis is the amount of articular cartilage damage within the joint. Partial and full thickness wear line and erosion formation of articular cartilage within the joint[3] will decrease the prognosis for return to successful athletic activity. More studies are needed to evaluate the efficacy of biologic therapies such as IRAP (Interleukin-1 Receptor Antagonist Protein), PRP (Platelet-rich Plasma, and mesenchymal stem cells on prognosis after removal of fragmentation.

Osteochondral Fracture

Osteochondral fractures, other than chip fragmentation of dorsal and palmar/plantar proximal phalanx, occur commonly in the fetlock joint in the first phalanx, third metacarpal/metatarsal bone, and proximal sesamoid bones. Although these fractures can be acute in nature, they are usually a result of chronic fatigue injury and accumulated damage. Cyclic fatigue loading can cause accumulation of microdamage and ultimately a complete fracture, causing clinical signs.

Clinical signs associated with osteochondral fracture are usually fairly significant; however, hairline fractures in the first phalanx and the distal third metacarpal/metatarsal condyles can induce subtle lameness, which requires advanced diagnostic imaging to fully characterize (Figure 21-1). Horses with incomplete fractures into the joint usually demonstrate synovial effusion, lameness, and positive response to flexion. Horses with complete fracture into the joint and out of the cortical bone or distal joints often have significant lameness, effusion, joint swelling, and pain on flexion. For these fractures routine radiography is usually used to characterize the injury.

Treatment

Subtle osteochondral fractures that can heal with conservative treatment may occur in the proximal dorsal aspect of P1 and in the distal third metacarpal/metatarsal condyles. These lesions are usually diagnosed with advanced imaging techniques such as nuclear scintigraphy or volumetric imaging and in some cases can respond well with 60 to 90 days of turnout. More advanced fractures that break into

the joint require lag screw fixation to reoppose the joint surface. This provides the best prognosis for healing and reduces the incidence of secondary osteoarthritis (OA). The management of these fractures is dealt with in detail in an arthroscopic surgery text.[1] For horses that are axially unstable, the limb should be stabilized in a Kimzey splint (for biaxial sesamoids fractures), bandage splint, or cast upon referral.

Fractures of the proximal sesamoid bone can be difficult to stabilize because of their inherently poor healing capability. Internal fixation in the form of lag screws is often preferred when fragmentation is too large to remove and athletic activity is sought. Circumferential wiring has been used but is unlikely to allow athletic activity in racehorses other than Standardbreds.

The prognosis for return to athletic use in horses with osteochondral fracture depends primarily on the amount of joint disruption and articular cartilage damage caused by the fractures. Meticulous realignment of the joint surface is needed to optimize joint health and return to athletic use.

Soft Tissue Injury

Any of the soft tissues within the fetlock joint can be injured. Synovitis and capsulitis are common as is injury to the collateral ligaments, intersesamoidean ligament, suspensory ligament branches, and distal sesamoidean ligaments. All these ligaments play a role in support of the fetlock joint and some of them communicate directly with the joint, injury of which causes clinical signs within the fetlock joint.

Diagnostic work-up of these cases is usually fairly straightforward in identifying pain within the joint; however, characterization of the injury using imaging techniques can be challenging. Radiographs are typically negative for identifying lesions within the joint; ultrasound can be useful but is usually best performed by an imager with significant experience. Volumetric imaging is the best technique for characterizing soft tissue lesions within the fetlock joint.

Treatment

The treatment of synovitis is best accomplished through intraarticular medication, which is described in Chapter 12. Because of its high motion nature, triamcinolone acetonide or betamethasone esters should be used in this joint rather than methylprednisolone acetate. The latter corticosteroid can lead to progressive damage to the articular cartilage and OA in the joint. Use of corticosteroids is covered separately in Chapter 12. Capsulitis is best treated through a combination of intraarticular medication and extracorporeal shockwave therapy (ESWT). These various treatment choices are detailed in Chapters 11 through 18. ESWT is best for treating joint capsule pain especially where the joint capsule inserts onto the bone. Tendon and ligament damage needs to be fully characterized to develop a treatment scheme for the structures. Biologic therapies are appropriate for these tissues, and their use is dictated by the site of injury, lesion characteristics, and access to the lesion (Chapter 16).

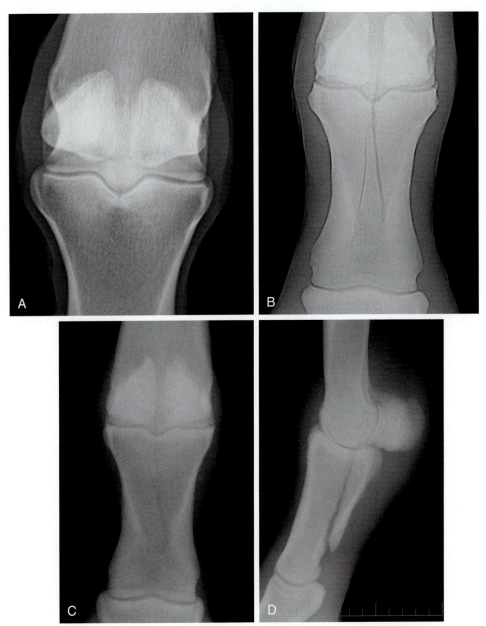

FIGURE 21-1 Fractures of proximal phalanx extending into the sagittal groove of the proximal phalanx. (A) Small "stress" fracture, (B) sagittal fracture extending distally for over half the distance of the proximal phalanx, (C) multiple fracture including a sagittal component (C) and a frontal component (D).

Subchondral Cystic Lesions

Subchondral cystic lesions can occur in the fetlock joint and are commonly seen on the weight-bearing surfaces of proximal phalanx and distal metacarpal/metatarsal condyles. These are typically developmental in nature, although recent cases have appeared to possibly be secondary to traumatic events. Injury to articular cartilage and underlying subchondral bone caused by high stress may be the cause.

If the cyst communicates with the joint, clinical signs of fetlock joint pain are similar to other diseases. However, for some subchondral cystic lesions lameness may be apparent without outward signs of fetlock joint disease. In these cases, diagnostic analgesia is needed to better characterize the site

of pain. As stated earlier for cystic lesions in the proximal first phalanx, lameness in these horses may improve with a palmar digital nerve block, thus becoming a diagnostic challenge. In these cases, advanced volumetric imaging is sometimes needed to best characterize the lesions.

The diagnosis of subchondral cystic lesions in the fetlock joint can usually be made using radiography; however, volumetric imaging techniques may sometimes be needed to best identify and characterize the disease.

Treatment

On occasion a subchondral cystic lesion may be an incidental finding and not lead to clinical disease. These are sometimes found on yearling radiographs made for sale. Most subchondral cystic lesions do lead to clinical disease and as such attempts are made to treat them. Conservative therapy using rest and intraarticular medication does not typically relieve the problem. If the cystic lesion can be reached arthroscopically, then cyst débridement is usually the most effective technique.[1] Refractory cases may be treated by osteostixis or osteochondral grafting.[5,6] Prognosis for return to performance for horses with third metacarpal subchondral cystic lesions is reported to be 80%.[6] Follow-up radiographs are necessary to update the prognosis based on healing of the cystic structure.

Osteochondritis Dissecans of the Fetlock Joint

Osteochondritis dissecans (OCD) is not uncommon in the fetlock joint, occurring on the sagittal ridge and condyles of the distal third metacarpus/metatarsus. Osteochondrosis-based fragments also occur on the proximal dorsal aspect of the proximal phalanx. Clinical signs are consistent with fetlock disease and care must be taken in assessing all four fetlock joints as it is not uncommon for this problem to be apparent in multiple fetlock joints. Radiographs are used to confirm the presence of the disease; however, clinical signs are not always apparent in horses that have radiographic appearance of lesions. These are most commonly encountered in radiographs of yearlings intended for sale. Sagittal ridge lesions can be one of three types. Type 1 OCD occurs when there is only flattening or defect on the sagittal ridge, type 2 OCD lesions occur when there is fragmentation within the area of flattening, and type 3 OCD is demonstrated by free or loose bodies within the joint.

Type 1 lesions are usually treated conservatively and clinical signs usually resolve.[7] Surgical débridement via arthroscopy is recommended for type 2 and type 3 lesions where fragmentation is present. Prognosis for type 1 lesions is good with conservative treatment but guarded for arthroscopic surgery needed for type 2 and type 3 lesions. Prognosis decreases with secondary signs of articular cartilage damage.

Traumatic Arthritis/Osteoarthritis of the Fetlock Joint

Osteoarthritis of the fetlock joint is common and can be insidious in onset and have no known causes. Known causes such as fragmentation, fracture, and luxation can ultimately lead to OA and treatments are aimed at preventing such a process. Insidious OA shows slow worsening of clinical signs including synovitis, capsulitis, reduced range of motion, and pain.

In athletes such as racehorses, the accumulation of damage over time likely leads to the insidious onset of OA. Progressive loss of articular cartilage can occur as can joint capsule fibrosis and limited range of motion. A wide spectrum of clinical signs can be apparent, and early signs include synovial effusion, reduced range of motion, and recurring lameness. However, it must be remembered that for disease processes that start within the subchondral bone, lameness may not be

associated with any outward signs of disease in the fetlock joint. These cases require more in-depth diagnostic work-up, as mentioned before. As the severity of disease worsens, synovial effusion will continue to be apparent but will be compounded by joint capsule thickening, soft tissue swelling, reduced range of motion (both passively and actively during movement), and pain.

Diagnosis of subtle injuries can be challenging and often require volumetric imaging to best characterize the pathologic process.

The treatment of OA depends on its stage of severity. Synovitis and capsulitis can be effectively treated through intraarticular medication and ESWT therapy. Mesenchymal stem cells are sometimes recommended at this stage to prevent worsening of articular cartilage damage. Their efficacy in preventing cartilage damage is unknown, but we have seen good results based on resolution of clinical symptoms. Proper hoof balance and joint alignment are necessary to minimize further abnormal forces on the joint.

For more advanced lesions, more continual therapy and strict management and oversight of exercise are often necessary to prolong the career and athletic ability of horses with fetlock OA. Occasionally diagnostic arthroscopy may be useful to débride cartilage lesions although this method of treatment is controversial. Use of stem cells may be needed, although efficacy correlated with severity of OA is unknown. In the most severe cases, fetlock arthrodesis may be needed to provide pain relief and prevent contralateral limb laminitis.

The prognosis for treating OA is mixed and dependent on joint damage severity, use of the horse, and expectations for the animal.

DIAGNOSTIC IMAGING OF THE EQUINE FETLOCK

Imaging Parameters

Radiographic evaluation is the most commonly performed diagnostic imaging modality for evaluating the fetlock joint. It is imperative that all five standard views (lateral, flexed lateral, dorso 15° to 30° palmar [DP], dorso 45° lateral-palmaromedial oblique [DLPMO], and dorso 45° medial-palmarolateral [DMPLO] oblique) be included for the most complete evaluation of possible changes in the joint (see Chapter 9). This includes a skyline image of the metacarpus improves detection of subchondral lysis and sclerosis of the dorsal metacarpal condyles. Angling distally on both the DP and oblique images elevates the sesamoid bones from the joint space and allows more accurate evaluation of the joint space and assessment of the subchondral bone. Improper positioning or excluding certain views can result in failure to detect relevant pathologic change. In particular, while obtaining a flexed lateral image on a young, untrained horse can be difficult, it is crucial that this view be included as this is often the only view that allows for detection of osteochondrosis defects of the sagittal ridge of the third metacarpal/tarsal bone.

Scintigraphy is a good screening tool for fetlock disease. Scintigraphic findings are typically followed up with radiographic evaluation and in some cases ultrasound or advanced imaging to better localize the areas of increased radiopharmaceutical uptake.

Ultrasound evaluation of the fetlock allows for evaluation of the periarticular soft tissues, dorsal articular cartilage, and osseous surfaces. A linear probe (8 to 12 mHz) can be used for the entire evaluation. A standoff pad is helpful for better conformation of the probe to the limb and for improved resolution of superficial structures. The skin on the dorsal aspect of the joint is typically thicker and can be callused, especially in horses that do not have deep stall bedding. Even in a horse that cannot be clipped, the area should be washed with warm water and coated in gel. Leaving the dorsal portion to the last part of the exam will allow the gel to soak in longer and should improve image quality. Often the probe frequency will need to be lowered to get adequate penetration of the dorsal aspect of the joint. The ultrasound examination should include both weight-bearing and non-weight-bearing images. Placing the dorsal aspect of the pastern on a farrier sling helps stabilize the limb, making the non-weight-bearing portion of the exam easier to perform.

Because of the limitations of radiography, advanced imaging can be quite valuable in evaluation of the pathologic changes of the fetlock joint. In particular, condylar damage is best assessed with advanced imaging, as radiography is not highly sensitive for condylar disease. When fractures are suspected, CT provides the best information for surgical planning. MRI allows for excellent evaluation of bone, articular cartilage, and soft tissue. Another advantage of advanced imaging is that the surrounding osseous and soft structures can be fully assessed as well, which is particularly useful in cases where the blocking pattern does not clearly show if the lameness is originating from intraarticular changes or adjacent structures, such as the digital sheath.

Osteochondrosis/Developmental Orthopedic Disease

Osteochondrosis is a common affliction of the fetlock joint and is most regularly manifested by osteochondral fragmentation. Osseous fragments can originate from the dorsoproximal aspect of the sagittal ridge, dorsoproximal aspect of the proximal phalanx, fragmentation or ununited palmar/plantar eminences of the proximal phalanx, and distal or proximal dorsal aspect of the proximal sesamoid bones.[8,9] Typically, radiographic diagnosis is sufficient for evaluation of these fragments. Palmar osteochondral fragments can occasionally be difficult to visualize because of superimposition and are often seen best on the lateral and occasionally flexed lateral view. Including proximal to distal oriented oblique images (dorsal 20 to 30 degrees, proximal 70 degrees, lateral-palmar distal medial oblique, and vice versa) can help determine laterality and improve visualization. Osteochondral fragments of the fetlock have been reported to both regress and develop up to 18 months of age.[10]

Ultrasound and MRI can be beneficial to determine the degree of involvement of the straight or cruciate sesamoidean ligaments in palmar/plantar fragmentation, as well as to try to determine whether a palmar fragment is intraarticular or not (Figure 21-2). Including a non-weight-bearing exam improves ultrasonographic evaluation of the distal palmar/plantar aspect of the fetlock, as this can be a difficult area to scan and the non-weight-bearing approach can improve access to the base of the fetlock. Resting the limb on a farrier sling can improve the ultrasound quality by minimizing the patient's movement and allowing a more comfortable position in which to perform the scan (Figure 21-3).

Subchondral lucencies, concavities, and osseous fragmentation can affect the sagittal ridge of the third metacarpal/metatarsal bone (Figure 21-4). Generally there is mild to moderate osseous sclerosis surrounding the defect. OCD lucencies of the distal aspect of the sagittal ridge are only visible on the flexed lateral image, which is why it is imperative that this be included in fetlock studies. It is a common normal radiographic variation to have a mild amount of smooth bone proliferation and/or a focal small concavity without adjacent sclerosis of the proximal dorsal aspect of the sagittal ridge, and this should not be confused with an osteochondrosis lesion.

Subchondral cystic lesions can occur in the distal metacarpus/tarsus and are generally radiographically apparent (Figure 21-5). If indicated, advanced imaging and/or ultrasound can be performed to determine whether there is articular involvement.

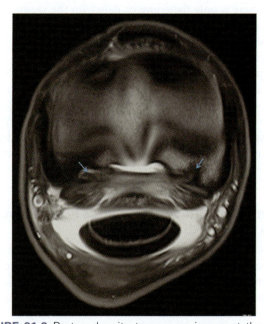

FIGURE 21-2 Proton density transverse image at the level of the fetlock joint in a 3-year-old Quarter horse. Biaxial osteochondral fragments are present on the medial and lateral palmar processes of the proximal phalanx (arrows). Although fragments are associated with the site of insertion of the cruciate and short sesamoidean ligaments, no significant ligamentous damage is present. There was no effusion of the fetlock joint. This patient had digital sheath effusion and a tear of the manica flexoria as well as degenerative changes of the navicular bone, which were considered the likely source of lameness.

Osteoarthritis

Osteoarthritic changes of the fetlock joint are not uncommon and can affect horses of many breeds and disciplines. Although known to be less sensitive in detecting degenerative changes in the joint compared with other modalities, radiography remains the typical first-line imaging modality for evaluation of the fetlock joint.

An early sign of joint disease, before development of osseous changes, is soft tissue swelling surrounding the joint. Although this can be caused by many factors external to the joint, including subcutaneous edema, suspensory ligament branch desmopathy, and digital sheath effusion, circumferential soft tissue swelling confined to the region of the joint visualized radiographically is most indicative of effusion and/or synovitis. Ultrasonography and MRI allow ready characterization of the degree of effusion and synovitis within the joint.[11,12] With chronic synovitis, palmar/plantar subchondral lysis occurs,[9,13] characterized by

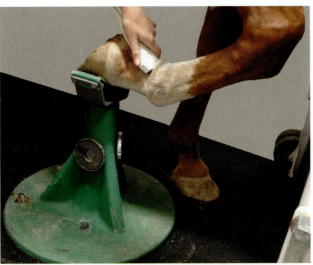

FIGURE 21-3 Resting the foot on a farrier sling helps to stabilize the limb, making the non-weight-bearing exam easier to perform. The probe is positioned for examining the palmar distal aspect of the joint and sesamoidean ligaments. This stand is helpful for examining the dorsal aspect of the joint as well.

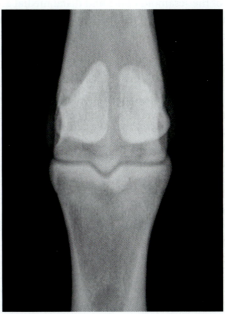

FIGURE 21-5 Subchondral cystic lesion in the distal metacarpus of a yearling Quarter horse found on a survey study. The horse did not exhibit lameness.

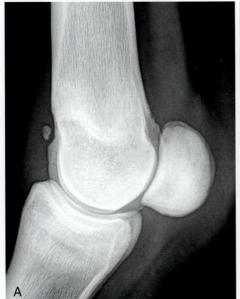

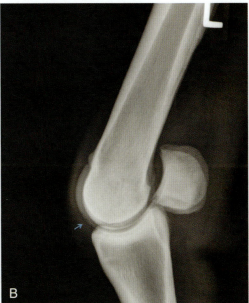

FIGURE 21-4 (A) Osteochondritis dissecans (OCD) type 2 lesion manifesting as a fragment at the proximal aspect of the sagittal ridge. (B) Flexed lateral view of the fetlock showing a concave defect and likely in situ fragment of the distal aspect of the sagittal ridge also consistent with an OCD lesion.

a smooth, scooped appearance just proximal to the MC/MT3 condyles (Figure 21-6). In more advanced cases, dorsal supracondylar lysis will occur as well. Although often a radiographic diagnosis, supracondylar lysis is readily evaluated with CT and MRI.

Periarticular osteophyte formation is generally one of the more obvious radiographic changes associated with OA. It is seen more frequently on the dorsal, dorsomedial, and dorsolateral aspects of the proximal phalanx,[9] followed by osteophytes on the dorsal distal and proximal articular margins of the sesamoid bones and distal medial and lateral aspects of the third metacarpal/tarsal bone. Articular cartilage degeneration generally first affects the dorsal aspect of the proximal phalanx, which is likely why osteophytes are often seen in this location earlier in the osteoarthritic process.[14] In some cases, the oblique views provide better evaluation of the dorsal periarticular osteophyte formation than the lateral view, as the osteophytes are generally located dorsomedially or dorsolaterally (Figure 21-7). Laterally and medially located osteophytes of the distal third metacarpal/tarsal bone and medial and lateral aspects of the proximal phalanx are best appreciated on the DP view. CT and MRI are superior to radiography in detection of osteophyte formation.[11,15]

Other radiographic findings associated with fetlock OA include subchondral bone sclerosis, flattening of the palmar/plantar aspect of the condyles, joint space narrowing, and joint capsule enthesopathy. Joint space narrowing can be seen diffusely throughout the joint or can be primarily located on the medial or lateral aspect and indicates severe diffuse loss of articular cartilage. Joint space narrowing is almost always accompanied by subchondral bone sclerosis and often subchondral lysis as well. The horse should be standing squarely

and bearing weight evenly to accurately assess the joint width radiographically.

Ultrasonographic evaluation of the osteoarthritic joint is useful for evaluation of periarticular osteophyte formation, osseous proliferation, and soft tissue assessment. The articular cartilage on the dorsal aspect of the joint can also be evaluated. Flexing the joint allows for greater visualization of the dorsal cartilage. Long-axis and transverse plane images of the dorsal sagittal ridge and dorsal condyles should be included. Care must be taken to avoid oblique transverse images, because if the image is accidentally obtained too proximally it can create the artificial appearance of cartilage thinning on one aspect of the joint. This dorsal approach also allows for concurrent evaluation of the dorsal joint capsule thickness and synovial pad.

Advanced imaging is superior to radiography and ultrasonography for evaluation of early or less severe osteoarthritic changes. Detection of periarticular osteophytosis, subchondral bone sclerosis, and lysis of the equine fetlock joint is improved using CT and MRI.[11,16] Additionally, MRI provides the best modality for evaluation of damage to the articular cartilage. The articular cartilage of the fetlock joint is thin, resulting in greater diagnostic difficulty in lesion assessment. The reliability of assessing articular cartilage using MRI will vary with multiple factors, including magnetic field strength, sequence selection, slice thickness, and other imaging parameters.[17,18] Low-field-strength magnets (≤0.3 T) and even the lower strength high-field magnets (1 T) are inferior to higher field strength for assessment of pathologic change to the articular cartilage of the fetlock joint.[16,18] The best sequences for evaluating cartilage

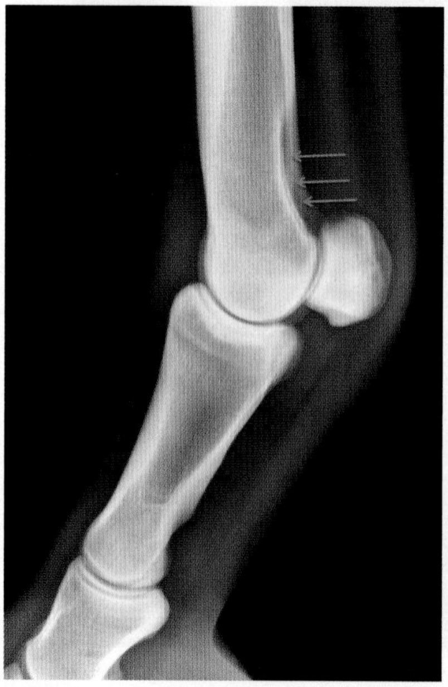

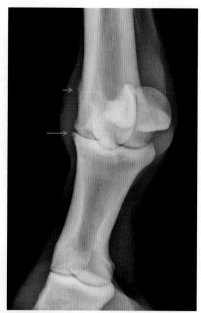

FIGURE 21-6 Palmar supracondylar lysis of the third metacarpal bone. This occurs secondary to chronic synovitis resulting in pressure resorption of the bone.

FIGURE 21-7 DLMPO view of the fetlock. A moderate periarticular osteophyte affects the dorsomedial aspect of the proximal phalanx (long arrow). Irregular bone formation on the distal aspect of the third metacarpal bone is consistent with chronic joint capsule enthesopathy. There is soft tissue swelling secondary to joint effusion.

damage are still being debated, but typically fat-saturated proton density (PDFS) and spoiled gradient echo (SPGR) sequences are the most frequently used. Including both in a study can improve lesion detection. Additionally, the use of three-dimensional fast spin echo sequences, which allow for submillimeter slice thickness and image reconstruction in any plane, may further enhance detection of subtle or thin longitudinal cartilage injuries. Further research specific to the equine fetlock joint is needed to substantiate this clinical impression. Using specialized dorsal oblique images that are tangential to the condyles can also improve lesion evaluation (Figure 21-8).

Damage to the articular cartilage can be seen at multiple sites within the joint, but it occurs most frequently in the mid-to-palmar aspect of the medial and lateral condyles of MC/MT3 and on the dorsal aspect of the proximal phalanx.[14,19] These lesions are most frequently identified on sagittal and dorsal plane images. The transverse sequence should not be overlooked; it is particularly useful for identification of cartilage and subchondral bone damage on the dorsal aspect of the condyles and sagittal ridge (Figure 21-9). Although reported less commonly, pathologic change dorsal to the midportion of the metacarpal condyles is not uncommon in sport horses and Western performance horses and should not be overlooked.[20,21]

Sensitivity of high-field MRI for detection of cartilage damage in the fetlock when compared with histopathologic analysis has been reported as moderate.[17,22] CT arthrography is another option for evaluation of articular cartilage, although its reported effectiveness in the equine fetlock has been variable and deserves further research.[16,22]

The presence of concurrent subchondral bone sclerosis, lysis, or bone edema can improve detection of cartilage damage by helping identify an area of pathologic change. In low-field MRI, direct evaluation of the articular cartilage is limited, but can sometimes be inferred by the surrounding subchondral bone damage, which is more readily assessed.[23]

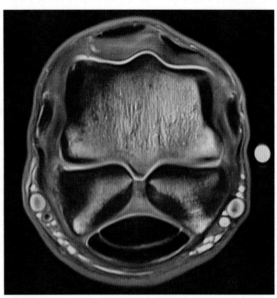

FIGURE 21-9 Transverse proton density image of the distal metacarpus. The dorsal medial condyle is sclerotic and there is a focal defect in the subchondral bone of the dorsal articular surface (arrow).

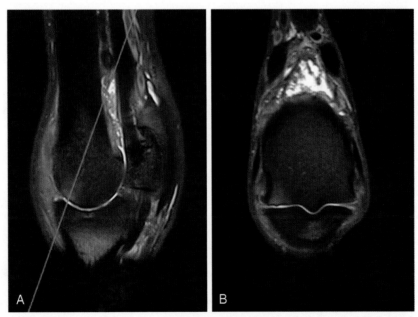

FIGURE 21-8 Sagittal (**A**) and dorsal oblique (**B**) proton-density, fat-saturated 3-dimensional FSE images of the fetlock. The line on the sagittal view indicates the plane of the oblique dorsal image. There is diffuse subchondral bone and cartilage damage throughout the joint. The obliquely oriented dorsal image is tangential to a defect on the dorsal medial condyle of the third metacarpal bone, which improves evaluation of this specific lesion. There is bone-edema-like signal of the condyle adjacent to the defect. A marked amount of soft tissue thickening and synovitis affects the joint and there is palmar supracondylar lysis.

Nuclear scintigraphy can also be a useful tool for identifying OA of the fetlock joint, although the results are not always easy to interpret, particularly in sport horses. Variable amounts of normal uptake can be seen in athletic horses and this must be differentiated from pathologic bone turnover. Additionally, mild OA may not result in increased radiopharmaceutical uptake (IRU).[24] Comparison of left and right can be helpful, although it is not uncommon for OA to be bilateral. If uptake is noted on the dorsal aspect of the joint, including a flexed lateral image can help differentiate dorsal condylar uptake from the proximal dorsal aspect of the proximal phalanx.

Distal Metacarpus/Metatarsus

Palmar/Plantar Osteochondral Disease, Osseous Stress Remodeling, and Fracture

Palmar/plantar osteochondral disease (POD) frequently affects racehorses, but can be seen in horses of other disciplines as well. Radiographs are frequently unreliable in diagnosing this disease. This is in part because of the degree of bone change that must occur to be detected radiographically as well as to the limited ability to obtain radiographs that isolate the condyles with minimal superimposition. Special views including a flexed dorsopalmar, and a 125° dorso-palmar view and metacarpal skyline view can improve visualization of the parasagittal groove and weight-bearing portion of the condyle,[25,26] thereby improving the likelihood of detecting nondisplaced condylar fractures. Additionally, the lateral 45° proximo-distal medial oblique (and opposite oblique) views improve visualization of the palmar condyles.

However, despite the use of these views, evaluation of this area is limited, and therefore the use of other imaging modalities is warranted when the radiographic findings are negative or equivocal.

When visualized, radiographic signs of POD include condylar sclerosis and flattening of the palmar/plantar condyles. Occasionally a central area of lucency with surrounding sclerosis is observed. This lucency can occur secondary to focal cartilage collapse and subsequent subchondral bone necrosis.[27] Condylar fractures can originate from the parasagittal groove or extend abaxially from the groove. Lateral condylar fractures are more commonly seen and tend to exit the lateral cortex in an oblique fashion.[28,29] Medial condylar fractures are more likely to spiral proximally; therefore, including radiographs of the entire metacarpus/metatarsus is necessary for complete evaluation.

Nuclear scintigraphy is frequently employed for evaluating condylar disease, particularly in racehorses. Scintigraphy is widely available and an excellent screening tool for stress fractures and condylar disease. It is of particular value in identifying radiographically occult osseous pathologic change. Because of the high amount of subchondral stress remodeling that occurs,[30,31] uptake is frequently seen in the condyles of racehorses, and IRU caused by adaptive remodeling must be distinguished from pathologic subchondral bone damage (Figure 21-10). Uptake is noted most frequently medially or biaxially in the palmar condyles of the forelimbs and laterally in the plantar condyles of the hind limbs.[31-33] Moderate to marked increased uptake has been associated with poorer performance outcome in racing Thoroughbreds

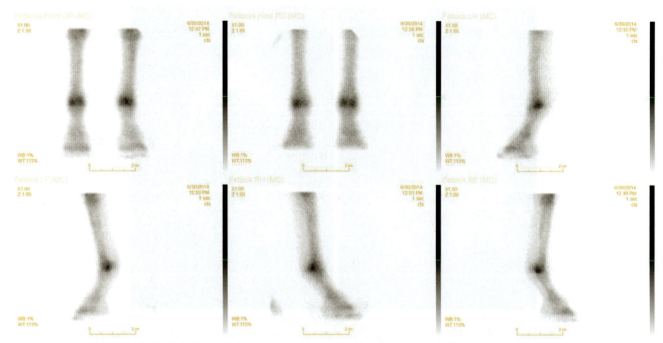

FIGURE 21-10 Scintigraphic images of all four fetlocks of a 3-year-old Thoroughbred colt with a short choppy gait and bilateral hind limb lameness that improves to a lateral plantar metatarsal nerve block. Radiographs were unremarkable. There is significant increased radiopharmaceutical uptake affecting the palmar/plantar condyles of all four fetlock joints. (Images courtesy of Dr. Michael Ross, University of Pennsylvania New Bolton Center.)

and Standardbreds.[32,33] Although a good screening tool for stress fractures, a distinct, discrete linear IRU to distinguish a lateral condylar fracture may not always be visualized with scintigraphy,[33,34] likely because of the concurrent adjacent bone remodeling and edema resulting in more diffuse uptake. Flexed dorsal images may help differentiate a fracture.[34] Recognizing abnormal uptake and allowing for appropriate management may help prevent the development of more substantial osseous damage.

CT and MRI provide the greatest anatomic and diagnostic details of the fetlock joint. If a fracture is suspected, general anesthesia may be contraindicated unless the situation is such that the patient can directly undergo surgical repair if necessary following the imaging study. CT provides excellent bone detail and can much more completely characterize the extent and severity of a condylar fracture.[35] Additionally, CT has been shown to provide superior trabecular bone detail, allowing for more comprehensive evaluation of subchondral stress remodeling. Quantitative CT has shown good correlation with bone density measurement in the distal metacarpus.[36] MRI also allows for evaluation of bone sclerosis, which is hypointense on all sequences, as well as focal bone edema-like signal in the areas of subchondral necrosis as part of the manifestation of POD. Additionally, with high-field MRI the degree of involvement of articular cartilage can be evaluated. Low-field standing MRI has also proven useful in evaluation of injuries associated with the fetlock joint in racehorses.[23] Standing MRI can help detect early condylar fissures or fractures without the risk of general anesthesia. These lesions are often surrounded by a significant amount of bone marrow edema-like signal.[23] Both low- and high-field MRI is useful for evaluation of concurrent soft tissue injury.

Proximal Phalangeal Fractures and Traumatic Fragmentation

Similar to other stress-related bone injuries, articular proximal phalangeal fractures and fragmentation are more common in racehorses, but they can occur in other disciplines as well. The most common injury is traumatic fragmentation of the dorsal proximal aspect of the proximal phalanx secondary to chronic bone stress secondary to hyperextension.[9,37] The fragments most commonly occur on the dorsomedial aspect of the joint. These fragments are typically readily identified radiographically and the oblique and/or DP views can be used to determine laterality. Further imaging is usually not required. Ultrasonography and/or MRI can be performed if indicated to evaluate for concurrent cartilage damage and evaluate the adjacent soft tissues.

Fractures can occur in a variety of configurations, with short, nondisplaced midsagittal fractures most common.[38,39] Other forms of sagittal fractures, dorsal plane fractures, and palmar/plantar eminence fractures also occur. Nondisplaced midsagittal fractures or fissures may be radiographically occult, or a faint linear lucency may be visualized extending distally from the sagittal groove on the DP radiograph. Fractures in this location will exhibit marked IRU which can then be compared with the radiographic evaluation.[40] On MRI, the linear hyperintense fracture line is often surrounded by bone marrow edema-like signal, and concurrent injuries of the distal metacarpus can occur.[40] Including a T1 gradient echo sequence can help improve fracture detection. However, in some cases a distinct fracture line is not visualized and only a small fissure with an associated articular cartilage defect and bone marrow edema-like signal is noted. These more subtle injuries typically will be best seen on fat-saturated fast spin echo sequences (Figure 21-11).

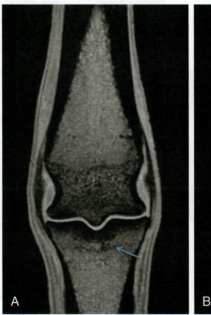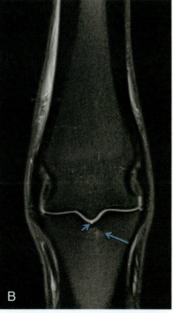

FIGURE 21-11 Dorsal VIBE **(A)** and PD three-dimensional fat-saturated fast spin echo sequence (FSE) **(B)**. On the PD three-dimensional FSE, a small, hyperintense fissure is present in the articular cartilage of the proximal phalanx (short arrow). There is mild bone edema in the subchondral trabecular l bone adjacent to the defect (long arrow). The articular cartilage defect is not visible on the VIBE image. The area of bone edema is seen as an area of low signal (arrow).

Even in cases in which the fracture line can be clearly visualized radiographically, CT can be helpful to further characterize the fracture before fixation. Simple fractures that have a somewhat curved configuration can create the artifactual radiographic appearance of multiple fracture lines (Figure 21-12), and conversely, radiographs can underestimate the extent of a comminuted fracture.

Proximal Sesamoid Bones

Injuries to the proximal sesamoid bones (PSB) include sesamoiditis, fracture, enthesopathy, and avulsion fragmentation. The definition of sesamoiditis is variable within the literature; however, radiographic findings commonly associated with sesamoiditis include dilated or rounded vascular channels, non-parallel vascular channels, lucencies, and bone production on the abaxial margin of the sesamoid bones.[41,42] The clinical relevance of such findings is contentious. Whether these lesions are active or not can be further assessed with nuclear scintigraphy. When evaluating the PSB scintigraphically, it is important to ensure that the horse is standing squarely. This is a particularly common issue in the hind limbs, where if a horse is standing toed-out, the lateral sesamoid will be closer to the gamma camera and will artifactually appear to have great IRU. Additionally, on MRI bone marrow edema-like signal can be seen in association with what are likely to be more active cases of sesamoiditis.

Fractures of the PSB are typically well visualized on standard radiographs, although including a lateral 45 degrees proximal-distal medial oblique (and vice versa) can improve visualization of PSB with decreased superimposition. Although the osseous damage is well characterized

radiographically, including an ultrasound exam before surgical fixation is very helpful for assessing the extent of soft tissue involvement as well as the degree of articular involvement. What may seem straightforward radiographically can actually be surprising in the exact extent and synovial and soft tissue involvement of the fracture fragment. Apical sesamoid fractures can result in damage to the suspensory ligament branches (Figure 21-13), and basilar sesamoid fractures can

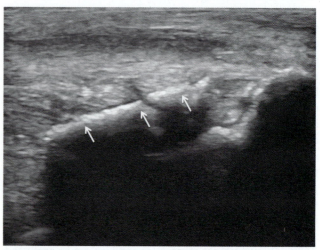

FIGURE 21-13 Long-axis ultrasound image of the insertion of the medial suspensory ligament branch on the sesamoid bone. Proximal is to the left. There is an apical sesamoid fracture that is displaced from the parent bone (arrows), resulting in marked disruption of the ligamentous fibers. The periarticular soft tissues are thickened and edematous.

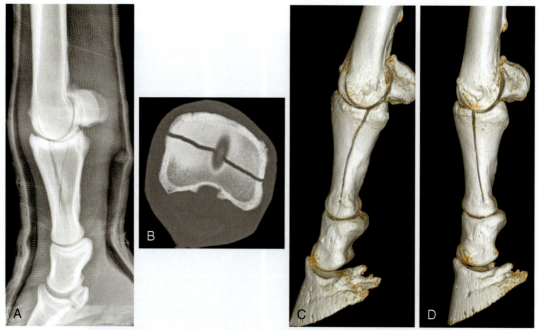

FIGURE 21-12 (A) Lateral radiograph of the fetlock with a cast in place. Multiple oblique fracture lines are present. The fracture is articular. Osteoarthritic changes are present in the fetlock joint. (B) Transverse CT and reconstructed three-dimensional CT images show that there is only a single, dorsal plane fracture line (C,D). Superimposition on the lateral radiograph creates the appearance of multiple fractures. The CT shows best the marked sclerosis of the proximal phalanx and periosteal proliferation and remodeling.

affect the straight, oblique, short, and cruciate sesamoidean ligament, depending on fracture location. Additionally, fractures that extend through the axial body of the sesamoid can result in disruption of the intersesamoidean ligament fibers (Figure 21-14). Including a non-weight-bearing exam will improve visualization of the base of the PSB.

Common abnormalities of the PSB noted on MRI include sclerosis, bone marrow edema-like signal, which can be either focal or diffuse, and enthesopathies. Enthesopathies can appear as focal areas of high signal, bone resorption, and bone proliferation and can affect the insertions of the suspensory ligament branches, distal sesamoidean ligaments, palmar/plantar annular ligament, and intersesamoidean ligament. Ligamentous tissue and cortical bone are both relatively low signal on fast spin echo sequences, which results in minimal contrast difference between the structures. Including a T1 GRE sequence can help delineate the interface between soft tissue and bone, improving recognition of pathologic change at these locations. Osteochondral damage of the palmar/plantar condyles can also result in adjacent articular cartilage and subchondral bone damage of the articular surface of the sesamoid bones, which is usually best appreciated on transverse images.

Periarticular Soft Tissues

Radiography can provide indirect evidence of soft tissue injury surrounding the fetlock joint. Direct evaluation of the periarticular soft tissues of the fetlock joint is most frequently performed using ultrasonography. Ultrasonography is often sufficient for detection of soft tissue lesions in this region, although MRI is excellent for evaluation of soft tissues and can be particularly useful in diagnosing more subtle cases of soft tissue injury. CT can be used as well, although the soft tissue detail is not ideal. Soft tissue phase nuclear scintigraphy can also be helpful to evaluate active injuries. Included structures that should be examined during a diagnostic scan of the fetlock include suspensory ligament branches, sesamoidean ligaments (straight, oblique, cruciate, and short), intersesamoidean (palmar/plantar) ligament, collateral ligaments, and joint capsule.

Suspensory ligament branch injuries are common and can affect many different breeds and disciplines. In performance horses, it is not uncommon to see chronic, mild changes to the ligament, generally characterized by a coarse fiber pattern, areas of mild alteration in echogenicity, possible thickening, and mild enthesopathy on ultrasound examination. These finding are often incidental and although they should not be overlooked, they should also not be overemphasized as significant pathologic changes unless there are concurrent clinical exam findings to support the diagnosis. Areas of discrete fiber tearing, moderate or marked enlargement with or without periligamentous thickening, moderate to severe enthesopathy, and avulsion fragments are common ultrasonographic findings that are more typically associated with lameness referable to this region. Evaluation of the chronicity of suspensory ligament branch changes is challenging because they generally do not regain a completely normal ultrasonographic

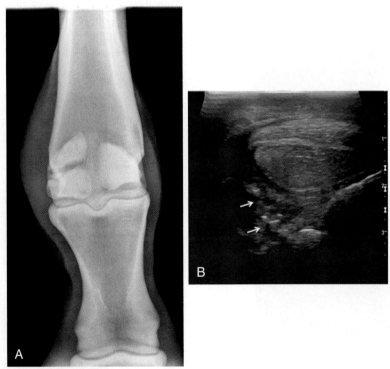

FIGURE 21-14 **(A)** DP radiograph of the left hind fetlock. A comminuted, transverse fracture extends through the lateral sesamoid bone. There is significant associated soft tissue swelling. **(B)** Ultrasound evaluation of the same horse: the transverse image at palmar axial surface of the sesamoid bones reveals marked osseous disruption of the lateral sesamoid bone with extensive fiber damage of the lateral aspect of the intersesamoidean ligament.

appearance after an injury, even once the injury has resolved clinically. Therefore, serial ultrasound examinations can be helpful to better stage the chronicity of a suspensory branch lesion. General indicators of a chronic lesion include periligamentous proliferative tissue, areas of hyperechogenicity within the ligament consistent with fibrosis, and dystrophic mineralization. Rounded avulsion fragments surrounded by fibrous tissue are typically chronic as well. Soft tissue phase nuclear scintigraphy can also be performed to help identify active cases of suspensory ligament branch desmopathy.

When evaluating tearing of the suspensory ligament branch, be it with ultrasonography or MRI, it is important to carefully evaluate the orientation and location of the tear. Tears that extend to the dorsal margin of the ligament can communicate with the fetlock joint (Figure 21-15). Lameness caused by this type of tearing may be improved or abolished with intraarticular analgesia of the fetlock joint. If there is associated effusion of the fetlock joint, joint fluid can be seen not only on the dorsal and axial margin of the suspensory ligament branch, but also, with more extensive effusion, palmar/plantar to the ligament as well. Although this is readily distinguished from digital sheath effusion on MRI, differentiation of digital sheath fluid from fetlock fluid located palmar/plantar to the branches can be more challenging with ultrasound.

Radiographically, the presence of osseous fragments at the palmar aspect of the fetlock joint originating from the distal aspect of the PSB and/or palmar proximal phalanx can be indirect indictors of damage or avulsion of the distal sesamoidean ligaments. More abaxially located PSB fragments are more likely to affect the oblique sesamoidean ligaments; whereas, more axially located fragments are more likely to affect the straight sesamoidean ligaments. Avulsion fragmentation of the axial aspect of the palmar processes of the proximal phalanx is associated with insertion of the short and cruciate sesamoidean ligaments and is of variable clinical significance.

Damage to the proximal aspect of the oblique sesamoidean ligaments in the absence of associated osseous abnormalities is often manifested by enlargement of the ligament and alteration of echogenicity or signal intensity. Normally the oblique sesamoidean ligaments have a mildly mixed echogenicity ultrasonographically, and their MRI appearance is characterized by hyperintense striations admixed with low-signal tissue. This normal mixed signal can make diagnosing subtle lesions more challenging and can lead to overinterpretation of mild changes. Comparing left and right sides is helpful for identifying more mild changes in size and fiber damage. Injuries to the oblique sesamoidean ligaments occur more frequently in the hind limbs.[43,44]

Pathologic change of the proximal aspect of the straight sesamoidean ligament can be difficult to identify ultrasonographically because of the difficulty in imaging the base of the fetlock and to the normal mild variability in echogenicity and shape. Including a non-weight-bearing approach can help, as can extending the limb caudally to open up the base of the fetlock. Damage to the straight sesamoidean ligament can be seen as increase in size, diffuse fiber damage, and focal, discrete tears. MRI is often useful for the diagnosis of these injuries, which are often underdiagnosed using ultrasound.[20,45,46] The straight sesamoidean ligament originates from the base of the sesamoid bones as well as intersesamoidean ligament.[43] Because of this relationship, it is possible to see tearing of the proximal aspect of the straight sesamoidean ligament to be confluent with the intersesamoidean ligament (Figure 21-16).

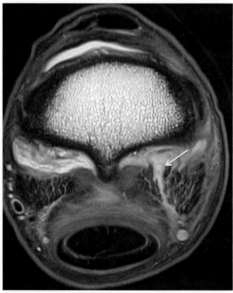

FIGURE 21-15 Proton density transverse image of the distal aspect of the suspensory ligament branches. A complete sagittally oriented tear affects the medial suspensory ligament branch. The tear communicates with the palmar recess of the fetlock joint. There is periligamentous thickening surrounding the branch. The joint is effusive with synovial proliferation and palmar supracondylar lysis of the third metacarpal bone.

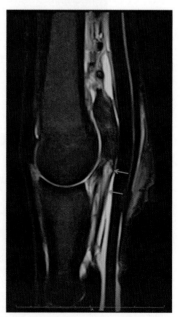

FIGURE 21-16 Sagittal STIR image. There is high-signal fiber tearing (arrows) of the straight sesamoidean ligament extending to the junction with the intersesamoidean ligament.

Tearing of the intersesamoidean ligament is generally seen in conjunction with fractures or osteomyelitis of the sesamoid bones.[47] However, this assumption may be somewhat skewed by the fact that diagnosis of intersesamoidean ligament desmopathy in the absence of associated osseous pathology can be challenging. Radiographically, irregular osseous margins and osteolysis of the axial borders of the sesamoid bones or transverse fractures can be indicators of intersesamoidean ligament damage. These changes are often best seen on the DP view of the fetlock and can be associated with osteomyelitis as well as nonseptic processes.[48] Ultrasonographically, damage to the intersesamoidean ligament is characterized by hypoechoic fiber disruption, often in conjunction with osseous lysis or irregularity of sesamoid bones. In chronic cases, increased echogenicity caused by fibrosis or mineralization can be seen. Diffuse thinning and even complete rupture have also been reported.[49] CT can be a valuable resource for more detailed assessment of the osseous changes of the PSB as well as evaluation of the soft tissues.

MRI is often the best modality to assess more subtle injuries to the intersesamoidean ligament, particularly in the absence of osseous changes.[45] The intersesamoidean ligament normally has intermediate signal intensity, particularly centrally, which should not be confused with desmopathy (Figure 21-17). Comparison images to the contralateral limb can be helpful to distinguish subtle injuries from normal variants. MRI findings consistent with intersesamoidean ligament injury include focal or diffuse increased signal and focal low signal, indicative of fibrosis. Concurrent osseous abnormalities of the sesamoid bones include irregularity or lysis of the axial margin and increased abnormal osseous fluid signal.

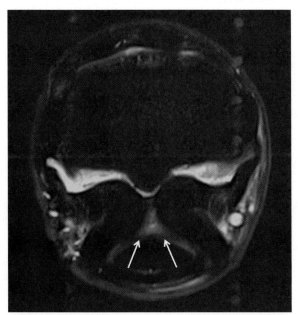

FIGURE 21-17 Transverse STIR image demonstrating normal intermediate signal intensity within the intersesamoidean ligament (arrows).

The collateral ligaments of the fetlock joint have two parts: a superficial (long) and a deep (short) portion. The superficial portion begins proximal to the condylar fossa and extends distally to the proximal phalanx. The deep portion begins in the condylar fossa and runs in a palmarodistal direction to insert on the proximal phalanx and proximal sesamoid bones.[50] Radiographic evidence of collateral ligament injury includes osseous proliferation at the origin or insertion and avulsion fragmentation. Stressed views can successfully demonstrate joint instability in cases of collateral ligament rupture.

Ultrasound evaluation of the collateral ligaments should be performed in long-axis and transverse planes. A standoff pad is generally needed unless there is a large amount of soft tissue swelling. Ultrasonographic evidence of collateral ligament injury can range from subtle fiber disruption and mild echogenicity changes to complete rupture of one or both portions. Evaluation of size is often best performed on the transverse images, and comparison of medial and lateral sides and the contralateral limb can help identify more subtle changes. Accompanying bone change can include osseous proliferation, focal lysis, incomplete fractures, and avulsion fragments.

MRI also will demonstrate desmopathy of the collateral ligaments. Because of the oblique orientation of the deep collateral ligament, it is susceptible to magic angle artifact. This will result in increased signal intensity of the ligament on PD and T1 images and should not be confused with desmopathy. Including a T2 sequence will minimize the magic angle effect and help distinguish true desmopathy from artifact. Most commonly, collateral ligament desmopathy will be manifested as enlargement and diffuse change in signal intensity, although focal discrete alteration in signal can also occur.[20,45] Concurrent bone proliferation, medullary sclerosis, or bone edema-like signal may be observed and can help improve detection of collateral ligament injuries. Comparison with the contralateral limb is helpful.

As mentioned previously, soft tissue swelling is often a primary indicator of pathologic changes within the joint. Ultrasound evaluation of the joint should include assessment of the degree of fluid distention, synovial proliferation, and joint capsule thickness. With chronic inflammation, the synovial folds will hypertrophy and become more prominent. Thickening of the dorsal synovial fold, also known as villonodular synovitis, is seen with chronic inflammation and has been defined as thickening of the synovial fold measuring greater than 4 mm.[47,51] Secondary smooth pressure resorption of the dorsal metacarpus/tarsus just proximal to the sagittal ridge and enthesophyte formation can accompany dorsal synovial proliferation. This should be assessed in both weight-bearing and non-weight-bearing flexed positions to minimize relaxation artifact.[50] Using MRI, the sagittal scan is often the most helpful for assessing dorsal synovial fold and joint capsule thickness. Generally the synovial fold thickness, amount of synovium in the plantar joint pouch, and degree of fluid is greater in the hind fetlock and should not be overly interpreted as synovitis. MRI may also demonstrate osseous sclerosis or focal bone edema-like signal at the level of the dorsal joint capsule attachment.

REFERENCES

1. McIlwraith CW, Nixon AJ, Wright IM. Diagnostic and surgical arthroscopy of the metacarpophalangeal and metatarsophalangeal joints. In: McIlwraith CW, Nixon AJ, Wright IM, et al., eds. *Diagnostic and surgical arthroscopy in the horse.* 4th ed. London: Elsevier; 2015:111–174.
2. Colon JL, Bramlage LR, Hance SR, et al. Qualitative and quantitative documentation of the racing performance of 461 Thoroughbred racehorses after arthroscopic removal of dorsoproximal first phalanx osteochondral fractures (1986-1995). *Equine Vet J.* 2000;32(6):475–481.
3. Kawcak CE, McIlwraith CW. Proximodorsal first phalanx osteochondral chip fragmentation in 336 horses. *Equine Vet J.* 1994;26(5):392–396.
4. Yovich JV, McIlwraith CW. Arthroscopic surgery for osteochondral fractures of the proximal phalanx of the metacarpophalangeal and metatarsophalangeal (fetlock) joints in horses. *J Am Vet Med Assoc.* 1986;188(3):273–279.
5. Bodo G, Hangody L, Modis L, et al. Autologous osteochondral grafting (mosaic arthroplasty) for treatment of subchondral cystic lesions in the equine stifle and fetlock joints. *Vet Surg.* 2004;33(6):588–596.
6. Hogan PM, McIlwraith CW, Honnas CM, et al. Surgical treatment of subchondral cystic lesions of the third metacarpal bone: results in 15 horses (1986-1994). *Equine Vet J.* 1997;29(6):477–482.
7. McIlwraith CW, Vorhees M. Management of osteochondritis dissecans of the dorsal aspect of the distal metacarpus and metatarsus. *Proc Am Assoc Equine Pract.* 1990;35:547–550.
8. Denoix JM, Jeffcott LB, McIlwraith CW, et al. A review of terminology for equine juvenile osteochondral conditions (JOCC) based on anatomical and functional considerations. *Vet J.* 2013;197(1):29–35.
9. Vanderperren K, Saunders JH. Diagnostic imaging of the equine fetlock region using radiography and ultrasonography. Part 2: the bony disorders. *Vet J.* 2009;181(2):123–136.
10. Jacquet S, Robert C, Valette JP, et al. Evolution of radiological findings detected in the limbs of 321 young horses between the ages of 6 and 18 months. *Vet J.* 2013;197(1):58–64.
11. Olive J, D'Anjou MA, Alexander K, et al. Comparison of magnetic resonance imaging, computed tomography, and radiography for assessment of noncartilaginous changes in equine metacarpophalangeal osteoarthritis. *Vet Radiol Ultrasound.* 2010;51(3):267–279.
12. Seignour M, Coudry V, Norris R, et al. Ultrasonographic examination of the palmar/plantar aspect of the fetlock in the horse: technique and normal images. *Equine Vet Educ.* 2011;24(1):19–29.
13. Kidd JA, Fuller C, Barr ARS. Osteoarthritis in the horse. *Equine Vet Educ.* 2001;13(3):160–168.
14. Brommer H, Weeren PR, Brama PAJ, et al. Quantification and age-related distribution of articular cartilage degeneration in the equine fetlock joint. *Equine Vet J.* 2003;35(7):697–701.
15. Conaghan PG, Felson D, Gold G, et al. MRI and non-cartilaginous structures in knee osteoarthritis. *Osteoarthritis Cartilage.* 2006;14(Suppl A):A87–94.
16. O'Brien T, Baker TA, Brounts SH, et al. Detection of articular pathology of the distal aspect of the third metacarpal bone in thoroughbred racehorses: comparison of radiography, computed tomography and magnetic resonance imaging. *Vet Surg.* 2011;40(8):942–951.
17. Olive J, D'Anjou MA, Girard C, et al. Fat-suppressed spoiled gradient-recalled imaging of equine metacarpophalangeal articular cartilage. *Vet Radiol Ultrasound.* 2010;51(2):107–115.
18. Werpy NM, Ho CP, Pease AP, et al. The effect of sequence selection and field strength on detection of osteochondral defects in the metacarpophalangeal joint. *Vet Radiol Ultrasound.* 2011;52(2):154–160.
19. Young BD, Samii VF, Mattoon JS, et al. Subchondral bone density and cartilage degeneration patterns in osteoarthritic metacarpal condyles of horses. *Am J Vet Res.* 2007;68(8):841–849.
20. King JNJ, Zubrod CJC, Schneider RKR, et al. MRI findings in 232 horses with lameness localized to the metacarpo(tarso)phalangeal region and without a radiographic diagnosis. *Vet Radiol Ultrasound.* 2012;54(1):36–47.
21. Sherlock CE, Mair TS, Ter Braake F. Osseous lesions in the metacarpo(tarso)phalangeal joint diagnosed using low-field magnetic resonance imaging in standing horses. *Vet Radiol Ultrasound.* 2009;50(1):13–20.
22. Hontoir F, Nisolle J-F, Meurisse H, et al. A comparison of 3-T magnetic resonance imaging and computed tomography arthrography to identify structural cartilage defects of the fetlock joint in the horse. *Vet J.* 2014;199(1):115–122.
23. Powell SE. Low-field standing magnetic resonance imaging findings of the metacarpo/metatarsophalangeal joint of racing Thoroughbreds with lameness localised to the region: a retrospective study of 131 horses. *Equine Vet J.* 2011;44(2):169–177.
24. Dyson S. Musculoskeletal scintigraphy of the equine athlete. *Semin Nucl Med.* 2014;44(1):4–14.
25. Kawcak CE, Bramlage LR, Embertson RM. Diagnosis and management of incomplete fracture of the distal palmar aspect of the third metacarpal bone in five horses. *J Am Vet Med Assoc.* 1995;206(3):335–337.
26. Hornof WJ, O'Brien TR. Radiographic evaluation of the palmar aspect of the equine metacarpal condyles: a new projection. *Vet Radiol.* 1980;21(4):161–167.
27. Norrdin RW, Kawcak CE, Capwell BA, et al. Subchondral bone failure in an equine model of overload arthrosis. *Bone.* 1998;22(2):133–139.
28. Ellis DR. Some observations on condylar fractures of the third metacarpus and third metatarsus in young Thoroughbreds. *Equine Vet J.* 1994;26(3):178–183.
29. Zekas LJ, Bramlage LR, Embertson RM. Characterisation of the type and location of fractures of the third metacarpal/metatarsal condyles in 135 horses in central Kentucky (1986-1994). *Equine Vet J.* 1999;31(4):304–308.
30. Kawcak CE, McIlwraith CW, Norrdin RW, et al. The role of subchondral bone in joint disease: a review. *Equine Vet J.* 2001;33(2):120–126.
31. Davidson EJ, Ross MW. Clinical recognition of stress-related bone injury in racehorses. *Clin Tech Equine Pract.* 2003;2(4):296–311.
32. Ross MW. Scintigraphic and clinical findings in the Standardbred metatarsophalangeal joint: 114 cases (1993-1995). *Equine Vet J.* 1998;30(2):131–138.
33. Trope GD, Anderson GA, Whitton RC. Patterns of scintigraphic uptake in the fetlock joint of Thoroughbred racehorses and the effect of increased radiopharmaceutical uptake in the distal metacarpal/tarsal condyle on performance. *Equine Vet J.* 2011;43(5):509–515.
34. Gaschen L, Burba DJ. Musculoskeletal injury in Thoroughbred racehorses: correlation of findings using multiple imaging modalities. *Vet Clin North Am Equine Pract.* 2012;28(3):539–561.

35. Morgan JW, Santschi EM, Zekas LJ. Comparison of radiography and computed tomography to evaluate metacarpo/metatarsophalangeal joint pathology of paired limbs of Thoroughbred racehorses with severe condylar fracture. *Vet Surg.* 2006;35(7):611–617.

36. Drum MG, Les CM, Park RD, et al. Correlation of quantitative computed tomographic subchondral bone density and ash density in horses. *Bone.* 2009;44(2):316–319.

37. Kawcak CE, McIlwraith CW. Proximodorsal first phalanx osteochondral chip fragmentation in 336 horses. *Equine Vet J.* 1994;26(5):392–396.

38. Ellis DR, Simpson DJ, Greenwood RE, et al. Observations and management of fractures of the proximal phalanx in young Thoroughbreds. *Equine Vet J.* 1987;19(1):43–49.

39. Markel MD, Richardson DW. Noncomminuted fractures of the proximal phalanx in 69 horses. *J Am Vet Med Assoc.* 1985;186(6):573–579.

40. Dyson S, Nagy A, Murray R. Clinical and diagnostic imaging findings in horses with subchondral bone trauma of the sagittal groove of the proximal phalanx. *Vet Radiol Ultrasound.* 2011;52(6):596–604.

41. O'Brien TR, Morgan JP, Wheat JD, et al. Sesamoiditis in the Thoroughbred: a radiographic study 1. *Vet Radiol Ultrasound.* 1971;12(1):75–87.

42. Spike Pierce DL, Bramlage LR. Correlation of racing performance with radiographic changes in the proximal sesamoid bones of 487 Thoroughbred yearlings. *Equine Vet J.* 2003;35(4):350–353.

43. Carnicer D, Coudry V, Denoix JM. Ultrasonographic examination of the palmar aspect of the pastern of the horse: sesamoidean ligaments. *Equine Vet Educ.* 2012;25(5):256–263.

44. Sampson SN, Schneider RK, Tucker RL, et al. Magnetic resonance imaging features of oblique and straight distal sesamoidean desmitis in 27 horses. *Vet Radiol Ultrasound.* 2007;48(4):303–311.

45. Gonzalez LM, Schramme MC, Robertson ID, et al. MRI features of metacarpo(tarso)phalangeal region lameness in 40 horses. *Vet Radiol Ultrasound.* 2010;51(4):404–414.

46. Smith S, Dyson SJ, Murray RC. Magnetic resonance imaging of distal sesamoidean ligament injury. *Vet Radiol Ultrasound.* 2008;49(6):516–528.

47. Vanderperren K, Saunders JH. Diagnostic imaging of the equine fetlock region using radiography and ultrasonography. Part 1: soft tissues. *Vet J.* 2009;181(2):111–122.

48. Vanderperren K, Bergman HJ, Spoormakers TJP, et al. Clinical, radiographic, ultrasonographic and computed tomographic features of nonseptic osteitis of the axial border of the proximal sesamoid bones. *Equine Vet J.* 2013;46(4):463–467.

49. Denoix JM, Busoni V, Olalla MJ. Ultrasonographic examination of the proximal scutum in the horse. *Equine Vet J.* 1997;29(2):136–141.

50. Denoix JM, Jacot S, Bousseau B, et al. Ultrasonographic anatomy of the dorsal and abaxial aspects of the equine fetlock. *Equine Vet J.* 1996;28(1):54–62.

51. Dabareiner RM, White NA, Sullins KE. Metacarpophalangeal joint synovial pad fibrotic proliferation in 63 horses. *Vet Surg.* 1996;25(3):199–206.

22

Carpus

Christopher E. Kawcak and Myra F. Barrett

The carpus is composed of three joints: the antebrachiocarpal (radiocarpal) joint, the middle carpal (intercarpal) joint, and the carpometacarpal joint. The proximal row of carpal bones is composed of the radiocarpal bone, the intermediate carpal bone, the ulnar carpal bone, and the accessory carpal bone. The distal row of carpal bones is composed of the second, third, and fourth carpal bones and occasionally the first carpal bone. These bones have been shown to move independently through strong intercarpal ligaments that help to dissipate the axial stress through the carpus.

Although the antebrachiocarpal joint is usually isolated from the other carpal joints, one report has documented a communication to the middle carpal and carpometacarpal joints.[1] The middle carpal and carpometacarpal joints communicate routinely and on occasion the antebrachiocarpal joint and the carpal sheath can communicate.[2] Of clinical significance is the fact that the carpometacarpal joint has distal palmar outpouchings that extend distally to the axial side of the second and fourth metacarpal bones. This area surrounds the proximal suspensory ligament; therefore, infusion of anesthetic into this area may inadvertently lead to anesthesia of the carpometacarpal and middle carpal joints. Conversely, injection of the middle carpal joint may lead to inadvertent desensitization of the proximal suspensory ligament area.[3]

Disease within the carpus often results from stress-induced fatigue damage that leads to osteochondral damage at consistent sites, especially in racehorses. Carpal disease can also result from acute damage that can lead to osteochondral damage at inconsistent sites or damage to the soft tissues, which can occur in all horses. Osteoarthritis (OA) is common in the carpus in all breeds and can manifest into progressive joint space narrowing, osteophyte and enthesophyte formation, restricted range of motion, and varus deformity.

Regardless of the site of pain within the carpus, horses with carpal pain will typically show limb abduction while moving at both the trot and the walk and consequently will have a very short gait. Although synovial effusion of the carpal joints is usually indicative of primary carpal pain, a lack of effusion can occur in cases of primary subchondral bone pain. Conversely, veterinarians must also be careful of swelling in structures other than the carpal joints such as the extensor tendon sheaths and acquired bursitis lesions such as

hygromas. Effusion in either structure can be mistaken for synovial effusion of the dorsal aspect of the carpal joints.

Arthrocentesis of the antebrachiocarpal and middle carpal joints is fairly straightforward (Figure 22-1). It is best accomplished through the dorsal aspect of the joints with the carpus in flexion. However, needles can be placed in the caudal aspects of the joints with the limb in weight bearing. The carpometacarpal joints typically communicate with the middle carpal joints, and therefore administration of therapeutics or blocking agents can diffuse into that joint. Care must be taken in differentiating carpal pain from pain in the proximal suspensory ligament region (proximal suspensory ligament origin) as the caudal outpouchings of the carpometacarpal joint typically surround the proximal suspensory ligament origin (Figure 22-2).

Developmental abnormalities of the carpus are one of the most common problems at birth in young horses. Any conformational abnormalities that affect the carpus should be addressed when the horse is young, although being overaggressive with treatments (as opposed to allowing the normal time frame for changes to occur) should be avoided. The types of developmental problems can be classified into four categories: angular limb deformities, although it should be noted that most foals are born slightly carpal valgus, which resolves over several months; flexural deformities; rotational deformities; and subchondral cystic lesions. Angular and flexural deformities may be pathologic in origin and sometimes require prompt therapy. However, rotational deformities are often conformational and the origin often occurs proximal to the carpus.

IMAGING PARAMETERS

A minimum of six to seven radiographic images is often needed to fully characterize the carpal joints, especially those with small fragmentation. This includes a lateral-medial, flexed lateral-medial, dorsopalmar (DP), dorso 45 degrees lateral-palmaromedial oblique (DLPMO), dorso 30 degrees medial-palmarolateral oblique, and dorsoproximal-dorsodistal (skyline) views of the proximal and distal row of carpal bones. The reason why the obliquity is less in the DMPLO view is that osseous fragmentation and pathologic changes occur more frequently on the dorsomedial aspect of the intermediate carpal bone, which is best highlighted by this degree of obliquity. Both limbs should be radiographed, since over 50% of all horses with osteochondral fragments will have them in both carpi.[4]

The third carpal skyline view is important for detecting sclerosis, lysis, and fracture, and it has been shown to give a good impression of third carpal bone density.[5] It is important to recognize that if the skyline view of the third carpal bone is not sufficiently dorsally protruded, either caused by inadequate flexion or inappropriate beam angle, the third carpal bone can look artifactually sclerotic and the corticomedullary distinction cannot be adequately assessed.

Ultrasound of the carpus is usually reserved for cases of suspected collateral ligament damage. Surrounding soft tissue diseases can be characterized, but for diseases specific to carpal joint disease, the collateral ligaments are the only articular soft tissues that can be visualized with ultrasound.

Because of the superimposition of carpal bones, and the relative insensitivity of radiographs to early bone loss, subchondral bone lysis within the cuboidal bones of the carpus may be underestimated or not visualized radiographically. As the disease progresses, lysis will then become visible radiographically, which justifies the use of subsequent radiographs to diagnose this problem once the bone in that area has resorbed. Volumetric imaging techniques such as computed tomography (CT) or magnetic resonance imaging (MRI) may also be needed (Figure 22-3).

Nuclear scintigraphy is an excellent modality for detecting bone remodeling (Figure 22-4). Although it is quite useful in the carpus to detect areas of osseous pathologic change, it is important to remember there can also be focal, marked increased radiopharmaceutical uptake (IRU) in cases of normal adaptive remodeling (most commonly in the radiocarpal and third carpal bones). Differentiating a pathologic process from normal remodeling requires correlation with lameness evaluation and, if possible, radiographic findings. In a study in Standardbreds, increased uptake was common in the middle carpal joint and most of this reaction was felt to be of clinical significance.[2] In addition, we have seen intense uptake in 2-year-old Quarter horses that were treadmilled for 6 months.[6] Therefore, one must be careful not to overinterpret the findings as uptake can occur in horses that are undergoing active exercise. Although standard scintigraphic images of the carpus include lateral and dorsal images, the addition of lateral, and occasionally dorsal, flexed images, can help better localize the area of uptake (Ross, personal communication).

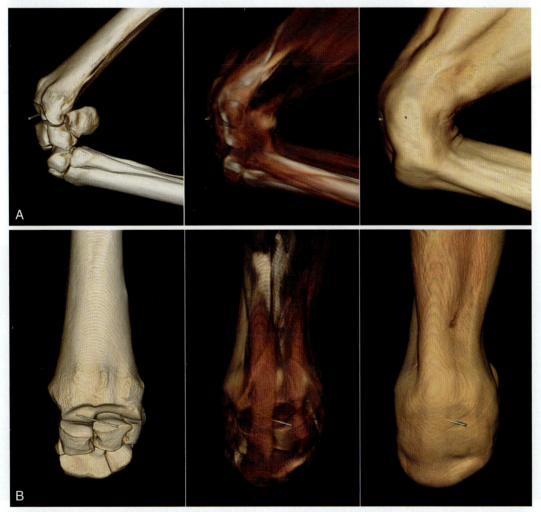

FIGURE 22-1 Three-dimensional rendering of needle placement in the antebrachiocarpal (A,B) and middle carpal joints. (Image courtesy of M. Ross, 2013.)

Continued

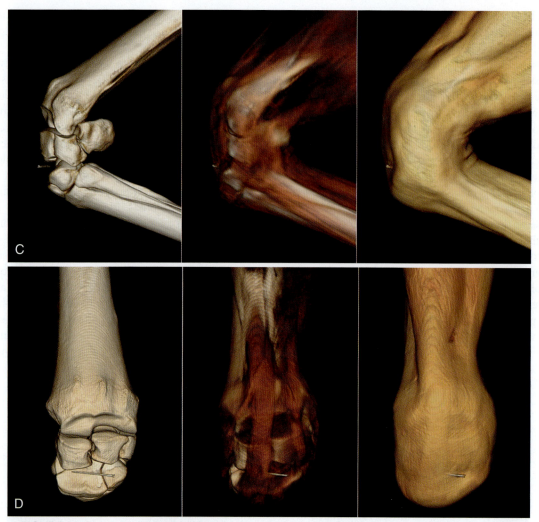

FIGURE 22-1, cont'd (C,D). Both the cranial and caudal approaches to each technique are demonstrated on the skeleton, with overlaid soft tissues, and with overlaid skin. The cranial approach is typically performed with the limb in flexion.

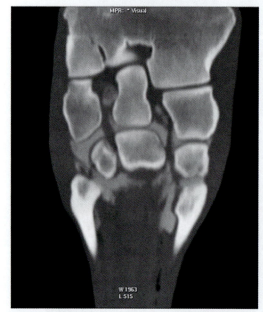

FIGURE 22-2 A frontal plane contrast computed tomographic image demonstrating contrast agent, administered in the middle carpal joint, that surrounds the proximal suspensory ligament origin.

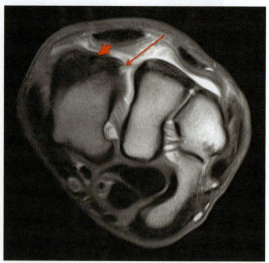

FIGURE 22-3 Transverse PD MR image of the distal radial carpal bone demonstrating moderate sclerosis (arrowhead), dorsal cortical proliferation and focal lysis of the radial carpal bone (arrow).

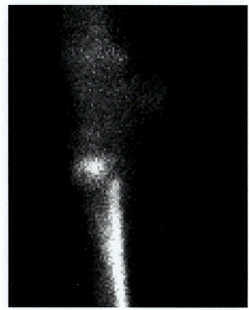

FIGURE 22-4 Nuclear scintigraphic image demonstrating significant uptake in the third carpal bone. This horse was grade II/V lame in the limb and would become sound with a lateral palmar nerve block. The horse subsequently became sound with intraarticular analgesia of the middle carpal joint.

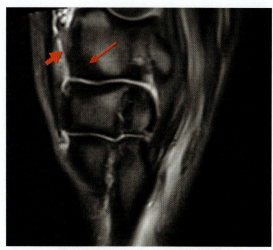

FIGURE 22-5 Fat-saturated PD sagittal MR image showing sclerosis (arrow), joint capsule enthesopathy (arrowhead) and mild subchondral lysis of the radial carpal bone.

CLINICAL SIGNS

Horses with fracture in the carpus can appear with various degrees of lameness, synovial effusion, soft tissue swelling, and carpal flexion during standing. If osteochondral damage is complete and enters the joint, synovitis typically results, which leads to clinical signs of joint effusion and pain. However, in rare occasions where subchondral bone damage alone occurs, synovitis leading to joint effusion may not be appreciated and the horse may or may not be positive to carpal flexion (Figure 22-5). Horses with small osteochondral carpal fragments are often only subtly lame with mild amounts of effusion and soft tissue swelling. However, the common characteristic of their movement is abduction of the forelimbs, which some have hypothesized is an attempt to minimize carpal flexion. Consequently this decreases their hoof height during flight. Horses with osteochondral damage are often flexion positive and in fact for some fractures, horses have intense pain even with passive flexion. Horses with fracture or fragmentation of the palmar aspect of the joints are often significantly responsive to flexion, which is reflective of the extensive soft tissue damage that can occur in this area. In more chronic stages of osteochondral fracture, there may be physical limitations to the amount of flexion in the carpus with or without pain. Horses with comminuted fractures of the carpus are often axially unstable and effusion may be associated with subcutaneous swelling. While flexed, if the horse can tolerate it, it is a good practice to palpate the dorsal aspect of the carpal bones as those horses with osteochondral damage often will demonstrate pain on palpation of certain bones. Often, if a significant amount of joint capsule is involved in the fragmentation, fibrous thickening of the

joint capsule can be appreciated. However, in these cases, one must rule out the presence of a hygroma or extensor sheath swelling.

If there are obvious signs of osteochondral fracture in the horse, it is often a good idea to perform a radiographic examination before performing intrasynovial analgesia. The concern here is that with loss of pain, the horse will no longer protect the limb, possibly leading to worsening of the damage. However, if a subtle lameness is present or radiographs are inconclusive, then often intraarticular analgesia is needed to confirm the site of pain. Again, with the absence of diagnostic imaging findings, a positive response to intraarticular analgesia could be a sign of proximal suspensory ligament origin pain and the two problems should be differentiated. For intraarticular analgesia of the carpal joints usually 5 to 7 mL of anesthetic is injected into the joint and the horse rechecked after 10 minutes and 30 minutes. Horses that have incomplete slab fractures that have not broken into the joint may not respond significantly to intraarticular anesthesia. The same may occur with horses that suffer from subchondral bone disease of the middle carpal joint. However, in these horses there may be subtle preexisting lameness that often will lead the clinician to further diagnostic imaging to characterize the problem.

SPECIFIC CONDITIONS

Osteochondrosis of the Carpus

Osteochondritis dissecans has been reported in the carpal bones although it is uncommon compared with other joints in the horse. Subchondral cystic lesions in some carpal bones are incidental and are often of questionable clinical significance. This is especially true with cysts within the second carpal bone in association with the presence of the first carpal bone and in the proximal aspect of the second metacarpal bone (Figure 22-6). However, subchondral cystic lesions in the radiocarpal bone and the distal aspect of the radius

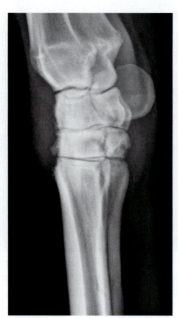

FIGURE 22-6 Radiograph of a subchondral cystic lesion in the second carpal bone.

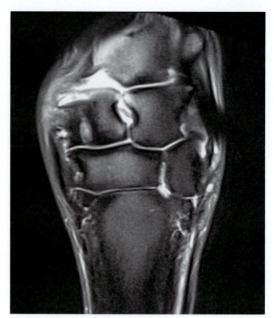

FIGURE 22-7 Dorsal plane PD fat saturated MR image showing an extensive subchondral bone cyst of the radial carpal bone with marked surrounding sclerosis (Courtesy of Dr. Jake Hersman, Animal Imaging, Irving, TX.)

(Figure 22-7) are often of clinical significance, and if they are felt to communicate with carpal joints, then arthroscopic surgery and débridement are warranted.

Soft Tissue Diseases
Synovitis/Capsulitis

Synovitis commonly occurs in the carpal joints without any grossly visible pathologic changes in the joints. This is typical in young racehorses as they begin their early training and speed work. Synovitis typically manifests as clinically detectable synovial effusion, which can be detected in both the cranial and palmar aspects of the joint. Nonclinical synovial effusion in which the horse is not lame or responsive to carpal flexion can occur, but in some cases mild lameness and response to carpal flexion are apparent. The presence of pain often dictates the need to treat the synovitis that occurs. Care must be taken to differentiate synovial effusion of the carpal joints from surrounding soft tissue swelling.

Capsulitis commonly occurs within the carpal joints without associated osteochondral changes. Acute capsulitis usually manifests as a combination of synovial effusion and soft tissue swelling along the joint capsule and often elicits a strong response to carpal flexion. Radiographs are often normal in these cases. However, on occasion radiographic signs of enthesophyte formation may be demonstrated 6 to 8 weeks later. It is not uncommon to see associated enthesophyte or osteophyte formation when osteochondral damage occurs within the joints. Treatment of capsulitis depends on the origin of the damage. Osteochondral damage must be treated if it is present. However, in the absence of ostechondral damage, capsulitis can be treated through local and systemic antiinflammatory medications.

Intercarpal Ligament Tearing

Injury to the intercarpal ligaments is not common with or without associated osteochondral damage. The dorsomedial intercarpal ligament attaches to the distal radiocarpal bone in the area in which osteochondral fragmentation typically occurs. The palmar intercarpal ligaments have been shown to provide considerable stability to the carpus. The medial and lateral palmar intercarpal ligaments allow abaxial translation of the carpal bones to dissipate axial forces through the carpus.[7]

Although tearing of the medial palmar intercarpal ligament is more readily diagnosed arthroscopically,[8] radiographically visible avulsion fractures of the palmar carpus are more commonly associated with the lateral palmar intercarpal ligament.[9] This is typically characterized as a focal area of concave lucency in the ulnar carpal bone with an adjacent ovoid fragment, best seen on the DP or DLPMO views. This can be a subtle finding, and easily overlooked. MRI evaluation of this lesion may show concurrent increased signal intensity within the lateral palmar intercarpal ligament.

Whitton et al. showed that there was no correlation of tearing of the palmar intercarpal ligaments with the severity of disease, other than the fact that severe tearing of these ligaments can lead to instability of the joint and hemarthrosis. Beinlich and Nixon reviewed the diagnosis and treatment of horses with avulsion fracture of the lateral palmar intercarpal ligament from the ulnar carpal bone.[9,10] They showed that the fragments were best demonstrated on the dorsopalmar and especially the dorsolateral palmar medial projections, which corresponded with arthroscopic findings in this group of horses. In addition, they found that arthroscopic removal of these fragments was more beneficial than rest alone, with 91% of operated horses returning to their intended use.[9,10] Primary tearing of the intercarpal ligaments can lead to lameness, which can improve with intraarticular analgesia and on occasion a lateral palmar nerve block. Associated synovial effusion may or may not occur in these cases (Figure 22-8).

Collateral Ligament Injury

Damage to the collateral ligaments of the carpus is relatively uncommon and not well described in the literature. Damage may be confined to the soft tissues or may occur in conjunction with osseous abnormalities. These injuries are typically a result of trauma. A complete rupture or transection of a collateral ligament of the carpus will result in severe joint instability that is manifested radiographically as widening of the joint spaces on the affected side of the limb. A stressed view showing marked disparity in joint width between medial and lateral is often sufficiently diagnostic for a collateral ligament injury. Some have described collateral ligament abnormalities in the carpus and its close association with OA.[11] The point here is that it is often not uncommon to diagnose the problem well after OA has already been established.

Less severe collateral ligament injuries of the carpus are best diagnosed ultrasonographically or with MRI (Figure 22-9). On MRI, the collateral ligaments can have a mildly heterogenous low-to-intermediate signal intensity at the origin. Recognition of this normal heterogenous appearance is important to avoid falsely diagnosing desmopathy.

Osteochondral Damage

Although most horses with intraarticular fracture of the carpus display acute-onset clinical signs, the damage is chronic in nature, at least in racehorses, and occurs at consistent sites in the dorsal aspect of the joints. This damage is caused by the end result of a chronic process in which stress-related subchondral bone damage occurs.[6] Acute fracture and fragmentation of the carpus can occur but typically in unusual locations, especially in the palmar aspect of the joints. Therefore, in equine athletes and especially racehorses, this damage occurs in predictable sites that lend themselves to more accurate prognosis with treatment.

Osteochondral Fragmentation

Osteochondral fragmentation typically occurs at consistent locations, which again are reflective of the chronic nature of the disease. Care must be taken in relying on these generalizations as fragmentation can occur anywhere within the carpi and the distribution may differ with different population bases. Although osteochondral fragmentation can occur anywhere in racing Thoroughbreds, Quarter horses, and Standardbreds, their most common distribution within the joints can be different.[12]

Osteochondral fragmentation of the carpus is typically readily diagnosed radiographically. The distal radiocarpal and proximal intermediate carpal bones are the most common sites of osteochondral fragmentation,[4] followed by the distal radius and third carpal bone. These fragments are generally

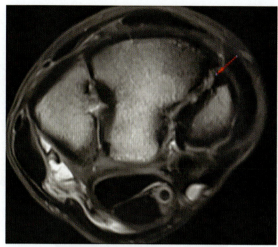

FIGURE 22-8 Magnetic resonance image of a 3-year-old horse showing mild damage to the intercarpal ligament (arrow). The horse was grade II/V lame in the limb, and became sound with a lateral palmar nerve block.

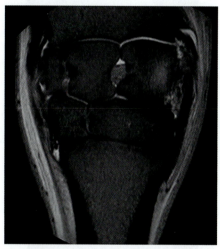

FIGURE 22-9 Magnetic resonance image of collateral ligament damage also showing subchondral bone edema.

best identified on the flexed lateral radiograph. Care must be taken to adequately image the dorsal aspect of the joints to best characterize subtle damage (Figure 22-10). Frequently there are concurrent pathologic changes to the affected joint, including evidence of effusion, subchondral sclerosis, and subchondral lysis. As mentioned above, it can occasionally be difficult to definitively differentiate an in situ osteochondral fragment from a periarticular osteophyte. However, as these areas are readily accessed arthroscopically, rarely is advanced imaging required to diagnose osteochondral fragmentation in the carpus.

Although fragmentation most frequently affects the dorsal aspect of the joint, palmar fragments can occur as well. These can be seen as either a result of osteochondral fragmentation, or, less commonly, avulsion of a palmar carpal ligament. In cases of osteochondral fragmentation, these are generally the result of acute trauma.[13] A thorough examination of the entire palmar aspect of the joint is required to

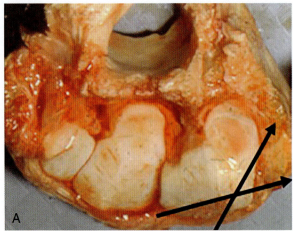

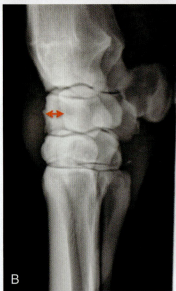

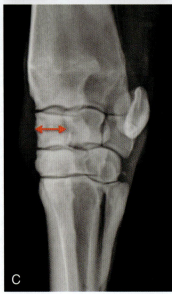

FIGURE 22-10 Gross image demonstrating a 30 degrees oblique, radiographic angle that is most apt to demonstrate subtle fragmentation, compared with a traditional 45 degrees oblique angle (**A**). DLPMO images demonstrating the 30 degrees oblique (**B**) versus the 45 degrees oblique image (**C**). Notice the change in overlap of bones in the images (arrows).

diagnose these fragments, although they are typically most visible on the lateral or flexed lateral images. Because they may concur with dorsal fragments, sometimes they are overlooked. The more readily apparent dorsal fragments may be the first abnormality recognized and may satisfy the evaluator's suspicion of the source of lameness, further emphasizing the need for a full radiographic evaluation of the entire carpus.

Fragmentation of the palmar aspect of the joint can be difficult to characterize and often requires subtle changes in the obliqueness of the images to best characterize the fragmentation (Figure 22-11). On occasion MRI or CT is needed to characterize the site of fragmentation.

Osteochondral Fracture

Slab fractures of the carpus usually occur completely through the bone and although most common in the radial facet of the third carpal bone, can occur in the intermediate and radial carpal bones as well. Slab fractures commonly occur in the third carpal bone of Thoroughbred and Standardbred racehorses and primarily affect the radial facet. These fractures can also occur on the intermediate facet, both facets, or in a sagittal orientation.[14-16] Radiographic characterization of osteochondral fractures is most commonly used; however, on occasion MRI is necessary to best characterize the damage (Figure 22-12).

Dorsal plane slab fractures of the carpus are often most easily seen on the standing dorsolateral-palmarmedial oblique projection as these fractures will often reduce in a flexed lateral position (Figure 22-13). However, in some cases, only the skyline views will allow for full appreciation of the extent of a fracture. Sagittal slab fractures typically occur on the medial aspect of the radial fossa of the third carpal bone, and either a third carpal bone skyline projection or a dorsomedial-palmar lateral oblique projection is needed to see this (Figure 22-14). Some surgeons feel there is a correlation between the amount of pain and the duration and displacement of the fragment. However, no objective studies have characterized this. Both the radial and intermediate facets of the third carpal bone may be involved in some cases (Figure 22-15), and lag screw fixation of both is needed. In cases of comminuted osteochondral fracture of the carpus, the third carpal bone is usually involved along with the radiocarpal and/or intermediate carpal bone. These can be difficult to characterize and subtle changes in the angles of the radiographic images may be needed. These horses are usually axially unstable and require emergency stabilization and usually some form of partial or pancarpal arthrodesis to be sound for breeding (Figure 22-16). Typically radiographs will help the surgeon to determine the type of arthrodesis procedure to perform; however, at times CT may be useful to best dictate the extent of damage in the joints to guide repair.

In addition to fragmentation and fracture of the carpus, it is not unusual to find subchondral bone sclerosis and lysis that leads to pain, typically in racehorses. This primarily occurs in older Standardbred racehorses because of chronic stress-induced disease within the subchondral bone.[2]

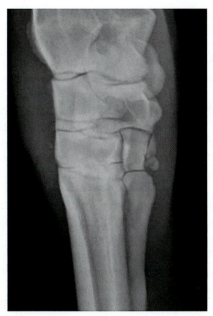

FIGURE 22-11 A radiograph demonstrating an osteochondral fragment from the palmar aspect of the carpus.

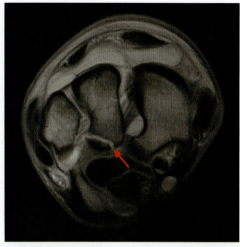

FIGURE 22-12 Dorsal plane slab fracture of the palmar aspect of the intermediate carpal bone.

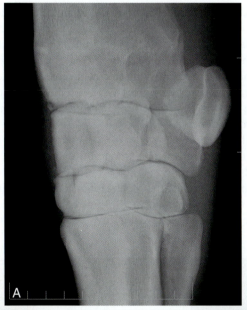

A

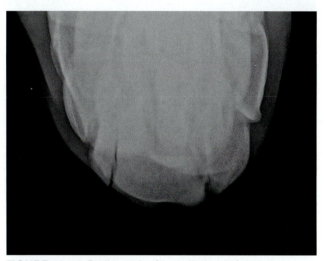

FIGURE 22-14 Radiograph of a sagittal slab fracture through the radial facet of the third carpal bone. (Images courtesy of Dr. CW McIlwraith.)

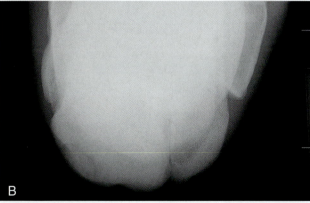

B

FIGURE 22-13 Radiographs of a slab fracture through the radial facet of the third carpal bone. (A) Dorsolateral-palmarmedial oblique projection. (B) Third carpal skyline projection. (Images courtesy of Dr. CW McIlwraith.)

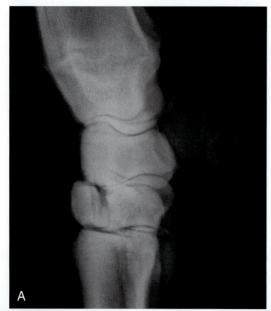

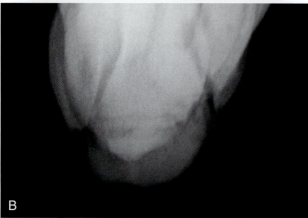

FIGURE 22-15 Radiographs of a slab fracture through the radial and intermediate facets of the third carpal bone. **(A)** Lateral-medial projection. **(B)** Third carpal skyline projection. (Images courtesy of Dr. CW McIlwraith.)

This syndrome will be discussed in the OA section of this chapter.

Treatment

Standard of care now dictates that any osteochondral damage should be arthroscopically removed to optimize the horse's chances of soundness and athletic potential. Arthroscopic surgery is the best method to fully characterize the disease process, treat the primary problem, and give an accurate prognosis for return to athletic use. Degeneration of articular cartilage and bone have been graded for severity and correlated with outcome[4,12]:

Grade 1: Minimal fibrillation or fragmentation at the edge of the defect left by the fragment, extending no more than 5 mm from the fracture line.

Grade 2: Articular cartilage degeneration extending more than 5 mm back from the defect and including up to 30% of the articular surface of that bone.

Grade 3: Loss of 50% or more of the articular cartilage from the affected carpal bone.

Grade 4: Significant loss of subchondral bone (usually distal radial carpal bone lesions).

Osteochondral fragments are removed and if the lesions are severe, then augmentative therapy such as microfracture or various intraarticular medications can be used. In the past there has been some concern about operating on horses after they have been recently injected with corticosteroids. The concern here is that the horses may be predisposed to postoperative synovial sepsis; however, this has not been shown to be of major concern.

Arthroscopic treatment for osteochondral damage, including osteochondral fragmentation and slab fractures, is best described elsewhere.[12]

Comminuted fractures require internal fixation or arthrodesis to restore axial stability to the limb and to give the horse a chance to become pasture sound.[17,18] The immediate stability

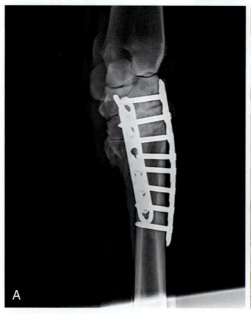

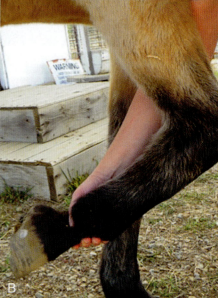

FIGURE 22-16 Partial carpal arthrodesis of the middle carpal joint and the carpometacarpal joint **(A)**. The horse still retains partial flexion of the carpus **(B)**.

gained from internal fixation improves the time to pain-free limb use and prevents overuse and consequent laminitis in the opposing limb. Conservative therapy with casting and/or splints results in more prolonged lameness, which can lead to cast sores within the limb and often laminitis within the opposing limb. Conservatively treated horses will sometimes heal with a deviation and significant chronic pain in the limb. It is unusual for a horse to achieve athletic soundness after such an injury, as the joint surface damage is often severe. Lag screw fixation can be used to stabilize individual fractures; however, in severely comminuted injuries internal fixation with plates may be necessary and partial or full arthrodesis needed.

Postoperative Care

Postoperative care of arthroscopically treated carpal joints has been completely described elsewhere.[12]

In addition to rehabilitation, most surgeons will often recommend some form of intraarticular therapy to reduce inflammation and speed healing, especially of articular cartilage. If intraarticular medication is needed, then the horses can be injected at the time of suture removal or after. The authors prefers the use of interleukin-1 receptor antagonist protein (IRAP) or polysulfated glycosaminoglycan/hyaluronic acid combination (with amikacin), typically give once weekly for 3 weeks starting 2 weeks after surgery. Treatment with IRAP is not uncommon, especially in those cases with severe joint damage, as the growth factor content in this product can be significant and theoretically can help with articular cartilage healing. Intraarticular hyaluronic acid and polysulfated glycosaminoglycan are thought to promote healing and decrease inflammation.[19] Some surgeons feel that intraarticular stem cell therapy is of some benefit, although an experimental study showed minimal benefit of intraarticular stem cell therapy in experimental osteochondral fragmentation. Theoretically, the potential for stem cells to promote release of growth factors into the joint could have some effect on articular cartilage healing of a defect.[19]

Some surgeons advocate the use of systemic medications. Most surgeons will medicate horses with carpal fractures with some form of systemic nonsteroidal antiinflammatory therapy, either in the form of phenylbutazone or Equioxx. Local application of Surpass has also been shown to be beneficial both clinically and experimentally.[19] Although in general systemic polysulfated glycosaminoglycan and intravenous hyaluronic acid therapies have shown modest effects, they may have some merit in maintenance of horses with carpal damage. Some have advocated the use of passive range of motion and swimming, which the author recommends if significant joint capsule damage is noted at the time of surgery. Potential problems postoperatively include sepsis and subcutaneous infection. Problems such as persistent effusion and osteophyte formation are usually a result of the primary disease process, although excessive débridement of the joint capsule can lead to enthesophyte formation.

Prognosis

The prognosis for osteochondal fragmentation, ostechondral fracture, and various bones within the carpal joints has been adequately described elsewhere.[12]

Osteoarthritis

Weather the OA is caused by previous injury or insidious in onset, the ultimate clinical response is similar. In those horses that are monitored closely, radiographic evidence of advancing OA in cases with a previous history of disease can be assessed and the horse treated. However, in insidious cases, problems are often not noticed until the limb begins to swell and lameness becomes obvious. Typically this occurs in pleasure or breeding horses in which athletic use no longer occurs and subtle lameness is not detected. In these latter cases, the farrier will often note that the horse will begin to resent flexion and manipulation of the limb. At this point, radiographs often will show some signs, and treatment can be helpful if started at this point.

Images should be evaluated for osteochondral damage that can be surgically addressed and for osteoarthritic changes, such as subchondral and trabecular bone sclerosis, subchondral lysis, osteophytosis, enthesophytosis, and joint space narrowing, that may have an impact on the prognosis for any surgical outcome. Radiographic evaluation of joint effusion, which commonly accompanies OA, is more accurately diagnosed in the carpus than many other equine joints because of the presence of well-defined dorsal fat pads. Dorsal displacement or loss of visualization of the dorsal fat pads is indicative of intraarticular effusion and helps differentiate extraarticular from intraarticular soft tissue swelling.

Common radiographic evidence of OA in the antebrachial and middle carpal joints includes osteophytosis of the distal or proximal aspects of the radial and intermediate carpal bones and distal radius, although any bone within the joint can be affected. The flexed lateral radiograph is useful for evaluating the proximal and distal margins of the intermediate and radial carpal bones with decreased superimposition. In some cases, it can be difficult to distinguish a distal margin osteophyte of the radiocarpal bone from an in situ fragment. If there is a thin lucent rim surrounding the distal projection of bone, it is likely to be an in-situ fragment, but in some cases, the diagnosis can only be made via advanced imaging or arthroscopic evaluation. Joint capsule enthesopathy is a common finding affecting the radial carpal bone and is manifested as dorsal cortical thickening and proliferation, which is often seen in conjunction with sclerosis of the radial carpal bone. This finding is best evaluated on the DLPMO view (Figure 22-17). Sclerosis of the third carpal bone can also be seen as a degenerative process, but can also be associated with adaptive remodeling[20]; the presence of other indicators of joint disease should be used to help differentiate the two processes.

Subchondral lysis and occasionally cystlike lesions will affect the cuboidal bones of the carpus, with the radiocarpal bone being frequently affected. Careful evaluation of the articular margin and subchondral bone density is necessary

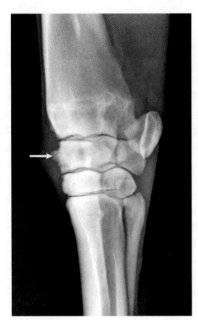

FIGURE 22-17 Radiographic appearance of dorsal cortical sclerosis and proliferation of the radiocarpal bone (arrow).

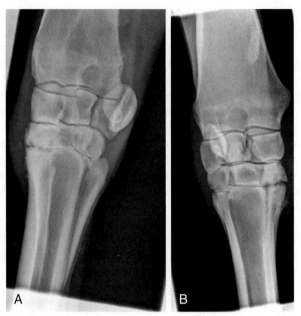

FIGURE 22-18 Radiographic images (A and B) of osteoarthritis in the carpometacarpal joint. (Images courtesy of Dr. L Goodrich.)

for detection of these lesions. Although the flexed lateral view is often the most helpful for evaluation, the DLPMO is invaluable for identification of pathologic changes of the radiocarpal bone. Additionally, in some cases, if the damage is located on the most dorsal aspect of the bone, the DP image will provide the best view for evaluation.

Osteoarthritis of the carpometacarpal joint is a separate syndrome that predominantly involves older Arabian horses.[21] The osteoarthritic changes manifest mostly at the articulation between the second carpal and second metacarpal bones, and like the distal tarsal joints, often manifest osteoarthritic changes as subchondral bone lysis in addition to periarticular osseous proliferation (Figure 22-18). Periarticular proliferation is most commonly seen on the medial aspect of the joint and can be quite extensive. In some cases, it can initially be difficult to distinguish a septic process from OA based purely on radiographs, and the horse's history, degree of lameness, and arthrocentesis must be correlated with the radiographic evaluation. Lameness is noted to be insidious in onset but can progress rapidly. The etiology of this problem is unknown, but there is a suggestion that an anatomic abnormality may exist between the second and third carpal bones.[21] Regardless of the cause, medical management of these cases can be frustrating over time as they typically become less responsive to treatment. Similar to OA at other sites, medical management is worth attempting until there is concern that the lameness could contribute to opposing limb laminitis. At this point, a partial carpal arthrodesis could be performed.

As with most joints, the degree and extent of osteoarthritic changes is most fully characterized by advanced imaging. CT has the advantage of being quick to perform, and it provides excellent bone detail. Detection of periarticular osteophytosis, subchondral lysis, subchondral and trabecular sclerosis, and evaluation of osseous fragments is unparalleled with CT imaging.

However, as with all other joints, CT is limited in the evaluation of articular cartilage damage and assessment of the intra- and periarticular soft tissue structures.

MRI provides the greatest overall evaluation of the joint. Subchondral sclerosis, lysis, and cystic lesions that may not be radiographically evident are easily identified with MRI. In addition, MRI allows for evaluation of abnormal fluid signal in the bone, that is, "bone edema-like" signal. The degree of increased fluid signal in the bone can sometimes help determine how active a pathologic process is and can help guide treatment and rehabilitation. A huge advantage of MRI is for evaluation of articular cartilage. Although articular cartilage can be indirectly assessed with CT via a contrast arthrogram, MRI remains the preferred modality for assessment of articular cartilage. Because the articular cartilage in the carpus is thin, a high field strength magnet (a minimum of 1.5 T) is required for complete evaluation of the cartilage. Interpretation of cartilage defects is aided by the fact that they are typically accompanied by subchondral bone sclerosis and sometimes subchondral lysis. Often during the osteoarthritic process, the joint capsule becomes thickened and there is synovial proliferation. These soft tissue changes are readily assessed with MRI.

Some early forms of OA can be treated with rest and systemic nonsteroidal antiinflammatory treatment. It appears that stall confinement is rarely helpful in management of horses with carpal OA, especially since strengthening of periarticular soft tissues is of benefit in other species, including humans.[22] Paddock turnout seems to help these horses, although it is important to monitor their activity and try and limit their exposure to other horses that may stimulate excessive exercise. Although surgery can be performed in those cases of OA to remove osteochondral fragments or to perform augmentative therapies such as microfracture and resurfacing, it is likely that the disease process will continue to progress postoperatively. In most cases the goal of surgery is to help relieve pain and the severity of disease progression. Intraarticular medication is meant to treat the synovitis component that often leads to pain and is of questionable efficacy for treating subchondral bone damage. Intraarticular corticosteroid and hyaluronic acid combinations may work for a short period of time but often these will stop working. Other considerations are intraarticular hyaluronic acid and polysulfated glycosaminoglycan combinations or IRAP. Although it has been advocated that only triamcinolone acetonide or betamethasone should be used in high motion joints such as the carpus, in some cases of severe OA methylprednisolone acetate may be the only thing that is effective. Even though it has been shown experimentally to result in progressive articular cartilage damage, in these cases management of pain is often considered the priority.

Medial collapse of the carpal joints is not uncommon in severe cases of OA and often dorsolateral breakover of the hoof in that limb is noticeable. (Figure 22-19) In between trimmings this becomes progressively worse and it is a subjective opinion that this can lead to worsening of pain. A mild lateral extension or a full shoe itself may help to alleviate some of this pain by slowing the dorsolateral breakover that occurs. In severe cases of OA, partial or pancarpal arthrodesis is often advocated to reduce the amount of chronic pain in the limb and prevent laminitis in the opposing limb. Occasionally, mineralization in the palmar aspect of the carpal joints will be appreciated. Some clinicians have attributed this to chronic corticosteroid injection; however, there is evidence to support that often this is caused by chronic damage within the dorsal aspect of the joints. This, in turn, leads to maceration of the fragments and migration to the palmar aspect of the joint. Generally there is concurrent significant OA and articular cartilage loss. Additionally, dystrophic mineralization can also often be differentiated by loss of mineral within the joint, based on the margination of the mineralization (typically more linear when dystrophic) and the movement of the mineral on different views.

Carpal Luxation

Luxation of the carpal joints is rare but can occur in any of the three joints. The medial collateral ligament is reportedly most commonly ruptured. However the lateral collateral ligament can be affected with or without carpal bone comminution. Avulsion fractures are also not uncommon. These are often caused by external trauma, such as foaling, jumping, falling, and slipping, or from kicks.

Clinically the horses are acutely lame with swelling around the joint and there may or may not be an angular limb deformity present depending on the severity of damage. Rarely will these luxations be open. Horses with carpal luxations may be axially unstable and crepitus may be palpable during manual deviation of the joint (Figure 22-20). Damage to the collateral ligament can also occur on its own.[11] Radiographs and ultrasound are often diagnostic for this; however, in some partial tears the horse will often need to be sedated and manual

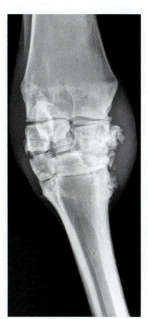

FIGURE 22-19 Radiograph demonstrating severe osteoarthritis of the carpus including acquired varus deformity.

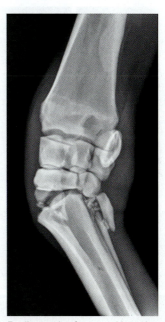

FIGURE 22-20 Radiograph of a carpal luxation due to fracture of the proximal aspect of the fourth metacapal bone.

deviation of the carpus imposed to see the subluxation on radiographs (stress radiographs) (Figure 22-21). In addition, dorsopalmar luxations can occur and radiographs should be assessed closely. Ultrasound is the best diagnostic method for characterizing full and partial thickness tears in the collateral ligaments, although with time, enthesophyte formation is usually appreciated radiographically (Figure 22-22).

Treatment for complete luxations often involves placing the horse under general anesthesia to achieve reduction. If joint damage occurs then arthroscopic surgery may be of value to débride damaged tissues. If the carpal bones

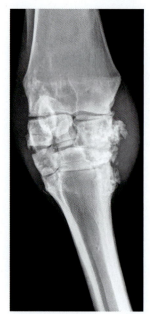

FIGURE 22-21 Stressed radiographic view demonstrating subluxation of the carpus.

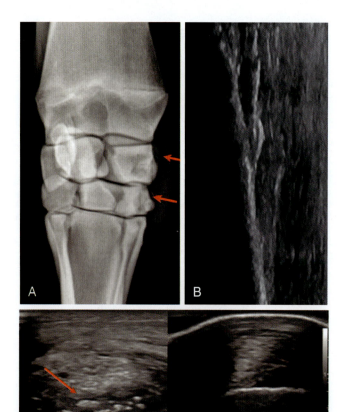

FIGURE 22-22 Radiograph of a carpus demonstrating fragmentation and enthesiophyte formation of the medial collateral ligament attachments of the middle carpal joints (**A**). Longitudinal ultrasound image of the fragmentation (**B** – arrow). Transverse ultrasound images of the fragmentation (arrow) compared to the opposite normal limb (**C**).

are not involved, then the luxation can be reduced. Otherwise, fractures may need to be débrided to facilitate reduction. Dorsopalmar luxations can be difficult to reduce, and sometimes manual fatiguing of the limb or surgery is needed to reduce the luxations. Once reduced, the limb can be put through rotational manipulation and if the limb is deemed to be rotationally stable, then a tube cast can be applied from the proximal aspect of the radius to the distal third metacarpus.[23] If the limb is deemed to be rotationally unstable, then a full limb cast should be used. Foals usually need to be casted for approximately 4 weeks and adults for 6 weeks. This will allow fibrosis to occur in the collateral ligament area and joint capsule. The horse may be transferred to a bandage and/or splint for several weeks but stall confinement for several months is necessary. If multiple fractures are present, then partial or pancarpal arthrodesis may be needed to stabilize the limb for breeding and pasture soundness. However, even if the limb can be reduced adequately, chronic OA and pain may necessitate arthrodesis to control pain and prevent contralateral limb laminitis. Soft tissue lesions can be augmented with stem cells, platelet-rich plasma, or extracorporeal shockwave therapy to help stimulate healing. Overall the prognosis is good for healing but guarded for athletic use.

REFERENCES

1. Ford TS, Ross MW, Orsini PG. Communications and boundaries of the middle carpal and carpometacarpal joints in horses. *Am J Vet Res.* 1988;49(12):2161–2164.
2. Ross MW. The carpus. In: Ross MW, Dyson SJ, eds. *Diagnosis and management of lameness in the horse.* Philadelphia, PA: Saunders; 2003:376–393.
3. Ford TS, Ross MW, Orsini PG. A comparison of methods for proximal palmar metacarpal analgesia in horses. *Vet Surg.* 1989;18(2):146–150.
4. McIlwraith CW, Yovich JV, Martin GS. Arthroscopic surgery for the treatment of osteochondral chip fractures in the equine carpus. *J Am Vet Med Assoc.* 1987;191(5):531–540.
5. Uhlhorn H, Ekman S, Haglund A, et al. The accuracy of the dorsoproximal-dorsodistal projection in assessing third carpal bone sclerosis in standardbred trotters. *Vet Radiol Ultrasound.* 1998;39:412–417.
6. Kawcak CE, McIlwraith CW, Norrdin RW, et al. Clinical effects of exercise on subchondral bone of carpal and metacarpophalangeal joints in horses. *Am J Vet Res.* 2000;61(10):1252–1258.
7. Bramlage LR, Schneider RK, Gabel AA. A clinical perspective on lameness originating in the carpus. *Equine Vet J Suppl.* 1988;(6):12–18.
8. McIlwraith CW. Tearing of the medial palmar intercarpal ligament in the equine midcarpal joint. *Equine Vet J.* 1992;24(5):367–371.
9. Beinlich CP, Nixon AJ. Prevalence and response to surgical treatment of lateral palmar intercarpal ligament avulsion in horses: 37 cases (1990-2001). *J Am Vet Med Assoc.* 2005; 226(5):760–766.
10. Beinlich CP, Nixon AJ. Radiographic and pathologic characterization of lateral palmar intercarpal ligament avulsion fractures in the horse. *Vet Radiol Ultrasound.* 2004;45(6):532–537.
11. Desmaizieres LM, Cauvin ER. Carpal collateral ligament desmopathy in three horses. *Vet Rec.* 2005;157(7):197–201.

12. McIlwraith CW, Nixon AJ, Wright IM. *Diagnostic and surgical arthroscopy in the horse.* 4th ed. London: Elsevier; 2014.

13. Wilke M, Nixon AJ, Malark J, et al. Fractures of the palmar aspect of the carpal bones in horses: 10 cases (1984-2000). *J Am Vet Med Assoc.* 2001;219(6):801–804.

14. Martin GS, Haynes PF, McClure JR. Effect of third carpal slab fracture and repair on racing performance in Thoroughbred horses: 31 cases (1977-1984). *J Am Vet Med Assoc.* 1988;193(1):107–110.

15. Schneider RK, Bramlage LR, Gabel AA, et al. Incidence, location and classification of 371 third carpal bone fractures in 313 horses. *Equine Vet J Suppl.* 1988;(6):33–42.

16. Stephens PR, Richardson DW, Spencer PA. Slab fractures of the third carpal bone in standardbreds and thoroughbreds: 155 cases (1977-1984). *J Am Vet Med Assoc.* 1988;193(3):353–358.

17. Bertone AL, Schneiter HL, Turner AS, et al. Pancarpal arthrodesis for treatment of carpal collapse in the adult horse. A report of two cases. *Vet Surg.* 1989;18(5):353–359.

18. Levine DG, Richardson DW. Clinical use of the locking compression plate (LCP) in horses: a retrospective study of 31 cases (2004-2006). *Equine Vet J.* 2007;39(5):401–406.

19. Kawcak CE, Frisbie DD, Werpy NM, et al. Effects of exercise vs experimental osteoarthritis on imaging outcomes. *Osteoarthritis Cartilage.* 2008;16(12):1519–1525.

20. Davidson EJ, Ross MW. Clinical recognition of stress-related bone injury in racehorses. *Clin Tech Equine Pract.* 2003;2(4):296–311.

21. Malone ED, Les CM, Turner TA. Severe carpometacarpal osteoarthritis in older Arabian horses. *Vet Surg.* 2003;32(3):191–195.

22. Bliddal H, Christensen R. The treatment and prevention of knee osteoarthritis: a tool for clinical decision-making. *Expert Opin Pharmacother.* 2009;10(11):1793–1804.

23. Bertone AL. Part 5: the carpus. In: Stashak TS, ed. *Adams' lameness in horses.* 5th ed. Baltimore, MD: Lippincot, Williams & Wilkins; 2002:830–863.

23

The Elbow and Shoulder

David D. Frisbie and Kurt Selberg

ELBOW

The elbow or cubital articulation is a hinge joint formed from the closely related articular surface of the distal aspect of the humerus and proximal aspect of the radius and ulna.[1]

Radiography is often the first line of defense in injuries that occur in the equine elbow. Radiographs provide a global picture to joint health; however an approximately 40% change in bone density is needed to visualize lesions. Nuclear scintigraphy is very sensitive for bone turnover and, when combined with anatomic imaging such as radiography, may increase disease detection. There are often radiographic clues to indicate soft tissue injury, such as enthesophyte formation or lysis at the insertion sites of tendons and ligaments. Ultrasonographic evaluation of these areas will further characterize the injuries and provide targeted treatment options for the soft tissue injuries. Additionally, ultrasound is very sensitive in bone margin change and may better characterize small osteophyte formation not seen on radiographs.

The articular surfaces of the joint are formed by the trochlear surface of the distal condyles of the humerus, trochlear notch of the unla, and fovea of the head of the radius. The articular surface of the condyles does not extend along the caudal aspect of the distal humerus; however, the groove for the trochlear notch (humeral trochlea) does, extending to the olecranon fossa. The only movements in the elbow are flexion and extension, with a typical range of about 60 degrees.

Radiography

A mediolateral projection of the equine elbow is obtained in a non-weight-bearing position. To achieve this radiographic projection, three people are often needed. The tuberosity of the lateral collateral ligament is easily palpated and can be used as reference for joint location. The x-ray detector is placed parallel with the long axis of the radius and ulna, centered over the elbow joint.

The cradiocaudal projection is obtained in a weight-bearing position with the edge of the x-ray detector placed 3 to 4 cm proximal to the olecranon. Then the elbow joint is centered in the x-ray detector, which may have to be slightly rotated to the body wall angle to increase the anatomy captured.

Nuclear Scintigraphy

The lateral image of the elbow is obtained with the protuberance for the collateral ligament centered on the gamma camera head. The cranial image is centered where the brachialis tendon is palpated. Counts at the elbow may range from 200,000 to 300,000. Lateral images are often the only view obtained. However, orthogonal images are needed to accurately triangulate areas of abnormal radiopharmaceutical uptake. The bone margins are less well delineated on the cranial images of the elbow caused by attenuation from the soft tissues and distance from the gamma camera.

Ultrasound

The complete ultrasonographic examination of the elbow has been reviewed elsewhere.[2] A complete examination includes evaluation of the joint margins, enthesis points of tendons for muscles (triceps brachii, tendon of ulnaris lateralis, brachialis, biceps brachii, extensor carpi radialis), joint recesses, and collateral ligaments. These areas should be examined in both long and short axis, and representative images of both normal and abnormal areas should be saved for the medical records. Ultrasonographic interrogation should use the highest megahertz possible and still be able to visualize the structure. Typically a variable megahertz linear transducer ranging from 7 to 14 is used with a scanning depth ranging from 2 to 6 cm. A microconvex transducer with a 6- to 10-MHz range may be employed to interrogate the medial and caudoproximal aspect of the elbow.

Lameness originating from the elbow is somewhat rare.[3] Three typical joint-related issues most commonly present when lameness is localized to the elbow: osteoarthritis (OA), collateral ligament damage, or subchondral bone cysts. The former two entities are thought to be traumatic in origin and, like other cystic lesions, subchondral bones cysts may be developmental or traumatic much like those that occur in the stifle.

Local anesthesia of the elbow joint can be achieved via placement of needles in various locations[4] but the author (DDF) prefers to use the caudal lateral approach to the elbow with an 18-gauge 3.5-inch spinal needle depositing 20 mL in the joint. Using 2 cm distal to the point of the elbow and

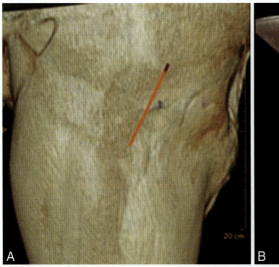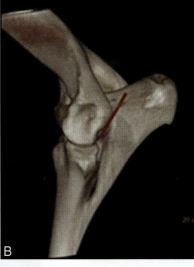

FIGURE 23-1 Caudal lateral approach to the elbow with an 18-gauge 3.5-inch spinal needle depositing 20 mL in the joint. (**A**) represents 3-D reconstruction of specimen showing desired needle placement (dark shading outside skin and lighter red inside skin) with soft tissues in place. (**B**) A 3-D reconstruction of needle placement with the soft tissues removed. Using a landmark 2 cm distal to the point of the elbow and 2 cm cranial with a 45 degree downward trajectory, the voluminous caudal pouch of the elbow joint can be accessed.

2 cm cranial with a 45 degree downward trajectory as a landmark, the voluminous caudal pouch of the elbow joint can be accessed (Figure 23-1).

Osteoarthritis

OA in the elbow is more often assumed to be associated with acute or chronic soft tissue injury, fracture, or developmental disease than with primary degeneration.[3,5,6] Typical early radiographic findings of osteoarthrosis are osteophyte formation along the medial and lateral aspects of the humerus or the cranial periarticular margin of the radial head. Late-stage disease may have concurrent joint space narrowing and subchondral bone sclerosis. The treatment of secondary OA in the elbow joint is much like that for all other joints with corticosteroids and hyaluronic acid (HA) the mainstays of initial treatment and response and duration of response the best indicators of prognosis. A corticosteroid-unresponsive joint that significantly improves with local anesthetic should be treated with intraarticular (IA) polysulfated glycosaminoglycan (Adequan) or biologics such as interleukin-1 receptor antagonist protein (IRAP) or platelet-rich plasma (PRP). The use of IA stem cells in cases of general OA of the elbow has been less rewarding in the authors' experience than in other joints.

Septic Arthritis

Joint infection in the adult horse is often a result of a deep laceration or penetrating wound and is somewhat uncommon. However, this is the most common indication for elbow arthroscopy.[7] In foals septic OA may occur via local spread from adjacent physeal infection from hematogenous spread and is relatively frequent.[8] Traumatic injury to the proximal radius may also result in a septic arthritis of the elbow.[8] Common radiographic findings in late stages are subchondral bone lysis, irregular periosteal proliferation, joint space narrowing, and osteophyte formation. Confirmation is generally made with cytology, culture, and sensitivity. Severe diffuse abnormal radiopharmaceutical uptake in the radius

and distal humeral condyle may also accompany the septic process. In foals, acute lameness that blocks out to the elbow joint followed by development of osteolysis in the olecranon is a common presentation for septic arthritis of the elbow. The treatment of choice is joint lavage, usually arthroscopically, to ensure that fibrin debris is not present within the joint, along with systemic and local antibiotics (around osteolytic areas). Because of the prolonged antibiotic treatment of the osteomyelitis, an aggressive attempt to obtain a culture and sensitivity of the organisms is undertaken.

Osteochondrosis/Cystlike Lesions

In the authors' practice, the incidence of subchondral osseous cystlike lesions is more common than generalized OA and often significantly improves with IA anesthesia. Common locations for cystlike lesions involving the elbow are the radial head[9] and distal humerus. The lesions are most often seen along the medial aspect of the joint. Radiographic findings may be a well-demarcated lucent area surrounded by variable degrees of sclerosis. Joint narrowing is possible if the elbow has concurrent late-stage degenerative changes. Cystic lesions can be seen in a variety of ages making the author conclude that both developmental and traumatic origins maybe involved. Although the author has had a limited number of cases in which a cyst cloacae could be visualized, arthroscopically that is typically not the case. In these cases the cyst lining was injected in a similar manner to that described for the medial femoral condyle, and similar good results have been achieved. However, most cysts must be reached via an extra-articular route. Although others have described complications to this approach,[10] it has not been the authors' experience (DDF). Because of the invasive nature of surgery when the author (DDF) uses an extraarticular approach, the cyst is curetted using a curved curette through a 4.0-mm drill hole, which limits the degree of débridement that can occur and then the void is filled with a combination of stem cells in an autologous fibrin glue (Figure 23-2). Follow-up on cases treated using this method is under way but has been very good to date. Drilling and/or disruption of the cyst lining might be as important as the cellular component. The low number of cases treated with any one method has hindered a clear definitive treatment plan.

Fractures/(Sub)Luxation

Fractures of the ulna and olecranon are most often caused by trauma. The mechanical result is the inability to extend the elbow and maintain the carpus in extension. Fracture typing in the ulna has been described in the ulna[11]; however, typing is often confusing and should be avoided. Common fracture configurations of the ulna are apophyseal, apophyseal that propagate to the articular margin, simple articular fractures, nonarticular fractures, and comminuted fractures, which may be articular, nonarticular, or oblique fractures at the distal extent of the olecranon.[11,12] Prognosis of the fracture depends on the fracture configuration. There is a reasonable chance for return to function with surgical intervention.[11-13] The degree of subsequent OA is most likely the best prognostic indicator for return to function. The severity of postfracture OA is thought to be directly related to the anatomic reconstruction of the joint surface. Luxation of the cuboidal joint is uncommon; however, it has been described in miniature ponies, foals, and horses with concurrent fractures of the radius or ulna.[14,15]

SHOULDER

Lameness associated with the shoulder region can have a variety of severities upon presentation. Localization to the shoulder region through flexion and palpation can be unrealizable and is nonspecific at best. Response to IA analgesia is the only reliable method although loss of supra- or infraspinatous musculature can help in focusing on the shoulder. Also, lameness that has a short swing arc with exaggerated head and neck movement as well as increased lameness observed on the outside of a circle is not dissimilar to elbow lameness.

Approaches to diagnostic analgesia of the shoulder joint have been nicely described elsewhere.[4] The author (DDF) prefers the cranial lateral approach, 2 cm proximal to the point of the shoulder and between the infraspinatous and supraspinatous muscles, perpendicular with the ground and angled caudomedial 45°. The joint capsule is thin in the shoulder and has been described as "leakier" than other capsules; thus, the author (DDF) uses a reduced volume of local anesthetic, 10 to 15 mL. Realizing the suprascapular nerve is in proximity to any anesthetic that leads or not deposited within the joint, sweeney (suprascapular nerve paralysis) is rare but not uncommon. For this reason the author (DDF) walks the horse with attention paid to any lateral luxation of the shoulder joint or change in gait characteristics for the first 5 minutes and then the horse is rested for an additional 5 minutes before reevaluation. Concurrent pain from the bicipital bursa is observed in approximately half the cases in the author's practice (DDF); thus, it is also blocked at the same time as the shoulder joint. If significant improvement is seen following

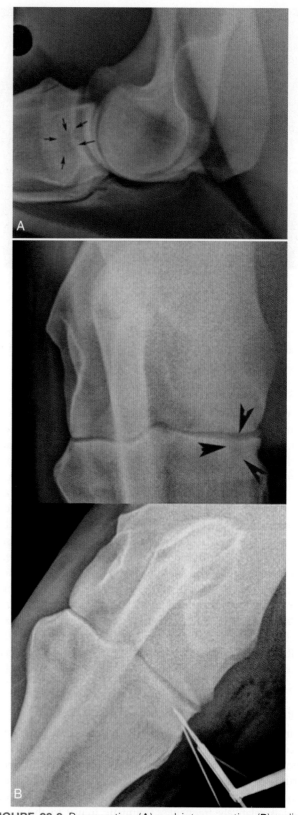

FIGURE 23-2 Preoperative (**A**) and interoperative (**B**) radiographs of a horse with a proximal medial radial bone cyst. Note the arrows outlining the preoperative cyst with a clear defect in the subchondral bone plate. The interoperative radiograph ensures correct area of débridement and placement of the MSC and fibrin.

analgesia, doing the blocks individually may be necessary if imaging does not make a definitive diagnosis. Approaches to blocking the bursa can be found elsewhere.[4]

Radiography

The shoulder or scapulohumeral joint is a ball and socket joint with the chief movement of extension and flexion. The articular surfaces are the glenoid cavity on the scapula and the humeral head. Four muscles and their tendinous attachments stabilize the shoulder: the supraspinatus, infraspinatus, subscapularis, and teres minor. Unlike joints with similar movement there are no collateral ligaments; instead, there are relatively small glenohumeral ligaments.[1] Although lameness related to the shoulder joint in horses is less common than that associated with the distal limb, when present it often causes significant lameness and decreased performance.[16,17] Radiography, ultrasound, and nuclear scintigraphic examinations of the shoulder joint provide important diagnostic information, support clinical suspicion of disease, and further direct a treatment plan.

The bicipital bursa facilitates sliding of the biceps brachii tendon over the biceps groove on the humerus. The bursa is situated between the humerus and biceps tendon. The synovium extends medially and laterally around the edges of the tendon to the superficial aspect of the tendon,[1] but it does not encompass the tendon.

As with most joints, the first diagnostic imaging of choice is often radiography. The standard radiographic views are the standing mediolateral, caudal 45 degree lateral-craniomedial oblique, and cranioproximal-craniodistal oblique "skyline."

When positioning for the lateral medial radiograph, the limb is slightly held in a cranial unweighted position. Ideally, the trachea is superimposed over the joint space. The subchondral bone of the glenoid is well demarcated. Cranially, there is a slight interruption in this subchondral bone corresponding to the glenoid notch. As the glenoid encompasses the humeral head, medially there is often summation with the humeral head. This interface causes a Mach line to be present over the mid-to-cranial aspect of the humeral head. This is may be confused with subchondral bone disease. The joint space should remain equidistant from cranial to caudal, if positioned correctly.

The oblique image of the shoulder is most easily obtained with the leg of interest placed slightly forward and the head pulled slightly to the opposite side. The x-ray generation is positioned caudally 45 degrees and centered approximately 3 to 4 cm caudal to the point of the shoulder. The x-ray detector is placed at an angle that is perpendicular to the x-ray beam, as close to the shoulder as possible. This method is slightly different from those previously described[18,19] and takes less personnel to obtain the same image. A well-positioned, caudal 45 degree lateral-craniomedial oblique image should separate and highlight the three tuberosities of the humerus.

The skyline image of the shoulder is often performed in flexed position with the edge of the plate held against the leg, perpendicular to the main gliding surface of the intertubercular grooves. The x-ray generator is positioned tangential to the intertubercular groove.

Nuclear Scintigraphy

Orthogonal images of the all body parts are recommended when feasible. The lateral image of the shoulder is obtained with the point of the shoulder centered on the gamma camera head. The cranial image is similarly centered at point of the shoulder. Counts at the shoulder may range from 200,000 to 300,000. Lateral images are often the only view obtained. However, orthogonal images are needed to accurately place areas of abnormal radiopharmaceutical uptake. The bone margins are often less well delineated on the cranial images of the shoulder caused by attenuation from the soft tissues and distance from the gamma camera.

Ultrasound

Complete ultrasonographic examination of the shoulder has been reviewed.[20,21] It includes evaluation of the joint margins, major enthesis for muscles (supraspinatus, infraspinatus, biceps, deltoid, and triceps), and joints recesses. These areas should be examined in both long and short axis, and representative images of both normal and abnormal areas should be saved for the medical records. Ultrasonographic interrogation of an area should use the highest megahertz possible and still be able to visualize the structure. Typically, a variable transducer ranging from 7 to 14 MHz is used with a scanning depth ranging from 4 to 8 cm. A macroconvex transducer with a megahertz range from 2 to 8 may be employed to interrogate the caudal aspect of the shoulder.

Osteoarthritis

Primary degenerative changes in the equine shoulder are somewhat rare but certainly occur. In a summary of shoulder lameness in horses, primary degenerative change is not listed as a cause in lame horses,[17] but in the authors' practice (DDF) it is estimated to occur in every 200 to 300 cases. There is minimal literature describing this as a primary disease process; however, it should be noted that miniature breeds, including Shetland ponies, are overrepresented.[22] Secondary degenerative changes associated with other pathologic changes are more common. Radiographic signs of OA included osteophyte production along the caudal aspect of the glenoid and the caudal aspect of the humeral head. Fragmentation along the caudal glenoid and sclerosis of the glenoid and humeral head have been reported in Shetland ponies.[22] Chronic effusion in the shoulder may present with a smooth concave margin, caudal to the tubercles (Figure 23-3). A series of cases speculated that cystlike lesions may also develop in the bicipital bursa as a result of altered biomechanics associated with shoulder OA.[23] Varying degrees of biceps injury were also seen in these cases.[23] Treatment of shoulder OA is not unlike other joints and the first line of therapy is corticosteroids and HA followed by biologic treatment in refractory cases.

Osteochondrosis/Cystlike Lesions of the Shoulder

As previously discussed at length, osteochondrosis is part of developmental orthopedic disease. However, trauma or degenerative cystlike lesions may aslso occur. Comparatively, the

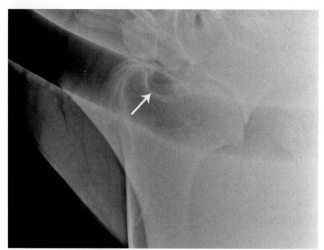

FIGURE 23-3 Lateral medial radiograph of the shoulder. A chronic, minimally displaced fracture of the supraglenoid tubercle is present. The cranial aspect of the humeral head has a smooth moderately concave margin (arrows). This is caused by chronic effusion and pressure resorption.

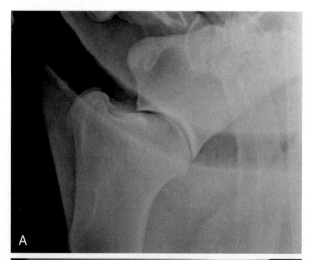

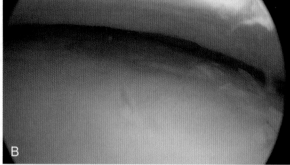

FIGURE 23-4 (A) Lateromedial radiograph. There are no abnormalities detected. (B) A circular area of cartilage thinning and irregularity is present along the caudal aspect of the humeral head. Concurrent cartilage scoring is present in the glenoid cavity.

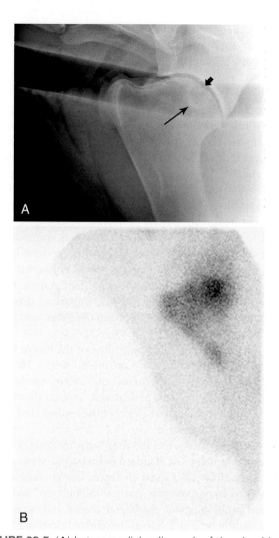

FIGURE 23-5 (A) Lateromedial radiograph of the shoulder. A well-demarcated subchondral bone defect is present in the midaspect of the humeral head. A concurrent articular defect is present (arrowhead). (B) Focal moderate radiopharmaceutical uptake is present in the medial aspect of the humeral head.

frequency of shoulder osteochondrosis is somewhat low.[17] Osteochondrosis in the shoulder often bears a poor prognosis for a career in racing; however, those horses intended for nonracing may have a reasonable chance to continue to their intended purpose.[24] Severity of the disease may also

dictate prognosis, and in the author's experience (DDF) is more useful than global statements that can be made from the current literature. Horses with subtle radiographic findings, such as a small central lucency in the subchondral bone of the glenoid, glenoid sclerosis, and minor alteration in the humeral head, that are young to middle aged have a favorable return to function.[24,25] However, similar lesions have been described in nonclinical horses.[17] In horses with a subtle lesion, radiography alone may be insufficient to diagnose the disease process (Figure 23-4).[25] Shoulders with more advanced osteochondrosis are often able to be diagnosed with radiographs alone (Figure 23-5); however, arthrography may provide better delineation of the lesion's dimensions[26] if diagnostic arthroscopy is not available. Similar outcomes for return to function may be achieved with conservative treatment and surgery,[24] and the author (DDF) uses duration of response to medical treatment as the outcome to proceed to surgical intervention. More specifically, horses that do not

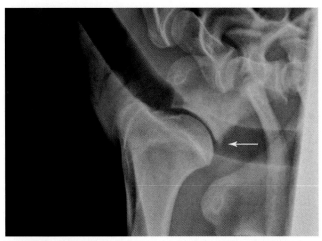

FIGURE 23-6 Lateromedial view of the left shoulder in a 3-year-old miniature horse. The glenoid cavity is shallow and flattened. Moderate osteophyte formation is present along the caudal articular margin of the glenoid (arrow). There was concurrent shoulder instability on physical examination.

respond to medical therapy but have more than 50% of their lameness abolished with IA analgesia of the shoulder go on to arthroscopic surgery as do those who respond to medical treatment but the response is less than 4 months in duration. Cystic lesions have similar presentations with respect to improvement following IA anesthesia based on degree of communication with the joint space as well as identification using bone scan. Treatment of these cystic lesions has been approached as described for the medial femoral condyle. Some consideration to additional IA injection of bone-derived culture-expanded mesenchymal stem cells (MSC) in the shoulder joint should be given because of the improved response in other joints with integral IA soft tissue structures.

Shoulder Dysplasia

Shoulder dysplasia is rare in large-breed horses. Shetland ponies are overrepresented. Shoulder dysplasia in ponies is likely related to the shape of the glenoid cavity in relation to the glenoid length (Figure 23-6).[27] This was characterized by flattening of the glenoid cavity evaluated on the lateromedial radiographic image in Shetland ponies compared with other breed types.[27] A sequela to dysplasia is luxation or subluxation of the shoulder, which often requires surgical intervention and arthrodesis in ponies.

Fractures

Multiple fracture configurations involving the scapulohumeral joint are possible, yet infrequent. Fractures of the distal scapula and proximal humerus have been described.[28,29] Although fractures affecting the shoulder are infrequent, the supraglenoid tubercle and greater tubercle are the most common locations.[17,28,29] Often the mediolateral radiographic projection is the most diagnostic for diagnosing supraglenoid tubercle fractures. The configuration of the fracture may be articular or nonarticular in nature. Generally, the articular configuration of the supraglenoid tubercle is considered poor

for return to athletics.[29] The distraction forces of the biceps and coracobrachialis muscles cause displacement of the supraglenoid fracture fragment in craniodistal fashion. Surgical intervention may require removal of the fracture fragment or internal fixation of the fragment.[30-32] Further discussion on fracture repair and prognosis can be found elsewhere.[33]

The greater tubercle has two parts, the cranial and caudal. The cranial portion serves as the insertion of the supraspinatus. The tendon of the infraspinatus overlies the caudal portion of the greater tubercle and may be injured when a fracture is present. The fracture configurations are most often long oblique in nature with mild proximocranial displacement.[28,29,34] These fractures are often best seen on the caudal 45 degree lateral-craniomedial oblique radiograph. However, the fracture can be difficult to identify, and ultrasound or nuclear scintigraphy can be used to confirm fracture. In addition to fracture confirmation, ultrasound will better characterize concurrent soft tissue injury. These fractures may be treated conservatively or surgically. Both treatments have a good prognosis for return to athletic performance.[28,29,31,34] Indications for surgical treatment include direct involvement of the shoulder joint, bicipital bursa, or significant pain that could not be managed with analgesics.[31]

Bicipital Bursitis

The bicipital bursa is positioned between the biceps brachii tendon and the proximal humerus or intubercular grooves. The synovial membrane extends to and around the abaxial margins of the biceps tendon.[1] Direct communication with the scapulohumeral joint exists in some horses[1] and should always be considered when blocking the shoulder joint. This may lead to false positives during IA diagnostic anesthesia. Injury involving the biceps bursa is rare.[17] Septic and nonseptic processes involving the bursa have been described.[35,36] Infected or septic biceps bursa often occur after sustaining a wound to the cranial aspect of the shoulder.[37] Additionally, septic processes in the shoulder may have osteomyelitis as a sequela. Septic processes in synovial structures often have thickened synovium,[38] which is often easily identified ultrasonographically. Nonseptic bicipital bursitis is characterized ultrasonographically as fluid accumulation along the abaxial aspects of the biceps, adjacent to the tubercles. Horses without other injuries such as biceps brachii tears often respond well to intrathecal corticosteroid administration, which typically consists of triamcinolone and HA. This may be achieved using both blind[4] and ultrasound-guided technique. Ultrasound-guided techniques are preferred to ensure correct placement of the medication with minimal collateral soft tissue damage.[39]

Trochlear and Intertrochlear Groove Abnormalities

Bicipital groove dysplasia is rare. Hypoplasia of the minor tubercle of the humeral has been described in the literature with concurrent biceps tendon dislocation in a Welsh pony and in large-breed horses.[40,41] These lesions are often suspected on radiographs. Specifically, the caudal 45 degree

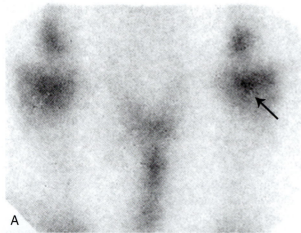

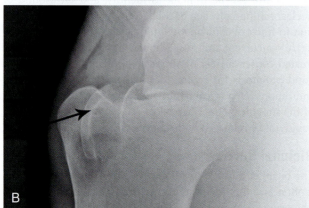

FIGURE 23-7 (A) Nuclear scintigraphic cranial view of the shoulders, with the left forelimb on the right. Focal moderate radiopharmaceutical uptake is present at the intermediate tubercle of the humerus (arrow). (B) Caudal 45 degree lateral-craniomedial oblique image. There is a focal well-demarcated cystlike lesion is the proximal aspect of the intermediate tubercle of the humerus (arrow).

lateral-craniomedial oblique should allow for differentiation of the tubercles. A cranioproximal-craniodistal oblique (skyline) has also proven useful to confirm hypoplasia and subchondral bone remodeling associated with the tubercle and biceps groove.[41] Ultrasound interrogation of the proximal humerus will also characterize bone margin morphology and presence of soft tissue abnormalities.[42] In the few reported cases with hypoplasia or minor tubercle of the humerus, return to athletic function is reasonably achievable.[41,42] Cystlike lesions also occur in the intertubercular grooves. These lesions are often documented with radiography and ultrasound (Figure 23-7).

Septic Arthritis

As with other shoulder-related injuries, septic arthritis is also a rarity and likely associated with traumatic wounds.[17,43] Radiographic evidence of a septic process may not be apparent early in the disease process.[17] Early treatment appears to have a good prognosis for return to athletic function.[17,43] In general, advanced septic arthritis often appears as subchondral and articular bone lysis surrounded by sclerosis.

REFERENCES

1. Sisson S, Grossman JD. In: *Sisson and Grossman's the anatomy of the domestic animals.* 5th ed. Philadelphia, PA: Saunders; 1975.
2. Tnibar MA, Auer JA, Bakkali S. Ultrasonography of the equine elbow technique and normal appearance. *J Equine Vet Sci.* 2001;21(4):177–187.
3. Dyson S. The shoulder and elbow. *Equine Vet J.* 1986;18:49–58.
4. Moyer W. In: *Equine joint injection and regional anesthesia.* 5th ed. Chadds Ford, PA: Academic Veterinary Solutions; 2011.
5. Chopin JB, Wright JD, Melville L, et al. Lateral collateral ligament avulsion of the humeroradial joint in a horse. *Vet Radiol Ultrasound.* 1997;38(1):50–54.
6. Wilson DG, Riedesel E. Nonsurgical management of ulnar fractures in the horse: a retrospective study of 43 cases. *Vet Surg.* 1985;14(4):283–286.
7. Nixon AJ. Elbow arthroscopy: indications, approaches and syndromes. *Equine Vet Educ.* 2012;24(4):176–181.
8. Swinebroad EL, Dabareiner RM, Swor TM, et al. Osteomyelitis secondary to trauma involving the proximal end of the radius in horses: five cases (1987-2001). *J Am Vet Med Assoc.* 2003;223(4):486–491.
9. Bertone AL, McIlwraith CW, Powers BE, et al. Subchondral osseous cystic lesions of the elbow of horses: conservative versus surgical treatment. *J Am Vet Med Assoc.* 1986;189(5):540–546.
10. McIlwraith CW, Nixon AJ, Wright IM. Diagnostic and surgical arthroscopy of the cubital (elbow) joint. In: McIlwraith CW, Nixon AJ, Wright IM, eds. *Diagnostic and surgical arthroscopy in the horse.* 4th ed. London: Elsevier; 2014.
11. Donecker JM, Bramlage LR, Gabel AA. Retrospective analysis of 29 fractures of the olecranon process of the equine ulna. *J Am Vet Med Assoc.* 1984;185(2):183–189.
12. Swor TM, Watkins JP, Bahr A, et al. Results of plate fixation of type 1b olecranon fractures in 24 horses. *Equine Vet J.* 2003;35(7):670–675.
13. Denny HR, Barr ARS, Waterman A. Surgical treatment of fractures of the olecranon in the horse: a comparative review of 25 cases. *Equine Vet J.* 1987;19(4):319–325.
14. Rubio-Martínez LM, Vázquez FJ, Romero A, et al. Elbow joint luxation in a 1-month-old foal. *Aust Vet J.* 2008;86(1-2):56–59.
15. Senior M, Smith M, Clegg P. Subluxation of the left elbow joint in a pony at induction of general anesthesia. *Vet Rec.* 2002;151:183–184.
16. Singer ER, Barnes J, Saxby F, et al. Injuries in the event horse: training versus competition. *Vet J.* 2008;175(1):76–81.
17. Dyson S. Shoulder lameness in horses—an analysis of 58 suspected cases. *Equine Vet J.* 1986;18(1):29–36.
18. Butler J, Colles C, Dyson S, et al. *Clinical radiology of the horse.* Wiley-Blackwell; 1993.
19. Fiske-Jackson AR, Crawford AL, Archer RM, et al. Diagnosis, management, and outcome in 19 horses with deltoid tuberosity fractures. *Vet Surg.* 2010;39(8):1005–1010.
20. Tnibar MA, Auer JA, Bakkali S. Ultrasonography of the equine shoulder: technique and normal appearance. *Vet Radiol Ultrasound.* 1999;40(1):44–57.
21. Whitcomb MB. How to perform a complete ultrasound exam of the equine shoulder. *Proc Am Assoc Equine Pract.* 2003:42–49.
22. Clegg PD, Dyson SJ, Summerhays GES, et al. Scapulohumeral osteoarthritis in 20 Shetland ponies, miniature horses and Falabella ponies. *Vet Rec.* 2001;148:175–179.

23. Little D, Redding WR, Gerard MP. Osseous cyst-like lesions of the lateral intertubercular groove of the proximal humerus: a report of 5 cases. *Equine Vet Educ.* 2009;21(2):60–66.

24. Jenner F, Ross M, Martin B, et al. Scapulohumeral osteochondrosis. A retrospective study of 32 horses. *Vet Comp Orthop Traumatol.* 2008;21(5):406–412.

25. Doyle PS, White II NA. Diagnostic findings and prognosis following arthroscopic treatment of subtle osteochondral lesions in the shoulder joint of horses: 15 cases (1996-1999). *J Am Vet Med Assoc.* 2000;217(12):1878–1882.

26. Nixon AJ, Spencer CP. Arthrography of the equine shoulder joint. *Equine Vet J.* 1990;22(2):107–113.

27. Boswell JC, Schramme MC, Wilson AM, et al. Radiological study to evaluate suspected scapulohumeral joint dysplasia in Shetland ponies. *Equine Vet J.* 1999;31(6):510–514.

28. Mez JC, Dabareiner RM, Cole RC, et al. Fractures of the greater tubercle of the humerus in horses: 15 cases (1986-2004). *J Am Vet Med Assoc.* 2007;230(9):1350–1355.

29. Dyson S. Sixteen fractures of the shoulder region in the horse. *Equine Vet J.* 1985;17(2):104–110.

30. Dart AJ, Snyder JR. Repair of a supraglenoid tuberosity fracture in a horse. *J Am Vet Med Assoc.* 1992;201(1):95–96.

31. Tudor R, Crosier M, Love NE, et al. Radiographic diagnosis: fracture of the caudal aspect of the greater tubercle of the humerus in a horse. *Vet Radiol Ultrasound.* 2001;42(3):244–245.

32. Baxter GM. The antebrachium, elbow and humerus. In: Baxter GM, ed. *Adams and Stashak's lameness in horses.* Wiley-Blackwell; 2011:687–705.

33. Nixon AJ, Watkins JP. Fractures of the humerus. In: Nixon AJ, ed. *Fracture repair in horses.* Philadelphia, PA: Saunders; 1996:242–253.

34. Yovich JV, Aanes WA. Fracture of the greater tubercle of the humerus in a filly. *J Am Vet Med Assoc.* 1985;187(1):74–75.

35. Gough MR, McDiarmid AM. Septic intertuberal (bicipital) bursitis in a horse. *Equine Vet Educ.* 1998;10(2):66–69.

36. Fugaro MN, Adams SB. Biceps brachii tenotomy or tenectomy for the treatment of bicipital bursitis, tendonitis, and humeral osteitis in 3 horses. *J Am Vet Med Assoc.* 2002;220(10):1508–1511.

37. Vatistas NJ, Pascoe JR, Wright IM, et al. Infection of the intertubercular bursa in horses: four cases (1978-1991). *J Am Vet Med Assoc.* 1996;208(9):1434–1437.

38. Easley JT, Brokken MT, Zubrod CJ, et al. Magnetic resonance imaging findings in horses with septic arthritis. *Vet Radiol Ultrasound.* 2011;52(4):402–408.

39. Schneeweiss W, Puggioni A, David F. Comparison of ultrasound-guided vs. "blind" techniques for intra-synovial injections of the shoulder area in horses: scapulohumeral joint, bicipital and infraspinatus bursae. *Equine Vet J.* 2012;44(6):674–678.

40. Heinen M-P, Busoni V, Petite A, et al. Bicipital groove dysplasia and medial dislocation of the biceps brachii tendon in a Welsh pony. *Vet Radiol Ultrasound.* 2002;44:235.

41. Coudry V, Allen AK, Denoix JM. Congenital abnormalities of the bicipital apparatus in four mature horses. *Equine Vet J.* 2005;37(3):272–275.

42. Lund CM, Ragle CA, Rice HC, et al. Bilateral hypoplasia of the minor tubercle of the humerus with medial luxation of the biceps tendon in two Quarter horses. *Equine Vet Educ.* 2014;26(9):467–472.

43. Schneider RK, Bramlage LR, Moore RM, et al. A retrospective study of 192 horses affected with septic arthritis/tenosynovitis. *Equine Vet J.* 1992;24(6):436–442.

24

Tarsus

Christopher E. Kawcak

The tarsus is unique in that it contains both high motion and low motion joints, each of which can undergo significant pathologic changes and lead to clinically relevant disease. The tarsus is made up of the tibia, talus, calcaneus, the central tarsal bone, the fused first and second tarsal bone, the third and fourth tarsal bones, and the second, third, and fourth metatarsal bones. The distal tibia and the proximal aspect of the talus articulate to form the tibiotarsal joint. The talus and calcaneus articulate to form the talocalcaneal joint. The talus and central tarsal bone articulate to form the proximal intertarsal joint (which is included in the tibiotarsal synovial pouch, making these two joints communicate); the central tarsal bone and the distal row of tarsal bones (fused first and second, third, and fourth tarsal bones) form the distal intertarsal joint; and the distal row of tarsal bones articulate with the proximal aspect of the metatarsal bones to form the tarsometatarsal joint.[1] The tibiotarsal joint has both cranial and caudal outpouchings, all of which can be used for arthrocentesis, especially when synovial effusion is present.

Numerous studies document the communication between the various joints within the tarsus. As mentioned, the tibiotarsal and proximal intertarsal joints communicate regularly and are considered one joint. The proximal intertarsal joint occasionally communicates with either the distal intertarsal joint or the tarsometatarsal joint.[2] Multiple studies document the frequency of communication between the distal intertarsal and tarsometatarsal joints, which varies from 8% to 38%.[2-4] In addition, medications injected into one joint have the potential to spread into others.[5] There is also evidence to support that medication or analgesic substances administered to the deep branch of the lateral plantar nerve may migrate into the tarsometatarsal joint.[6] Consequently, interpreting the results of diagnostic analgesia in the horse can be fraught with problems, often necessitating volumetric imaging to determine the exact site of pain.

There are many different pathologic processes that can lead to disease within the tarsus. Acute traumatic injuries can result in acute fractures in any of the bones including the tibia and proximal metatarsus. Soft tissue injuries can occur from traumatic incidents including damage to the collateral ligaments and the intraarticular ligaments within the distal tarsal joints. Developmental orthopedic disease is common in the tarsus and includes osteochondritis dissecans lesions,

especially within the tibiotarsal joint and subchondral cystic lesions within all bones of the tarsus. In addition, similar to other joints, athletic horses can suffer from fatigue-related injuries of the tarsus. Fragmentation, fracture, and subchondral bone disease within the distal tarsal joints are common in horses of all disciplines, especially sport horses and Western performance horses. These joints will readily suffer from osteoarthritis (OA), often necessitating medical and/or surgical treatment. OA can also occur in the tibiotarsal and talocalcaneal joints but is rare yet debilitating.

Horses that suffer from pain within the tarsus typically present in one of two ways. Diseases within the tibiotarsal joint typically manifest with significant synovial effusion and variable degrees of lameness. Diseases within the proximal intertarsal joint typically manifest with significant synovial effusion of the tibiotarsal joints because those two joints communicate; however, proximal intertarsal joint disease can occur without synovial effusion (Figure 24-1). In most cases of distal tarsal joint injury, horses typically demonstrate variable degrees of lameness and have shortened stride with worsening of the lameness on the inside of a circle. Synovial effusion is not palpable in these joints, and capsular swelling can sometimes be appreciated. Synovitis and various degrees

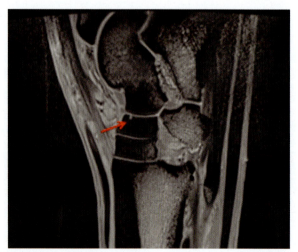

FIGURE 24-1 Magnetic resonance image of a tarsus demonstrating articular changes within the proximal intertarsal joint (arrow) in a horse with no synovial effusion.

of OA in the distal tarsal joints usually occur bilaterally and consequently a shuffling, short-strided lameness is evident. The lameness in these horses is typically worse with the limb on the inside of a circle and positive to full-limb flexion. Occasionally pain will be palpable on the medial side of the distal tarsal joints. Osteochondral damage in the form of fragmentation or fracture in the distal tarsal joints is not uncommon and those horses will typically have a significant unilateral lameness that is moderately to severely responsive to full-limb flexion. Synovial effusion is not palpable in the proximal intertarsal, distal intertarsal, and tarsometatarsal joints, although, significant injury can lead to soft tissue swelling of this area.

Arthocentesis of the tarsus can range from easy to very difficult. The tibiotarsal joint is most easily aspirated from the large dorsomedial pouch. Care should be taken to avoid the saphenous vein, which is often easily identifiable in the standing horse (Figure 24-2). The caudal aspect of the tarsocrural joint can also be aspirated or injected especially if there is a laceration on the cranial aspect of the joint. Care must be taken that swelling in this area is truly effusive and not soft tissue swelling, which can typically occur in Western performance horses especially on the caudal lateral aspect of the joint. Usually upon further palpation, this swelling is firm and associated synovial effusion is not present in the other outpouchings. This is likely an adaptive response within the joint

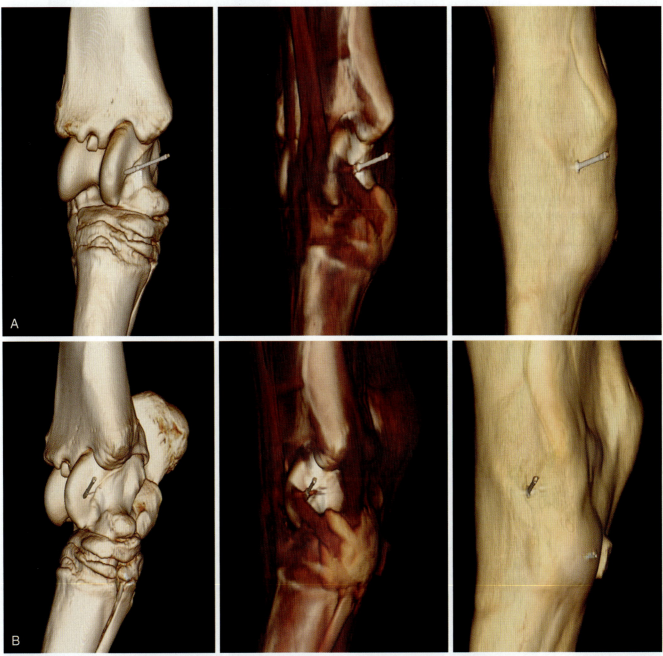

FIGURE 24-2 A computed tomography rendering demonstrating needle placement in the dorsomedial aspect of the tarsocrural joint (**A** and **B**).

because of the tremendous workload placed on the hind limbs of Western performance horses. Disease within the proximal intertarsal joint is typically characterized with diagnostic analgesia and treated by injecting the tibiotarsal joint. Precise placement of a needle into the proximal intertarsal joint is difficult and if necessary can be done under radiographic guidance. The distal intertarsal joint is difficult to aspirate and inject even under normal circumstances. The medial approach can be used based on palpation and in a horse with a minimal amount of radiographic change, can often be done consistently by the experienced practitioner (Figure 24-3). This injection is typically performed from the opposite side of the horse with the limb in weight-bearing position. The goal for injecting at this site is to direct a needle in the joint space between the fused first and second tarsal bones, the third tarsal bone, and the central tarsal bone. There are a number of landmarks to use, which have been described previously, and a medial approach has been advocated for many decades.[7-9] From the medial side a small depression can be felt with the fingernail just distal to the cunean tendon. Ultrasound can also be used to guide needle placement at the side of the joint. A 1-inch 22- to 25-gauge needle is directed perpendicular to the joint surface at this site.[7] Rarely is fluid acquired and the ease of injection subjectively allows the clinician to feel confident in the injection. Although this technique has been used for years and many practitioners swear by it, it can still be inconsistent for the administration of analgesics. Therapeutics administered through this site may be effective because of diffusion into and around the joint. Another technique for injection of the distal intertarsal joint is through a dorsal lateral approach. The clinician stands on the same side of the horse with the horse in full weight bearing. The injection site is on the craniolateral aspect of the joint approximately halfway between

the distal end of the lateral trochlear ridge and the head of the fourth metatarsal bone. Radiographic guidance of the technique is often needed to ensure proper placement of the needle (Figures 24-3 and 24-4). A 1.5-inch 20-gauge needle is typically used and directed plantar medially at an angle of 70 degrees to the sagittal plane until bone is contacted. A digital radiograph can be taken at this point to be sure that the needle is in the distal intertarsal joint and analgesic or medication is injected. At times this injection technique is easier as there

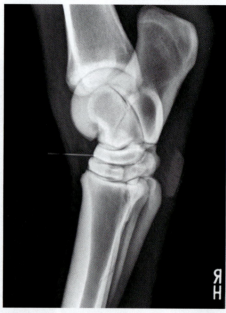

FIGURE 24-4 A radiographic image showing proper placement of the needle into the distal intertarsal joint from the dorsal lateral approach.

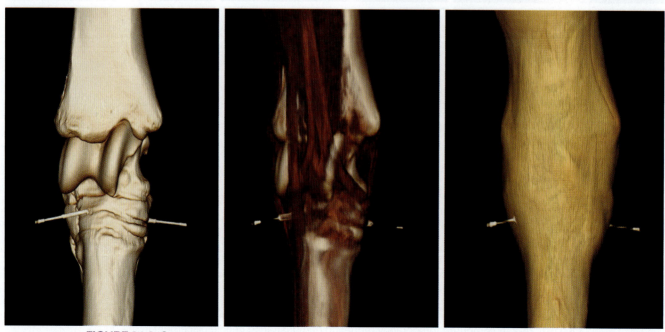

FIGURE 24-3 Computed tomographic rendering of the medial and dorsolateral approaches to the distal intertarsal joint.

may be less periarticular bone formation on the craniolateral aspect of the joint compared with the medial aspect.[10] The tarsometatarsal joint is considered one of the most commonly injected joints and with experience can be relatively simple to perform as it is easily entered with a 20-gauge 1.5-inch needle aimed in a caudolateral to craniomedial direction downward 30 degrees into the joint approximately 1 cm proximal to the head of the lateral splint bone (Figure 24-5). The site for injection is on the caudal lateral aspect of the limb just proximal to the most proximal aspect of the fourth metatarsal bone. A 1.5-inch needle is typically inserted in the depression approximately 1 cm proximal to the head of the fourth metatarsal bone. The head of the needle is typically brought 30 degrees lateral from midsagittal plane and 30 degrees proximal from a midtransverse plane, approximately 1 cm proximal to the head of the fourth metatarsal bone. Synovial fluid is often observed especially in cases with synovitis.[7]

Conformational abnormalities in the tarsus are not uncommon and in fact some breeds prefer a slight tarsal valgus conformation for optimized athletic potential. This is typically seen in the Standardbred and not uncommon in the cutting horse industries. Tarsal varus and rotational abnormalities to the tarsus are not uncommon and abnormalities to the cuboidal bones are common. Subtle abnormalities in the cuboidal bones of the distal tarsus are thought to result in early-onset OA that has been termed juvenile spavin.

IMAGING PARAMETERS

Radiographic examination of the tarsus is performed with the axis to the limb perpendicular to the ground and the horse bearing full weight. Four radiographic views are typical of a routine examination: the lateral medial, dorsal plantar, dorsolateral-plantaromedial oblique, and dorsomedial-plantarolateral oblique. In some practices the lateral oblique is shot more in a plantarolateral-dorsomedial oblique direction for ease of use. In some cases a flexed lateral medial projection is needed, and for cases of suspected calcaneal damage a flexed proximal plantar-distal plantar image is needed. For a lateral medial view of the tarsal joints, the beam should be centered at the talus and the image should demonstrate superimposition of the lateral and medial trochlear ridges. As a side note, the plantar aspect of the third metatarsal bone diverges from a caudolateral to a dorsomedial orientation at approximately 30 degrees; therefore, for assessment of the caudal aspect of the third metatarsal bone the angle should be in the

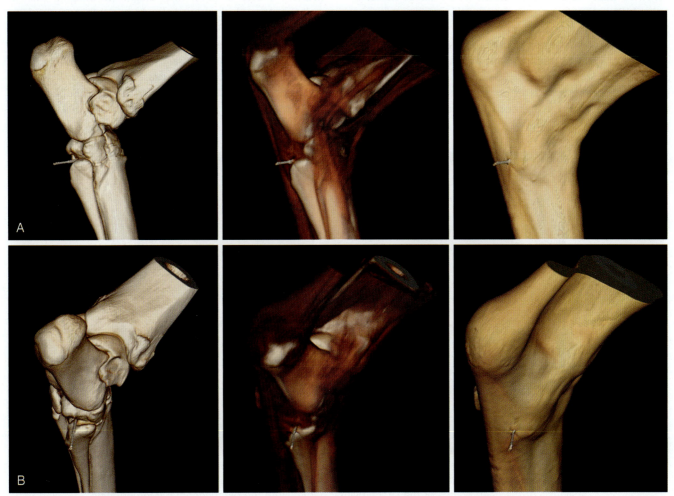

FIGURE 24-5 Computed tomographic rendering of needle placement for injection of the tarsometatarsal joint. **(A)** View from the lateral aspect. **(B)** View from a proximal perspective, which is the typical position where a clinician would perform the procedure.

30 degrees plantarolateral-dorsomedial oblique projection for superimposition of the second and fourth metatarsal bones. For the dorsal plantar view the beam should be centered on the distal aspect of the talus and shot in a true sagittal plane. However, for more precise imaging of the medial malleolus, the x-ray generator should be moved approximately 10 degrees laterally to give a 10 degree dorsolateral-plantaromedial oblique projection. The opposite is true for more precise imaging of the lateral malleolus.[11] Subtle changes in the obliquity of the images may be needed especially in cases of acute lameness in which osteochondral damage is suspected. For horses in which subtle abnormalities indicative of OA are seen, radiographic imaging of the opposite limb is suggested since most disease in this joint is bilateral in nature.

Ultrasound of the tarsus is usually reserved for suspected cases of collateral ligament damage. Surrounding soft tissue diseases can be characterized, but the collateral ligaments are the only articular structures that can be visualized using ultrasonography.[12]

Although in many cases subchondral bone sclerosis and lysis can be identified radiographically, characterization of subtle lesions often requires volumetric imaging such as magnetic resonance imaging (MRI) or computed tomography (CT). In many cases, subtle lesions in the tarsus detected using MRI or CT often occur when there is suspicion of proximal suspensory ligament injury. In these cases, horses typically go into the MRI or the CT unit for suspicion of proximal suspensory ligament origin lesions, and the tarsal lesions are often seen incidentally (Figure 24-6).[13,14]

Nuclear scintigraphy is an excellent modality for detecting tarsal diseases involving the subchondral bone. Although some horses will have significant increased radiopharmaceutical uptake (IRU) caused by normal bone adaptation from exercise, unlike the carpus, diseases and pain within the tarsus typically show specific IRU in the lower tarsal joints.[15]

CLINICAL SIGNS

For diseases of the tarsocrural joint in which synovial effusion and/or swelling around the tarsocrural joint are apparent, the area should be meticulously palpated to try and best characterize whether the swelling caused entirely by synovial effusion or if isolated swelling around the soft tissues is identified. It is important to discern synovial effusion from joint capsule swelling. Both lameness and response to full limb flexion should be characterized. Because synovial effusion of the tarsocrural joint is not uncommon in some athletes, those horses with persistent swelling should be blocked with intraarticular analgesia of the tarsocrural joint to confirm the site of pain. Even with a negative response to diagnostic analgesia, it may still be important to image the joint, not to characterize the immediate source of pain but to characterize the source of synovial effusion. If the tarsocrural joint is identified as the primary source of pain, then diagnostic imaging such as radiography and ultrasound should be performed. In those cases where it is deemed necessary, volumetric imaging such as MRI and CT should be performed. In some cases, diagnostic arthroscopy is necessary to visualize the joint surfaces to characterize and treat the cause of lameness. It must be remembered in these cases that both the front and the back of the joints should be scoped to completely examine the area.[16]

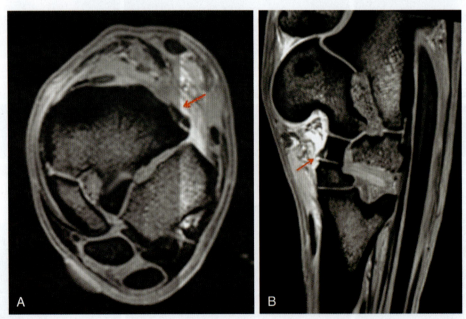

FIGURE 24-6 Magnetic resonance image of a tarsus in a horse suspected of proximal suspensory ligament injury. The lameness in this specific horse improved significantly with diagnostic analgesia of the deep branch of the lateral plantar nerve. Note the osteochondral fragmentation in the tarsus. The linear hyperintense artifact that extends through the image is secondary to transverse reconstruction of this three-dimensional image. (**A**) Transverse view; (**B**) Sagittal view.

The diagnostic workup for characterizing distal intertarsal and tarsometatarsal joint disease is more difficult. As mentioned earlier, outward swelling may not be appreciated and the horse shows a unilateral or bilateral lameness with positive response to full limb flexion. Although some clinicians feel they can discern hock pain from stifle pain with isolated flexions, it is not uncommon for horses with distal intertarsal and tarsometatarsal joint pain to respond to all flexions of the hind limb. Intraarticular analgesia of the tarsometatarsal and distal intertarsal joints should be performed to document the site of pain. In some cases, even with a radiographically guided technique, a certain percentage of horses will improve with diagnostic analgesia of the distal intertarsal and tarsometatarsal joints even though the primary pain may be outside of the joint. In most cases this is caused by pain in the proximal suspensory ligament origin. However, it is difficult to know whether that is the primary source of pain or if there is pain at both sites. It is not uncommon to see horses that have signs of chronic proximal suspensory desmitis improve with medication into the distal intertarsal and tarsometatarsal joints. However, in these cases it is difficult to know whether it is the joint, the suspensory origin, or both that are causing pain.

SPECIFIC CONDITIONS

Osteochondrosis of the Tarsus

Osteochondrosis of the tarsus is typically clinically relevant when there is tibiotarsal joint effusion or when the lesions are found on radiographs of young horses that have yet to go into training. The latter lesions are considered significant when it is predicted that they may influence future athletic endeavors. Lameness may or may not be present in these cases but the presence of tibiotarsal joint effusion signifies the clinical significance of the lesions. Osteochondritis dissecan lesions are common within the tibiotarsal joint and typically seen on the distal intermediate ridge of the tibia, the lateral trochlear ridge, and the medial trochlear ridge within the cranial aspect of the joint.[16] On occasion lesions can be in the caudal aspect of the joint. Osteochondritis dissecans is not uncommonly seen on the axial side of the medial malleolus.[16] Radiographic characteristics of the lesion include presence of a separated boney fragment from the distal intermediate ridge of the tibia, either trochlear ridge or the lateral or medial malleolus (Figure 24-7). Boney irregularity and fragmentation at the distal aspect of the medial trochlear ridge are often not of clinical significance (Figure 24-8). Subtle irregularities in the subchondral may or may not be of clinical significance especially in the absence of synovial effusion. For these particular cases, ultrasonographic examination of the area may be beneficial in identifying separated articular cartilage. However, in these cases synovial effusion will often be present. Because of the high incidence of bilateral lesions, detection of osteochondritis dissecan lesions in one tarsus makes it mandatory to perform radiographic investigation of the opposite tarsus.

Occasionally an osteochondritis dissecans lesion can be seen in the caudal aspect of the joint. Although there have been reports of treating osteochondritis dissecans conservatively with intraarticular medication, there is concern that many of the these horses can ultimately develop OA.[17] Typical cysts have been found in specific locations within the tarsocrural joint.[18,19] Although some of these can be caused by osteochondrosis or sepsis, trauma must also be considered as an etiology.

Horses with mild signs typically do well with arthroscopic débridement of these cysts; however, those with more significant lameness and damage within the joint often have a limited prognosis.[18,19]

Soft Tissue Diseases
Synovitis/Capsulitis

Synovitis/capsulitis of the tarsus is not uncommon. It is assumed in most cases of lower tarsal joint pain with no radiographic abnormalities that synovitis/capsulitis plays a major role in causing pain. However, this is difficult to document. Synovitis of the distal intertarsal (DIT) and tarsometatarsal (TMT) joints is common in the athletic horse, and there is often poor correlation between lameness and radiographic signs of disease. Cases in which radiographic signs of disease are nonexistent or mild, in which the horse blocks to the DIT and TMT joints or responds positively to intraarticular medication, can be treated effectively over a long period of time. However, horses that fail to respond to medication, either initially or over time, should be reexamined or the joint reassessed with intraarticular analgesia. More advanced imaging may be needed to best characterize the site of pain and the pathologic process that is occurring.

Septic arthritis of the tibiotarsal joint is common in foals and often is the result of septic physitis of the distal tibia (Figure 24-9). Septic arthritis is covered in more detail in Chapter 7.

Synovitis and OA of the proximal intertarsal joint are rare, but when it does occur signs typically manifest in the tibiotarsal joint. In these cases, facilitated ankylosis is not an option because of concern about the status of the tibiotarsal joint with which it communicates. Long-term intraarticular medication is usually necessary to best manage the horse for use.

Synovitis/capsulitis in the tibiotarsal joint is common and can have significant ramifications. Synovitis is common when an osteochondritis dissecans lesion is present. As long as the lesion is treated promptly after the presence of effusion, the synovitis typically resolves after removal of the fragment. However, in cases that are considered chronic, removal of the fragment may not resolve the synovitis since the tibiotarsal joint seems to be prone to synovitis once it becomes chronic. Various medications can be used to try to resolve the synovitis; however, chronic effusion synovitis can be difficult to control. Synovitis can occur in the tibiotarsal joint without a primary cause of disease, and this is not uncommon in sport horses and Western performance

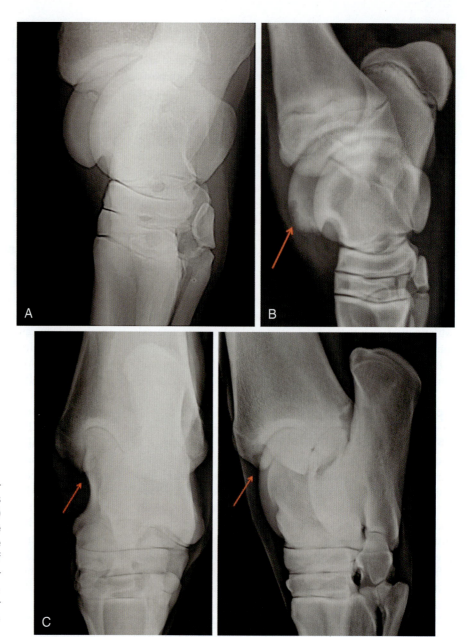

FIGURE 24-7 Typical radiographic lesions of osteochondritis dissecans (OCD) within the tibiotarsal joint. **(A)** OCD lesion of the distal intermediate ridge of the tibia. **(B)** OCD lesion of the lateral trochlear ridge. **(C)** OCD lesion of the medial malleolus of the tibia. (Reproduced from McIlwraith CW, Nixon AJ, Wright IM. (2014). Diagnostic and Surgical Arthroscopy in the Horse, 4th ed. London, Elsevier.)

horses that are in active work. Capsulitis is not uncommon in the tibiotarsal joint and sometimes can be associated with soft tissue damage in the collateral ligaments. Chronic synovial and capsular change within the tarsus can lead to significant clinical signs and be difficult to treat. These horses typically have synovial effusion and persistent soft tissue swelling around the joint, which does not resolve with bandaging. They also typically have limited range of motion and significant pain on flexion.

Idiopathic synovitis of the tibiotarsal joint is becoming uncommon with the evolution of advanced imaging techniques. Damage within or around the tibiotarsal joint can lead to either primary or secondary synovitis leading to lameness. Idiopathic tibiotarsal septic arthritis has been described in cases in which there is no history of injection or laceration to contaminate the joint.[20] In most cases

tarsocrural joint synovitis is caused by a primary cause, either within the joint or extraarticular. Intraarticular damage can be in the form of osteochondral fragmentation or primary articular cartilage damage. Osteochondral fragmentation can typically be seen radiographically and in most cases is caused by some form of osteochondritis dissecans. However, primary traumatic articular cartilage damage, which requires arthroscopic visualization and treatment, can occur. For horses with significant lameness in association with severe synovitis, care must be taken to acquire radiographic images highlighting subtle osteochondral fractures. Damage to collateral ligaments and extraarticular structures can also lead to tarsocrural synovitis. Whether this occurs primarily because of damage to the structure or secondary to instability is unknown. However, in many cases the site of disease is first identified

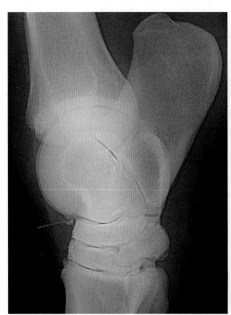 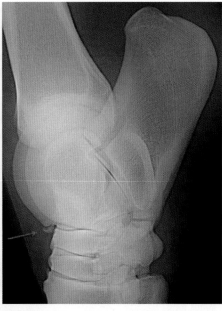

FIGURE 24-8 Radiographic image of the tarsus demonstrating a clinically insignificant fragment at the distal aspect of the medial trochlear ridge (arrow).

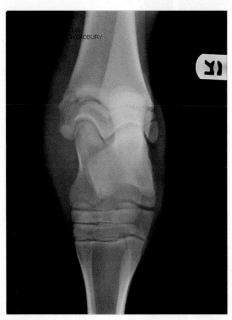

FIGURE 24-9 Radiographic image of the tarsus of a foal demonstrating a lytic lesion on the medial aspect of the distal tibial physis indicative of septic physitis. The foal presented with severe lameness and effusion of the tibiotarsal joint. The distal medial tibial physis was painful to palpation.

through significant tarsocrural joint effusion. In these cases radiographs and ultrasound are necessary to best characterize the site and severity of pain. In those cases in which radiographic and ultrasonographic images are unremarkable, volumetric imaging using MRI or CT is necessary. At that time definitive treatment can be initiated. The prognosis for horses with tarsocrural synovitis is dependent on the primary disease process and response to treatment. Regardless of the cause of tarsocrural synovitis, the development of joint capsule fibrosis and restricted range

of motion can in itself be limiting to normal movement and athletic potential of the horse. Residual synovitis and capsular thickening are not uncommon in the tarsocrural joint and efforts must be made to reduce the chance of this occurring even after the primary disease is resolved.

Osteoarthritis

OA of the distal intertarsal and tarsometatarsal joints is one of the most common clinical manifestations in equine practice. OA of the distal tarsal joints can be very mild to very severe; however, in this area facilitated ankylosis can be used as an ultimate therapy to decrease clinical symptoms. Radiographic signs of mild OA include periarticular osteophyte and enthesophyte formation, mild narrowing of the joint space, and subchondral bone sclerosis. With advancing severity of OA, osteophytes and enthesophytes can become larger, periarticular lysis can become evident, and subchondral bone sclerosis can become progressive. In severe cases, joint space narrowing can be significant with associated subchondral bone sclerosis and lysis. Horses with these latter lesions are typically very lame and response to intraarticular analgesia can be limited, likely because of significant subchondral bone pain (Figure 24-10).

The clinical presentation of horses with OA of the distal intertarsal and tarsometatarsal joints is not too dissimilar from that in horses with proximal suspensory origin pain. There is evidence to show that diagnostic analgesia of the tarsometatarsal joint can result in elimination of pain in the proximal suspensory region,[3] and it has been shown that diagnostic analgesia of the proximal suspensory ligament (PSL) area (PSL infusion, high 4-point, and deep branch of the lateral plantar nerve) can lead to decrease in pain from the lower hock joints.[6] Consequently, if therapeutic management of distal tarsal OA or PSL origin pain is unsuccessful, then volumetric imaging of this area is recommended to specifically identify the site of pain. On many occasions, the volumetric imaging may find something other than the suspected lesion, leading to a change in management (Figure 24-11).

In some cases OA may set in and the joint become less responsive to intraarticular medication. In those cases in which horses fail to respond to intraarticular medication or extracorporeal shock wave therapy, facilitated ankylosis can be considered. Since the DIT and TMT joints have low motion, facilitated ankylosis has a good chance of returning these horses to use pending the absence of lesions around this area.[21-23]

Facilitated ankylosis can be achieved in a number of ways. The most consistent treatment is by surgical forage of the DIT and TMT joints. This technique is described elsewhere.[24] Intraarticular application of monoiodoacetate has been advocated by some; however, a handful of horses in those studies have shown proximal intertarsal joint OA well after the

lower hock joints have fused.[25,26] Intraarticular administration of ethanol has also been advocated. The DIT and TMT joints are injected under contrast radiographic guidance; 70% ethanol is then injected into the joints.[27] The benefits of this technique are that it eliminates the need for surgery and general anesthesia, is less expensive, and may have some immediate effect in relieving pain so as to continue exercise. In some cases the joint needs to be redosed. Laser energy using an Nd:YAG or gallium-aluminum-arsenide-diode laser may be effective in relieving DIT and TMT pain.[21] With this technique, horses have been reported to return to work within a couple of weeks. The exact mechanism that achieves this soundness is unknown. In two experimental studies, laser application to the DIT and TMT joints did not create consistent joint fusion and stability.[22,23] It could be that the laser is

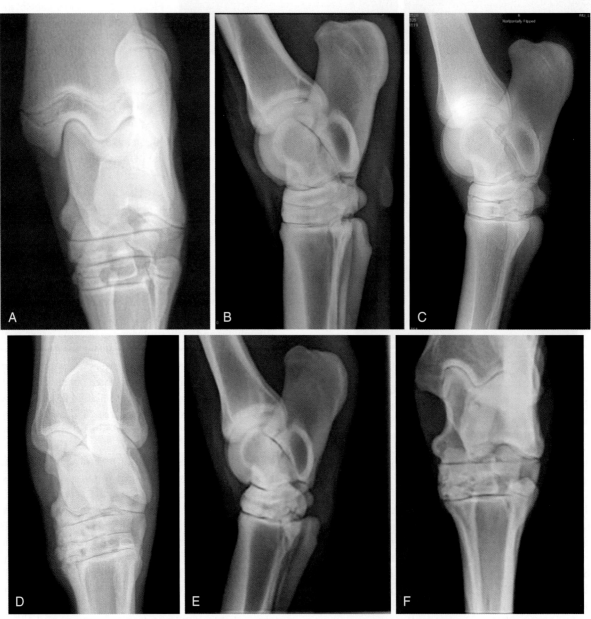

FIGURE 24-10 Variable degrees of radiographically evident osteoarthritis typical of horses. (A) Shows a relatively normal joint. (B) and (C) demonstrate mild changes, including subchondral bone sclerosis and joint space narrowing. OA progression worsens in (D) and becomes severe in (E) and (F).

illuminating fibrous joint capsule response caused by "boiling" of the intrasynovial fluid. However, care must be taken in case selection as there is some concern that horses with extensive subchondral bone necrosis may not be as responsive to the laser technique. The techniques for application of the laser to the DIT and TMT joints are described elsewhere.[21]

Overall treatment of horses with synovitis or OA of the DIT and TMT joints can be rewarding. The most difficult part of dealing with these problems is developing an effective management plan. The other difficult decision is when to perform facilitated ankylosis. This depends on the effectiveness of medical management, the horse's show schedule, and the owner's ability and desire to rehabilitate the horse during this time.

OA of the tibiotarsal joint can cause significant effusion and joint capsule swelling, limited range of motion, and significant lameness. Horses with OA of the tibiotarsal joint are often resentful of full-limb flexion. Radiographic signs of osteophyte and enthesophyte formation, subchondral bone sclerosis and lysis, and joint space narrowing are typical. In some cases in which subtle subchondral bone damage may be present and not radiographically apparent, MRI may be necessary to characterize those changes (Figure 24-12). OA of the talocalcaneal joint is occasionally seen and has distinguishing radiographic changes (Figure 24-13). Horses with these lesions do not typically have significant joint swelling but are lame. Treatment options for this disease are limited.

OA of the proximal intertarsal joint is rare and in most cases manifests with clinical signs in the tibiotarsal joint (Figure 24-14). Similar to OA of the tibiotarsal joint, the only option is medical therapy. On occasion fragmentation of the proximal intertarsal joint can be arthroscopically removed but in some cases those fragments lie within the joint capsule, making removal difficult if not impossible.

Intertarsal Ligament Tearing

Figure 24-15 illustrates an example of intertarsal ligament tearing. Identification of this injury is difficult and often requires volumetric imaging, namely MRI for proper diagnosis. Clinical signs can appear similar to horses with diseases of the lower hock joints.

Collateral Ligament Injury

Injury to the collateral ligaments of the tarsus is uncommon; however, when they do occur they can lead to significant pain

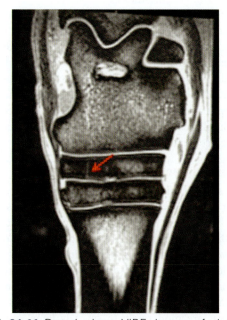

FIGURE 24-11 Dorsal plane VIBE image of the tarsus. Marked sclerosis of the central tarsal bone with a bi-articular slab fracture (red arrow). This horse had acute onset of 3/5 lameness that was localized to the PSL via regional anesthesia. Only mild changes noted in the PSL on the MRI.

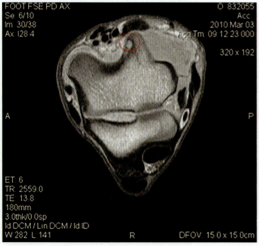
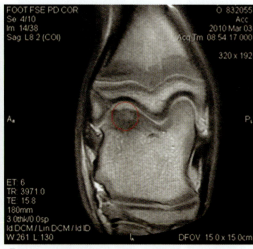

A   B

FIGURE 24-12 Magnetic resonance images of a yearling Quarter horse in which no outward swelling was apparent but the horse had moderate unilateral lameness and significant pain on full-limb flexion. The images demonstrate subchondral bone edema within several areas of the talus and calcaneus (white arrows). (A) Transverse image; (B) Frontal plane image.

and swelling. Not only will synovitis of the tibiotarsal joint be present, but typically periarticular swelling will also occur especially in the area of the collateral ligaments. Pain on palpation may be evident and on occasion radiographs may demonstrate an avulsion fracture at the origin of the particular ligament. It is recommended that diagnostic ultrasonography be used to best characterize the location and severity of damage to the collateral ligament (Figure 24-16). On occasion MRI is needed to best characterize the site and severity

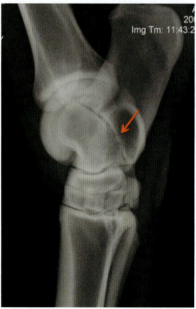

FIGURE 24-13 Radiographic image of the tarsus demonstrating subchondral bone sclerosis and lysis in the talocalcaneal joint indicative of osteoarthritis.

of the lesion especially when they are subtle (Figure 24-17). Depending on the severity of the lesion and pain, these lesions can usually be treated conservatively. If the lesion is severe and joint instability is present, then a sleeve cast or a bandage cast can be applied until stability is acceptable. Intralesional therapy may also be appropriate. Cases in which avulsion fractures are present often require surgery to remove the avulsed piece of bone and to prevent ongoing joint disease.

Osteochondral Damage
Osteochondral Fragmentation

Osteochondral fragmentation can occasionally occur in the lower tarsal joints and can be traumatic in nature. On occasion these fragments may be difficult to see on radiographs, and volumetric imaging such as CT or MRI may be necessary to fully characterize the disease (see Figure 24-6). These lesions are difficult to treat, as they are not amenable to arthroscopic removal. Medical therapy can be used to help manage the clinical signs but in some cases facilitated ankylosis may be needed to remove the pain.

Osteochondral Fracture

Fractures of the central and third tarsal bones can affect any breed but are most common in the racing breeds.[28-30] The exact causes of these fractures are unknown; however, considering their high prevalence in racing breeds an "overstress or adaptive mechanism" must be considered.

Complete osteochondral fracture/slab fracture of the lower tarsal bones is not uncommon. In most instances these can be diagnosed radiographically (Figure 24-18). Typically these horses are moderately to severely lame and severely

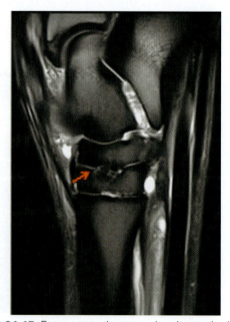

FIGURE 24-15 Fat-saturated proton density sagittal MR image showing marked sclerosis and osseous proliferation of the fossa of the intertarsal ligament with a loss of the normal signal or fiber pattern of the intertarsal ligament. Compare to the normal fossa of the tarsometatarsal ligament.

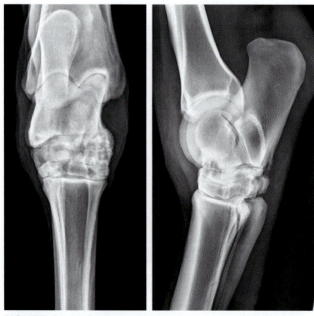

FIGURE 24-14 Radiographic images demonstrating severe osteoarthritic changes to the proximal intertarsal joint.

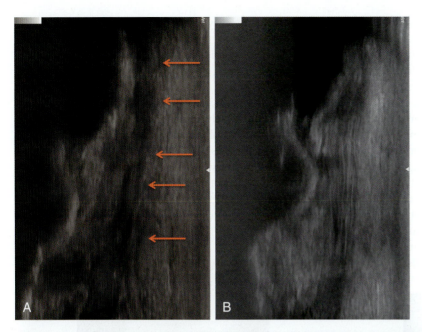

FIGURE 24-16 Ultrasonographic imaging of the collateral ligament demonstrating a lesion (A - arrows). Compare to the collateral ligament from the normal limb (B). (Images courtesy of Dr. Kurt Selberg)

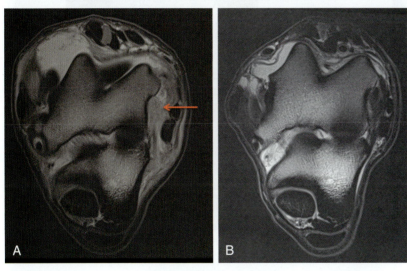

FIGURE 24-17 Magnetic resonance image of a damaged collateral ligament in the tarsus (A - arrow). Compare to the MRI from the normal limb (B).

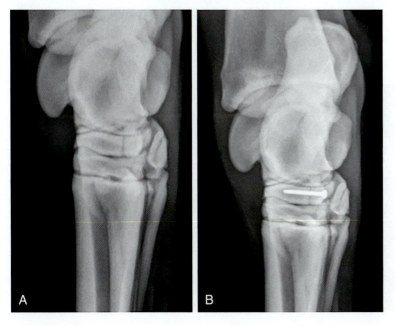

FIGURE 24-18 Radiographic image of a complete slab fracture of the central/third tarsal bone of the horse before (A) and after lag screw fixation (B).

positive to full-limb flexion. Pain may be palpable in the area of the fracture. On occasion, when radiographs are negative, volumetric imaging such as CT or MRI may be useful to fully characterize the lesion (Figure 24-19). Lag screw fixation of the fracture usually provides the best chance for the horse to return to performance.[28,29] The approach to repair using lag screw fixation has been reported elsewhere.[29] Conservative treatment has been reported, although fewer Thoroughbreds appear to return to work compared with Quarter horses, and horses with fracture of the central tarsal bone had significantly poorer prognosis than those with third tarsal bone fracture.[30]

Osteochondral fracture of the distal tibia, talus, and metatarsal bones are not uncommon and involve the joints of the tarsus. The basic principles of accurate joint alignment and internal fixation should be used to optimize future performance and comfort. On occasion, these fractures may be difficult to see and may only be present on radiographs after 10 to 14 days of rest or may be acutely present on volumetric imaging techniques (Figures 24-20 and 24-21).

Tarsal Luxation

Luxation of the tarsal joints is uncommon; however, care should be taken to appropriately diagnose this so that appropriate therapy can be initiated. Collateral ligament and joint capsule damage is typical of these lesions. In addition to routine radiographs of the tarsus, stress views should be used to further document the luxation. In addition, ultrasound examination may be useful to better characterize the soft tissue lesions. For unstable cases in which the proximal intertarsal, distal intertarsal, or

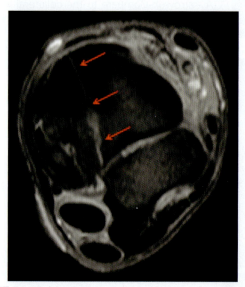

FIGURE 24-19 Magnetic resonance image of a slab fracture through the third tarsal bone (arrows).

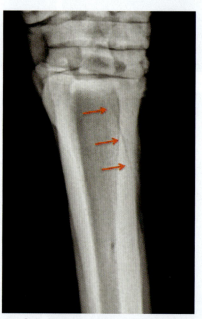

FIGURE 24-21 Subsequent radiographs did demonstrate the presence of the fracture once fracture line resorption occurred.

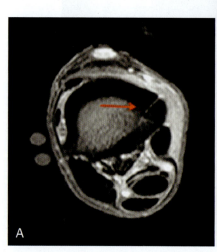

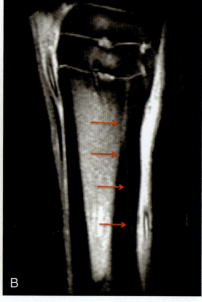

FIGURE 24-20 Proximal third metatarsal fracture is apparent on these magnetic resonance images in a horse that was only mildly lame and on which the fracture was not apparent on initial radiographs. **(A)** Transverse plane image; **(B)** Sagittal plane image.

tarsometatarsal joints are involved, internal fixation can be used to stabilize those joints. However, for the tibiotarsal joint conservative management using tube casting or splinting may be appropriate once the joint is fully reduced.[31]

REFERENCES

1. Kainer RA, Fails AD. *Functional anatomy of the equine musculoskeletal system. In: Adam's and Stashak's lameness in horses.* 6 ed. West Sussex, UK: Wiley Blackwell; 2011 (pp. 43–49).
2. Kraus-Hansen AE, Jann HW, Kerr DV, et al. Arthrographic analysis of communication between the tarsometatarsal and distal intertarsal joints of the horse. *Vet Surg.* 1992;21(2):139–144.
3. Dyson SJ, Romero JM. An investigation of injection techniques for local analgesia of the equine distal tarsus and metatarsus. *Equine Vet J.* 1993;25(1):30–35.
4. Bell BTL, Baker GJ, Foreman JH, et al. In vivo investigation of communication between the distal intertarsal and tarsometatarsal joints in horses and ponies. *Vet Surg.* 1993;22(4):289–292.
5. Serena A, Shoemaker J, Schramme MC, et al. Concentration of methylprednisolone in the central distal joint after administration of methylprednisolone acetate in the tarsometatarsal joint. *Equine Vet J.* 2005;37(2):172–174.
6. Contino EK, King MR, Valdes-Martinez A, et al. In vivo diffusion characteristics following perineural injection of the deep branch of the lateral plantar nerve with mepivacaine or iohexal in horses. *Equine Vet J.* 2015;47(2):230–234.
7. Moyer W. *Equine joint injection and regional anesthesia.* 5th ed. Chadds Ford, P.A: Academic Veterinary Solutions; 2011.
8. Sack WO, Orsini PG. Distal intertarsal and tarsometatarsal joints in the horse: communication and injection sites. *J Am Vet Med Assoc.* 1981;179(4):355–359.
9. Baxter GM, Stashak TS. Perineural and intrasynovial anesthesia. In: *Adam's and Stashak's lameness in horses.* 6th ed. West Sussex, UK: Wiley Blackwell; 2011(pp. 195–196).
10. Just EM, Patan B, Licka TF. Dorsolateral approach for arthrocentesis of the central distal joint in horses. *Am J Vet Res.* 2007;68(9):946–952.
11. The tarsus. In: Butler JA, Colles CM, Dyson SJ, et al. eds. *Clinical radiology of the horse.* 3rd ed. Wiley Blackwell; 2008. (pp. 321–361).
12. Raes EV, Vanderperren K, Pille F, et al. Ultrasonographic findings in 100 horses with tarsal region disorders. *Vet J.* 2010;186(2):201–209.
13. Daniel AJ, Judy CE, Rick MC, et al. Comparison of radiography, nuclear scintigraphy, and magnetic resonance imaging for detection of specific conditions of the distal tarsal bones of horses: 20 cases (2006-2010). *J Am Vet Med Assoc.* 2012;240(9):1109–1114.
14. Raes E, Bergman HJ, Van Ryssen B, et al. Computed tomographic features of lesions detected in horses with tarsal lameness. *Equine Vet J.* 2014;46(2):189–193.
15. Murray RC, Dyson SJ, Weekes JS. Scintigraphic evaluation of the distal tarsal region in horses with distal tarsal pain. *Vet Radiol Ultrasound.* 2005;46(2):171–178.
16. McIlwraith CW, Nixon AJ, Wright IM. *Diagnostic and surgical arthroscopy in the horse.* 4th ed. London: Elsevier; 2014.
17. Peremans K, Verschooten F. Results of conservative treatment of osteochondrosis of the tibiotarsal joint in the horse. *J Equine Vet Sci.* 1997;17(6):322–326.
18. Garcia-Lopez JM, Kirker-Head CA. Occult subchondral osseous cyst like lesions of the equine tarsocrural joint. *Vet Surg.* 2004;33(5):557–564.
19. Montgomery LJ, Juzwiak JS. Subchondral cyst-like lesions in the talus of four horses. *Equine Vet Educ.* 2009;21(12):629–637.
20. Schneider RK, Bramlage LR, Moore RM, et al. A retrospective study of 192 horses affected with septic arthritis/tenosynovitis. *Equine Vet J.* 1992;24(6):436–442.
21. Hague BA, Guccione A. Clinical impression of a new technique utilizing a Nd: YAG laser to arthrodese the distal tarsal joints. *Vet Surg.* 2000;29:464.
22. Scruton C, Baxtor GM, Cross MW, et al. Comparison of intra-articular drilling in diode laser treatment for arthrodesis of the distal tarsal joints in normal horses. *Equine Vet J.* 2005;37(11):81–86.
23. Zubrod CJ, Schneider RK, Hague BA, et al. Comparison of three methods for arthrodesis of the distal intertarsal and tarsometatarsal joints in horses. *Vet Surg.* 2005;34(4):372–382.
24. Dechant JE, Baxter GM, Southwood LL, Crawford WH, Jackman BR, Stashak TS, Trotter GW, Hendrickson DA. Use of a three-drill-tract technique for arthrodesis of the distal tarsal joints in horses with distal tarsal osteoarthritis: 54 cases (1990-1999). *J Am Vet Med Assoc.* 2003;223:1800–1805.
25. Dowling BA, Dart AJ, Matthews SM. Chemical arthrodesis of the distal tarsal joints using sodium monoiodoacetate in 104 horses. *Aust Vet J.* 2004;82:38–42.
26. Bohanon TC, Schneider RK, Weisbrode SE. Fusion of the distal intertarsal and tarsometatarsal joints in the horse using intraarticular sodium monoiodoacetate. *Equine Vet J.* 1991;23:289–295.
27. Shoemaker RW, Allen AL, Richardson CE, Wilson DG. Use of intra-articular administration of ethyl alcohol for arthrodesis of the tarsometatarsal joint in healthy horses. *Am J Vet Res.* 2006;67:850–857.
28. Tulamo RM, Bramlage LR, Gabel AA. Fractures of the central and third tarsal bones in horses. *J Am Vet Med Assoc.* 1983;182(11):1234–1238.
29. Winberg FG, Pettersson H. Outcome in racing performance after internal fixation of third and central tarsal bone slab fractures in horses: a review of 20 cases. *Acta Vet Scand.* 1999;40(2):173–180.
30. Murphy ED, Schneider RK, Adams SB, et al. Long-term outcome of horses with a slab fracture of the central or third tarsal bone treated conservatively: 25 cases (1976-1993). *J Am Vet Med Assoc.* 2000;216(12):1949–1954.
31. Reeves MJ, Trotter GW. Tarsocrural joint luxation in a horse. *J Am Vet Med Assoc.* 1991;199:1051–1053.

25

Stifle

Myra F. Barrett and David D. Frisbie

The equine stifle consists of three compartments: femoropatellar, medial femorotibial, and lateral femorotibial. Communication of the femoropatellar and medial femorotibial joints has been found 60% to 70% of the time, although inflammation, anatomic variation, and unidirectional flow affect this communication. Communication between the lateral femorotibial joint and either the femoropatellar or medial femorotibial joint is thought to be rare. For practical purposes, the clinician should assume that the compartments of the stifle do not communicate. Approximately 20 to 30 mL of local anesthetic is used to block each of the compartments. Although there are multiple methods to perform diagnostic anesthesia on the stifle joints,[1] the author's (DDF) method of choice is described here. A single skin entry point to block all three compartments of the stifle helps to rule in or rule out stifle involvement. This can be followed by individual desensitization of the each compartment if warranted. This approach uses an 18-gauge 8.9-cm spinal needle that is placed 2 cm proximal to the tibial plateau between the lateral and middle patellar ligament. Access to the femoropatellar joint is obtained by directing the needle in a proximal and slightly caudal direction to place the needle tip between the patella and trochlea in the area of the trochlear grove (Figure 25-1). Access to the medial femorotibial joint is obtained by withdrawing the needle to a point close to the entry area but still in the subcutaneous tissues and directing in a medial (45 degrees) caudal direction from perpendicular with the limb and horizontal with the tibial plateau until gentle contact with the medial condyle is made (Figure 25-2). Access to the lateral femorotibial joint is obtained by withdrawing the needle to a point close to the entry area but still in the subcutaneous tissues. The needle is then directed in a caudal direction to gently contact the lateral condyle (Figure 25-3). A small amount (1 to 2 mL) of local anesthetic can also be used to desensitize the subcutaneous tissue but the author rarely uses the "skin" block.

There are differing opinions on the duration of time to wait after intraarticular (IA) anesthesia before reevaluation of lameness. The author (DDF) considers 10 minutes and an improvement of more than 50% to be indicative of significant pathology in the stifle joint. Multiple methods have been described to flex the stifle area and some have been suggested to be diagnostic for stifle disease; this has not been

the author's (DDF) experience. The findings of an increase in pain after full limb flexion and effusion in one of the stifle joints have been useful in suspecting stifle lesions, although in a small number of cases stifle pathology exists with no palpable joint effusion.

DIAGNOSTIC IMAGING OF THE STIFLE

Imaging Parameters

Because of the size, proximal location of the stifle, and surrounding muscle mass, diagnostic imaging evaluation is limited compared with the more distally located joints. Radiography, followed by ultrasound, is currently the mainstay of stifle imaging. A minimum standard radiographic evaluation should include a lateral view, caudocranial (CC), and caudo 45 degrees lateral-craniomedial oblique (CLO). It is important that the patella be included in the lateral image. Occasionally in large horses the entire stifle cannot be included in a single image, in which case two lateral images, one proximally and one distally located, should be obtained. Portable x-ray equipment is generally sufficient for evaluation of the stifle, although lower output generators may not produce enough power to obtain high-quality images, particularly on the CC view. Higher output portable generators and in-house high mA generators are ideal for imaging thicker body parts, such as the stifle.

Ultrasound evaluation of the stifle is useful in patients that respond to IA diagnostic analgesia of the stifle, regardless of whether there are radiographic abnormalities or not. Even in cases where there are clear radiographic abnormalities, ultrasonography provides information about any concurrent intraarticular or periarticular soft tissue injuries. A high-quality diagnostic scan requires an experienced ultrasonographer to detect more subtle lesions and more confidently differentiate artifact, normal variants, and true pathologic change. Most of the stifle ultrasound can be performed with a linear probe, in the range of 8 to 12 mHz. A microconvex probe can be helpful for evaluating the cranial aspect of the joint, particularly the lateral cranial meniscal ligament, as its smaller footprint fits more easily between the patellar ligaments than the linear probe. A lower frequency macroconvex probe (3 to 5 mHz) is generally required for the caudal aspect of the stifle, although on smaller or less

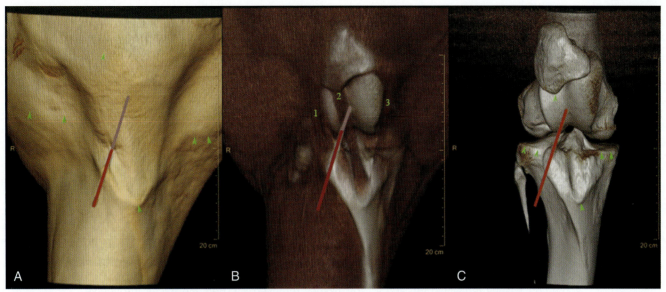

FIGURE 25-1 CT renditions of the equine stifle joint with skin present (A), skin removed and some soft tissues remaining (B), and all soft tissues removed (C). Green arrowheads represent similar landmarks on all renditions. Red line traces the needle path for optimal placement in the FP joint with more transparent portion of line crossing under depicted structures. Numbers 1, 2, and 3 represent lateral, middle, and medial patellar ligaments, respectively.

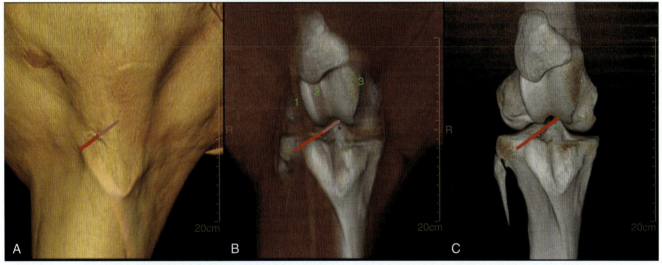

FIGURE 25-2 CT renditions of the equine stifle joint with skin present (A), skin removed and some soft tissues remaining (B), and all soft tissues removed (C). Red line traces the needle path for optimal placement in the medial femorotibial joint with more transparent portion of line crossing under depicted structures but in front of medial tibia eminence (*) to contact the axial non-weight-bearing portion of the medial condyle. Numbers 1, 2, and 3 represent lateral, middle, and medial patellar ligaments, respectively.

muscled horses a microconvex probe (6 to 8 mHz) may be sufficient.

Availability of advanced imaging of the stifle remains limited. There are several institutions with open low-field magnetic resonance imaging (MRI) systems in the United States and Europe that are capable of imaging stifles.[2] High-field MRI of the stifle remains a challenge because of the size of the bore of the magnet. Increasing availability of wide, short-bore MRI units may allow for greater opportunities in evaluating

the equine stifle with high-field MRI in the future. Although more expensive to buy and maintain than low-field MRI systems, high-field MRI systems provide superior image quality and are better for detection of cartilage injuries and more subtle soft tissue damage in the authors opinion.

Computed tomography (CT) evaluation of the stifle is routinely performed in some practices, particularly in Europe, but remains of limited availability. Helical, multislice CT improves the scan quality, reduces scan time, and allows

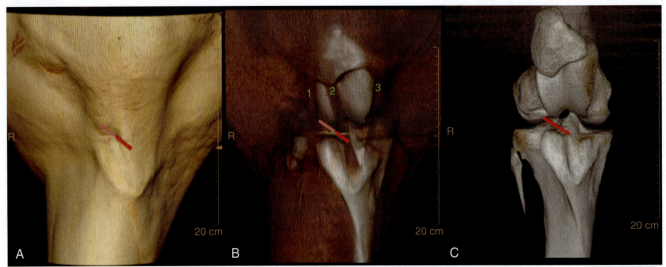

FIGURE 25-3 CT renditions of the equine stifle joint with skin present (**A**), skin removed and some soft tissues remaining (**B**), and all soft tissues removed (**C**). Red line traces the needle path for optimal placement in the medial femorotibial joint with more transparent portion of line crossing under depicted structures to contact the lateral condyle. Numbers 1, 2, and 3 represent lateral, middle, and medial patellar ligaments, respectively.

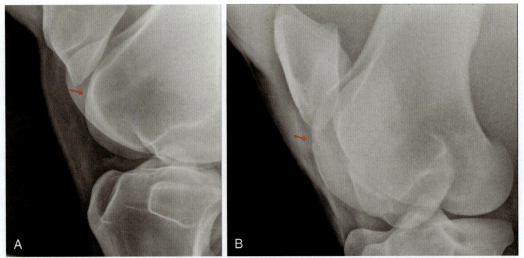

FIGURE 25-4 Lateral (**A**) and caudolateral oblique (**B**) radiographs of the stifle. A small flattening and subchondral irregularity is present on the lateral trochlear ridge. There is a minimally displaced osteochondritis dissecans fragment, which can only be seen on the caudolateral oblique image.

for high-quality multiplanar reconstructions. Although CT provides excellent bone detail, because the soft tissue detail and contrast is limited, CT arthrography (CTR) is generally performed for better evaluation of the IA soft tissues. CTR is particularly helpful for evaluating IA soft tissue structures that cannot be fully evaluated with ultrasound, such as the cruciate ligaments.

SPECIFIC CONDITIONS

Osteochondrosis

The lateral trochlear ridge is the most common site of osteochondrosis (OC) and osteochondritis dissecans lesions in the

stifle.[3] Radiographically, the appearance can range from subtle flattening of the lateral trochlear ridge to multiple osseous fragments and marked change in the normal contour of the trochlea. The lesions are often found adjacent to the distal aspect of the patella. Although these changes are generally readily apparent on the lateral view, in some subtle cases, the defect is best (or only) seen on the CLO (Figure 25-4). Less commonly, OC is found in the medial trochlear ridge, trochlear groove, and patella. The articular surface of the patella should be closely examined for subchondral defects, which more frequently occur in conjunction with OC of the lateral trochlear ridge.[4] OC of the patella can be radiographically occult, and a negative radiographic finding does not necessarily rule out the presence of disease. Lesions of the trochlear groove can be subtle and can occur in conjunction with other changes or, less commonly, in isolation. They are usually seen as focal disruption of the outline of the groove. Ultrasound also allows for accurate assessment of OC of the trochlear ridges, which is particularly helpful in cases in which the radiographic findings are equivocal, and provides greater detail about the size and extent of the lesion.[5] If OC of the lateral trochlear ridge is detected in foals at 6 months of age or less, radiographically monitoring these lesions up to 18 months of age in nonlame horses is recommended, as these lesions have a moderate chance of resolving or improving in that time as long as pain/lameness is not consistently present.[6]

Subchondral Bone Defects and Cystlike Lesions

Subchondral cystlike lesions (SCLs) of the medial femoral condyle (MFC) can be found in young horses as a result of abnormal endochondral ossification and are considered a form of OC (more details on SCLs are available in Chapter 6). It should be noted that acquired SCL, which form from a different pathologic process and are related to trauma, can be found in horses of all ages, including young horses.[7-9] This makes the etiology of the SCL somewhat unclear in many cases. Diagnostic imaging modalities cannot distinguish the two forms of SCL, as both types have the same radiographic and ultrasonographic appearance. When other evidence of joint disease is present and the horse is over 2 years of age, a traumatic etiology is generally considered more likely.

Multiple differing grading systems have been published to characterize the types of MFC subchondral defect.[10-12] Changes can range from a simple flattening of the MFC with no associated subchondral bone sclerosis to concave defects within the articular surface and subchondral bone to varyingly sized subchondral cystic lesions. Flattening of the medial femoral condyle in the absence of subchondral sclerosis is considered incidental. The clinical significance of small subchondral defects as well as subchondral cystic lesions is variable, and with all radiographic lesions must be interpreted in conjunction with clinical signs.

Although the CC and CLO views are most frequently used for evaluating subchondral defects of the MFC, including a flexed latero 10-20° cranio 10° disto-mediocaudoproximal oblique (flexed lateral oblique) view is extremely helpful for assessing changes to the MFC free from superimposition. The cranial-caudal length of a lesion, subtle lesions, and sclerosis are also often best detected using this projection (Figure 25-5).[13]

Ultrasound is also a widely available and useful tool for evaluating subchondral cystic lesions.[14] Ultrasound is particularly useful in cases in which the radiographic findings are equivocal. To image the weight-bearing articular surface of the MFC (where cystic lesions typically occur), the limb must be in a flexed position. The foot can be rested on a stand or held flexed. It is not sufficient flexion for the horse to be incompletely non-weight-bearing with the weight shifted onto the toe or dorsum of the hoof. Ultrasonography provides excellent visualization of the dimension of the articular portion of the subchondral bone defect, in greater detail than appreciated radiographically. However, if there is a narrow cloaca leading to a subchondral cystic lesion, the entire depth of the cystic structure may not be appreciated. The overlying articular cartilage generally is thickened. Concurrent meniscal injuries may also be appreciated. The degree of articular cartilage damage after cyst débridement has been associated with outcome in nonraced Thoroughbreds when radiographic change was not.[15] The ultrasound appearance related to outcome in nondébrided cysts is unknown.

Subchondral cystic lesions also affect the proximal tibia, although they are much less common. Isolated cystlike lesions of the lateral proximal tibia in the absence of other evidence of joint disease have been reported to be a result of osteochondrosis.[16] The other type of tibial cysts is considered a degenerative condition and is generally found in conjunction with advanced osteoarthritic changes and may have a concurrent cystic lesion of the MFC (Figure 25-6). Meniscal disease may also be present. Subchondral cystic lesions of the tibia are generally difficult to visualize with ultrasound.

Advanced imaging can be useful to identify earlier subchondral bone sclerosis, lysis, and cystlike lesions of the femoral and tibial condyles that may remain radiographically occult (Figure 25-7).[2] The degree of associated cartilaginous injury can be evaluated with high-field MRI, and, in a limited fashion, with low-field MRI. In addition, MRI is useful to assess the presence of bone marrow lesions in the bone. High signal on fat-suppressed images can indicate edema, inflammation, fibrosis, contusions and/or osteonecrosis, among other differentials. These lesions are a potential source of pain and lameness that cannot be completely characterized with other imaging modalities.

Scintigraphic evaluation of the stifle is of variable value, and it is not uncommon to have lameness localized to the stifle that does not show uptake on a bone scan, independent of the etiology of the lameness. Defects of the subchondral bone of the medial femoral condyle can have variable increased radiopharmaceutical uptake (IRU), depending on the degree of active bone remodeling (Figure 25-8). Additionally, because of the thicker soft tissues surrounding this joint compared with the distal limb, subtle IRU may be less apparent, particularly the caudal view. Although the caudal view can often seem unrewarding because of the soft tissue attenuation, particularly in thickly muscled horses such as Quarter horses, it should always be included in the exam. Localizing IRU to the medial femoral condyle requires the caudal view, because there is not the superimposition of the condyles that occurs on the lateral view. Because the findings are often subtle, the scintigraphic images must be closely evaluated for changes. Questionable areas of uptake are best further evaluated with IA analgesia and radiographic examination.

Treatment of clinically significant subchondral cystic lesions is typically surgery. Three basic techniques are discussed here. The first is the débridement of the cystic contents including the cystic lining; the latter produces cytokines thought to propagate the disease process and impede natural bone healing.[17] Débridement has the disadvantage of leaving a significant cartilage defect, which as the size of the cartilage defect increases, the prognosis decreases.[15] Depending on the breed/discipline of the patients, prognosis has ranged from 40% to 80%; a more detailed discussion of this can been found in a recent publication.[18] The second procedure that has been recently described involves the placement of a lag screw across the cyst.[19,20] Although this technique has gained some publicity, neither the effects

of drilling through the cyst lining nor the long-term outcomes in clinical cases have been adequately evaluated; thus, the authors do not recommend this technique at the present time. The final and recommended technique in most clinical cases is the injection of the cyst lining with triamcinolone acetonide, which provides a good prognosis even in older patients with a short (30- to 60-day) convalescent period.[21] It should be noted that technique, convalescent period, and preexisting osteoarthritis (OA) all appear to significantly affect the return to performance. Further, injection of the cyst lining using imaging (ultrasound and radiographic guidance) techniques has been less successful

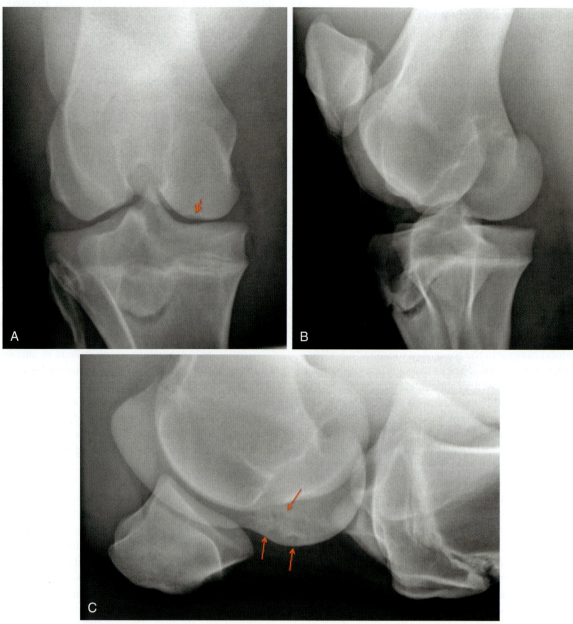

FIGURE 25-5 (A) Caudocranial view of the stifle. A smooth, concave bone defect is present on the distal articular surface of the medial femoral condyle (arrow). (B) Caudolateral oblique image shows only a faint subchondral defect of the MFC. (C) Flexed lateral oblique image of the stifle. The defect is much more extensive than appears on the other images. In addition to the surface defect, areas of osteolysis and sclerosis extend well into the subchondral trabecular bone (arrows).

than direct visualization.[22] Direct visualization also helps in the diagnosis of other associated lesions (such as an OC flap) that might be concurrently present. The reader should be cautioned that presence of a cystic lesion in the femur (as well as other locations) is not definitive confirmation of clinical pain and often the reestablishment of an intact

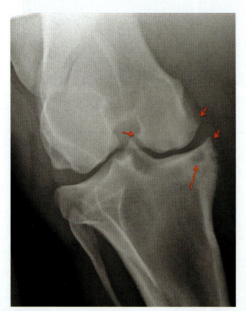

FIGURE 25-6 Caudocranial view of a horse with advanced degenerative changes of the stifle joint. There is a subchondral bone defect and cystic lesion of the medial femoral condyle as well as cystic lesion of the proximal medial tibia with marked surrounding sclerosis (long arrow). There is osteophyte formation of the medial tibial condyle and axial and abaxial aspects of the medial femoral condyle (short arrows).

subchondral bone plate is associated with clinical soundness (Figure 25-9).

Osteoarthritis

Radiography is the primary means of assessing for osteoarthritic changes of the stifle. The most commonly recognized finding is periarticular osteophyte formation on the medial tibial condyle on the CC view. Depending on the angle of the radiograph, the normal marginal curvature of the medial tibial condyle can appear prominently and be mistaken for an osteophyte. Repeat CC radiographs at a different angle, confirmation of the presence of osteophyte on the CLO view, and comparison to the opposite limb are all means by which this finding can be further evaluated. Osteophytes can also be found on the axial and abaxial periarticular margins of the MFC as well as on the medial intercondylar eminence of the tibia. These are more difficult to identify radiographically than the tibial osteophytes. The abaxially located MFC osteophytes are easily identified with ultrasound evaluation, and, if large, can be seen deforming or displacing the medial meniscus (Figure 25-10). Larger axially located MFC osteophytes can be identified radiographically with excellent positioning to minimize superimposition in the intercondylar fossa; they cannot be well visualized with ultrasound (see Figure 25-6). Less commonly osteophytes can be found on the lateral periarticular margins, associated with OA of the lateral femoral tibial joint.

Unlike in human and canine patients, equine periarticular osteophyte formation is not commonly found on the trochlear ridges when there is femoropatellar OA. The distal articular margin of the patella will undergo remodeling and osteophyte formation in some cases of femoropatellar OA.

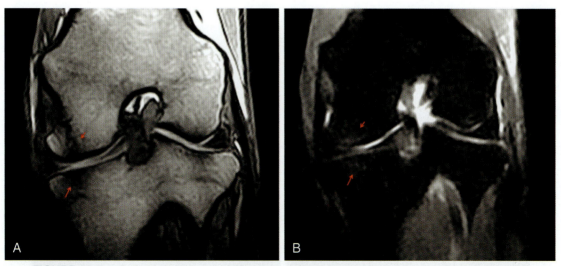

FIGURE 25-7 Low-field dorsal plane MR images of a 6-year-old Tennessee Walking horse with mild right hind lameness. **(A)** Three-dimensional GE T1 (0.9-mm) and **(B)** STIR (5-mm) images. There is a subchondral bone defect of the medial femoral condyle with an opposing lesion on the proximal tibia. The increased signal on STIR images indicates bone edema, hemorrhage, and/or bone necrosis among other differential diagnoses. Images courtesy of Dr. Alexia McKnight and Delta Equine Center, Vinton, LA.

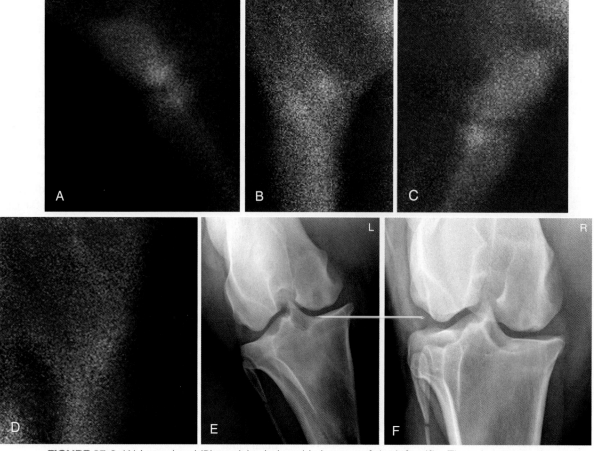

FIGURE 25-8 (A) Lateral and (B) caudal scintigraphic images of the left stifle. There is increased radiopharmaceutical uptake in the region of the medial femoral condyle. (C) Lateral and (D) caudal scintigraphic images of the left stifle. The left stifle is scintigraphically normal. (E) Caudocranial (CC) view of the left stifle. A large subchondral cystlike lesion is present in the medial femoral condyle, and chronic osteoarthritic remodeling affects the medial femoral tibial joint. (F) CC view of the right stifle. The image is mildly oblique. A subchondral cystlike lesion and articular defect is present in the medial femoral condyle with marked surrounding sclerosis. There is chronic osteoarthritic remodeling affecting the medial femoral tibial joint. Abnormal increased uptake was not associated with these lesions on the bone scan.

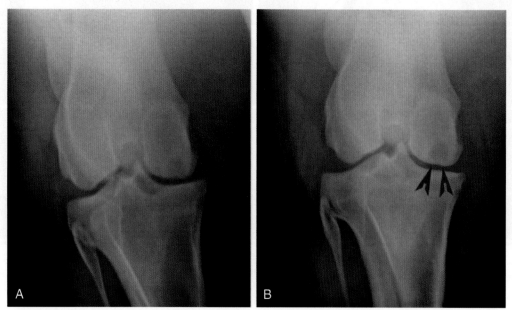

FIGURE 25-9 Radiograph showing a clinically painful subchondral cystic lesion (A) before surgery and reestablishment of the subchondral bone plate in the same horse with no clinical pain after injection of cyst lining with corticosteroids (B).

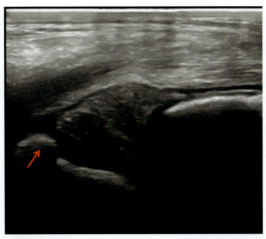

FIGURE 25-10 Ultrasound image of the medial meniscus. Proximal is to the left. There is an osteophyte of the medial femoral condyle (arrow) that is displacing the meniscus, and the meniscus is protruding beyond the joint margin.

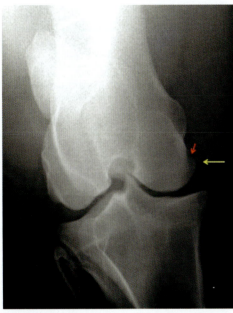

FIGURE 25-11 Caudocranial view of the stifle. There is a scooped appearance to the medial femoral epicondyle (small arrow) secondary to chronic effusion/synovitis. An osteophyte is present on the abaxial periarticular margin of the medial femoral condyle (large arrow).

Chronic synovitis and capsulitis can result in supracondylar lysis of the medial femoral epicondyle; a similar pathologic process is found in the fetlock joint. Radiographically this is characterized by a scooped, concave appearance to the medial femoral epicondyle on the CC view, often with a concurrent periarticular medial femoral condylar osteophyte (Figure 25-11). Mild obliquity of the CC view can obscure this finding. This smooth bone resorption is readily identified with ultrasound, and often more subtle cases can be identified with ultrasound when

compared with radiography. Additionally, ultrasound allows for concurrent evaluation of degree of joint capsule distention, synovial proliferation, and joint capsule thickening. Regularly comparing ultrasound and radiographic findings improves one's ability to detect the more subtle changes on radiographs when they are confirmed ultrasonographically.

Central osteophyte formation is osseous production within a joint, on the articular surface, rather than the periarticular margin. Central osteophyte formation is a common osteoarthritic manifestation in human knees associated with full-thickness articular cartilage defects.[23] Central osteophytes are not frequently detected radiographically on the femoral condyles of horses. Ultrasonographic evaluation of the MFC sometimes reveals proliferative bone adjacent to a subchondral bone defect. In a study in which small concave subchondral bone defects were created on the medial trochlear ridge of the equine stifle, central osteophyte formation adjacent to the defect was not an uncommon radiographic abnormality.[24] The fact that they are not regularly radiographically found on the femoral condyles could be reflected by the limited resolution of radiography at this location.

Although joint space narrowing is noted radiographically in other joints as a manifestation of diffuse cartilage loss associated with advanced OA, narrowing of the femorotibial joints secondary to diffuse cartilage loss is rare. This is because the presence of the medial and lateral meniscus separates the joint space sufficiently that the several millimeter loss of articular cartilage will not be evident. Generally, to have radiographically evident joint space narrowing of the femorotibial joints, there must be concurrent marked meniscal disease. Conversely, diffuse loss of articular cartilage in the femoropatellar joint, particularly on the articular surface of the patella, can result in radiographically evident joint space narrowing, often with concurrent subchondral bone sclerosis (Figure 25-12).

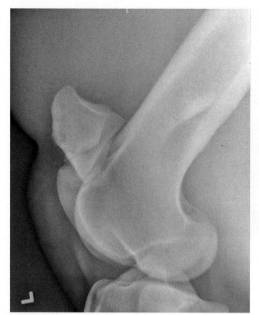

FIGURE 25-12 Lateral radiograph of a Thoroughbred racehorse with an unknown medical history. The horse was 4/5 lame with severe femopatellar effusion. There is marked narrowing of the patellofemoral articulation, particularly medially, with subchondral bone sclerosis. There is also moderate osseous proliferation and osteophyte formation of the distal medial aspect of the patella.

Both CT and MRI allow for more complete evaluation of osteoarthritic changes when compared with radiography.[25-28] CT and MRI are superior to radiography in the detection of osseous abnormalities, including periarticular and central osteophyte formation, subchondral lysis, and sclerosis. MRI is particularly useful, because it provides excellent information regarding cartilage, soft tissues, and presence or absence of bone marrow lesions (bone edema-like syndrome). Evaluation of the soft tissues is particularly important in the stifle because damage to the medial meniscus and/or cruciate ligaments can result in joint instability that leads to OA.

Currently, the availability of advanced imaging for evaluation of cartilage of the equine stifle is poor. As mentioned previously, the majority of the MR scanners in use for evaluation of the equine stifle are low-field units, which are limited for evaluation of cartilage lesions. Although full-thickness defects may be more readily detected, particularly in conjunction with concurrent subchondral bone injury, partial-thickness cartilage loss, fissuring, fraying, and alteration in signal caused by chondromalacia are changes that cannot be reliably assessed with low-field MRI. Additionally, although three-dimensional gradient echo sequences can be run at 1 mm or submillimeter slice thickness, the rest of the sequences (fast-spin echo and STIR) typically are performed with 4- to 5-mm slice thickness. Therefore, it is quite likely that smaller full-thickness defects could be missed as well. At the time of this writing, there are two high-field MRI scanners in the United States that are being used on occasion to scan stifles; case selection is limited to horses of a certain size and

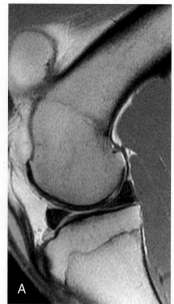

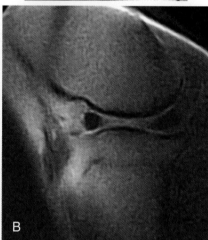

FIGURE 25-13 Sagittal proton density-weighted magnetic resonance images of the medial aspect of the joint. **(A)** High-field (1.5 T) and **(B)** low-field (0.2 T) images. The resolution and signal-to-noise ratio are superior with the high-field image.

conformation and the more proximal aspect of the stifle may be truncated (Figure 25-13).

CT arthrography has been described for evaluation of the equine stifle joint, but faces limitations in evaluation of articular cartilage. Articular cartilage is not readily visible without iodinated IA contrast. The articular cartilage appears as a hypoattenuating (dark) line between the hyperattenuating (bright) subchondral bone and IA contrast material. Defects in the articular cartilage will be apparent as an area of contrast filling in the space where the articular cartilage is absent. Unfortunately, because of the marked extension that the limb must be in to fit into the CT gantry, it is difficult to get even contrast distribution to the weight-bearing articular surface of the MFC, limiting evaluation of articular cartilage defects in this area. When using arthroscopy as the gold standard, CT had 60% sensitivity for detection of articular cartilage lesions of the medial femoral condyle.[29]

Ultrasonographically, articular cartilage is well visualized as an anechoic rim overlying subchondral bone. To evaluate the articular cartilage of the weight-bearing surface of the medial femoral condyle, the limb must be in flexion. Although articular cartilage defects that occur in conjunction with subchondral bone defects are readily detected, articular cartilage defects in the absence of subchondral bone damage can be difficult to detect on the MFC.[30] Fissuring, fraying, and surface irregularities of the MFC are not readily identified ultrasonographically. This is likely caused in part by inherent limitations in spatial and contrast resolution of ultrasound. Even more diffuse changes, such as cartilage thinning, can often be difficult to detect on the MFC. This can be attributed in part to the fact that, when the ultrasound beam is not perfectly tangential to the articular cartilage, the cartilage will appear thicker than it truly is.[31] On a rounded surface, such as the MFC, there is a limited portion of the condyle that can be positioned to be directly tangential to the ultrasound beam. Therefore, a normal ultrasonographic appearance of the articular cartilage does not rule out pathologic changes that could be detected with a different modality, such as arthroscopy.

Recently, standing diagnostic arthroscopy has improved the ability to diagnose some of these more subtle lesions that have been hard to definitively detect with routine imaging.[18,32] This modality has helped in defining what is most likely the primary cause of the secondary OA changes such as osteophyte formation. Diagnosis of cruciate lesions, articular cartilage chondromalacia, fissuring, and fibrillation as well as meniscal lesions has become more routine, and the ability to diagnose and treat earlier may potentially lead to better outcomes. Surgical lesions are covered elsewhere.[18] Medical treatment of the stifle is similar to other joints, and these options are presented in detail in Chapters 11 through 17. Because of the increased volume of the stifle, though, doses 2× greater than those used in a smaller joint such as the fetlock are often used.

Soft Tissue Injuries

The stifle is particularly complex because of the large number of associated intraarticular and periarticular soft tissue structures. Injuries to the soft tissues may occur in isolation or in conjunction with osseous damage. Soft tissue injuries can lead to joint instability that contributes to the development of OA.

Meniscus and Meniscal Ligaments

Injuries to the menisci and meniscal ligaments are not uncommon, with the majority of the pathologic processes occurring in the medial femorotibial articulation.[33] Although the majority of injuries have been reported to affect the cranial horn and cranial meniscal ligament, this perception is likely affected in part by the fact that this is the most readily visible area arthroscopically.

Although radiography provides little direct evidence of pathologic changes of soft tissues, indirect evidence can support the radiographic diagnosis of more severe or advanced

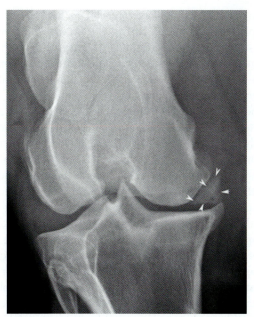

FIGURE 25-14 Radiograph of an equine stifle joint showing severe mineralization of the medial meniscus (arrowheads).

meniscal injuries. The two most reliable radiographic indications of meniscal injury are meniscal mineralization and femorotibial joint space narrowing. Soft tissue mineralization within the stifle cannot always be definitively localized; however, when the mineralization occurs within the femorotibial joint space, it is likely to be associated with the meniscus. This typically is found in conjunction with other degenerative changes in the joint. Meniscal mineralization is readily confirmed with ultrasonographic evaluation but can be seen on radiographs in severe cases (Figure 25-14).

Joint space narrowing is best appreciated on the CC view and can occur secondary to severe meniscal protrusion/extrusion with associated extensive degenerative changes of the meniscus. Meniscal extrusion has been reported secondary to acute trauma.[34] When assessing joint width, it is important to assess the symmetry of the medial and lateral femorotibial joint space. Improper radiographic technique can easily create the artifactual appearance of joint space narrowing; however, this will affect both the medial and lateral aspect of the joint. Conversely, true joint space narrowing secondary to meniscal disease will result in asymmetric, unilateral narrowing of the joint. If there is a concern that the appearance is caused by artifact, repeat CC views at a different angle are indicated (Figure 25-15).

Ultrasonography is the most commonly used diagnostic imaging modality for evaluation of the meniscus. Ultrasound allows for complete visualization of the menisci, from the cranial to caudal horns, including the meniscal ligaments.[35] The shape of the meniscus and its location are readily assessed. Normally the majority of the meniscus should not extend beyond the periarticular margins of the joint, although very mild protrusion can be a normal variant in Quarter horses. When assessing the degree to which the meniscus is protruding, it is important to evaluate what the joint margin should be, and not include periarticular osteophyte formation as part of the normal joint margin, as this will falsely underestimate the degree of protrusion (Figure 25-16). Moderate to large periarticular osteophytes of the MFC can cause deformation of the femoral abaxial border of the medial meniscus.

Fiber damage to the medial meniscus can present as discrete tearing or more diffuse injury. Discrete tears are frequently found in the horizontal plane, dividing the meniscus into proximal and distal portions.[36] These horizontal tears pose a particular diagnostic challenge, as they can sometimes be difficult to distinguish from a prominent, but normal, meniscal striation. Including a non-weight-bearing exam can help to distinguish the two, as a striation will not change in shape but a tear often will widen when the patient is not weight-bearing. Additionally, abnormalities in the position or shape of the meniscus can help distinguish a tear from a striation (Figure 25-17). Tears can also have an oblique orientation or may radiate longitudinally from the cranial or caudal horn. In more severe, diffuse injury, much of the meniscus can have a heterogeneous, hypoechoic appearance. The majority of the ultrasound evaluation occurs in a transverse plane to the meniscus (long-axis to the limb). It is worthwhile to include imaging of the fibers in long-axis to the meniscus; however, the presence of tibial osteophytes often precludes complete visualization of the meniscus in this plane. Visualizing tears of the axial aspect of the meniscus can be difficult. It is important to appropriately adjust the frequency and focal zones of the ultrasound unit to maximize visualization of the entire meniscus, including the deep axial margin.

To adequately visualize the cranial horn and cranial meniscal ligaments, the patient must be non-weight-bearing. Evaluation of the medial structures is easier than the lateral. In particular, the insertion of the lateral cranial meniscal ligament can be difficult to image because of the overlying patellar ligaments and peroneus tertius, inhibiting full transducer contact. In some cases, the image is more readily obtained with a microconvex transducer; however, the trade-off is decreased resolution when compared with a linear transducer.[37] It is important that the cranial meniscal ligaments be evaluated in both the transverse and long-axis planes. Lesions include longitudinal tears, core-type lesions, and diffuse shape change. Mild fraying, which is readily evaluated arthroscopically, is not easily detected ultrasonographically.[35] Osseous proliferation or resorption can accompany tearing

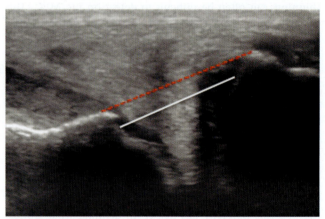

FIGURE 25-16 Ultrasound image of the medial meniscus, with proximal to the left. There is significant periarticular osteophyte formation of the medial femoral and tibial condyles, which is resulting in an abnormal extension of the joint margin. The white line denotes where the normal joint margin should be. The dotted line denotes the expanded articular margin secondary to osteophyte production. By evaluating the true joint margin, this indicates that there is moderate protrusion of the medial meniscus from the joint. The meniscus is compressed and misshapen.

FIGURE 25-15 Caudocranial radiographs of the same horse. On (**B**), the beam angle is not tangential to the joint space, creating the appearance of joint space narrowing. When joint space narrowing is suspected, repeating the radiographs with a slightly different beam angle and comparing the medial and lateral joint widths should be performed to verify if the joint is truly narrowed or a positioning artifact (**A**).

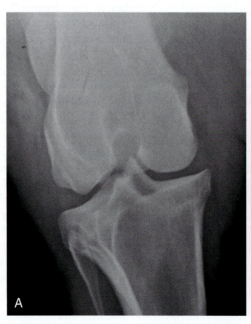
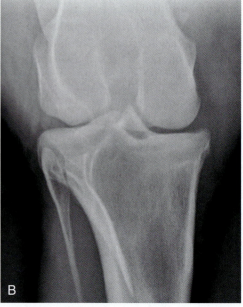

of the cranial meniscal ligaments; this is readily assessed ultrasonographically.

The evaluation of meniscus and meniscal ligament injuries using CT requires the use of IA contrast agents. In order for the lesion to be visualized, the tearing must communicate with the synovial fluid and fill with contrast. Therefore, a limitation of CT is the detection of intrasubstance meniscal tears or degeneration. CT is very good for evaluating osseous changes at the insertion of the cranial or caudal meniscal ligaments. Detection of caudal meniscal ligament tears is improved with CT when compared with ultrasound.[38]

In people, MRI is the gold standard for imaging meniscal injuries. High-field MRI has been shown to be highly accurate in detection of meniscal tears and superior to ultrasound for detection of both medial and lateral meniscal injuries.[39-42] Low-field MRI has also been shown to have good sensitivity and specificity for medial meniscal tears, but has not been as effective for detecting lateral meniscal lesions in people.[43] Although there has not been a direct study examining the correlation of ultrasound, MRI, arthroscopy, and histopathologic results in the equine patient, it is likely that MRI would provide a relatively accurate assessment of meniscal injuries if the stifle could be placed in the MRI unit. In contrast to CT, MRI does not require the lesion to communicate with the joint, improving detection rates. With increasing availability of MRI of the equine stifle, validation in the horse is needed.

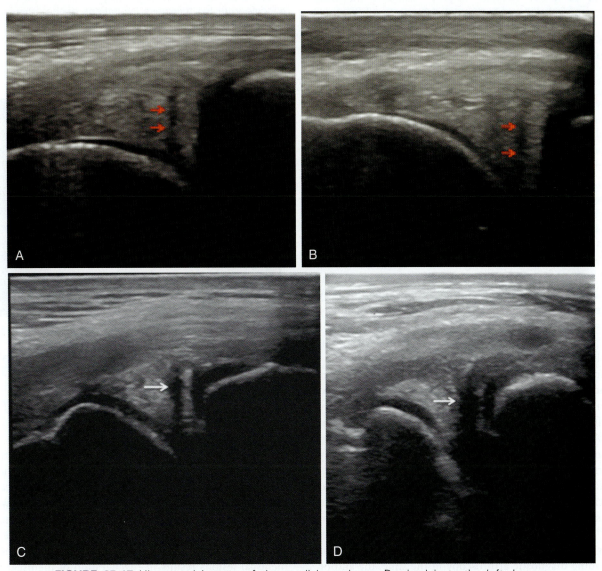

FIGURE 25-17 Ultrasound images of the medial meniscus. Proximal is to the left. Images A and B are of the same horse and images C and D are of the same horse. Images A and C were obtained in a weight-bearing position and B and D in non–weight-bearing. The horse in images A and B has a prominent striation within the medial meniscus that does not change when weight-bearing. The meniscus is normal. The horse in images C and D has a horizontally oriented meniscal tear that increases in size when non-weight-bearing (D). There is periarticular osteophyte formation and the medial meniscus protrudes from the joint space.

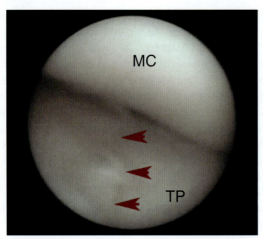

FIGURE 25-18 Arthroscopic image of mild axial meniscal tearing (arrows) without concurrent damage to other structures. This image comes from the standing needle scope, hence the lower resolution. Medial femoral condyle (MC) and tibial plateau (TP).

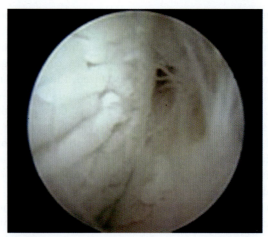

FIGURE 25-19 Arthroscopic image of the medial femoral condyle with full thickness lacerations of the articular cartilage but no surface fibrillation. Not visualized in the picture is the primary meniscal injury in this case.

The use of standing arthroscopy offers additional promise in early detection of meniscal injury in the cranial and caudal compartments by visualizing subtle lesions not observed by other imaging modalities (Figure 25-18). In general, arthroscopy (standing diagnostic or routine) is often limited in diagnosing midbody or axial lesions unless they are severe enough to extend to the periphery of the menisci. Other factors, most likely secondary, are often suggestive of meniscal insufficiency such as full-thickness fissures of the articular cartilage on either condyle without concurrent fibrillation (Figure 25-19). It has also been noted that fraying of the cranial ligament of the medial meniscus is associated with other lesions identified by imaging. This most likely is caused by the vast majority of this ligament being outside the synovial cavity and this fraying, most likely from stretching, is a secondary sign of pathology.

Currently the treatment of most meniscal injuries revolves around partial meniscectomy to decrease the continued inflammation by the loose, damaged tissues. More recently the author (DDF) has combined arthroscopic débridement with IA treatment with bone-derived culture-expanded stem cells and realized a significant improvement in the ability of horses with meniscal injuries to return to performance. Specifically, there was a two to three times greater return to performance depending on the degree of injury, where the more severe injuries were improved the most by use of stem cells.[44] This is in contrast to previous publications suggesting a guarded prognosis for sport horses.[45] Since the advent of standing diagnostic arthroscopy in the stifle, the author (DDF) has had occasion to observe horses that appear to have meniscal issues based on ultrasound but do not have lesions that are amenable to arthroscopic treatment, most likely because of central, midbody lesions or laxity reasons. These cases have included horses with nonfibrillated articular cartilage fissures that have been treated after diagnosis of

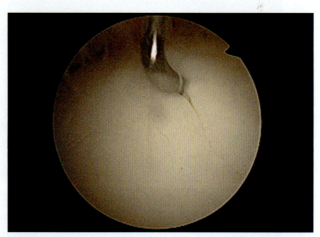

FIGURE 25-20 Arthroscopic image of medial condyle with single full-thickness fissure and no surface fibrillation of the articular cartilage. Ultrasound demonstrated a moderate dynamic tear in the medial meniscus that could not be visualized arthroscopically. The horse was treated with IA stem cells free in the joint and went on to a more than 3-year national career in reining.

nonsurgical lesions with stem cells alone and have returned to athletic performance without requiring other medical treatments within the joint (Figure 25-20). Thus, accurate diagnosis and débridement of abnormal tissues followed by IA stem cells in the postinflammatory phase is the author's (DDF) current recommendation for meniscal lesions. As noted in the Chapter 17 (Stem Cells), IA treatment of meniscal lesions results in regeneration of meniscal tissue in both experimental (goat, rat, and rabbit) and human clinical cases. Cases that present with a history of improving with IA anesthesia of the stifle and no or shortened (<6 week) response to therapy and no significant imaging findings should have meniscal injury high on the differential diagnosis list.

Cruciate Ligaments

The cranial cruciate ligament originates on the caudoaxial margin of the lateral femoral condyle and inserts on the axial aspect of the medial intercondylar eminence of the tibia. The caudal cruciate ligament originates on the caudal medial aspect of the tibia and inserts on the cranioaxial margin of the medial femoral condyle. These sites should be closely inspected radiographically for evidence of bone resorption, sclerosis, or fracture fragments. Osseous fragmentation of the medial intercondylar eminence can be associated with avulsion of the cranial cruciate ligament, but this is not definitive as fragmentation of the eminence can occur proximal to the ligamentous insertion. Including a caudomedial-craniolateral oblique view improves visualization of the origin of the cranial cruciate ligament (Figure 25-21).[46] Mineralization within the intercondylar fossa can be associated with dystrophic mineralization and/or avulsion fragmentation of the cranial cruciate ligament.

Ultrasonographically, evaluation of the cruciate ligaments is limited. Approximately the distal third of the cranial cruciate ligament can be visualized, but its deep location limits resolution. Although more severe damage of the cranial cruciate ligament may be visible, mild or moderate tearing is not likely to be recognized. Tearing that occurs within the region of the intracondylar fossa cannot be seen. Using the caudal approach to the stifle, the origin of the cranial and caudal cruciate ligaments can be visualized. Because of the thick hamstring muscle tissue on the caudal aspect of the limb, these structures are imaged at a much greater depth than the cranial structures of the stifle, which limits resolution and hinders lesion detection. Concurrent enthesopathies of the origin of the cruciate ligaments will improve detection rates of ligamentous injuries.

Advanced imaging provides a much better means for evaluation of the cruciate ligaments. Whereas in human and canine patients, the clinical evaluation may be sufficient for the diagnosis of a cranial cruciate ligament injury,[47] it is difficult to demonstrate joint laxity secondary to cruciate ligament injury in the clinical exam of the equine patient. Therefore, diagnostic imaging remains the noninvasive manner of diagnosing cruciate ligament tears in the horse. With further availability of advanced imaging in the horse, it is likely that we will appreciate a greater number of cruciate ligament injuries than has been traditionally reported.

Currently in the horse caudal and cranial cruciate ligament tears are more frequently diagnosed with CT than with ultrasound, and a negative ultrasound exam has been reported to be frequently associated with cruciate ligament injuries found on CT.[38,48] Concurrent medial meniscal injuries have been reported to occur not infrequently with both caudal and cranial cruciate ligament injuries.[38] This is thought to occur in part because of acute trauma to the joint as a whole, thereby damaging multiple structures and often not just a single entity. Damage to the cruciate ligaments is typically seen as margin fraying or midsubstance

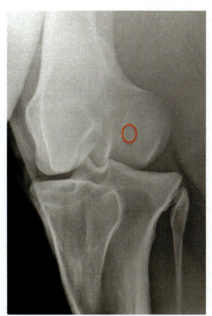

FIGURE 25-21 Caudomedial-craniolateral oblique view of the stifle. This view highlights the site of the origin of the cranial cruciate ligament (red circle).

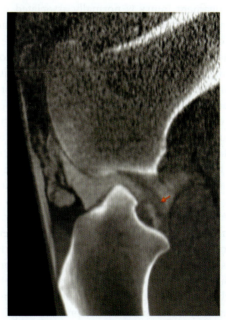

FIGURE 25-22 Reconstructed, sagittally formatted CT arthrogram of the stifle. There is a thin line of contrast within the caudal cruciate ligament (arrow), indicating a linear tear with surface communication. (Image courtesy of Dr. Brad Nelson, Orthopaedic Research Center, Colorado State University.)

tearing with surface communication (S.M. Puchalski, personal communication, 2014) (Figure 25-22).[49] In an evaluation of 141 horses that underwent clinical CT evaluation of the stifle, 78 were found to have abnormalities of the cruciate ligaments. Of these horses, 17 went to postmortem, where the lesions were confirmed. Damage to the caudal cruciate ligament most frequently occurred at the proximal aspect of the ligament; whereas, the cranial cruciate ligament injuries occurred at multiple locations with similar frequency.[38] Similar to the meniscus, the tears of the cruciate ligaments must communicate with the synovial fluid of the joint to fill with contrast and be visible on CT. More subtle thickening and shape changes without contrast-filled tears can also be appreciated. In these cases there may be intrasubstance tearing that does not communicate with the joint, but is resulting in a visible shape change. The full extent of cruciate injuries is most likely yet to be realized.

MRI is an excellent modality for the assessment of cruciate ligament injuries in people.[41,50] In a retrospective evaluation of 61 clinical cases that underwent low-field MRI evaluation of the stifle, 36 (59%) had evidence of pathologic changes of the cranial and/or caudal cruciate ligaments including discrete tearing, intrasubstance lesions, and ruptures. This review did not report the number of cases in which the findings were confirmed with arthroscopy or postmortem evaluation.[51] Again, a large advantage of MRI over CT is that lesions do not need to communicate with the surface to be detected, therefore increasing the detection rate of intrasubstance tearing and diffuse degeneration.

As with other soft tissue injury and trauma to the stifle, cruciate ligament injury is normally associated with joint effusion and pain following upper limb flexion. Other manipulations of the limb to indicate specific injury to the cruciate ligaments are thought by most, including the authors, to be nonspecific. Postdiagnosis treatment of cruciate injuries follows a similar path as for meniscus, including débridement of the damaged tissue and often treatment of the joint with IA stem cells. In people other methods of stimulating healing through use of a laser or mechanical penetration of the ligaments have been described but widespread acceptance has not been realized. In the horse many of the cruciate injuries appear to be relatively severe when diagnosed and often seem to be related to trauma and injury to multiple structures of the joint, thus carrying a generally poor prognosis. The literature suggests that moderate to severe injury to the cruciate ligaments is associated with less than 50% pasture soundness.[52,53] Walmsley et al. even reported that horses diagnosed with minor superficial changes had only a 62% chance of soundness. They obtained follow-up on 7 cases with cruciate injury as the primary diagnosis. The diagnosis was confirmed arthroscopically and torn aspects of the ligament that could be reached arthroscopically were resected; the horses were then treated with IA stem cells. The low number of cases precluded a breakdown by injury severity; however, 71% of the horses were able to return to athletic work.[44] As diagnostic methods improve, better prognoses may be realized because of less severe and earlier diagnoses. However, currently, when the authors diagnose cruciate injury, we assume that other soft tissues within the joint have been damaged. The ideal treatment is a complete diagnostic exploration and débridement of damaged tissue followed by IA MSCs 4 weeks after surgery. Typically, a 4- to 6-month rehabilitation protocol is followed for returning the horse to full work.

Collateral Ligaments

Collateral ligament injuries of the equine stifle are not frequently reported. Complete rupture is rare and generally occurs secondary to trauma. Concurrent meniscal extrusion can occur in conjunction with a collateral ligament rupture. A complete rupture could present radiographically as a marked asymmetry in medial and lateral joint space widths when stress views are acquired. If there has been avulsion of the ligament, osseous fragments will be appreciated radiographically.

Less severe injury such as discrete tearing or thickening can occur throughout the ligament, with the medial collateral ligament more frequently affected. Ultrasonographic evaluation should be performed in two planes, both long and short axis. The origin of the medial collateral ligament is most easily assessed when the patient rests the limb, as this unweighted position allows for the transducer to be better positioned tangentially to the origin. Osseous irregularity can occur at the origin or insertion of the collateral ligament. Bone proliferation of the tibia adjacent to the insertion of the medial collateral ligament is not uncommon, and is often seen without concurrent changes to the ligament. This is generally an incidental finding.

Reports of collateral ligament injuries detected with CT and MRI are also relatively low. In a review of low-field clinical stifle MRIs, 6 of 61 horses were found to have desmopathy of a collateral ligament.[51] In 24 horses that underwent both ultrasound and CT evaluation of the stifle, desmopathy of the medial collateral ligament was diagnosed in 5 horses with CT and 4 horses with ultrasound. However, in only 2 horses was the diagnosis made by both modalities, indicating limitations of each modality for accurate lesion detection. CT is limited by the fact that only a small portion of the medial collateral ligament is IA.

Enthesopathy of the collateral ligaments can sometimes be appreciated as a focal area of IRU on a bone scan. This is more commonly noted on the lateral aspect. However, it is important not to confuse the normal area of increased uptake associated with superimposition of the head of the fibula with enthesopathy of the insertion of the lateral collateral ligament. Ultrasound evaluation of this area can be performed after scintigraphy to further evaluate findings.

Much like the other soft tissue injuries, nonspecific signs such as joint effusion and pain to full limb flexion can be observed. Also, other injuries to joint structures are assumed to often occur when damage to the collateral ligaments is observed. However, in people with discrete medial collateral ligament injuries, a good prognosis for full return to function following rest alone is seen with conservative treatment of all but complete ruptures. The author (DDF) has also had similar experience in horses when involvement of other structures was not identified. One of the authors (DDF) has used extracorporeal shockwave to injured collateral ligaments with success, but no definitive follow-up has been performed comparing this with rest alone. Thus it appears that the prognosis following injury to the collateral ligaments may be related more to other involved structures than to the ligaments themselves.

Patellar Ligaments

Patellar ligament injuries are readily diagnosed with ultrasound. Damage to the middle patellar ligament is most common.[54] Middle patellar ligament injuries are often manifested as obliquely oriented, well-defined, or diffuse tearing (Figure 25-23). The middle patellar ligament normally has a mildly heterogeneous, striated appearance at the distal aspect, which should not be confused with desmopathy. Tears of the middle patellar ligament often occur in conjunction with upward fixation of the patella, but can be found in horses without a history of patellar fixation. Middle patellar ligament tears can occur anywhere, but the midbody is most frequently affected. Concurrent enthesopathy at the origin on the patella or insertion on the tibia can occur, but many times the bone is not affected. Enthesopathy can generally be appreciated radiographically as osseous proliferation, most commonly on the distocranial aspect of the patella. IRU of the tibia has been reported in conjunction with middle patellar ligament enthesopathy.[54] However, as there is normally increased uptake of tibial tuberosity, it is important that this is not confused with pathologic change.

Medial patellar ligament injuries are not common. Horses that have previously undergone desmoplasty of the medial patellar ligament for treatment of upward fixation of the patella will generally have a significantly thickened ligament with a loss of normal fiber pattern, because of the surgically induced desmopathy. The proximal aspect of the medial patellar ligament has a strong fibrocartilagenous union with the patella, minimizing enthesopathy of the origin. Sagittal-oriented medial patellar fractures, usually secondary to trauma,[55,56] generally result in avulsion and disruption of the medial patellar ligament. These fractures are generally assessed with a skyline radiograph of the patella and the associated soft tissue damages evaluated ultrasonographically.

Lateral patellar ligament injuries most frequently occur secondary to trauma and may be associated with an external wound.[57] With traumatic injuries such as kicks, concurrent fractures, or partial avulsions of the tibial tuberosity can occur. A combination of ultrasound and radiography is generally used to evaluate the osseous and soft tissue injury.

It is important to recognize that patellar ligaments will often have some degree of persistent decreased echogenicity and irregular fiber pattern, even when tearing has resolved clinically. Therefore, an abnormal ultrasonographic appearance does not necessarily indicate an active or clinically significant lesion, and the finding must be clinically correlated.

The treatment of horses with patellar ligament injury is not unlike other ligaments with respect to choice of treatment and rehabilitation. Shockwave, PRP, and stem cells are among the common treatment modalities. In the acute-phase, systemic NSAIDs and a decrease in exercise are used, with controlled exercise increasing if clinical signs of lameness are no longer present.

In summary, although diagnostic imaging evaluation of the equine stifle is limited in comparison to more distal joints, using a combination of multiple imaging modalities and experienced equine imagers will result in the greatest diagnostic information. In the future, we are likely to see greater availability of advanced imaging, which will greatly improve the diagnostic capabilities and understanding of pathologic changes and normal variants of the equine stifle. This will continue to provide better specificity with our treatment selections.

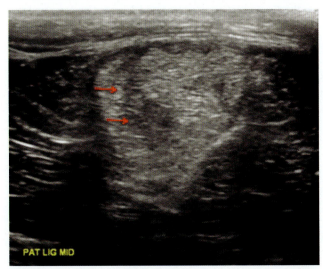

FIGURE 25-23 Transverse ultrasound image of the middle patellar ligament with an obliquely oriented, hypoechoic tear (arrows).

REFERENCES

1. Moyer W. *Equine joint injection and regional anesthesia.* 5th ed. Chadds Ford, PA: Academic Veterinary Solutions; 2011.
2. McKnight AL. MRI of the equine stifle—61 clinical cases. *J Equine Vet Sci.* 2012;32(10):672.
3. McIlwraith CW. Surgical versus conservative management of osteochondrosis. *Vet J.* 2013;197(1):19–28.
4. Foland JW, McIlwraith CW, Trotter GW. Arthroscopic surgery for osteochondritis dissecans of the femoropatellar joint of the horse. *Equine Vet J.* 1992;24(6):419–423.
5. Bourzac C, Alexander K, Rossier Y. Comparison of radiography and ultrasonography for the diagnosis of osteochondritis dissecans in the equine femoropatellar joint. *Equine Vet J.* 2009;41(7):685–692.
6. Jacquet S, Robert C, Valette JP, et al. Evolution of radiological findings detected in the limbs of 321 young horses between the ages of 6 and 18months. *Vet J.* 2013;197(1):58–64.
7. Denoix JM, Jeffcott LB, McIlwraith CW, et al. A review of terminology for equine juvenile osteochondral conditions (JOCC) based on anatomical and functional considerations. *Vet J.* 2013;197(1):29–35.
8. Jeffcott LB, Kold SE, Melsen F. Aspects of the pathology of stifle bone cysts in the horse. *Equine Vet J.* 1983;15(4):304–311.
9. Ray CS, Baxter GM, McIlwraith CW, et al. Development of subchondral cystic lesions after articular cartilage and subchondral bone damage in young horses. *Equine Vet J.* 1996;28(3):225–232.
10. Contino EK, Park RD, McIlwraith CW. Prevalence of radiographic changes in yearling and 2-year-old Quarter horses intended for cutting. *Equine Vet J.* 2011;44(2):185–195.

11. Howard RD, McIlwraith CW, Trotter GW. Arthroscopic surgery for subchondral cystic lesions of the medial femoral condyle in horses: 41 cases (1988-1991). *J Am Vet Med Assoc.* 1995;206(6):842–850.

12. Wallis TW, Goodrich LR, McIlwraith CW, et al. Arthroscopic injection of corticosteroids into the fibrous tissue of subchondral cystic lesions of the medial femoral condyle in horses: a retrospective study of 52 cases (2001-2006). *Equine Vet J.* 2010;40(5):461–467.

13. Barrett M. How to obtain flexed lateral oblique radiographs of the equine stifle. *Proc Am Assoc Equine Pract.* 2012;58:383–387.

14. Jacquet S, Audigie F, Denoix J-M. Ultrasonographic diagnosis of subchondral bone cysts in the medial femoral condyle in horses. *Equine Vet Educ.* 2007;19(1):47–50.

15. Sandler EA, Bramlage LR, Emberston RM, et al. Correlation of lesion size with racing performance in Thoroughbreds after arthroscopic surgical treatment of subchondral cystic lesions of the medial femoral condyle: 150 cases (1989-2000). *Proc Am Assoc Equine Pract.* 2002;48:255–256.

16. Textor JA, Nixon AJ, Lumsden J. Subchondral cystic lesions of the proximal extremity of the tibia in horses: 12 cases (1983-2000). *J Am Vet Med Assoc.* 2001;218(3):408–413.

17. Von Rechenberg B, McIlwraith CW, Luetenegger C, et al. Fibrous tissue of subchondral bone cyst lesions (SCL) in horses produce inflammatory mediators and neutral metalloproteinases and caused bone resorption in vitro. *Vet Surg.* 1998;27:520.

18. McIlwraith CW, Frisbie DD. Diagnostic and surgical arthroscopy of the femoropatellar and femorotibial joints. In: McIlwraith CW, Nixon AJ, Wright IM, eds. *Diagnostic and surgical arthroscopy in the horse.* 4th ed. London: Elsevier; 2014.

19. Bonilla AG, Williams JM, Litsky AS, et al. Ex vivo equine medial tibial plateau contact pressure with an intact medial femoral condyle, with a medial femoral condyle defect, and after placement of a transcondylar screw through the condylar defect. *Vet Surg.* 2014. http://dx.doi.org/10.1111/j.1532-950X.2014.12242.x. Epub ahead of print.

20. Santschi EM, Williams JM, Morgan JW, et al. Preliminary investigation of the treatment of equine medial femoral condylar subchondral cystic lesions with a transcondylar screw. *Vet Surg.* 2014. http://dx.doi.org/10.1111/j.1532-950X.2014.12199.x. Epub ahead of print.

21. Wallis TW, Goodrich LR, McIlwraith CW, et al. Arthroscopic injection of corticosteroids into the fibrous tissue of subchondral cystic lesions of the medial femoral condyle in horses: a retrospective study of 52 cases (2001-2006). *Equine Vet J.* 2008;40(5):461–467.

22. Foerner JJ, Rick MC, Juzwiak JS, et al. Injection of equine subchondral bone cysts with triamcinolone: 73 horses (1999-2005). *Proc 52nd AAEP.* 2006;52:412–413.

23. McCauley TR, Kornaat PR, Jee W-H. Central osteophytes in the knee. *Am J Roentgenol.* 2001;176(2):359–364.

24. Frisbie DD, McCarthy HE, Archer CW, et al. Evaluation of articular cartilage progenitor cells for the repair of articular defects in an equine model. *J Bone Joint Res.* 2014;97(6):484–493.

25. Kornaat PR, Ceulemans RYT, Kroon HM, et al. MRI assessment of knee osteoarthritis: Knee Osteoarthritis Scoring System (KOSS)—inter-observer and intra-observer reproducibility of a compartment-based scoring system. *Skel Radiol.* 2005;34(2):95–102.

26. Conaghan P. Is MRI useful in osteoarthritis? *Best Pract Res Clin Rheumatol.* 2006;20(1):57–68.

27. Conaghan PG, Felson D, Gold G, et al. MRI and non-cartilaginous structures in knee osteoarthritis. *Osteoarthritis Cartilage.* 2006;14(Suppl A):A87–94.

28. Guermazi A, Zaim S, Taouli B, et al. MR findings in knee osteoarthritis. *Eur Radiol.* 2003;13:1370–1386.

29. Nelson B, Kawcak CE, Goodrich LR, et al. Use of CT and CT arthrography as a multimodal diagnostic approach to stifle disease in quarter horses. *Proc Am Coll Vet Surg.* 2013:E102.

30. Adrian AM, Barrett M, Werpy NM, et al. The use of arthroscopy and ultrasonography for identification of pathologic changes in the equine stifle. *Proc Am Coll Vet Surg.* 2013:E82.

31. Barthez PY, Bais RJ, Vernooij JCM. Effect of ultrasound beam angle on equine articular cartilage thickness measurement. *Vet Radiol Ultrasound.* 2007;48(5):457–459.

32. Frisbie DD, Barrett MF, McIlwraith CW, et al. Diagnostic stifle joint arthroscopy using a needle arthroscope in standing horses. *Vet Surg.* 2014;43(1):12–18.

33. Walmsley JP, Phillips TJ, Townsend HGG. Meniscal tears in horses: an evaluation of clinical signs and arthroscopic treatment of 80 cases. *Equine Vet J.* 2003;35(4):402–406.

34. ter Woort F, De Busscher V, Riley CB. Ultrasonographic diagnosis of acute extrusion of the lateral meniscus in a competing quarter horse. *J Equine Vet Sci.* 2011;31(2):53–56.

35. Barrett MF, Frisbie DD, McIlwraith CW, et al. The arthroscopic and ultrasonographic boundaries of the equine femorotibial joints. *Equine Vet J.* 2011;44(1):57–63.

36. De Busscher V, Verwilghen D, Bolen G, et al. Meniscal damage diagnosed by ultrasonography in horses: a retrospective study of 74 femorotibial joint ultrasonographic examinations (2000-2005). *J Equine Vet Sci.* 2006;26(10):453–461.

37. Whitcomb MB. Ultrasound of the equine stifle: basic and advanced techniques. *Proc Am Assoc Equine Pract Focus on Hindlimb Lameness 1-10.* 2012. www.phenix-veterinaire.com/download/file1345_AAEP_Lameness_Hindlimb_2012_article10.pdf.

38. Puchalski SM, Bergman EH. Computed tomography arthrography for the diagnosis of equine femorotibial lameness in 137 horses: 2007 to 2012. *Proc Am Assoc Equine Pract.* 2013:228.

39. De Smet AA, Tuite MJ. Use of the "two-slice-touch" rule for the MRI diagnosis of meniscal tears. *Am J Roentgenol.* 2006;187(4):911–914.

40. Unlu EN, Ustuner E, Saylisoy S, et al. The role of ultrasound in the diagnosis of meniscal tears and degeneration compared to MRI and arthroscopy. *Acta Medica Anatolia.* 2014;2(3):80–87.

41. Manoj MK, Brijesh Ray RS, Jose F. Correlation between MRI and arthroscopic findings in injuries of knee joint. *Kerala J Orthop.* 2014;27(1):18–21.

42. Sladjan T, Zoran V, Zoran B. Correlation of clinical examination, ultrasound sonography, and magnetic resonance imaging findings with arthroscopic findings in relation to acute and chronic lateral meniscus injuries. *J Orthop Sci.* 2013;19(1):71–76.

43. Lee CS, Davis SM, McGroder C, et al. Analysis of low-field magnetic resonance imaging scanners for evaluation of knee pathology based on arthroscopy. *Orthop J Sports Med.* 2013;1(7). http://dx.doi.org/10.1177/2325967113513423.

44. Ferris DJ, Frisbie DD, Kisiday JD, et al. Clinical outcome after intra-articular administration of bone marrow derived mesenchymal stem cells in 33 horses with stifle injury. *Vet Surg.* 2014;43(3):255–265.

45. Walmsley JP. The stifle. In: Ross MW, Dyson SJ, eds. *Diagnosis and management of lameness in the horse.* 2nd ed. Philadelphia, PA: Elsevier Saunders; 2011.

46. Conway JD, Goodrich LR, Valdés-Martínez A. How to radiographically localize the entheses of the equine stifle joint. *Proc Am Assoc Equine Pract*. 2012:388–391.

47. Rayan F, Bhonsle S, Shukla DD. Clinical, MRI, and arthroscopic correlation in meniscal and anterior cruciate ligament injuries. *Intern Orthop*. 2008;33(1):129–132.

48. Puchalski SM. Advances in equine computed tomography and use of contrast media. *Vet Clin North Am Equine Pract*. 2012;28(3):563–581.

49. Valdés-Martínez A. Computed tomographic arthrography of the equine stifle joint. *Vet Clin North Am Equine Pract*. 2012;28(3):583–598.

50. Sampson MJ, Jackson MP, Moran CJ, et al. Three Tesla MRI for the diagnosis of meniscal and anterior cruciate ligament pathology: a comparison to arthroscopic findings. *Clin Radiol*. 2008;63(10):1106–1111.

51. McKnight AL. Magnetic resonance imaging of the equine stifle: 61 clinical cases. *Equine Vet*. 2012:6–15.

52. Dyson SJ. Normal ultrasonographic anatomy and injury of the patellar ligaments in the horse. *Equine Vet J*. 2002;34(3):258–264.

53. Prades M, Grant BD, Turner TA, et al. Injuries of the cranial cruciate ligament and associated structures: summary of clinical, radiographic arthroscopic and pathological findings from 10 horses. *Equine Vet J*. 1989;21(5):354–357.

54. Sanders-Shamis M, Bukowiecki CF, Biller DS. Cruciate and collateral ligament failure in the equine stifle: seven cases (1975-1985). *J Am Vet Med Assoc*. 1988;193(5):573–576.

55. Dik KJ, Nemeth F. Traumatic patella fractures in the horse. *Equine Vet J*. 1983;15(3):244–247.

56. Dyson S, Wright I, Kold S, et al. Clinical and radiographic features, treatment and outcome in 15 horses with fracture of the medial aspect of the patella. *Equine Vet J*. 1992;24(4):264–268.

57. Gottlieb R, Whitcomb MB, Vaughan B, et al. Ultrasonographic appearance of normal and injured lateral patellar ligaments in the equine stifle. *Proc Am Assoc Equine Pract*. 2013:226–227.

26

The Hip

David D. Frisbie and Kurt Selberg

Lameness originating from the hip joint can be considered a relatively rare condition. This is in part because of most clinicians' lack of comfort with diagnostic analgesia of this joint. It appears to the author (DDF) that diagnoses of lesions in the hip are increasing in conjunction with increased attention. The author prefers ultrasonographic guidance (2- to 6-mHz curvilinear transducer) of the needle into the hip joint, which facilitates placement of an 18-gauge, 8- to 10-inch spinal needle in the mid- to cranial aspect of the hip joint. The ultrasound probe is oriented in long axis in relation to the femoral neck, often with the concave slope of the greater tubercle included in the image. The joint margin is more easily seen in this orientation. The needle may be placed on either end of the ultrasound transducer (toward midline or lateral). If the needle is placed toward midline, the angle of the needle is more perpendicular to the floor. With the lateral approach, the needle is more parallel with the floor. Fifteen mL of local anesthetic is administered and the horse walked for 5 minutes, followed by standing for 5 minutes before reevaluation (Figure 26-1).

RADIOGRAPHY

The hip or coxofemoral joint is a ball and socket joint with the greatest range of motion in extension and flexion. The articular surfaces are the acetabulum and the femoral head. The articular surface is divided by a well-demarcated notch that serves as the insertion for the round and accessory ligaments.[1] Epidemiologic data on lameness originating from the hip are scarce. This likely relates to the infrequency of injury to this area. Radiography, ultrasound, and nuclear scintigraphic examinations of the hip joint provide important diagnostic information, support clinical suspicion of disease, and further direct a treatment plan.

Radiographic examination of the hip may be challenging and is often limited in the field by the size of the available generator and horse. Standing radiographic views are becoming more widely used. These include ventrodorsal and lateral 30 degrees dorsal-lateroventral oblique views. Anesthetized ventrodorsal images may also be obtained.

When positioning for the ventrodorsal radiograph, the generator is typically positioned ventral to the contralateral side being imaged and angled 10 to 15 degrees lateral, toward the hip. The plate is placed in a holder and positioned such that the great trochanter is toward the bottom of the x-ray detector. The articular margins should be congruent.

Depending on the angle of the x-ray generator, the notch dividing the femoral head may be clearly seen.

The lateral 30 degrees dorsal-lateroventral oblique image of the hip is most easily obtained with the rectum void of feces and distended with gas.[2] The gas distention usually occurs well enough as the rectum is evacuated. The x-ray detector is positioned vertically against the hip under examination. The x-ray panel is positioned with the greater trochanter in the caudodorsal corner. The x-ray tube is angled approximately 30 degrees ventrally from horizontal.

ULTRASOUND

An ultrasonographic examination of the pelvis including the hip has been reviewed.[3-5] A complete evaluation includes evaluation of the joint margins, muscles, and joints recesses. These areas should be examined in both long and short axis and representative images of both normal and abnormal areas should be saved for the medical records. Ultrasonographic interrogation of an area should use the highest megahertz possible and still be able to visualize the structure. Typically, a variable megahertz transducer ranging from 2 to 6 MHz is used with a scanning depth ranging from 12 to 18 cm used to interrogate the hip.

NUCLEAR SCINTIGRAPHY

Orthogonal images of the all body parts are recommended when feasible. The lateral image of the hip superimposes the femoral neck and partially the greater trochanter. It is recommended that the lateral images of the hip be obtained slightly oblique, with the camera head angled 20 to 30 degrees in a dorsomedial to ventrolateral fashion to eliminate superimposition. Counts at the hip may range from 200,000 to 300,000 if obtained in static mode. However, there is often motion degradation. Motion correction images may render better images in this region. Caudal images with the tail on the detector are also obtained to evaluate the hips. The hips are often faint because of attenuation of the large muscles of the pelvis and distance from the detector.

OSTEOARTHRITIS

Primary degenerative changes in the equine hip are rarely diagnosed, with minimal literature describing this as a primary

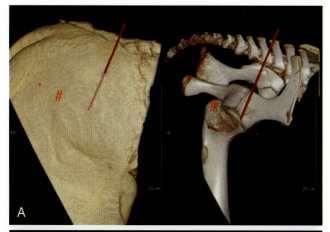

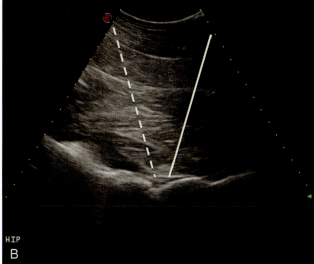

FIGURE 26-1 (A) Computed tomography renditions of an ultrasonographic-guided placement of a needle in the hip joint. The ischium (*) and greater trochanter (#) are used as palpable landmarks for commencing the ultrasound exam and locating the hip joint. The specimen shown is a foal and has less of the needle within the tissue (lighter color on needle) than would be expected in an adult. (B) Ultrasound image of the left hip. Medial is to the left. During arthrocentesis, needles may be directed from the medial aspect of the ultrasound transducer, toward midline (dashed line) or laterally (solid line).

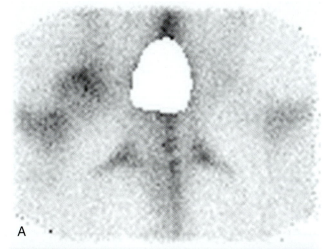

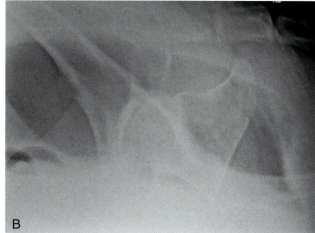

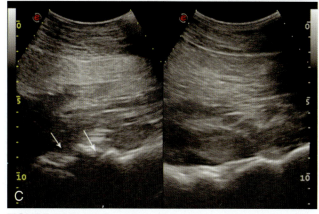

FIGURE 26-2 (A) Caudal nuclear scintigraphic image of the pelvis of a 20-year-old Paint horse. Moderate diffuse radiopharmaceutical uptake is present in the femoral head and acetabulum. Curvilinear radiopharmaceutical uptake is present along the articular margin. (B) Standing 30 degrees oblique of the left hip. The femoral head is mildly subluxated with widening of the ventrocranial aspect of the joint. Moderate osteophyte formation is present along the dorsal aspect of the acetabular rim. (C) Transverse plane ultrasound image of the left and right hips (the left hip is on the left). Medial is to the left. Moderate irregular bone proliferation is present along the dorsal aspect of the left actebabular rim and articular margin of the femoral head (arrows). The normal right hip is included for comparison.

disease process.[6] Secondary degenerative changes associated with other pathologic changes such as articular fractures, luxation, or fraying/rupture of the round ligament are more common, yet still considered rare.[7,8] Radiographic signs of osteoarthrosis include varying degrees of osteophyte production along the acetabular rim, joint space widening, and subchondral bone sclerosis (Figure 26-2). In the field, radiography may not be possible because of the constraints of the x-ray generator. However, similar osteophyte formation is typically seen well on ultrasound interrogation. Additionally, in some horses a large ventrocranial synovial outpouching may develop. The hip typically has concurrent diffuse moderate increased radiopharmaceutical uptake (see Figure 26-4).

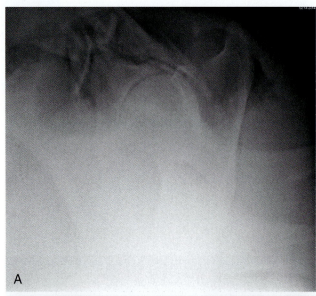

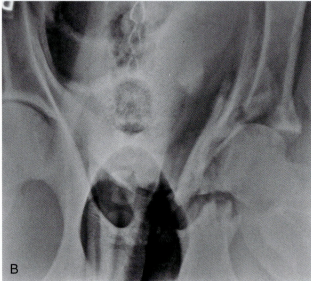

FIGURE 26-3 (A) Standing 30 degrees oblique radiograph of the left hip in an adult horse. There is a highly comminuted, articular fracture of the ilium. (B) Standing ventrodorsal radiograph of the hip in an adult horse with a segmental, medially displaced, articular fracture of the left ilium.

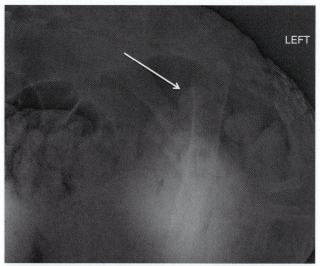

FIGURE 26-4 Left lateral image of the pelvis in a 20-year-old donkey. The left femoral head is dorsally luxated (arrow).

OSTEOCHONDROSIS/HIP DYSPLASIA

Few reports in the literature suggest that osteochrondrosis is rare in this hip. Subchondral bone cystlike lesions are described in both the acetabulum and the femoral head.[9-11] Radiographic findings range from irregular-lucent articular margins with or without sclerotic borders and secondary osteoarthrosis. Treatment is not unlike cystic lesions in the medial femoral condyle, although the location must be relatively lateral to be reached arthroscopically.[12]

The main features in dysplasia of the coxofemoral joint are acetabular and femoral head malformation.[13] The femoral head may also be subluxated.

In the foal, radiographic features of septic arthritis and hip dysplasia may overlap. Arthrocentesis should be performed to rule out septic processes.

FRACTURES/LUXATION

Multiple fracture configurations involving the pelvis are described (Figure 26-3).[14,15] A retrospective study including 100 pelvic fractures describes 23 involving the acetabulum.[14] This configuration often bears a poor prognosis for return to athletic function. However, many horses have a fair prognosis for breeding. Decisions on prognosis should be made based on degree of displacement and response to extended stall rest, as the author (DDF) has seen minimally displaced articular fractures go back to race training 12 months after injury. To date, fixation of fracture is extremely limited and conservative management is normally applied.[16]

Luxation of the hip can occur, albeit rarely (Figure 26-4). The large surrounding musculature and supporting ligaments make luxation difficult. Most luxations of the femoral head are dorsal. Ponies are more frequently affected with this disease.[17] Clinical reports of an aged, large-breed horse exist in the literature with concurrent osteoarthritis and acetabular rim fractures.[8]

SEPTIC ARTHRITIS

Hematogenous spread is the most likely cause of septic arthritis in the hip. This is most frequently seen in foals and is rare in adult horses. In these cases, the proximal femoral physis and epiphyses are the most common anatomic regions affected.[18] Common radiographic findings are irregular zones of lysis and adjacent sclerosis. Routine lavage, often using arthroscopy, is undertaken along with antibiotic treatment with reasonably successful outcomes.

REFERENCES

1. Sisson S, Grossman JD. In: *Sisson and Grossman's the anatomy of the domestic animals*. 5th ed. Philadelphia, PA: Saunders; 1975.
2. Barrett EL, Talbot AM, Driver AJ, et al. A technique for pelvic radiography in the standing horse. *Equine Vet J*. 2006;38(3):266–270.
3. Rottensteiner U, Palm F, Kofler J. Ultrasonographic evaluation of the coxofemoral joint region in young foals. *Vet J*. 2012;191(2):193–198.
4. Tomlinson JE, Sage AM, Turner TA, et al. Detailed ultrasonographic mapping of the pelvis in clinically normal horses and ponies. *Am J Vet Res*. 2001;62(11):1768–1775.
5. Geburek F, Rotting AK, Stadler PM. Comparison of the diagnostic value of ultrasonography and standing radiography for pelvic-femoral disorders in horses. *Vet Surg*. 2009;38(3):310–317.
6. Lamb CR, Morris EA. Coxofemoral arthrosis in an aged mare. *Equine Vet J*. 1987;19(4):350–352.
7. Bennett D, Campbell JR, Rawlinson JR. Coxofemoral luxation complicated by upward fixation of the patella in the pony. *Equine Vet J*. 1977;9(4):192–194.
8. Brenner S, Whitcomb MB. Ultrasonographic diagnosis of coxofemoral subluxation in horses. *Vet Radiol Ultrasound*. 2009;50(4):423–428.
9. Nixon AJ, Adams RM, Teigland MB. Subchondral cystic lesions (osteochondrosis) of the femoral heads in a horse. *J Am Vet Med Assoc*. 1988;192(3):360–362.
10. Rose JA, Rose EM, Smylie DR. Case history: acetabular osteochondrosis in a yearling thoroughbred. *J Equine Vet Sci*. 1981;1(5):173–175.
11. Nixon AJ. Diagnostic and operative arthroscopy of the coxofemoral joint in horses. *Vet Surg*. 1994;23(5):377–385.
12. McIlwraith CW, Nixon AJ, Wright IM. Diagnostic and surgical arthroscopy of the coxofemoral (hip) joint. In: *Diagnostic and Surgical Arthroscopy in the Horse*. 4th ed. London: Elsevier; 2014:308–316.
13. Speirs VC, Wrigley R. Case of bilateral hip-dysplasia in a foal. *Equine Vet J*. 1979;11(3):202–204.
14. Rutkowski JA, Richardson D. A retrospective study of 100 pelvic fractures in horses. *Equine Vet J*. 1989;21(4):256–259.
15. Shepherd MC, Pilsworth RC. The use of ultrasound in the diagnosis of pelvic fractures. *Equine Vet Educ*. 1994;6(4):223–227.
16. Ducharme NG. Pelvic fracture and coxofemoral luxation. In: Nixon AJ, ed. *Equine fracture repair*. Philadelphia, PA: Saunders; 1996:294–298.
17. Amitrano FN, Gutierrez-Nibeyro SD, Joslyn SK. Radiographic diagnosis of craniodorsal coxofemoral luxation in standing equids. *Equine Vet Educ*. 2014;26(5):255–258.
18. Schneider RK, Bramlage LR, Moore RM, et al. A retrospective study of 192 horses affected with septic arthritis/tenosynovitis. *Equine Vet J*. 1992;24(6):436–442.

27

Equine Joint Disease: Present and Future Directions in Research

C. Wayne McIlwraith, David D. Frisbie, Christopher E. Kawcak,
Laurie R. Goodrich, and P. René van Weeren

Principal joint diseases of clinical relevance in the horse are traumatic arthritis (including focal traumatic loss of articular cartilage, intraarticular (IA) fractures, meniscal and ligamentous injuries, synovitis, and capsulitis), osteoarthritis (OA), osteochondral fractures and fragmentation, osteochondrosis, subchondral cystic lesions, and septic arthritis. These are different disorders with different needs for improvement of diagnosis and therapy. IA fractures and their management have been dealt with separately in another textbook.[1]

Some of these equine conditions, with articular cartilage defects and OA being the most prominent, are of great clinical importance in human medicine as well. Much research effort is therefore dedicated to research on these joint disorders worldwide, and substantial progress can be expected in some areas in the relatively near future. Joint diseases continue to plague performance horses and result in decreased performance and loss of use.[2,3] All of the conditions listed above and detailed in various chapters in this book emphasize the need for early diagnosis as well as effective treatments for the numerous conditions that lead to OA.

In discussing present and future directions in research, we will divide this chapter into three areas: attempts to improve (early) diagnosis of joint disease, including advances in imaging and biomarker research; research into improvement of medication and delivery routes for other treatments (both symptom-modifying and disease-modifying); and attempts at regenerating deteriorated parts of joints that aim at anatomic or at least durable functional repair. In addition, prevention of joint disease is an item that has received more attention recently.

(EARLY) DIAGNOSIS OF JOINT DISEASE

This is most important for traumatic arthritis progressing to posttraumatic OA as well as subchondral bone-based diseases such as incipient IA fractures. Work is currently ongoing with the authors but needs to continue in the areas discussed below.

Further Development of Joint Imaging

Rapid advancements are currently being made in volumetric imaging of joints. Magnetic resonance imaging (MRI) and computed tomography (CT) are the basic imaging techniques that are being manipulated to enhance information about tissue status and physiology. Most importantly, newer techniques are being developed to improve clinicians' ability to predict the chances that an individual will undergo joint injury.

MRI has improved significantly over the last several decades and improvements continue to be made in both device enhancements and sequence development.[4] MRI units with high magnetic strength are now commonly used in the clinic. 3T magnets are commonly seen clinically and the resolution and amount of information that come from these units is significant. Device enhancements will likely continue, allowing for more robust imaging of joints. At the same time, newer sequences are constantly being developed that enhance certain aspects of tissues for better characterization of disease processes. Sequences can also be manipulated to determine effective physiologic status of tissues. For instance, T2 mapping is now commonly used.[5] In addition, contrast agents can be injected into the joint such as with the dGEMRIC technique in which proteoglycan content can be objectively assessed.[6] These techniques allow for more objective assessment of cartilage metabolism, response to treatment, and predisposition to injury.

CT assessment of joints has gained a fair bit of attention over the last several years. Newer devices in which hard and soft tissue resolution is improved although radiation dose is lowered have been developed.[7,8] At the same time, the price of digital plates has decreased, making the use of CT economically favorable. CT requires relatively short scan times (30 to 60 seconds) and delivers information in all three planes that can be manipulated with postprocessing. CT imaging of hard tissues has long been established and resolution of clinical scanners is currently at 90 to 100 μ. Dual-energy techniques with CT have also been developed that can be used to detect fluid in the subchondral bone whether from edema or contusion.[9] Spectral CT techniques that can improve the detection of various chemical signatures within the tissues and allow for enhanced resolution of tissues are currently being developed.[10]

The biggest criticism of CT for diagnosis of joint disease has been poor resolution and characterization of soft tissues. Dual-energy and spectral CT techniques are now being developed to allow better characterization of soft tissues. In addition, cone beam technology has been modified to allow better characterization of soft tissue morphology. Contrast agents have been and are currently being developed to enhance soft tissue and articular cartilage visualization within the joints. Anionic contrast agents can be injected into the joint and diffuse into articular cartilage and meniscal and ligamentous defects within the joints.[11] The only requirement for using this technique is that those lesions communicate with the joint space so that the contrast agent can highlight the diseased area. A cationic contrast agent that can incorporate into the articular cartilage has been developed.[12] The amount of cationic contrast taken up into the articular cartilage can be assessed through determination of Hounsfield units. There has been good correlation between uptake of cationic contrast into articular cartilage and the proteoglycan content, thus giving more objective measures of articular cartilage metabolism.

Periarticular soft tissues can also be characterized using anionic contrast agents administered intraarterially.[13,14] Soft tissue lesions can be detected upon administration of contrast and during a delayed phase in which contrast remains in the lesion after the arterial flow of contrast has dissipated.

Although generally anesthesia is currently required for CT assessment of the lower limbs, extremity units are currently being developed that can be used in the standing, sedated horse. There is some indication that high-field standing MRI units are currently being developed, but the status of that effort is unknown.

Although radiography and ultrasound are essential components of diagnostic imaging in daily equine practice, volumetric imaging is being used more and more, and recent developments are bringing the price down, making the approach more affordable for the equine industry and hence increasing its use.

Developments in Arthroscopy and Associated Techniques

The most direct way of assessing the status of articular cartilage in vivo is visual inspection during arthroscopy. As the interpretation of what is observed is based on clinical judgment, the technique is inherently subjective. However, it is to be recognized that grading, albeit subjectively, can be consistent and has been used to correlate the amount of damage in equine joints when clinical arthroscopy in the horse is being performed.[1,15-17]

In attempts to mitigate subjectivity, various scales have been developed that guide the observer towards a semiquantitative outcome, such as the ICRS (International Cartilage

Repair Society) scale.[18] It has been pointed out that even with grading, traditional visual arthroscopic evaluation is not optimal, as interoperator and intraoperator reproducibility has been reported to be poor.[19] It is also recognized that in clinical cases conventional arthroscopy does not provide information on the depth of lesion, cartilage thickness, or internal structure of the articular cartilage. These limitations are recognized by most clinical surgeons, but many subchondral bone disease problems can be recognized arthroscopically.

Several techniques have been introduced to overcome the above-mentioned disadvantages and shortcomings of visual arthroscopic assessment. Arthroscopic indentation devices provide quantitative information on alterations in mechanical properties of the articular cartilage. An indenter device for the assessment of cartilage was first developed for ex vivo use,[20] but later adapted for arthroscopic application.[21] In the horse, indenter data appeared to correlate well with glycosaminoglycan content of the cartilage but was not indicative of collagen content.[22] A more sophisticated indenter featuring a spherical endplate was used to test the relationship between indenter data and cartilage stiffness.[23] The study showed that the reproducibility of the technique was adequate, but accuracy was limited with the device identifying degeneration-associated decreases in cartilage stiffness only if the mechanical properties of the cartilage were considerably changed. It was concluded that the instrument had limited use in the initial phase of OA-like cartilage degeneration, but might yield important information in more advanced OA.

An inherent problem associated with plain indenters is that they do not measure cartilage thickness, which is related to stiffness. This problem has been solved by the integration of a miniature ultrasound transducer at the tip of the instrument, enabling simultaneous determination of the cartilage thickness at the location under scrutiny and thus providing much better data for the accurate determination of mechanical characteristics.[24,25]

Quantitative ultrasound imaging can also generate information on intrinsic structural properties of cartilage and has already been used in vivo to characterize cartilage injuries and degeneration in humans.[26] However, the technique assumes that the speed of sound is constant, which is not the case in pathologically altered cartilage, possibly affecting reliability of the measurements.[27] Further, the visual information on cartilage structure is restricted because of the limited resolution of ultrasound images.

Optical coherence tomography (OCT) is a relatively new imaging method. It is based on the measurement of reflection and backscattering of near infrared light and has superior visualization capacities compared with ultrasound. The technique produces cross-sectional digital images at resolutions comparable to that of low-power microscopy.[28] OCT is already being clinically used in cardiovascular surgery and ophthalmology,[29] and its potential usefulness for articular cartilage diagnosis has been evaluated in an in vitro setting using bovine cartilage[30] and in situ as well as ex vivo using human knee cartilage.[31] It has better penetration depth than ultrasound (Figure 27-1). Equine cartilage was used to compare the sensitivity of OCT versus ultrasound in an ex vivo setting[32] using normal cartilage and repair tissue that had formed in artificially created chondral and osteochondral lesions. In that study spontaneously repaired tissue could be quantitatively discerned from intact tissue with both techniques. There were several correlations between ultrasound and OCT parameters with the superior resolution of OCT providing a better measurement of surface roughness and the ultrasound backscattering from the inner structures of the cartilage matching better with the histologic findings. In another study using equine material, arthroscopically guided OCT provided more detailed and quantitative information on the morphology of articular cartilage lesions than conventional arthroscopy.[33] OCT was able to visualize a spectrum of lesions, including cavitation, fibrillation, superficial and deep clefts,

erosion, ulceration, and fragmentation, which could not be or only partially be detected by conventional arthroscopy (Figure 27-2). Not unimportantly, when applied in the equine fetlock joint, the arthroscopically inaccessible area between the dorsal third metacarpal bone and the proximal phalanx appeared to be reachable in some cases thanks to the small diameter of the OCT probe. OCT therefore certainly has potential value for clinical use as an adjunct to arthroscopy for (early) detection of cartilage lesions and degeneration.

Near infrared spectroscopy is a type of vibrational spectroscopy using near infrared light (NIR), generating spectral feedback when the NIR light is applied to a sample via a probe. Biochemical features that can be visualized within a typical

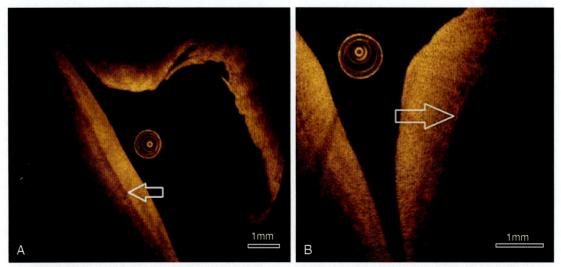

FIGURE 27-1 Optical coherence tomography images of normal cartilage of the sagittal ridge of the third metacarpal bone (**A**) and the dorsal eminence of the proximal phalanx (**B**). The interface between cartilage and subchondral bone is clearly visible (arrows). (From: Te Moller N.C.M., Brommer H., Liukkonen J., et al. (2013). Arthroscopic optical coherence tomography provides detailed information on cartilage lesions in horses. Vet J 197(3):589-595.)

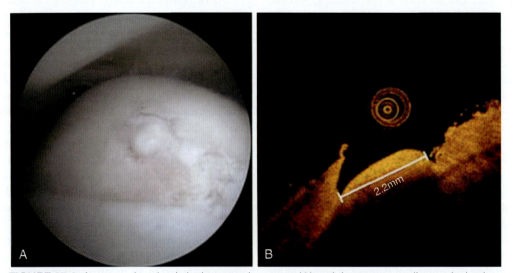

FIGURE 27-2 An osteochondrosis lesion on arthroscopy (**A**) and the corresponding optical coherence tomography (OCT) image (**B**). Based on the OCT image the fragment is still attached to the subchondral bone and the diameter of the lesion is 2.2 mm. (From: Te Moller N.C.M., Brommer H., Liukkonen J., et al. (2013). Arthroscopic optical coherence tomography provides detailed information on cartilage lesions in horses. Vet J 197(3):589-595.)

spectrum are CH, NH, OH, and SH bonds, which are the fundamental building blocks of organic materials, including cartilage, and varying in concentration with tissue type and (disease) state of the tissue.[34] The method is sensitive to both microscopic and macroscopic properties of tissue and penetrates deep into biologic tissues, beyond full-depth articular cartilage thickness, permitting simultaneous quantitative evaluation of both cartilage and subchondral bone.[34,35] At the time of writing, the technique is still under development and not clinically available, but it is one of the new arthroscopically applicable nondestructive tissue assessment techniques that has great potential, especially because of its penetration depth and its capacity to assess both cartilage and subchondral bone simultaneously.

The nondestructive cartilage (and/or subchondral bone) assessment techniques that can be used as an adjunct to direct visual arthroscopic assessment add substantially to the objectivity and repeatability of joint health evaluations. Further, most of them can visualize areas that cannot be seen by simple visual inspection. Some of the techniques are already on the market and available for clinical uses; others are expected to enter the market in the foreseeable future. As all techniques have their strengths and limitations, they are to a large extent complementary. It lies at hand, therefore, that a multimodal approach will produce maximal information and will be the path to follow for future equipment development, as suggested by Virén et al.[32]

Developments in Synovial Fluid and Serum Biomarkers

The current status of synovial fluid and serum biomarkers is detailed in Chapter 10. That chapter concludes that biomarker research has so far produced some exciting and promising data, but the implementation of these data into a commercially viable platform that is available to the equine practitioner and the patient has yet to be realized. There is still room to overcome the limitations of synovial fluid and serum biomarker measurements whenever they are employed for the investigation of disease or response to treatment.

Extensive work with biomarkers of articular cartilage and bone as well as biomarkers of joint inflammation and pain in both human and equine OA patients has yielded promising results. Accurate and earlier diagnosis with fluid biomarkers can potentially lead to identification of OA before irreversible changes occur within joint tissues. At the moment the potential for such earlier diagnosis has been depicted in a research setting through measuring levels of molecular signals and (by)products of tissue turnover as indicators of disease, but we have yet to develop clinical platforms. A second indication that has been explored with promise in the horse is the ability to predict early subchondral bone disease to identify risk of severe fracture and/or catastrophic injury.[36]

A summary of the Dorothy Russell Havemeyer Foundation Workshop on Equine Musculoskeletal Biomarkers (2009) was recently published,[37] and further details can be found online.* In that summary, biomarkers were defined and the ideas of

* http://CSU-CVMBS.colostate.edu/documents/research-equine-musculoskeletal-biomarkers-white-paper.pdf.

the equine biomarker sample bank initiated. At that workshop the following biomarkers were discussed: protein biomarkers, genetic biomarkers, postgenomic technologies and biomarkers (transcriptomics, proteomics, metabolomics), and imaging biomarkers.

At the 3rd Dorothy Russell Havemeyer Biomarker Foundation Symposium in 2014, the state of biomarkers for human OA was summarized and pitfalls and needs for both human and equine biomarkers were discussed. The current position, including steps towards further validation for human OA biomarkers, has been published.[38,39] At this symposium, Dr. Virginia Kraus stated that, to make advances in the field of OA research and new treatment opportunities, it is necessary to accelerate the development, validation, quantitation, and regulatory approval of OA-related biomarkers for clinical trials and clinical use.[40] She also pointed out that this process will be aided by a robust disease paradigm and a consensus on nomenclature to define the disease. At the moment the U.S. Food and Drug Administration (FDA) states that they "currently use disease classifications systems that define disease as primarily on the basis of their signs and symptoms."[41] As a result many disease subtypes with distinct molecular causes are still classified as one disease, although multiple different diseases that share a common molecular cause are not properly linked. Dr. Kraus also stated that the National Academy of Science has called for the creation of a "new taxonomy" of disease that is designed to advance our understanding of disease pathogenesis and improve health, which defines and describes diseases on the basis of their intrinsic biology in addition to traditional signs and symptoms.[42] Biomarkers form the cornerstone of a new taxonomy for all diseases, including OA. To aid the advance of this taxonomy, Dr. Kraus and others have proposed standardizing the nomenclature describing OA disease (molecular, anatomic, and physiologic aspects) and illness.

At the same symposium Dr. Stefan Lohmander asked pertinent questions (and gave answers) on the current state of biomarkers for human OA[43]:

1. What do we have? Many candidate markers, but few, if any, results are consistently replicated in independent laboratories, studies, and populations. Also, there is inconsistent and insufficiently transparent reporting of research findings. The answer is that the community needs to agree on guidelines for transparent reporting for biomarker research and authors and journals should follow them.
2. What are we getting? More candidate markers, some of which are now being tested in the Osteoarthritis International (OAI) subset and this will yield important experience. Any "positives" will need to be replicated in independent populations and phenotype subsets.
3. Sensitivity, specificity, and positive and negative predictive values? Receiver operated characteristics (ROC) as a measure for the performance of binary classification methods?
4. What do biomarkers add to other (easily) obtained risk factors such as age, BMI, history of injury, symptoms, clinical examination, family history, structural change, and joint shape. Care needs to be taken that the marker is also sufficiently verified as a correct signal originating from appropriate sources and is in the pathway of action.

5. To what extent does biomarker change reliably predict clinical outcome? Small effects are difficult to distinguish from biases.

6. A major bottleneck in OA biomarker validation is lack of large, stringently annotated, longitudinal sample collections.

7. We need markers to enrich clinical trial populations for disease progression and markers to provide early indication of treatment response in clinical trials.

Where to with Equine Biomarkers?

The above comments from leaders in the human OA biomarker field certainly apply to us in the equine world as we have the same goals. Some specific proposals for equine biomarker research follow:

1. Biomarker development should be based on purpose. The previously described "BIPEDS" biomarker classification (burden of disease, investigative, prognostic/predictive efficacy of intervention, diagnostic, safety)[44] is a good system to follow. These technologies should be value added to clinical expertise and imaging biomarkers.

2. What other technologies have a viable chance at commercialization? There is considerable work to be done here to engage companies to commercialize the technologies. We not only need to understand how the technology works but also its pros and cons versus other technologies.

3. Protein/epitopes are still good but we are dealing with kits that are 10 to 15 years old. Monoclonal antibodies are not going to be the screening tool but are okay for specific tests.

4. We need to qualify and define usefulness for the next-generation biomarkers; for example, biomarkers based on proteomics, genomics, posttranslational modification of protein, or specific inflammatory manifestations of OA. Several proteomic techniques have been tested in the horse and provide a catalog of potential biomarkers in aging and disease as well as a number of neopeptides, which may be distinct between conditions and tissues.[45]

5. Discovery platforms such as infrared spectroscopy, metabolomics, and transcriptomics need to be compared and their "state of readiness" for commercial use evaluated.

6. Biobank collaboration is critical and is planned. There is considerable promise for Fourier transform infrared spectroscopy (FTIR) as a diagnostic and screening tool.[46]

7. We need to consider the current level of qualification to determine what biomarkers to pursue and what data are needed.[47]

8. Statistical analysis of biomarkers is an important area for further definition. For example, principal component analysis (PCA) has its advocates versus kernel alignment and support vector machine (SVM) or discriminate analysis to get more specific information from data.

THERAPIES (BOTH SYMPTOM-MODIFYING AND DISEASE-MODIFYING)

The following are recent ongoing developments as well as further needs for investigation:

1. Testing of anti-nerve growth factor (anti-NGF) therapies in both experimental models and horses.

2. Regional delivery of medications using gels, microspheres, and regional perfusion.

3. Controlled-release medications as an approach to treat inflammation and infection.

4. Developments in IA disease-modifying drugs. There needs to be continued pursuit of disease-modifying osteoarthritic drugs (DMOADs) that can result in decreased loss of structure or promotion of healing response in the articular cartilage. The combination of a DMOAD and a symptom-modifying osteoarthritic drug (SMOAD) is logical. As has been pointed out, interventions focused exclusively on nourishing, replenishing, or replacing articular cartilage have little chance of providing long-term symptomatic relief unless they also simultaneously relieve strain on other affected structures whether the intervention is dietary, pharmacologic, or surgical.[48] This same author also notes that a more logical approach is to assess the function of the entire joint organ and direct the intervention to reduce pain and physical limitations on all moving parts.

   In various studies using the equine carpal fragmentation-exercise model, we have demonstrated DMOAD properties with the corticosteroid triamcinolone acetonide (and of course predictable SMOAD properties occurred in the same study). We have also demonstrated DMOAD effects with intramuscular pentosan polysulfate, IA hyaluronan, oral avocado-soy, and particularly impressive SMOAD and DMOAD effects with gene therapy with adenoviral-equine IL-1ra. The latter technique remains the gold standard for DMOAD treatment in the horse but of course is not yet clinically available (see gene therapy discussed later).

5. Developments in IA medication with biologic therapies (including modifications of autologous conditioned serum products, platelet-rich plasma (PRP), and metalloproteinase inhibitors). Biologic therapies have been previously presented in Chapter 16. The principal ones discussed in equine joint disease are autologous conditioned serum (ACS) and PRP products. ACS has been used clinically since the mid-2000s. In a published survey of equine practitioners, 54% of the 791 respondents indicated that they had used ACS and 22% said they used it frequently.[49] The original ACS product for horses, IRAP®, was tested in the equine fragment-exercise model,[50] and treatment improved synovial membrane inflammation and also significantly decreased the degree of gross articular cartilage fibrillation compared with placebo treatment, indicating a disease-modifying property of ACS treatment. There was also a continued increased level of presumably endogenous IRAP in the synovial fluid 3 weeks after the first treatment, which remained significantly elevated at study endpoint, indicating a prolonged beneficial effect. A newer product IRAP II® (Arthrex Vet Systems), has since been developed. In a comparison of the cytokine profiles of the two products, the concentration of IL-1ra was significantly higher

with IRAP II compared with IRAP and the ratio of IL-1ra/IL-1β was also significantly higher in IRAP II compared with IRAP. Equally importantly there was a significant increase in TNF-α with IRAP compared with IRAP II, which is of concern. The levels of IGF-1 and TGF-β were not significantly different between products.[51]

PRP was discussed in Chapter 16. There have also been a number of review articles. One comprehensive review of the literature supported the potential use of PRP both nonoperatively and intraoperatively in human orthopedics but highlighted the absence of large clinical studies and the lack of standardization between method, product, and clinical efficacy.[52] Findings from clinical trials that were reviewed suggested that PRP may have the potential to fill cartilage defects to enhance cartilage repair, attenuate symptoms of OA, and improve joint function with an acceptable safety profile.[53] There is also some evidence favoring PRP over hyaluronan for the treatment of OA, but the efficacy of PRP therapy remains unpredictable because of the highly heterogeneous nature of reported studies and the various compositions of the PRP preparations.

The question that needs to be answered is the relative value of single- versus double-centrifugation systems as this also relates to white blood cell (WBC) concentration. It has been shown that high WBC counts in association with high platelet count in PRP preparations can increase the presence of catabolic signaling proteins in vitro.[54] This was further supported by work in our laboratory evaluating the influence of a high- versus a low-platelet product on anabolic and catabolic activities in equine cartilage and meniscal implants.[55]

In five human clinical studies where PRP was compared with HA, significantly improved functional outcomes were shown for a minimum of 24 weeks with PRP compared with HA.[56] In another systematic review of data from 1543 patients, no discrepancy in effectiveness between groups using different centrifugation methods or activation agents could be identified, but single centrifugation and lack of activation overlapped with a range of ineffective treatments.[57] The relative value of a high WBC concentration versus a low WBC concentration requires further clarification.

There is very little published work on the IA use of PRP in horses. The relative values of the various systems need to be clarified. Many techniques are being used, and for a large part, they are based on protocols developed for human use, which is not necessarily optimal for the horse and yields widely varying concentrations of growth factors.[58] One study showed that either no activation or calcium chloride to activate the platelets yielded the least clinical reaction in the joint, the best growth factor profile (TGF and PDGF), and the lowest endogenous WBC release into the synovial fluid.[59] Up until now there have been only anecdotal reports and no Medline-indexed publications describing the use of PRP in the joints of horses with clinical disease. There has been a publication

on the processing of blood using a proprietary system but the authors use the term autologous protein solution, rather than PRP.[60] The product concentrates WBC (12-fold), platelets (1.6-fold), and various proteins (>3-fold) and in 40 client horses there was a significant reduction in lameness at 14 days after treatment. There was also satisfaction based on client-assessed parameters at 12 and 52 weeks.

6. Advances in IA therapies with mesenchymal stem cells (MSCs) are presented in Chapter 17. The current state of use, limitations, and knowledge have also been reviewed in the literature.[61] When direct injections of MSCs into the joint space are used, cells have been shown to populate both the articular cartilage and the synovial membrane. Enhancement of healing of microfractured chondral defects with IA MSCs has already been described,[62] and superiority of bone marrow-derived MSCs over the adipose-derived stromal vascular fraction has been demonstrated with experimental equine OA. In a clinical study 33 horses with stifle injury showed improved repair of grade 3 meniscal lesions with IA injection of 20 million MSCs 4 weeks after arthroscopic surgery.[63] This is in contradiction to insinuations that early administration of stem cells is more advantageous than attempting treatment when fibrous scar tissue has formed.[61] Areas that need further investigation include:

a. Better markers to describe cell types; current methods of describing cell surface markers are incomplete and we do not know all the cell surface markers that exist or the function of each of the receptors.

b. Specific studies assessing the dose of MSCs to be used in the equine joint have not been published; however, the range of doses used in studies with successful outcomes has been roughly 10 to 50 million in a 10- to 50-mL joint.

c. Timing and number of treatments have also yet to be definitively assessed. In studies of IA MSCs as well as studies of tendon injury, better long-term outcomes may occur when delaying the MSC treatment past the inflammatory phase of the disease.

d. Impending changes in regulatory laws by the U.S. FDA threaten to limit the use of some or all types of equine stem cells, at least in the U.S.[64,65]

e. Although there is strong evidence in the literature that MSCs have antiinflammatory and immunomodulatory properties, there is variable evidence regarding whether or not equine MSCs incite an immune response if used allogenically, especially if administered repeatedly. Work from Cornell using MHC-haplotyped horses revealed that passage to bone marrow-derived-MSCs (BM-MSCs) is highly heterogeneous in the MSC class II expression (range 0% to 98% positive) and that increasing MHC II expression is directly related to increasing response to T-cell proliferation in vitro.[62] However, when examining the immunoregulatory ability of equine bone marrow-derived-MSCs on mismatched MHC lymphocytes and their influence on the T-cell subsets in an in vitro system, equine bone marrow-derived-MSCs were able to suppress the proliferation of stimulated peripheral blood mononuclear cells as the Carboxy Fluorescein Succinimidyl Ester (CFSE) profile showed a reduction of the generation of lymphocytes and the stimulation decreased in the presence of bone marrow-derived-MSCs. The immunosuppression occurred in a dose-dependent manner being the most marked at the 1:10 ratio, and at this ratio CD8[+] T cell inhibition was detected although the CD4[+] cells in the novel CD4/CD8-positive lymphocyte population were slightly modified.[66] Such results encourage performing in vivo clinical studies.

f. The most suitable cell source still needs to be clarified but current equine research favors bone marrow-derived-MSCs.

g. There are ongoing challenges to the technical logistics of cell manufacturing and supply and delivery.

h. There may be a need for serum-free and animal protein-free culture systems that will remove the dependency of fetal bovine serum.[67] This has been proposed as an issue of safety relating to the risk of disease transmission associated with products of bovine origin, as well as to limited supplies of these materials.

i. There is always room for new and more efficient isolation methods that are biologically specific and more reproducible. This need is related to a proposed risk associated with plastic adherence as a method of isolating MSCs from tissues, as this is associated with marked heterogenicity. An example is a method that involves prospective isolation using antibody selection.[67]

j. There is a need for further studies on the mechanisms of action including molecular signals by which the cells communicate with the host within the injury niche. It has been suggested this will require both probing the phenotype of cells delivered in the injured joint and sophisticated experiments in cell tracking and retrieval. With regard to cell tracking in the horse, a recent study described labeling equine umbilical cord blood-derived and bone marrow-derived MSCs with an ultrasmall supermagnetic iron oxide (SPIO) contrast agent and detecting the labeled MSCs with MRI.[68] This is an example of being able to do labeling studies on cells without need to sacrifice. However, the proliferative capacity of the cells was decreased after labeling. Further investigations of cell function with regard to immune modulation and cell lineage differentiation potential in vitro and the biologic effect of labeling, label load, and effect of labeled cells on host tissue in vivo remain to be performed.

7. Developments in gene therapy. The field of gene therapy for treating joint disease has been rapidly evolving over the last 2 decades. The implantation of cells into the synovial cavity or chondral and osteochondral defects offers a mechanism by which genetic manipulation of transferred cells may enhance cell signaling or provide a strategy where cells can be "preprogrammed" to progress down a desired cell lineage. The development of improved gene vectors that have longer-term expression of therapeutic proteins has resulted in significant optimism within this field as it relates to orthopedics and specifically joint

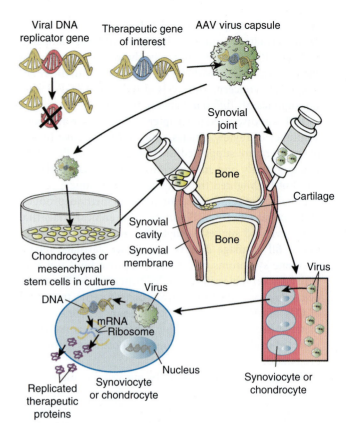

FIGURE 27-3 A pictorial depiction of in vivo or ex vivo gene therapeutic approaches. DNA encoding for a wild-type vector capsid with replicating sequences is initially utilized. The replicating DNA (DNA that allows the virus to replicate and be wild type) is then removed and replaced with DNA of a therapeutic gene (IGF-I, IL-1ra, etc.). A viral capsule with the therapeutic gene is then either injected directly into the joint (in vivo gene therapy) or cells in culture are transduced and then directly injected into the joint cavity or placed in a cartilage defect within a scaffold or biomaterial (ex vivo gene therapy). Once transduced, synoviocytes, chondrocytes, or mesenchymal stem cells are transduced by the gene therapeutic vector, the vector capsid releases its DNA, and transcription/translation occurs to produce the therapeutic DNA. (Modified from McIlwraith C.W. (2005). AAEP Proceedings, with permission.)

disease. Further, with important advances in scaffold development and cell transfer techniques, a niche for gene therapeutic applications has been realized. Because gene therapy has not been presented in detail in this text previously (and that is because it is still not a clinical treatment in the horse), an introduction of the principles follows.

a. Strategies for gene therapy in joint disease: Gene therapy is the transfer of therapeutic genes to cells of a joint for the purposes of augmenting healing by increasing anabolic proteins or decreasing (or blocking) inflammatory mediators.[69] Two approaches are in vivo or ex vivo administration (Figure 27-3). The in vivo approach involves direct injection of gene therapeutic vectors into the synovial cavity. This method of administration is straightforward but does not delineate which tissues become transduced. The ex vivo approach involves

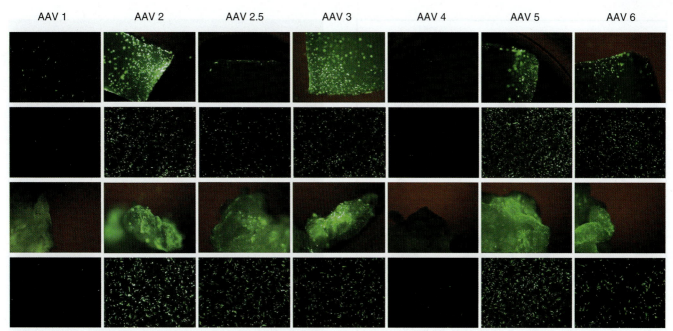

AAV 1   AAV 2   AAV 2.5   AAV 3   AAV 4   AAV 5   AAV 6

FIGURE 27-4 Photomicrograph of Green Fluorescent Protein (GFP) transduction of various self-complimentary adeno-associated virus (scAAV) serotypes in cartilage explants (top row), chondrocytes (second row), synovial explants (third row), and synoviocytes (bottom row). scAAV2, 2.5, 3, 5, and 6 appear to be the most efficient in transduction of these tissues (From: Hemphill D.D., McIlwraith C.W., Samulski R.J., et al. (2014). Adeno-associated viral vectors show serotype specific transduction of equine joint tissue explants and cultured monolayers. Sci Rep 4:5861.)

genetic manipulation of cells destined to be either injected into the joint or implanted into a defect often within a scaffold such as a fibrin matrix or within a biomaterial.[71-72] Although both nonviral and viral capsids have been used for gene therapy, decades of vector development have led to viral vectors being the most efficient and best at producing proteins for extended periods of time, which is crucial for success in orthopedic indications. Adenoviral and retroviral[73] vectors offered proof of concept in early gene therapy studies on joint disease, but the optimal vector that appears safest and produces protein for extended periods of time is adeno-associated virus (AAV).[74-77] Further, recent modifications to this vector have allowed rapid production of protein (within 3 days) because of a self-complementary aspect, which converts the vector's single-stranded DNA into double-stranded segments allowing for quick transcription and translation.[78] In joint tissues several different serotypes appear to be appropriate and result in long-term expression (Figure 27-4).

b. Therapeutic proteins delivered by gene therapy mechanisms: Both anabolic proteins beneficial to cartilage healing and anticatabolic proteins have been used to enhance collagen and matrix synthesis and block detrimental effects of inflammatory molecules, respectively. Gene sequences used within gene therapy vectors include insulin-like growth factor I (IGF-I),[70,79] bone morphogenic proteins 2 and 7 (BMP 2, 7),[71,80] transforming growth factor-β (TGF-β),[81,82] and fibroblast growth factor (FGF).[83,84] Alternatively a strong anticatabolic

approach has been to insert the gene sequence encoding for interleukin receptor antagonist (IL-1ra) into a gene vector. This molecule has shown great promise in preclinical studies in the horse and human clinical trials of gene therapy for cartilage repair, OA, and rheumatoid arthritis.[74,77,85-89] Using a dual approach of enhancing anabolism and blocking catabolism will likely result in maximal benefits to repairing cartilage and reversing OA progression (Figure 27-5). Indeed, work at CSU demonstrated that a gene therapy approach using both anticatabolic gene transfection (IL-1ra) and anabolic gene transfection (IGF-I) significantly enhanced quality of articular cartilage repair in horses.[90] Further, with recent advances in maximal cartilage transduction efficiency, delivery of these factors is realistic and will be an important clinical entity[77] (Figure 27-6).

c. The future strategies of gene therapy: As safety and efficacy studies offer promising advances in gene therapy approaches, this field will continue to develop and vectors will be further perfected that both reduce dosages and maximize therapeutic benefits. Work that is currently under way includes: 1) vector capsid modifications that reduce immunity to injections and increase the efficiency of cell transduction,[91] 2) combining both anabolic and anticatabolic genes that have dual roles in repairing tissues and reducing inflammation,[92] 3) genetic modifications to DNA promoters that result in "on/off" switches that can control protein production[72,93]; and 4) biomaterials that allow controlled release of gene therapeutic vectors by slow, controlled

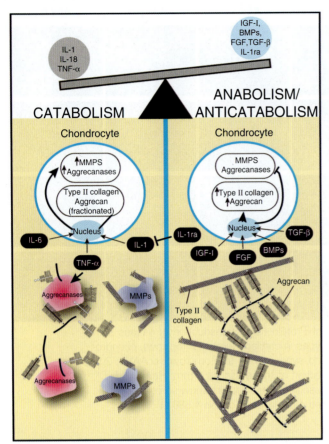

FIGURE 27-5 A pictorial demonstration of the effects of therapeutic proteins on both anabolism and catabolism of cartilage. All proteins in this cartoon can be delivered with gene therapeutic vectors. (Reprinted from Goodrich LR. Gene therapy and tissue engineering. In: Biologic Knee Reconstruction: A Surgeon's Guide, BJ Cole, JD Harris (eds), SLACK Inc., Thorofare, NJ, 2015 pp233-239.)

release of therapeutic vectors as the biomaterials are slowly degraded.[72,93] These advances will lead to a tailored gene therapy approach. Exciting research in the areas of tissue engineering such as multilayered implants and bioreactors that can "precondition" genetically modified cells offer a unique arena to apply gene therapeutic applications. The future of this technology in orthopedics remains bright.

8. What is to be expected from nutraceuticals in the future? The current knowledge with nutraceuticals has been presented in Chapter 19. The biggest need for future research in this area is further controlled clinical studies as exemplified by the randomized, double blinded, placebo controlled study on the efficacy of green lipped mussel in horses with chronic fetlock lameness attributed to OA.[94] Realizing the difficulties with such clinical studies, the study with Sasha's Equine Powder (SEQ) demonstrating that intraarticular IL-1β injections did not induce significant increases in synovial fluid PGE2 and GAG concentrations compared to untreated horses can provide valuable in vivo support as well.[95]

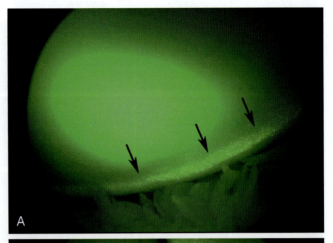

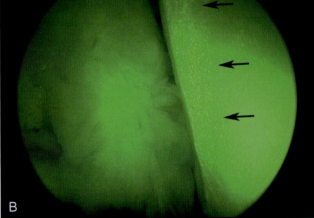

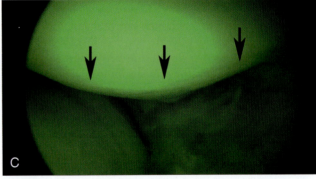

FIGURE 27-6 Arthroscopic images revealing in situ transduction of chondrocytes 4 months after in vivo injection with scAAVGFP gene vectors. **(A)** reveals the edge of a cartilage surface with intense transduction of chondrocytes producing GFP (arrows); **(B)** reveals intense transduction of surface chondrocytes (also producing GFP); **(C)** is the cartilage surface from the joint injected with saline. (Reprinted from Goodrich LR. Gene therapy and tissue engineering. In: Biologic Knee Reconstruction: A Surgeon's Guide, BJ Cole, JD Harris (eds), SLACK Inc., Thorofare, NJ, 2015 pp233-239.)

ARTICULAR CARTILAGE HEALING (REPAIR)

There is much ongoing research in improving articular cartilage repair. Because this text is focused on current diagnosis and treatment of equine clinical joint conditions, the reader is referred elsewhere for details on the history and advances in this field; except, when techniques have reached clinical use in the horse as detailed in various preceding chapters. This section of the chapter briefly describes the current state of knowledge with certain techniques that are being used in the horse as well as areas for further research.

Developments in Surgical Techniques

Surgical options in cartilage repair have been divided into three categories: 1) palliative (arthroscopic débridement and lavage, 2) reparative (marrow stimulation techniques) and 3) restorative (osteochondral grafting, autologous chondrocyte implantation [ACI] and, more recently, augmentation with MSCs).[96] The goals of repair of articular cartilage defects from a clinical point of view include restoration of clinical function (including pain relief) and prevention, or at least, delay of the onset of OA.[97] These goals can potentially be achieved by replacement of damaged or lost articular cartilage with a substance capable of functioning under normal physiologic environments for an extended period as well as integration of the repair tissue to the surrounding articular cartilage and the subchondral bone. The limitations of this repair process have long been recognized.[98-99]

The current standard of care for the surgical treatment of articular cartilage defects in both humans and horses is débridement of the affected area followed by microfracture. Various experimental studies of microfracture have been performed in the horse. They were initially commenced to validate microfracture in humans, which led to development of the first model of articular cartilage repair in horses simulating femorotibial defects in humans.[100] Multiple equine models of articular cartilage healing have been developed both to simulate the human situation and to evaluate better techniques for horses.[62] Studies in the equine femorotibial model have demonstrated a significant increase in amount of repair tissue with full-thickness defects treated with microfracture versus débridement alone[100] and an increase in type II collagen mRNA expression at 8 weeks with microfracture.[101] In addition, removal of the calcified cartilage layer was critical to optimal repair in microfractured defects.[102]

Clinical assessment in human patients receiving microfracture versus ACI showed that both methods had acceptable short-term clinical results with satisfactory Short Form 36-item (SF-36) physical component score at 2 years postoperatively, but microfracture was significantly better than ACI in that parameter although histologic evaluation and biopsies were comparable.[103] Patient satisfaction with functional outcome was good in top-level alpine skiers following microfracture of full-thickness chondral defects in the knee.[104] In general, short-term outcome of microfracture in humans is reported to be good to excellent with a high level of patient satisfaction.[105] In a review of cartilage repair techniques, long-term outcome was less certain,[106] and this was proposed as caused by functional inferiority of the repair tissue resulting in the development of OA in the long run.

In a systematic analysis of microfracture, including 28 studies describing 3122 patients, the average follow-up was 41 months with 5 studies reporting 5 years or more.[107] Microfracture effectively improved knee function in all studies during the first 24 months following it, but reports on durability of the initial functioning improvement were conflicting. Shortcomings included limited hyaline repair tissue, variable repair cartilage volume, and possible functional deterioration; the conclusion was that further well-designed studies are needed.[107] A review of clinical results and complications with microfracture concluded that clinical results in humans with resolution or improvement in pain are promising and last an average of 2 to 3 years, although equine studies indicate that repair tissue continues to remodel toward chondrogenesis for at least a year but longer-term results are not available to gain insight into the mechanism of microfracture function or failure over time.[108] The issue of central or intralesional osteophytes was also addressed, and there was some suggestion that it may be stimulated by excessive débridement rather than microfracture per se. This is certainly an area that requires further investigation.

The first three authors of this chapter routinely use microfracture when encountering full-thickness defects with an intact subchondral plate in the horse. Although anecdotal impressions are positive, there are no clinical studies with solitary defects undergoing microfracture. Cohen et al.[109] were unable to demonstrate an association between the use of microfracture and any measure of long-term outcome in a study of 44 horses. However, this population was very heterogeneous and many animals suffered from more complex lesions than cartilage lesions alone. Given the similarity between human and equine cartilage, at least in the femorotibial articulation,[110,111] it is logical that results with microfracture, at least in those articulations, would be similar. Although limitations in the quality of the repair tissue after microfracture (principally fibrocartilage) are recognized in experimental equine studies, the repair tissue has withstood a high level of athletic exercise over a long-term period.[100,102] Studies have also been done augmenting the response to microfracture with both gene therapy[90] and IA MSCs.[62] Most recently a study at the Orthopaedic Research Center at Colorado State University in collaboration with the Massachusetts Institute of Technology tested the ability of an injectable self-assembling peptide hydrogel to augment cartilage repair with or without microfracture.[112] Treatment with hydrogel alone further caused further improvement in clinical symptoms and improved filling compared with empty defects without microfracture as well as protecting against radiographic changes versus microfracture-treated defects. Microfracture of full-thickness defects improved clinical symptoms compared with nonmicrofractured defects, and the repair tissue contained increased amounts of aggrecan and type II collagen compared with hydrogel alone-treated defects. Microfracture also protected against synovial fibrosis compared with empty and hydrogel alone-treated defects.

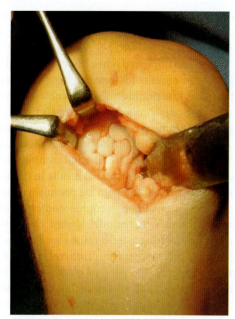

FIGURE 27-7 Miniarthrotomy mosaicplasty on the medial femoral condyle for osteochondritis dissecans in a human patient. (From: Hangody L., Dobos J., Baló E., et al. (2010). Clinical experiences with autologous osteochondral mosaicplasty in an athletic population: a 17-year prospective multicenter study. Am J Sports Med 38(6):1125-1133.)

Mosaicplasty

This surgical method, also called osteochondral autologous transplantation, was developed in Hungary in the 1990s by Hangody et al.[113,114] It uses cylindrical osteochondral autografts that are harvested from a nonaffected and non-weight-bearing donor site and subsequently implanted in the recipient site, which is created at the site of the cartilage defect that is to be treated (Figure 27-7). Long-term clinical results in humans are reported as good to excellent for small- to medium-sized defects (1 to 4 cm^2), in both the general patient population[113,115] and athletes.[116] The limitations are potential donor site morbidity, possible graft site mismatch leading to altered joint biomechanics (when surfaces are not flush), inability to treat large defects, and lack of integration with the surrounding tissue.[105]

In the horse, the technique has been used to fill a subchondral cystic lesion.[117] It has recently been further explored in an experimental study in which osteochondral plugs were harvested from the cranial surface of the medial femoral trochlea and used to fill defects on the weight-bearing surface of the contralateral medial femoral condyle, using either an arthrotomy or an arthroscopic approach. During follow-up arthroscopy at 12 months when biopsies were also taken, the transplanted areas looked congruent and smooth. In 5 of 10 biopsies, hyaline cartilage was seen, but remaining biopsies showed loss of glycosaminoglycans and change in the architecture of the transplanted cartilage.[118]

Autologous Chondrocyte Implantation and Matrix-Induced Autologous Chondrocyte Implantation

Autologous chondrocyte implantation (ACI) was initially demonstrated to be useful in rabbits by Grande et al.[119] Briefly, chondrocytes are harvested from non-weight-bearing cartilage, expanded in vitro, and implanted in the defect during a second surgical procedure.[120] The technique has evolved over the years. First-generation ACI used a periosteal flap to cover the defect and keep the implanted chondrocytes in place. However, this led to hypertrophy of the flap in certain cases.[121]

Second-generation ACI used various membranes on which cells were cultured (Figure 27-8). Overall, the clinical outcome of ACI has been shown to be quite satisfactory with a randomized clinical trial in 100 patients showing more favorable results 10 years postoperatively than with mosaicplasty.[122] In comparison to microfracture, ACI showed better clinical and structural outcome in some studies,[123,124] although in another study both methods had acceptable short-term clinical results and microfracture was significantly better than ACI in SF-36 physical component score at 2 years.[103] Further, the recovery time needed for maturation of the neotissue that is formed is relatively long (6 to 12 months), thus leading to long rehabilitation periods.[125]

A further development is the use of three-dimensional biodegradable materials in which the chondrocytes are seeded before implantation to allow them to develop in a three-dimensional environment, which is a well-known prerequisite to prevent dedifferentiation of chondrocytes. This third-generation ACI is also called matrix-assisted autologous chondrocyte implantation (MACI) and typically uses specially developed collagen (type I and III) membranes that permit low friction at one side and chondrocyte infiltration at the other. The matrix is then implanted in the defect with the cell-laden side against the subchondral bone and the other one at the side of the articular surface. Advantages of MACI are easier and better filling of the defect and a shorter rehabilitation period owing to better graft stability.[125] Disadvantages are the same as for conventional ACI. Clinical results thus far seem promising[126] and large randomized clinical trials are under way,[127] but long-term results have not yet been published.

A modified MACI technique has been tested in the horse with defects on the medial trochlear ridge of the femur with chondrocytes cultured on a collagen membrane and implanted with PDS/PGA staples.[128] Good repair was shown at 18 months with MACI compared with collagen membrane alone and empty cartilage defect groups.

The future with these techniques probably resides with 1-step techniques such as the cartilage autologous implantation system, which has demonstrated efficacy in the horse.[129] After preclinical studies in the horse, this technique was used in a human prospective clinical safety trial with 2 years' follow-up with positive results.[130] Unfortunately, the phase III study was halted at the decision of the company (business decision).

The Use of Seeded/Unseeded Scaffolds of Various Types and Three-Dimensional Bioprinting

Although techniques like ACI and MACI generally have good clinical outcomes, they are not the definitive answer for the repair of (osteo)chondral defects for both technical and

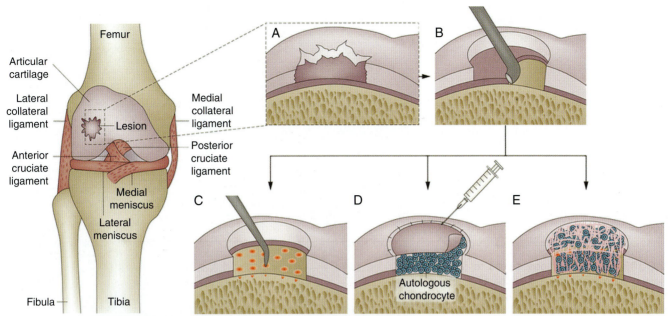

FIGURE 27-8 (A) A full-thickness focal chondral lesion. **(B)** The lesion is débrided to ensure healthy, stable margins for integration of the host tissue with the neotissue. **(C)** Microfracture. Channels are created using a 45° awl, spaced 3 to 4 mm apart and 3 to 4 mm deep to penetrate the subchondral bone, allowing MSCs to migrate from the marrow to the cartilage defect. **(D)** ACI. The débrided lesion is filled with 12 to 48 million autologous chondrocytes and covered with a periosteal flap or mixed collagen type I and type III membrane. **(E)** MACI. The autologous chondrocyte population is expanded in vitro and then seeded for 3 days onto an absorbable three-dimensional (collagen types I and III or hyaluronic acid) matrix before implantation. The cell-seeded scaffold is then secured into the lesion with fibrin glue. *ACI,* Autologous chondrocyte implantation; *MACI,* matrix-assisted autologous chondrocyte implantation; *MSC,* mesenchymal stem cell. (From: Makris E.A., Gomoll A.H., Malizos K.N., et al. (2014). Repair and tissue engineering techniques for articular cartilage. Nat Rev Rheumatol 11(1):21-34.)

practical reasons. Technically, none of the above-mentioned techniques results in the restoration of hyaline cartilage that is functionally equal to the original tissue; hence long-term prognosis is still guarded. In a more practical sense, ACI and MACI are two-stage procedures, meaning they present a heavy burden for the patient, carry some increased risk, and entail considerable costs. The latter factor is important at present owing to huge increases in healthcare budgets, in part caused by the aging population and by the introduction of innovative but expensive techniques (such as ACI and MACI). For these reasons, there is an ongoing quest for novel techniques that are more efficacious and less expensive.

Extracellular Matrix-Based Scaffolds. Most of the current research in this area focuses on the development of biocompatible scaffolds to fill the osteochondral defects. The scaffolds can be derived from biologic material or may consist of artificial components or combinations of the two and may be cell-seeded or not. The idea is that they temporarily fill the defect and allow for the formation of the best possible quality of repair tissue. Ideally, there is a simultaneous process of degradation of the implanted scaffold and formation of neotissue, resulting in functionally optimal tissue once this process is completed. Apart from biocompatibility, important issues related to this concept are the biomechanical stability of the scaffold, integration with the surrounding tissue,

determination of the optimal cell source (if seeded), and final quality of the neotissue and related long-term durability.

Several tissue engineering techniques use scaffolds based on the natural extracellular matrix (ECM) of a variety of tissues, which are decellularized and otherwise processed before being implanted. The idea is that the ECM in the natural situation provides a unique, tissue-specific three-dimensional environment containing both structural and functional molecules, which, in interaction with the resident cells, determines tissue homeostasis. Therefore, natural ECM-derived scaffolds are thought to be better prepared to form a basis for functional matrices than entirely artificial scaffolds.[131] This type of scaffold is already being used clinically in several applications, such as the regeneration of heart valves.[132] In the form of a decellularized organ, the concept has been used for the regeneration of trachea.[133] Many more applications for organ regeneration are being developed or foreseen.[134] For these applications matrices derived from either bladder or small intestinal submucosa are often used.

Although the use of osteochondral plugs (as in mosaicplasty) can in theory be considered to be an ECM-based technique, as bone and cartilage matrix are directly transplanted, the use of more sophisticated variants of ECM-based scaffolds is still a new approach in cartilage tissue engineering. In a recent review, several ways in which ECM-based

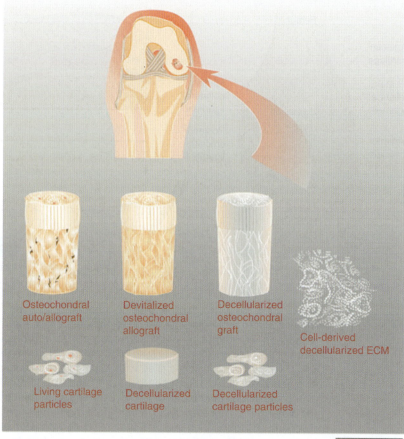

Osteochondral auto/allograft

Devitalized osteochondral allograft

Decellularized osteochondral graft

Cell-derived decellularized ECM

Living cartilage particles

Decellularized cartilage

Decellularized cartilage particles

TRENDS in Biotechnology

FIGURE 27-9 Various possibilities for matrix-based approaches to (osteo)chondral repair: osteochondral defects can be filled with fresh, devitalized, or decellularized osteochondral grafts, which can be from autologous or allogeneic origin. Defects can be treated with allogeneic living cartilage particles, a decellularized cartilage graft, or decellularized cartilage particles. In addition, use of in vitro produced cell-derived decellularized matrix is also being actively explored. (From: Benders K.E., van Weeren P.R., Badylak S.F., et al. (2013). Extracellular matrix scaffolds for cartilage and bone regeneration. Trends Biotechnol 31(3):169-176.)

scaffolds could be used for (osteo)chondral repair were outlined[131] (Figure 27-9). The use of such scaffolds holds great promise in osteochondral repair, but several issues need to be addressed. These include the recapitulation of the zonal structure of natural cartilage by these scaffolds, the question of which tissue might form the ideal basis for this type of scaffold (decellularized cartilage is rich in collagen type II although other tissues yield predominantly collagen type I-rich scaffolds), and the question of how to generate neotissue with biphasic character (cartilage and bone), although minimizing the risk of overgrowth of the latter.[131] Whereas mosaicplasty has been reported in the horse, as mentioned earlier,[118] the use of a decellularized cartilage scaffold for osteochondral repair has only been reported in a single pilot study in which an artificial defect was created.[131] Short-term (8-week) outcome seemed favorable (Figure 27-10), but no data on long-term performance were available. The technique is promising, though. In a study in rabbits, adipose-derived stem cell-loaded cartilage ECM scaffolds showed excellent results, yielding repair tissue that was comparable to native cartilage in terms of mechanical properties and biochemical components.[135]

Artificial Scaffolds. Artificial scaffolds have the advantage over tissue-derived scaffolds in that the composition is more reproducible, immune-related problems are less likely to occur, and regulatory approval will be easier and quicker to obtain. However, they need extensive in vitro testing, and

functionalization may require adding extra components, such as certain enzymes, cytokines, and growth factors that can already be naturally present in ECM. Hydrogels prepared from natural and synthetic polymers are usually the principal component of these scaffolds, as they are biocompatible and can exhibit swelling and lubricating behavior comparable to articular cartilage. They also offer an excellent environment for chondrocytes or other cells, such as stem cells.[136] Several types of hydrogels have been used for cartilage tissue engineering. Of these, gelatin methacrylamide (gelMA) hydrogels have received much attention recently, as they have been shown to have excellent chondrogenic potential,[137] which can be further modified by the addition of specific ECM components, such as hyaluronan (HA).[138]

A disadvantage of this and other hydrogels is their low intrinsic stiffness, which is far below the stiffness of natural cartilage. There are various ways to address this problem, such as photo crosslinking and/or the use of chemicals.[139,140] Another technique to improve biomechanical properties is the fabrication of a hybrid scaffold in which the hydrogel is combined with a much stiffer other material. This approach to a certain extent mimics the natural situation in which the collagen network has definitely different biomechanical properties than the glycosaminoglycan matrix. Poly(ϵ)caprolactone (PCL) is a polymer that is frequently used to complement hydrogels in hybrid scaffolds,[141] but silk-derived and electrospun fibers have also been used.[142,143]

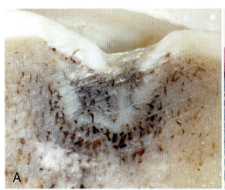
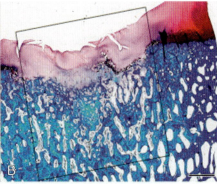
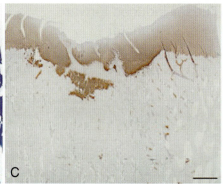

TRENDS in Biotechnology

FIGURE 27-10 Osteochondral repair in a horse using decellularized cartilage. **(A)** Macroscopic overview of osteochondral repair tissue after 8 weeks of implantation. Both **(B)** glycosaminoglycan-rich (Safranin-O, Fast Green) and **(C)** collagen type II-rich neotissue was found after 8 weeks, with clear distinction between the cartilage and bone phase. Scale bars represent 2 mm; the box approximates the osteochondral defect created. (From: Benders K.E., van Weeren P.R., Badylak S.F., et al. (2013). Extracellular matrix scaffolds for cartilage and bone regeneration. Trends Biotechnol 31(3):169-176.)

Three-Dimensional Bioprinting. Three-dimensional bioprinting is based on additive manufacturing and is a rapidly developing field in regenerative medicine.[144,145] The three-dimensional printing technology was originally developed for nonbiologic applications by its inventor Charles Hull, who patented a method in which sequentially printed layers of a material that could be cured with UV light served to build a three-dimensional structure.[146] Later, the technique was applied to biologic materials, first using modified industrial inkjet printers and more recently custom-built bioprinters (Figure 27-11).

Currently, three main types of bioprinters are discerned according to their dispersing system.[147] Two of these produce serial droplets of the material to be printed, which are generated either by laser technology, heat, or piezoelectric pulses; the third technique, called robotic dispensing, generates a continuous strand of material, driven by mechanical or pneumatic forces (Figure 27-12).

Materials need to meet specific requirements for use in bioprinters.[144,148] These include printability characteristics, such as rheologic properties, biocompatibility (no cytotoxicity or immunogenicity), possession of appropriate degradation kinetics (depending on the rate of generation of the neotissue with ideally simultaneous degradation and replacement), and possession of appropriate structural and biomechanical properties (in relation to the tissue that is substituted and to the degradation rate). Further, there may be specific requirements for tissue architecture, such as porosity or multicomposite composition, depending again on the (functionality of the) tissue that is replaced. Normally, a certain amount of so-called biomimicry (resemblance to the natural tissue) is desired.

Materials that are printed may, depending on their nature, contain cells or not. In the latter case, the scaffolds will need to be populated by migrating cells from surrounding tissues or by homing cells from a systemic source. As this is unlikely to occur in large defects and is impossible when organ replacement is envisaged, many (bio)printing approaches use

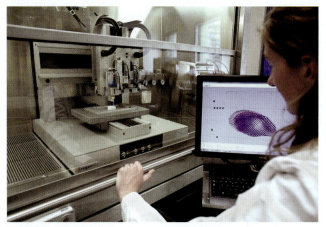

FIGURE 27-11 Three-dimensional bioprinter based on robotic dispensing technology. (Image courtesy of the Utrecht Biofabrication Facility.)

cell-laden materials. There are several possible cell sources. The principal choice is between primary cells pertaining to the tissue to be replaced and more stem cell types of cells; there are several factors that may influence the cell type(s) chosen.[144] An important requirement is that cells must be robust enough to survive the manipulations to which they are exposed during the printing process. Challenges may be several and include mechanical, toxic, and heat stress. In vitro testing can give information about the degree to which cells can cope with these factors. For instance, when alternatingly printing a thermoplastic polymer (polycaprolactone), dispersed at about 100° C, and a chondrocyte-laden sodium alginate hydrogel, dispersed at room temperature, cell viability was only marginally below viability of control cells at day 1 after printing and not significantly affected at day 3, indicating the absence of any negative thermal effect.[148] Another factor to take into account when selecting the cell source is the capacity of the cells to retain their phenotype and functional profile during and after the printing process (if using

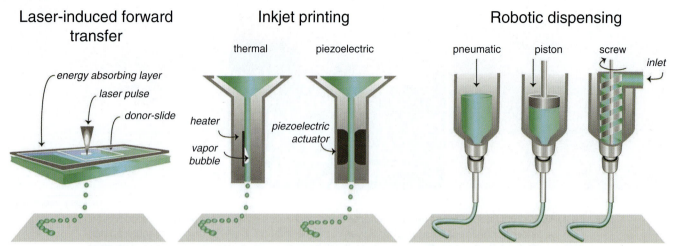

Laser-induced forward transfer

Inkjet printing

Robotic dispensing

FIGURE 27-12 Schematic drawings of the three major dispersion systems used in bioprinters. Laser-induced forward transfer technology uses laser pulses that are focused on an absorbing substrate containing the bioink to generate a pressure that will propel the ink (cell-laden or not) onto the substrate. Inkjet printing relies on electric heating of the nozzle of the printer that will produce air-pressure pulses, forcing droplets from the nozzle, or acoustic pressure pulses generated by ultrasound or a piezoelectric actuator that do the same. Robotic dispensing, also called microextrusion, uses pneumatic or mechanical devices to extrude the material from the nozzle. (From: Malda J., Visser J., Melchels F.P., et al. (2013). 25th anniversary article: engineering hydrogels for biofabrication. Adv Mater 25(36):5011-5028.)

primary cell sources). For stem cells, it is important they have the capacity to convert into or to induce a resident cell type that can be instrumental in tissue regeneration, which is apt to maintain regular tissue homeostasis once a stable situation has been achieved. Additionally, any type of multipotent or pluripotent cell should differentiate into the desired direction and not in others. In cartilage it is of special importance that no bone formation occurs.

Bioprinting offers several advantages for application in tissue engineering of osteochondral defects. The additive character of the technique easily allows for the fabrication of biphasic, that is, osseous and cartilaginous, constructs through the manipulation of scaffold composition and cell type[149,150] (Figure 27-13). It also allows for the mimicking of the zonal structure of cartilage by either changing the relative proportions of the extracellular matrix components that are printed or by functionalizing layers of the cartilage using different bioactive molecules (Figure 27-14). The field is developing quickly and novel applications are being developed; in a recent study microcarriers were used to fabricate constructs with high cell concentrations and to improve the compressive modulus of the hydrogel constructs.[150]

Although there are no regulatory-approved clinical applications of bioprinted osteochondral constructs yet, much research is being conducted in the area and progress is fast. A large variety of potential ECM components, such as hydrogels and reinforcement materials, are being tested, and cells of various sources are being combined with them. The research is slowly passing from the in vitro phase and testing in small laboratory species to large animal models, and the horse is one of the best models for OA.[151] Significant breakthroughs are to be expected in the coming years.

Intralesional versus Intraarticular Use of MSCs in Repair of Articular Cartilage, Meniscus, and Ligaments

Initial research using GFP labeled bone marrow-derived-MSCs has confirmed their ability to localize and participate in repair of damaged joint structures, including cruciate ligaments menisci and cartilage lesions.[152] There have been a number of studies using both intraarticularly injected MSCs as well as intralesional placement to evaluate their potential in the repair of articular cartilage, meniscus and ligaments. The in vivo study in a goat OA model involving anterior cruciate ligament (ACL) transection and medial meniscectomy producing regrowth of meniscal tissue as well as a decrease in OA[153] has led to evaluation of this technique in the horse.

A clinical equine study with intraarticular bone marrow-derived equine cultured MSCs in 33 horses with stifle injury has been reported.[154] All cases had mean follow-up posttreatment time of 44 months and were all cases that had previously failed routine treatments, had moderate to severe damage and the damage was confirmed with arthroscopic surgery. The overall success rate for returning to work was 72.5%. Of particular interest were 62.5% of horses with Grade 3 damage returning to work, which was considerably superior to two other studies with Grade 3 meniscal damage showing 0% and 35%. In an experimental study with defects created on the medial femoral condyle, a single injection of 20 million bone marrow-derived-MSCs four weeks after creation of the defects showed increased firmness of repair tissue as well as increased aggrecan content compared to microfractured defects alone.[62]

On the other hand, placement of MSCs in fibrin or fibrin composites has not been as successful in demonstrating enhanced repair. A study with bone marrow-derived-MSCs in fibrin in full thickness articular defects on the lateral

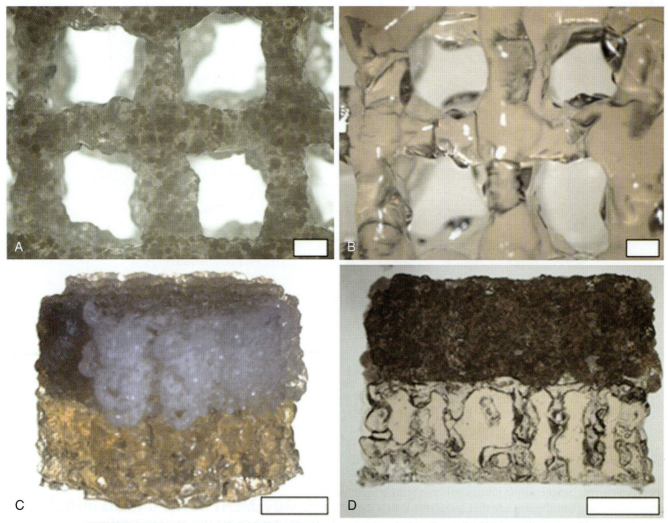

FIGURE 27-13 Bilayered GelMA-GG cylindrical osteochondral graft model (16 mm diameter, 1 cm height). (**A**) Microcarrier (MC)-laden layer top view. (**B**) Gelatin methacrylamide Gellan Gum (GelMA-GG) layer top view. (**C**) Perspective. (**D**) Cross-section. Scale bars are 400 μm for **A** and **B** and 4 mm for **C** and **D**. (From: Levato R., Visser J., Planell J.A., et al. (2014). Biofabrication of tissue constructs by 3D bioprinting of cell-laden microcarriers. Biofabrication 6:035020.) © IOP Publishing. Reprovided with permission. All rights reserved.

trochlear ridge of the femur suggested enhancement of repair at one month but no significant difference at eight months.[155] A laboratory study done after this at CSU evaluating the effect of fibrin concentration on MSC migration out of autologous and commercial fibrin or hydrogels showed that migration from a 25% autologous hydrogel dilution was 7.3, 5.2, and 4.6-fold higher than migration from 100%, 75%, and 50% autologous hydrogels, respectively.[156] In another in vivo study with full thickness defects on the equine femoral trochlear ridge, BMSCs in a fibrin/PRP hydrogel showed inferior repair compared to the fibrin/PRP injected controls, and there was bone formation in 4/12 of the BMSCs fibrin/PRP defects.[157]

New Developments in the Diagnosis and Treatment of Subchondral Cystic Lesions of the Medial Femoral Condyle

The definition of a subchondral cystic lesion (SCL) has evolved. In early reports, cases of SCLs had lameness, and radiographs usually showed an obvious lesion. With the advent of digital radiographs and survey radiographs at yearling sales, more attention is now paid to "traditional" SCLs but also to subchondral defects and even flattening. Current radiographic definitions include five different lesions.[158] There has been some modification of this in evaluating radiographic changes in yearling and 2-year-old Quarter horses intended for cutting.[159] A challenge that has emerged is determining when a radiographic lesion becomes significant. This has been addressed in both Thoroughbred racehorses and Quarter horses bred for cutting and needs further elucidation with large numbers.

A treatment algorithm has been reported recently.[1] For a typical SCL where there is clinical lameness on radiographs, arthroscopic evaluation determines if the cyst has stable margins (probe and no penetration or collapse of margins) or unstable margins and/or collapsed margins (cartilage collapses at the margins). In the former case the first line of

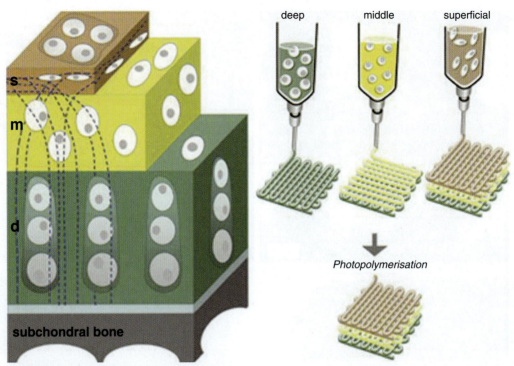

FIGURE 27-14 Schematic representation of how the zonal organization of cartilage featuring a superficial, middle and deep layer could be reconstructed using three-dimensional bioprinting. (From: Klein T.J., Rizzi S.C., Reichert J.C., et al (2009). Strategies for zonal cartilage repair using hydrogels. Macromol Biosci 9(11):1049-1058.)

treatment is intralesional triamcinolone acetonide injection under arthroscopic observation. If there is no response or there is recurrent lameness in an immature horse, arthroscopic evacuation and débridement are then performed. In a cyst with unstable or collapsed margins in an immature horse, arthroscopic evacuation and débridement are performed and if the horse is 3 years of age or older arthroscopic débridement plus augmentation is recommended. Results have been published with these techniques and are summarized in the previously cited book.[1]

Since that time, a transcondylar screw technique has been described; its rationale is that it alters SCL strain, which is then believed to promote trabecular bone formation and remodeling. Results with this technique have been recently published.[160] This was a retrospective study of 20 horses with lameness attributed to an MFC (medial femoral condyle) SCL. A 4.5-mm screw was inserted in lag screw fashion across the SCL. Treatment was considered successful if lameness was eliminated and the radiographic area of the SCL on a caudocranial projection decreased greater or equal to 50% by 120 days. Lameness was reduced by 1 to 2 grades by 60 days after surgery in 18 horses and was eliminated in 15 horses by 120 days at which time the SCL area had decreased greater or equal to 50% and work had resumed without lameness (mean follow-up 12 months). Treatment was less successful in horses older than 3 years of age. The conclusion was that lameness could be eliminated in approximately 75% of horses by 120 days. This is no better than previously described techniques, but the ability to

improve radiographic density dictates further research and clinical evaluation of this technique.

IMPROVEMENT IN THE UNDERSTANDING OF PATHOGENESIS OF EXERCISE-INDUCED TRAUMATIC DISEASE

Catastrophic injury is a major problem in the equine athletic industry, closely followed by severe wastage of racehorses because of nonfatal injuries. The pathologic sequence of events that lead to most injuries in athletes is becoming known. Much information has been gained by following exercising horses with imaging techniques including CT, MRI, and nuclear scintigraphy as sentinels of early damage. However, the equine industry lacks an easy-to-use, relatively inexpensive diagnostic method that can be used repeatedly to identify horses prone to injury. A CT system with rapid acquisition time that could be used on the extremities of horses under sedation would be ideal for monitoring athletes. Work is under way to develop such a device. Once such a device is developed, large, prospective studies can be performed so that epidemiologic data can be used to identify factors that can lead to injury. More recent modeling studies based on CT have revealed differences in joint shape of horses suffering condylar fractures. This type of protocol has been developed in humans.[161-163] Similar to these human studies, large epidemiologic studies would be needed to characterize shape and density distribution as factors that could lead to injury in horses. It is likely that shape variations in joints occur during development and early training, both of which could be characterized once standing CT imaging is available. Results of these studies will then help to guide optimum development and growth in foals so as to reduce the incidence of injury.

Currently, there are a few studies that correlate limb conformation with the incidence of injury later in life.[164,165] More of these studies are needed, specifically for limb conformation with specific disease entities. There may be a place for volumetric conformation assessment of the limbs, which could be correlated to specific disease entities. Three-dimensional assessment of the limbs can be performed through kinematic studies and their movement assessed with inertial measurement units.

REHABILITATION AND PHYSICAL THERAPY

Continued validation of rehabilitation and physical therapy techniques for musculoskeletal disease in the horse is urgently needed. These treatments are a newer focus and objective assessment has commenced but needs to continue. The research in this area up until this time in the horse has been presented in Chapter 18.

Because very little research has been done in the horse there is great opportunity to expand knowledge. A controlled study with equine OA has been done with underwater treadmilling[167] but there are numerous other rehabilitation techniques that could benefit from controlled studies as well as long-term epidemiologic studies with a prospective allotment of cases.

Another area of interest includes management practices influencing joint disease later in life (including management of foal and yearling limb conformation).

Breeding and Selection Practices for Osteochondrosis

The genetic background of osteochondrosis (OC) is complex, which is to a large extent caused by the dualistic character of the disorder in which lesions originate in the early juvenile phase in the foal and for the major part subsequently heal. As screening for OC usually takes place after this active period, the phenotype is based on the end result of two different processes (the generation of lesions and the healing of these), which are both certainly polygenic and most likely unrelated to each other. This background may partially explain the low effectiveness of even the strictest selection methods against OC that have been tested up to this time. Another factor may be the fact that possible effects of selecting against OC may be counteracted by breeding pressure in favor of certain conformational traits, of which height at the withers and high growth rate are the most important, that are highly valued in the modern sport horse and known to be associated with development of OC (detailed in Chapter 5).

The description of the horse genome and the following molecular genetic studies have not yet brought a solution, as loci associated with some form of OC have been found on 22 of the 33 chromosomes of the horse.[166] Although this explains the large variation in heritability (h^2) for equine OC

as described in the literature and also the variation in h^2 per joint and even per predilection site within a joint or clinical manifestation of OC (e.g., flattening versus fragmentation), it also means that the hope for a few marker genes for equine OC was in vain.

Genomic selection is a possible and likely future avenue for the selection against OC in the horse. In genomic selection, genome-wide single nucleotide polymorphism (SNP) genotype information is combined with pedigree and phenotypic data to produce genomic-estimated breeding values. The major limitations for the implementation of these techniques, until recently, were the large number of markers required and the cost of genotyping. At present, in many species in which the genome has been determined, high-density SNP chips are now available and these limitations have been overcome. In several commercial species, such as dairy livestock, genomic selection is now a reality.[168] A limitation of genetic selection is that large reference populations are needed to obtain highly accurate estimated breeding values. This is relatively easy in cattle, but less so in horses. It has been shown, however, that in case of a limited number of phenotypic records the same individuals should be phenotyped and genotyped, rather than genotyping parents and phenotyping their progeny, as is often done in commercial livestock breeding. On the condition that the generation interval is substantially shortened (which is possible when using genomic selection), genomic selection can then be more effective than classic breeding schemes based on either a phenotypically recorded performance or the performance of progeny.[169] It should be realized, however, that in equine OC environmental factors contribute more to the phenotype than genetic influences (see also Chapter 5) and that progress in selection is less with a lower h^2. Even when using sophisticated molecular genetic techniques, the strategy to reduce the incidence of OC must remain multifocal.

REFERENCES

1. McIlwraith CW, Nixon AJ, Wright IM. *Diagnostic and surgical arthroscopy in the horse.* 4th ed. Philadelphia, PA: Elsevier; 2014.
2. Caron JP, Genovese RL. Principles and practices of joint disease treatments. In: Ross MW, Dyson SJ, eds. *Diagnosis and management of lameness in the horse.* Philadelphia, PA: Elsevier; 2003.
3. National Animal Health Monitoring Systems: lameness in laminitis in US horses. Fort Collins, CO: USDA, APHIS, Veterinary Services—Centers for Epidemiology and Animal Health; 2000.
4. Li X, Majumdar S. Quantitative MRI of articular cartilage and its clinical applications. *J Magn Reson Imaging.* 2013;38(5):991–1008.
5. Hesper T, Hosalkar HS, Bittersohl D, et al. T2* mapping for articular cartilage assessment: principles, current applications and future prospects. *Skeletal Radiol.* 2014;43(10): 1429–1445.
6. Jazrawi LM, Alaia MJ, Chang G, et al. Advances in magnetic resonance imaging of articular cartilage. *Am Acad Orthop Surg.* 2011;19(7):420–429.

7. Kokkonen HT, Suomalainen JS, Joukainen A, et al. In vivo diagnostics of human knee cartilage lesions using delayed CBCT arthrography. *J Orthop Res.* 2014;32(3):403–412.

8. Larheim TA, Abrahamsson AK, Kristensen M, et al. Temporomandibular joint diagnostics using CBCT. *Dentomaxillofac Radiol.* 2015;44(1):20140235.

9. Nicolaou S, Liang T, Murphy DT, et al. Dual-energy CT: a promising new technique for assessment of the musculoskeletal system. *AJR Am J Roentgenol.* 2012;199(5 Suppl):S78–S86.

10. Yveborg M, Danielsson M, Bornefalk H. Theoretical comparison of a dual energy system and photon counting silicon detector used for material quantification in spectral CT. *IEEE Trans Med Imaging.* 2014;34(3):796–806.

11. Hontoir F, Nisolle JF, Meurisse H, et al. A comparison of 3-T magnetic resonance imaging and computed tomography arthrography to identify structural cartilage defects of the fetlock joint in the horse. *Vet J.* 2014;199(1):115–122.

12. Stewart RC, Bansal PN, Entezari V, et al. Contrast-enhanced CT with a high-affinity cationic contrast agent for imaging ex vivo bovine, intact ex vivo rabbit, and in vivo rabbit cartilage. *Radiology.* 2013;266(1):141–150.

13. Vallance SA, Bell RJ, Spriet M, et al. Comparison of computed tomography, contrast enhanced computed tomography and standing low field magnetic resonance imaging in horses with lameness localized to the foot. Part I: anatomical visualization scores. *Equine Vet J.* 2012;44(1):51–56.

14. Vallance SA, Bell RJ, Spriet M, et al. Comparison of computed tomography, contrast enhanced computed tomography and standing low field magnetic resonance imaging in horses with lameness localized to the foot. Part II: lesion identification. *Equine Vet J.* 2012;44:149–156.

15. McIlwraith CW, Yovich JV, Martin GS. Arthroscopic surgery for the treatment of osteochondral chip fractures in the equine carpus. *J Am Vet Med Assoc.* 1987;191(5):531–540.

16. Kawcak CE, McIlwraith CW. Proximodorsal first phalanx osteochondral chip fragmentation in 336 horses. *Equine Vet J.* 1994;26(5):392–396.

17. Walmsley JP, Philips TJ, Townsend HGG. Meniscal tears in horses: an evaluation of clinical signs and arthroscopic treatment of 80 cases. *Equine Vet J.* 2003;35(4):402–406.

18. Brittberg M, Winalski CS. Evaluation of cartilage injuries and repair. *J Bone Joint Surg.* 2003;85(A Suppl 2):58–69.

19. Spahn G, Klinger HM, Baums M, et al. Reliability in arthroscopic grading of cartilage lesions: results of a prospective blinded study for evaluation of inter-observer reliability. *Arch Orthop Trauma Surg.* 2011;131(3):377–381.

20. Lane JM, Chisena E, Black J. Experimental knee instability: early mechanical property changes in articular cartilage in a rabbit model. *Clin Orthop Rel Res.* 1979;140:262–265.

21. Lyyra T, Jurvelin J, Pitkanen P, et al. Indentation instrument for the measurement of cartilage stiffness under arthroscopic control. *Med Eng Phys.* 1995;17(5):395–399.

22. Brama PA, Barneveld A, Karssenberg D, et al. The application of an indenter system to measure structural properties of articular cartilage in the horse. Suitability of the instrument and correlation with biochemical data. *J Vet Med A Physiol Pathol Clin Med.* 2001;48(4):213–221.

23. Brommer H, Laasanen MS, Brama PA, et al. In situ and ex vivo evaluation of an arthroscopic indentation instrument to estimate the health status of articular cartilage in the equine metacarpophalangeal joint. *Vet Surg.* 2006;35(3):259–266.

24. Laasanen MS, Töyräs J, Hirvonen J, et al. Novel mechano-acoustic technique and instrument for diagnosis of cartilage degeneration. *Physiol Meas.* 2002;23(3):491–503.

25. Kiviranta P, Lammentausta E, Töyräs J, et al. Indentation diagnostics of cartilage degeneration. *Osteoarthritis Cartilage.* 2008;16(7):796–804.

26. Liukkonen J, Hirvasniemi J, Joukainen A, et al. Arthroscopic ultrasound technique for simultaneous quantitative assessment of articular cartilage and subchondral bone: an in vitro and in vivo feasibility study. *Ultrasound Med Biol.* 2013;39(8):1460–1468.

27. Töyräs J, Laasanen MS, Saarakkala S, et al. Speed of sound in normal and degenerated bovine articular cartilage. *Ultrasound Med Biol.* 2003;29(3):447–454.

28. Brezinski ME, Tearney GJ, Bouma B, et al. Optical biopsy with optical coherence tomography. *Ann N Y Acad Sci.* 1998;838:68–74.

29. Fercher AF. Optical coherence tomography—development, principles, applications. *Z Med Phys.* 2010;20(4):251–276.

30. Huang YP, Saarakkala S, Toyras J, et al. Effects of optical beam angle on quantitative optical coherence tomography (OCT) in normal and surface degenerated bovine articular cartilage. *Phys Med Biol.* 2011;56(2):491–509.

31. Chu CR, Lin D, Geisler JL, et al. Arthroscopic microscopy of articular cartilage using optical coherence tomography. *Am J Sports Med.* 2004;32(3):699–709.

32. Virén T, Huang YP, Saarakkala S, et al. Comparison of ultrasound and optical coherence tomography techniques for evaluation of integrity of spontaneously repaired horse cartilage. *J Med Eng Technol.* 2012;36(3):185–192.

33. Te Moller NCM, Brommer H, Liukkonen J, et al. Arthroscopic optical coherence tomography provides detailed information on cartilage lesions in horses. *Vet J.* 2013;197(3):589–595.

34. Afara I, Prasadam I, Crawford R, et al. Non-destructive evaluation of articular cartilage defects using near-infrared (NIR) spectroscopy in osteoarthritic rat models and its direct relation to Mankin score. *Osteoarthritis Cartilage.* 2012;20(11):1367–1373.

35. Afara IO, Prasadam I, Crawford R, et al. Near infrared (NI) absorption spectra correlates with subchondral bone micro-CT parameters in osteoarthritic rat models. *Bone.* 2013;53(2):350–357.

36. Frisbie DD, McIlwraith CW, Arthur RM, et al. Serum biomarker levels for musculoskeletal disease in two- and three-year-old racing Thoroughbred horses: a prospective study of 130 horses. *Equine Vet J.* 2010;42(7):643–651.

37. McIlwraith CW, Clegg PD. Science in brief: report on the Havemeyer Foundation workshop on equine musculoskeletal biomarkers—current knowledge and future needs. *Equine Vet J.* 2014;46(6):651–653.

38. Hunter DJ, Nevitt M, Losina E, et al. Biomarkers for osteoarthritis: current position and steps towards further validation. *Best Pract Res Clin Rheum.* 2014;28(1):61–71.

39. Kraus VB, Burnett B, Coindreau J, et al. Application of biomarkers in the development of drugs intended for treatment of osteoarthritis. *Osteoarthritis Cartilage.* 2011;19(5):515–542.

40. Kraus VB. (2014). Current state of the art in osteoarthritis biomarkers. Havemeyer Symposium (abstract)

41. U.S. Department of Health and Human Services. U.S. Food and Drug Administration. *Paving the way for personalized medicine: FDA's role in a new era of medical product development*. Silver Spring, MD: U.S. Food and Drug Administration; 2013 (pp. 1–61).

42. Desmond-Hellmann S, Sawyers C, Cox D, et al. *Toward precision medicine: building a knowledge network for biomedical research and a new taxonomy of disease*. Washington, DC: National Academy of Sciences; 2011.

43. Lohmander S. (2014). Looking forward what do we need. Keynote presentation at 3rd Dorothy Russell Havemeyer Foundation Workshop on Equine Skeletal Biomarkers. Steamboat Springs, CO.

44. Bauer DC, Hunter DJ, Abramson SB, et al. Classification of osteoarthritis biomarkers: a proposed approach. *Osteoarthritis Cartilage*. 2006;14(8):723–727.

45. Peffers MJ, Beynon RJ, Clegg PD. Absolute quantification of selective proteins in the human osteoarthritic secretome. *Int J Mol Sci*. 2013;14:20658–20681.

46. Fijar N, Som M, Riley CB, et al. Use of infrared spectroscopy for diagnosis of traumatic arthritis in horses. *Am J Vet Res*. 2006;67(8):1286–1292.

47. Wagner JA, Williams SA, Webster CJ. Biomarkers and surrogate endpoints for fit for purpose development and regulatory evaluation of new drugs. *Clin Pharmacol Ther*. 2007;81(1):104–107.

48. Hunter DJ. Are there promising biologic therapies for osteoarthritis? *Curr Rheumatol Rep*. 2008;10(1):19–25.

49. Ferris DJ, Frisbie DD, McIlwraith CW, et al. Current joint therapy usage in equine practice: a survey of veterinarians 2009. *Equine Vet J*. 2011;43(5):530–535.

50. Frisbie DD, Kawcak CE, Werpy NM, et al. Clinical, biochemical, and histologic effects of intra-articular administration of autologous conditioned serum in horses with experimentally induced osteoarthritis. *Am J Vet Res*. 2007;68(3):297–304.

51. Hraha TH, Doremus KM, McIlwraith CW, et al. Autologous conditioned serum: the comparative cytokine profiles of two commercial methods (IRAP and IRAP II) using equine blood. *Equine Vet J*. 2011;43(5):516–521.

52. Metcalf KB, Mandelbaum BR, McIlwraith CW. Application of platelet-rich plasma to disorders of the knee joint. *Cartilage*. 2013;4(4):295–312.

53. Xie X, Zhang C, Tuan RS. Biology of platelet-rich plasma and its clinical application in cartilage repair. *Arthritis Res Ther*. 2014;16:204.

54. Sundman EA, Cole BJ, Fortier LA. Growth factor and catabolic cytokine concentrations are influenced by the cellular composition of platelet-rich plasma. *Am J Sports Med*. 2011;39(10):2135–2140.

55. Kisiday JD, McIlwraith CW, Rodkey WR, et al. Effects of platelet-rich plasma composition on anabolic and catabolic activities in equine cartilage and meniscal explants. *Cartilage*. 2012;3:245–254.

56. Khoshbin A, Leroux T, Wasserstein D, et al. The efficacy of platelet-rich plasma in the treatment of symptomatic knee osteoarthritis: a systematic review with quantitative synthesis. *Arthroscopy*. 2013;29(12):2037–2048.

57. Chang K-V, Hung C-Y, Aliwarga F, et al. Comparative effectiveness of platelet-rich plasma injections for treating knee joint cartilage degenerative pathology: a systematic review and meta-analysis. *Arch Phys Med Rehab*. 2014;95(3):562–575.

58. Hessel LN, Bosch G, van Weeren PR, et al. Equine autologous platelet concentrates: a comparative study between different available systems. *Equine Vet J*. 2015;47(3): 319–325.

59. Textor JA, Tablin F. Intra-articular use of a platelet-rich product in normal horses: clinical signs and cytologic responses. *Vet Surg*. 2013;42(5):499–510.

60. Bertone AL, Ishihara A, Zekas LJ, et al. Evaluation of a single intra-articular injection of autologous protein solution for treatment of osteoarthritis in horses. *Am J Vet Res*. 2014;75(2):141–151.

61. Schnabel LV, Fortier LA, McIlwraith CW, et al. Therapeutic use of stem cells in horses: which type, how, and when? *Vet J*. 2013;197(3):570–577.

62. McIlwraith CW, Fortier LA, Frisbie DD, et al. Equine models of articular cartilage repair. *Cartilage*. 2011;2(4):317–326.

63. Ferris DJ, Frisbie DD, Kisiday JD, et al. Clinical outcome after intra-articular administration of bone marrow derived mesenchymal stem cells in 33 horses with stifle injury. *Vet Surg*. 2014;43(3):255–265.

64. Nobert KM. The regulation of veterinary regenerative medicine and the potential impact of such regulation on clinicians and firms commercializing these treatments. *Vet Clin North Am Equine Pract*. 2011;27(2):383–391.

65. Yingling GL, Nobert KM. Regulatory considerations related to stem cell treatment in horses. *J Am Vet Med Assoc*. 2008;232(11):1657–1661.

66. Ranera B, Antzcak D, Miller D, et al. Donor-derived equine mesenchymal stem cells suppress proliferation of mismatched lymphocytes. *Equine Vet J*. 2015. http://dx.doi.org/10.1111/evj.12414. [Epub ahead of print).

67. Murphy M, Barry F. Cellular chondroplasty: a new technology for joint regeneration. *J Knee Surg*. 2015;28(1):45–50.

68. Bourzac CE, Koenig JB, Link KA, et al. Evaluation of ultra-small super magnetic iron oxide contrast agent labeling of equine cord blood and bone marrow mesenchymal stromal cells. *Am J Vet Res*. 2014;75:1010–1017.

69. Evans CH, Robbins PD. Possible orthopaedic applications of gene therapy. *J Bone Joint Surg Am*. 1995;77(7):1103–1114.

70. Goodrich LR, Hidaka C, Robbins PD, et al. Genetic modification of chondrocytes with insulin-like growth factor-1 enhances cartilage healing in an equine model. *J Bone Joint Surg Br*. 2007;89(5):672–685.

71. Hidaka C, Goodrich LR, Chen CT, et al. Acceleration of cartilage repair by genetically modified chondrocytes over expressing bone morphogenetic protein-7. *J Orthop Res*. 2003;21(4):573–583.

72. Glass KA, Link JM, Brunger JM, et al. Tissue-engineered cartilage with inducible and tunable immunomodulatory properties. *Biomaterials*. 2014;35(22):5921–5931.

73. Brunger JM, Huynh NP, Guenther CM, et al. Scaffold-mediated lentiviral transduction for functional tissue engineering of cartilage. *Proc Natl Acad Sci U S A*. 2014;111(9):E798–E806.

74. Kay JD, Gouze E, Oligino TJ, et al. Intra-articular gene delivery and expression of interleukin-1Ra mediated by self-complementary adeno-associated virus. *J Gene Med*. 2009;11(7):605–614.

75. Hemphill DD, McIlwraith CW, Samulski RJ, et al. Adeno-associated viral vectors show serotype specific transduction of equine joint tissue explants and cultured monolayers. *Sci Rep*. 2014;4:5861.

76. Goodrich LR, Choi VW, Carbone BA, et al. Ex vivo serotype-specific transduction of equine joint tissue by self-complementary adeno-associated viral vectors. *Hum Gene Ther.* 2009;20(12):1697–1702.

77. Goodrich LR, Phillips JN, McIlwraith CW, et al. Optimization of scAAVIL-1ra in vitro and in vivo to deliver high levels of therapeutic protein for treatment of osteoarthritis. *Mol Ther Nucleic Acids.* 2013;2:e70.

78. McCarty DM, Monahan PE, Samulski RJ. Self-complementary recombinant adeno-associated virus (scAAV) vectors promote efficient transduction independently of DNA synthesis. *Gene Ther.* 2001;8(16):1248–1254.

79. Goodrich LR, Brower-Toland BD, Warnick L, et al. Direct adenovirus-mediated IGF-I gene transduction of synovium induces persisting synovial fluid IGF-I ligand elevations. *Gene Ther.* 2006;13(17):1253–1262.

80. Palmer GD, Steinert A, Pascher A, et al. Gene-induced chondrogenesis of primary mesenchymal stem cells in vitro. *Mol Ther.* 2005;12(2):219–228.

81. Jin XB, Sun YS, Zhang K, et al. Tissue engineered cartilage from hTGF beta2 transduced human adipose derived stem cells seeded in PLGA/alginate compound in vitro and in vivo. *J Biomed Mater Res B.* 2008;86(4):1077–1087.

82. Ulrich-Vinther M, Stengaard C, Schwarz EM, et al. Adeno-associated vector mediated gene transfer of transforming growth factor-beta1 to normal and osteoarthritic human chondrocytes stimulates cartilage anabolism. *Eur Cell Mater.* 2005;10:40–50.

83. Cucchiarini M, Madry H, Ma C, et al. Improved tissue repair in articular cartilage defects in vivo by rAAV-mediated overexpression of human fibroblast growth factor 2. *Mol Ther.* 2005;12(2):229–238.

84. Hiraide A, Yokoo N, Xin KQ, et al. Repair of articular cartilage defect by intraarticular administration of basic fibroblast growth factor gene, using adeno-associated virus vector. *Hum Gene Ther.* 2005;16(12):1413–1421.

85. Evans CH, Ghivizzani SC, Robbins PD. Arthritis gene therapy and its tortuous path into the clinic. *Transl Res.* 2013;161(4):205–216.

86. Evans CH, Ghivizzani SC, Robbins PD. Getting arthritis gene therapy into the clinic. *Nat Rev Rheumatol.* 2011;7(4):244–249.

87. Wehling P, Reinecke J, Baltzer AW, et al. Clinical responses to gene therapy in joints of two subjects with rheumatoid arthritis. *Human Gene Ther.* 2009;20(2):97–101.

88. Ghivizzani SC, Gouze E, Gouze JN, et al. Perspectives on the use of gene therapy for chronic joint diseases. *Current Gene Ther.* 2008;8(4):273–286.

89. Frisbie DD, Ghivizzani SC, Robbins PD, et al. Treatment of experimental equine osteoarthritis by in vivo delivery of the equine interleukin-1 receptor antagonist gene. *Gene Ther.* 2002;9(1):12–20.

90. Morisset S, Frisbie DD, Robbins PD, et al. IL-1ra/IGF-1 gene therapy modulates repair of microfractured chondral defects. *Clin Orthop Relat Res.* 2007;462:221–228.

91. Asokan A, Schaffer DV, Samulski RJ. The AAV vector toolkit: poised at the clinical crossroads. *Mol Ther.* 2012;20(4):699–708.

92. Chen B, Qin J, Wang H, et al. Effects of adenovirus-mediated bFGF, IL-1Ra and IGF-1 gene transfer on human osteoarthritic chondrocytes and osteoarthritis in rabbits. *Exp Mol Med.* 2010;42(10):684–695.

93. Vermeij EA, Broeren MG, Bennink MB, et al. Disease-regulated local IL-10 gene therapy diminishes synovitis and cartilage proteoglycan depletion in experimental arthritis. *Ann Rheum Dis.* 2014. http://dx.doi.org/10.1136/annrheumdis-2014-205223.

94. Cayzer J, Hedderley D, Gray S. A randomized, double-blinded, placebo-controlled study on the efficacy of a unique extract of green-lipped mussel (perna cuniculus) in horses with chronic fetlock lameness attributed to osteoarthritis. *Equine Vet J.* 2012;44(4):393–398.

95. Pearson W, Orth MW, Lindinger MI. Evaluation of inflammatory responses induced via intraarticular injection of interleukin-1 in horses receiving a dietary nutraceutical and assessment of the clinical effects of long-term nutraceutical administration. *Am J Vet Res.* 2009;70(7):848–861.

96. Cole BJ, Pascual-Garrido C, Grumet RC. Surgical management of articular cartilage defects in the knee. *J Bone Joint Surg Am.* 2009;91(7):1778–1790.

97. O'Driscoll SW. Preclinical cartilage repair: current status and future perspective. *Clin Orthop Relat Res.* 2001;391(Suppl):S397–S401.

98. Hunter W. Of the structure and diseases of articulating cartilages. *Phil Trans R Soc London.* 1743;9:514–521.

99. McIlwraith CW, Nixon AJ. *Joint resurfacing: Attempts at repairing articular cartilage defects. Joint Disease in the Horse.* WB Saunders; 1996. 317–334.

100. Frisbie DD, Trotter GW, Powers BE, et al. Arthroscopic subchondral bone plate microfracture technique augments healing of large chondral defects in the radial carpal bone and medial femoral condyle of horses. *Vet Surg.* 1999;28(4):242–255.

101. Frisbie DD, Oxford JT, Southwood L, et al. Early events in cartilage repair after subchondral bone microfracture. *Clin Orthop Relat Res.* 2003;407:215–227.

102. Frisbie DD, Morisset S, Ho CP, et al. Effects of calcified cartilage on healing of chondral defects treated with microfracture in horses. *Am J Sports Med.* 2006;34(11):1824–1831.

103. Knutsen G, Engebretsen L, Ludbigsen TC. Autologous chondrocyte implantation compared with microfracture in the knee. *J Bone Joint Surg.* 2004;86A(3):455–464.

104. Steadman JR, Hanson CM, Briggs KK, et al. Outcomes after knee microfracture of chondral defects in alpine ski racers. *J Knee Surg.* 2014;27(5):407–410.

105. Clanton TO, Johnson NS, Matheny LM. Outcomes following microfracture in grade 3 and 4 articular cartilage lesions of the ankle. *Foot Ankle Int.* 2014;35(8):764–770.

106. Mollon B, Kandel R, Chahal J, et al. The clinical status of cartilage tissue regeneration in humans. *Osteoarthritis Cartilage.* 2013;21(12):1824–1833.

107. Mithoefer K, McAdams T, Williams RJ, et al. Clinical efficacy of the microfracture technique for articular cartilage repair in the knee: an evidence-based systematic review. *Am J Sports Med.* 2009;37(10):2053–2063.

108. Fortier LA, Cole BJ, McIlwraith CW. Science and animal models of marrow stimulation for cartilage repair. *J Knee Surg.* 2012;25(1):3–8.

109. Cohen JM, Richardson DW, McKnight AL, et al. Long-term outcome in 44 horses with stifle lameness after arthroscopic exploration and debridement. *Vet Surg.* 2009;38(4):543–551.

110. Frisbie DD, Cross MW, McIlwraith CW. A comparative study of articular cartilage thickness in the stifle of animal species used in human pre-clinical studies compared to articular cartilage thickness in the human knee. *Vet Comp Orthop Traumatol.* 2006;19. 142e6.

111. Malda J, Benders KE, Klein TJ, et al. Comparative study of depth-dependent characteristics of equine and human osteo-chondral tissue from the medial and lateral femoral condyles. *Osteoarthritis Cartilage.* 2012;20(10):1147–1151.

112. Miller RE, Grodzinsky AJ, Barrett MF, et al. Effects of the combination of microfracture and self-assembling peptide filling on the repair of clinically-relevant troch-lear defect in an equine model. *J Bone Joint Surg Am.* 2014;96(19):1601–1609.

113. Hangody L, Vásárhelyi G, Hangody LR, et al. Autologous osteochondral grafting—technique and long-term results. *Injury.* 2008;39(Suppl 1):S32–S39.

114. Hangody L, Kárpáti Z. New possibilities in the management of severe circumscribed cartilage damage in the knee. *Magy Traumatol Ortop Kezseb Plasztikai Seb.* 1994;37(3):237–243.

115. McCoy B, Miniaci A. Osteochondral autograft transplanta-tion/mosaicplasty. *J Knee Surg.* 2012;25(2):99–108.

116. Hangody L, Dobos J, Baló E, et al. Clinical experiences with autologous osteochondral mosaicplasty in an athletic popula-tion: a 17-year prospective multicenter study. *Am J Sports Med.* 2010;38(6):1125–1133.

117. Bodó G, Hangody L, Szabó Z, et al. Arthroscopic autologous osteochondral mosaicplasty for the treatment of subchondral cystic lesion in the medial femoral condyle in a horse. *Acta Vet Hung.* 2000;48(3):343–354.

118. Bodó G, Vásárhelyi G, Hangody L, et al. Mosaic arthroplasty of the medial femoral condyle in horses—an experimental study. *Acta Vet Hung.* 2014;62(2):155–168.

119. Grande DA, Pitman MI, Peterson L, et al. The repair of experimentally produced defects in rabbit articular cartilage by autologous chondrocyte transplantation. *J Orthop Res.* 1989;7(2):208–218.

120. Brittberg M, Lindahl A, Nilsson A, et al. Treatment of deep cartilage defects in the knee with autologous chondrocyte transplantation. *N Engl J Med.* 1994;331(14):889–895.

121. Peterson L, Minas T, Brittberg M, et al. Two- to 9-year outcome after autologous chondrocyte transplantation of the knee. *Clin Orthop Relat Res.* 2000;374:212–234.

122. Bentley G, Biant LC, Vijayan S, et al. Minimum ten-year results of a prospective randomised study of autologous chondrocyte implantation versus mosaicplasty for symptom-atic articular cartilage lesions of the knee. *J Bone Joint Surg Br.* 2012;94(4):504–509.

123. Saris DB, Vanlauwe J, Victor J, et al. Characterized chon-drocyte implantation results in better structural repair when treating symptomatic cartilage defects of the knee in a randomized controlled trial versus microfracture. *Am J Sports Med.* 2008;36(2):235–246.

124. Saris DB, Vanlauwe J, Victor J, et al. Treatment of symptom-atic cartilage defects of the knee: characterized chondrocyte implantation results in better clinical outcome at 36 months in a randomized trial compared to microfracture. *Am J Sports Med.* 2009;37(Suppl 1):10S–19S.

125. Makris EA, Gomoll AH, Malizos KN, et al. Repair and tissue engineering techniques for articular cartilage. *Nat Rev Rheu-matol.* 2014;11(1):21–34.

126. Aldrian S, Zak L, Wondrasch B, et al. Clinical and radiological long-term outcomes after matrix-induced autologous chondrocyte transplantation: a prospective follow-up at a minimum of 10 years. *Am J Sports Med.* 2014;42(11):2680–2688.

127. Saris D, Price A, Widuchowski W, et al. Matrix-applied char-acterized autologous cultured chondrocytes versus microfrac-ture: two-year follow-up of a prospective randomized trial. *Am J Sports Med.* 2014;42(6):1384–1394.

128. Frisbie DD, Bowman SM, Colhoun HA, et al. Evaluation of autologous chondrocyte transplantation via a collagen mem-brane in equine articular defects' results at 12 and 18 months. *Osteoarthritis Cartilage.* 2006;16(6):667–679.

129. Frisbie DD, Lu Y, Kawcak CE, et al. In vivo evaluation of autolo-gous cartilage fragment-loaded scaffolds implanted into equine articular defects and compared with autologous chondrocyte implantation. *Am J Sport Med.* 2009;37(Suppl 1):S71–S80.

130. Cole BJ, Farr J, Winalski CS, et al. Outcomes after a single-stage procedure for cell-based cartilage repair: a prospective clinical safety trial with 2-year follow-up. *Am J Sports Med.* 2011;39(6):1170–1179.

131. Benders KE, van Weeren PR, Badylak SF, et al. Extracellular matrix scaffolds for cartilage and bone regeneration. *Trends Biotechnol.* 2013;31(3):169–176.

132. D'Onofrio A, Cresce GD, Bolgan I, et al. Clinical and hemo-dynamic outcomes after aortic valve replacement with stented and stentless pericardial xenografts: a propensity-matched analysis. *J Heart Valve Dis.* 2011;20(3):319–325.

133. Macchiarini P, Jungebluth P, Go T, et al. Clinical transplantation of a tissue-engineered airway. *Lancet.* 2008;372(9655):2023–2030.

134. Badylak SF, Weiss DJ, Caplan A, et al. Engineered whole organs and complex tissues. *Lancet.* 2012;379(9819):943–952.

135. Kang H, Peng J, Lu S, et al. In vivo cartilage repair using adipose-derived stem cell-loaded decellularized cartilage ECM scaffolds. *J Tissue Eng Regen Med.* 2014;8(6):442–453.

136. Spiller KL, Maher SA, Lowman AM. Hydrogels for the repair of articular cartilage defects. *Tissue Eng Part B.* 2011;17(4):281–299.

137. Schuurman W, Levett PA, Pot MW, et al. Gelatin-methacryl-amide hydrogels as potential biomaterials for fabrication of tissue-engineered cartilage constructs. *Macromol Biosci.* 2013;13(5):551–561.

138. Levett PA, Melchels FP, Schrobback K, et al. A biomimetic extracellular matrix for cartilage tissue engineering centered on photocurable gelatin, hyaluronic acid and chondroitin sulfate. *Acta Biomater.* 2014;10(1):214–223.

139. Wang H, Zhou L, Liao J, et al. Cell-laden photocrosslinked GelMA-DexMA copolymer hydrogels with tunable mechani-cal properties for tissue engineering. *J Mater Sci Mater Med.* 2014;25(9):2173–2183.

140. Suo H, Xu K, Zheng X. Using glucosamine to improve the properties of photocrosslinked gelatin scaffolds. *Biomater Appl.* 2014;29(7):977–987.

141. Mintz BR, Cooper Jr JA. Hybrid hyaluronic acid hydrogel/ poly(ε-caprolactone) scaffold provides mechanically favorable platform for cartilage tissue engineering studies. *J Biomed Mater Res A.* 2014;102(9):2918–2926.

142. Mirahmadi F, Tafazzoli-Shadpour M, Shokrgozar MA, et al. Enhanced mechanical properties of thermosensitive chitosan hydrogel by silk fibers for cartilage tissue engineering. *Mater Sci Eng C Mater Biol.* 2013;33(8):4786–4794.

143. Gomez-Sanchez C, Kowalczyk T, Ruiz De Eguino G, et al. Electrospinning of poly(lactic acid)/polyhedral oligomeric silsesquioxane nanocomposites and their potential in chondrogenic tissue regeneration. *J Biomater Sci Polym Ed.* 2014;25(8):802–825.

144. Murphy SV, Atala A. 3D bioprinting of tissues and organs. *Nat Biotechnol.* 2014;32:773–785.

145. Derby B. Printing and prototyping of tissues and scaffolds. *Science.* 2012;338(6109):921–926.

146. Hull CW. Apparatus for production of three-dimensional objects by stereolithography. U.S. patent 4,575,330, 1986.

147. Malda J, Visser J, Melchels FP, et al. 25th anniversary article: engineering hydrogels for biofabrication. *Adv Mater.* 2013;25(36):5011–5028.

148. Schuurman W, Khristov V, Pot MW, et al. Bioprinting of hybrid tissue constructs with tailorable mechanical properties. *Biofabrication.* 2011;3(2):021001.

149. Fedorovich NE, Schuurman W, Wijnberg HM, et al. Biofabrication of osteochondral tissue equivalents by printing topologically defined, cell-laden hydrogel scaffolds. *Tissue Eng Part C Methods.* 2012;18(1):33–44.

150. Levato R, Visser J, Planell JA, et al. Biofabrication of tissue constructs by 3D bioprinting of cell-laden microcarriers. *Biofabrication.* 2014;6(3):035020.

151. McIlwraith CW, Frisbie DD, Kawcak CE. The horse as a model of naturally occurring osteoarthritis. *Bone Joint Res.* 2012;1(11):297–309.

152. Agung M, Ochi M, Yanada S, et al. Mobilization of bone marrow-derived mesenchymal stem cells into the injured tissues after intraarticular injection and their contribution to tissue regeneration. *Knee Surg Sports Traum Arthrosc.* 2006;14:1307–1314.

153. Murphy JM, Fink DJ, Hunziker EB, et al. Stem cell therapy in a caprine model of osteoarthritis. *Arthritis Rheum.* 2003;48:3464–3474.

154. Ferris DJ, Frisbie DD, Kisiday JD, et al. Clinical outcome after intra-articular administration of bone marrow derived mesenchymal stem cells in 33 horses with stifle injury. *Vet Surg.* 2014;43:255–265.

155. Wilke MM, Nydam DV, Nixon AJ. Enhanced early chondrogenesis in articular defects following arthroscopic mesenchymal stem cell implantation in an equine model. *J Orthop Res.* 2007;25:913–925.

156. Hale BW, Goodrich LR, Frisbie DD, et al. Effect of scaffold dilution on mesenchymal stem cell migration from fibrin hydrogels. *Am J Vet Res.* 2012;73:313–318.

157. Goodrich LR, Chen A, Werpy NM, et al. Autologous platelet enhanced fibrin (APEF) scaffolds supports in situ repair in the equine model. In, Proceedings ICRS, Izmir, Turkey 2013.

158. Wallis TW, Goodrich LR, McIlwraith CW, et al. Arthroscopic injection of corticosteroids into the fibrous tissue of subchondral cystic lesions in the medial femoral condyle in horses: a retrospective study of 52 cases (2001-2006). *Equine Vet J.* 2007;40(5):461–467.

159. Contino EK, Park RD, McIlwraith CW, et al. Prevalence of radiographic changes in yearling and 2-year-old Quarter horses intended for cutting. *Equine Vet J.* 2012;44(2):185–195.

160. Santschi EM, Williams JM, Morgan JW, et al. Preliminary investigation of the treatment of equine medial femoral condylar subchondral cystic lesions with a transcondylar screw. *Vet Surg.* 2015;44(3):281–288.

161. Bredbenner TL, Mason RL, Havill LM, et al. Fracture risk predictions based on statistical shape and density modeling of the proximal femur. *J Bone Min Res.* 2014;29(9):2090–2100.

162. Nicolella DP, Bredbenner TL. Development of a parametric finite element model of the proximal femur using statistical shape and density modeling. *Comput Methods Biomech Biomed Engin.* 2012;15(2):101–110.

163. Bredbenner TL, Eliason TD, Potter RS, et al. Statistical shape modeling describes variation in tibia and femur surface geometry between control and incidence groups from the osteoarthritis initiative database. *J Biomech.* 2010;43(9):1780–1786.

164. Anderson TA, McIlwraith CW. Longitudinal development of equine conformation from weanling to three-years-of-age in the Thoroughbred. *Equine Vet J.* 2004;36(7):563–570.

165. Anderson TA, McIlwraith CW, Douay P. The role of conformation in musculoskeletal problems in the racing Thoroughbred. *Equine Vet J.* 2004;36(7):571–575.

166. Distl O. The genetics of equine osteochondrosis. *Vet J.* 2013;197:13–18.

167. King MR, Haussler KK, Kawcak CE, et al. Effect of underwater treadmill exercise on postural sway in horses with experimentally induced carpal joint osteoarthritis. *Am J Vet Res.* 2013;74:971–982.

168. Stock KF, Reents R. Genomic selection: status in different species and challenges for breeding. *Reprod Domest Anim.* 2013;48(Suppl 1):2–10.

169. Van Grevenhof EM, Van Arendonk JA, Bijma P. Response to genomic selection: the Bulmer effect and the potential of genomic selection when the number of phenotypic records is limiting. *Genet Sel Evol.* 2012;44:26.

Page numbers followed by *b, t,* and *f* indicate boxes, tables, and figures, respectively.